Contents

Osteoarchaeology
A Guide to the Macroscopic Study of Human Skeletal Remains

Efthymia Nikita

AMSTERDAM • BOSTON • HEIDELBERG • LONDON • NEW YORK • OXFORD • PARIS
SAN DIEGO • SAN FRANCISCO • SINGAPORE • SYDNEY • TOKYO

Academic Press is an imprint of Elsevier

Academic Press is an imprint of Elsevier
125 London Wall, London EC2Y 5AS, United Kingdom
525 B Street, Suite 1800, San Diego, CA 92101-4495, United States
50 Hampshire Street, 5th Floor, Cambridge, MA 02139, United States
The Boulevard, Langford Lane, Kidlington, Oxford OX5 1GB, United Kingdom

Notices
Knowledge and best practice in this field are constantly changing. As new research and experience broaden our understanding, changes in research methods, professional practices, or medical treatment may become necessary.

Practitioners and researchers must always rely on their own experience and knowledge in evaluating and using any information, methods, compounds, or experiments described herein. In using such information or methods they should be mindful of their own safety and the safety of others, including parties for whom they have a professional responsibility.

To the fullest extent of the law, neither the Publisher nor the authors, contributors, or editors, assume any liability for any injury and/or damage to persons or property as a matter of products liability, negligence or otherwise, or from any use or operation of any methods, products, instructions, or ideas contained in the material herein.

Library of Congress Cataloging-in-Publication Data
A catalog record for this book is available from the Library of Congress

British Library Cataloguing-in-Publication Data
A catalogue record for this book is available from the British Library

ISBN: 978-0-12-804021-8

For information on all Academic Press publications
visit our website at https://www.elsevier.com/

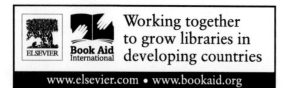

Working together
to grow libraries in
developing countries

www.elsevier.com • www.bookaid.org

Publisher: Sara Tenney
Acquisition Editor: Elizabeth Brown
Editorial Project Manager: Joslyn Chaiprasert-Paguio
Production Project Manager: Lisa Jones
Designer: Maria Ines Cruz

Typeset by TNQ Books and Journals

Preface

When I read Larsen's *Bioarchaeology* as an undergraduate student of archeology, I knew that this was the specialization I wanted to follow. The problem was that I had no idea how to perform the fascinating analyses described in the case studies that Larsen presented. Over the following months, more excellent books piled up on my bookshelves. White and Folkens' *Human Osteology*, Katzenberg and Saunders' *Biological Anthropology of the Human Skeleton*, and Cox and Mays' *Human Osteology in Archeology and Forensic Science* are only a few of the most recent titles. Every book gave me an even better understanding of the potentials of human skeletal analysis but at the same time it made me realize how much more there was to learn on a practical level to actually engage in such a study. When I discovered the Buikstra and Ubelaker *Standards for Data Collection from Human Skeletal Remains* it felt like a big barrier had been finally lifted, and indeed the information provided by the contributors of this seminal volume was pivotal in the completion of my M.Phil. in Biological Anthropology. Nevertheless, given the advances that had occurred in the discipline since the date of publication of this volume (1994), important aspects of human skeletal analysis, such as the calculation of cross-sectional geometric properties of long-bone diaphyses or the performance of geometric morphometric analysis, were missing.

The current book attempts to provide the practical guidance required so that the reader can perform a thorough macroscopic study of human skeletal remains starting from bone identification and progressing to advanced analyses, such as biodistance estimation. Microscopic, biomolecular, and biochemical methods have intentionally been omitted despite their prominent role in osteoarchaeological research. The reason was that the aim of this book is to present methods that the reader can use on his or her own without any particularly specialized equipment required. Several other books discuss the use of such specialized techniques in detail.

Before the structure of the book is outlined, a brief clarification on terminology is in need. There is currently no single universally agreed-upon term to describe the study of human skeletal remains from archaeological contexts. The term *bioarchaeology* is frequently adopted for this purpose; however, by definition this term covers all remains of a biological nature, not solely human skeletal material. Similarly, *osteoarchaeology* is another common term used to denote human skeletal analysis, but again, by definition this term also covers the study of animal skeletal remains. Owing to the lack of a generally accepted term, *osteoarchaeology* is used in the current book to refer exclusively to the study of human skeletal material, acknowledging the limitations of this choice.

This book is structured in nine chapters. Chapter 1 presents the adult human skeleton and provides identification tips for each bone and tooth, and Chapter 2 outlines the main taphonomic factors that affect the preservation of human skeletal remains. Chapter 3 describes methods for assessing the sex and ancestry of an individual based on various skeletal elements. The methods presented are mostly designed for adult material because sex and ancestry assessment in juveniles is problematic for reasons explained in the relevant sections. However, brief mention is also made of methods for sex and ancestry assessment in subadults. Age estimation standards for adults and juveniles are given in Chapter 4. Chapter 5 focuses on biodistance analysis by means of metric and nonmetric traits. Descriptions of cranial measurements and landmarks are provided, along with definitions of cranial and dental nonmetric traits. A number of appendices describe in detail the steps to be followed, from data collection to preprocessing and the actual calculation of biodistances. Chapter 6 outlines the utility of growth pattern studies. In this context, methods for stature and body mass estimation are also provided, along with an appendix illustrating postcranial measurements. Chapter 7 presents skeletal markers of activity, namely cross-sectional geometric properties of long-bone diaphyses, entheseal changes, and dental wear. Instructions for how to calculate cross-sectional geometric properties using a nondestructive method are provided, as well as recording protocols for entheseal changes. With regard to dental wear, both ordinal scoring schemes and a method for calculating the area of exposed dentine are described. Chapter 8 briefly presents the main pathological conditions that may be identified on human skeletal remains. Considering the large number of excellent textbooks on paleopathology, the focus of this chapter is on listing the lesions commonly associated with pathological conditions that frequently affect the skeleton. Finally, Chapter 9 offers step-by-step instructions for the statistical analysis of human osteological data using SPSS and, secondarily, Excel. Descriptive and inferential statistics are presented and numerous case studies are given to cover simple tests but also more advanced multivariate analyses.

The emphasis in all chapters is on the practical implementation of each method, which resulted in a very limited reference to background theoretical information or published case studies. This was a necessary compromise but the reader may find ample information regarding the context of use of each described method in already published osteology books and scientific papers. Note that even though there is limited reference to published case studies, case studies based on artificial and actual data sets are used throughout this book to demonstrate the steps of data acquisition, processing, and results interpretation.

As its title suggests, this book has been written primarily for osteoarchaeologists. Nevertheless, forensic anthropologists are also expected to find most sections of it useful. Specifically, the methods described in Chapters 1−4 are practically identical to those used in forensic contexts. Similarly, the stature and body mass estimation methods described in Chapter 6 are among the main approaches used in the identification of unknown individuals, along with sex, age, and ancestry. Finally, although the trauma section in Chapter 8 is brief, it may be useful in the forensic analysis of the manner of death of an individual. The remaining chapters and sections are also potentially useful in the study of forensic material but more marginally.

To facilitate the use of the methods described in this book, a series of macros is provided in the companion website of this book, available on http://textbooks.elsevier.com/web/Manuals.aspx?isbn=9780128040218. The most important of these may be used for (1) the calculation of the number of individuals in commingled assemblages; (2) the pretreatment of cranial landmarks and nonmetric traits for the calculation of biodistances; (3) the actual calculation of biodistances based on continuous, ordinal, and binary data; (4) the estimation of sex, age, stature, and body mass; (5) the generation of artificial data sets; and (6) statistical analysis.

This book would not have been completed without numerous people who, directly or indirectly, contributed to its creation. First of all, I would like to thank my editor, Elizabeth Brown, for believing in this book and supporting its publication despite my rather young academic age. Similarly, Joslyn Chaiprasert-Paguio and Lisa Jones offered important help with practical issues toward the final stages of the submission and publication. I would also like to express my gratitude to other personnel at Elsevier with whom I never had direct contact and who contributed to the production of this book. Furthermore, I would particularly like to thank the four reviewers of my book proposal, namely Dr. Elizabeth DiGangi, Dr. Megan Moore, Dr. Christina Papageorgopoulou, and Dr. Jay Stock, for approving it as well as for their valuable comments. In addition, I would like to acknowledge the contributions of Dr. Charlotte Henderson, Olivia Jones, Ria Kiorpe, Anna Lagia, Effrossyni Michopoulou, Dr. Marin Pilloud, and Dr. Emma Pomeroy in reviewing various chapters before my final submission and providing useful suggestions for their improvement. My mother, Malamati Nikita, patiently proofread all chapters, and Dr. Victoria Ling also proofread a few of the chapters in their early stages of preparation and kindly sent me certain publications that I could not access in Greece. Finally, my father, Professor Panos Nikitas, provided valuable guidance during the creation of the macros given as online material.

Unless otherwise specified, all photographs were obtained by the author from the Athens Collection, housed at the Division of Animal and Human Physiology, Department of Biology, National and Kapodistrian University of Athens. I am deeply grateful to Professor Efstratios Valakos for granting me permission to use this material for the current publication, as well as to Professor Sotiris Manolis, Dr. Costas Eliopoulos, and Anna Lagia for setting up this important collection. Image processing was sort of a family business, as my father and sister, Margarita, spent endless hours preparing the illustrations of each chapter. Moreover, Professor David Mattingly kindly provided me a photo from his personal records for the taphonomy chapter, and France Casting gave me permission to use photos I took of their Suchey−Brooks casts free of charge. Similarly, I am grateful to Dr. Chris Dudar for allowing the use of screenshots of the Osteoware software and Professor Dennis Slice for permitting the use of screenshots of Morpheus et al. Finally, the Leicester Arts and Museums Service, and Laura Hadland in particular, generously allowed me to use photographs I had obtained from material from Medieval Leicester, without which the paleopathology chapter would have been notably poorer.

My Ph.D. supervisor, Dr. Marta Lahr, and all my colleagues and tutors at the Leverhulme Center for Human Evolutionary Studies, University of Cambridge, played a major role in shaping my research interests and way of thinking. The same applies to my colleagues in Greece, primarily Dr. Sevi Triantaphyllou, Professor Kostas Kotsakis, and all members of the Fitch Laboratory at the British School at Athens. I feel very lucky to have worked with all of them. Finally, I would like to thank my employers and colleagues at the Cyprus Institute for being particularly supportive during the preparation of this book.

On a more personal level, I would like to thank my dear friend and colleague Anita Radini for granting me access to a rich collection of skeletal material from Leicester and permitting the publication of selected photographs from the Southwell material. My friend Eleftheria Bousaki spent several hours translating Martin's (1928) definitions of postcranial measurements from German to English, which was quite an admirable task! Finally, my family and friends have supported me in every step of this endeavor. At this point, special thanks must be addressed to my husband for his endless patience and encouragement at all times.

I am hoping that this book will complement existing textbooks used in upper-level undergraduate and graduate courses on osteoarchaeology, human osteology, and, to some extent, forensic anthropology. The book is also addressed to professional osteologists. It must be stressed that the methods presented here are by no means the only way to approach each research question. Various recording protocols, data processing methods, and statistical tests may provide equally valid results. The methods described here are those that I have had the opportunity to apply myself and found to perform well. However, they are aimed at acting as a starting point and equipping the reader with a basic understanding required for a thorough human skeletal study so that he or she subsequently feels confident enough to experiment with different techniques. Every effort has been made to avoid mistakes and present an updated review of the literature. Given the volume of this book, it is inevitable that some major publication will have been missed, and some errors must have found their way in. I apologize in advance and I would be very grateful if you could contact me directly to point out any mistakes or omissions or share suggestions for the future improvement of this book.

Chapter 1

The Human Skeleton

Chapter Outline

Chapter Objectives

By the end of this chapter, the reader will be able to:

- understand the function, structure, and composition of the human skeleton;
- use proper terminology to describe skeletal anatomy;
- define the terms of orientation for the human skeleton;
- identify the major bones of the adult human skeleton in complete and fragmentary states; and
- identify all permanent maxillary and mandibular teeth.

This chapter outlines the function, structure, and composition of the human skeleton; presents basic anatomical terminology; and offers images and brief descriptions for all skeletal elements and the permanent dentition. The emphasis is on adult skeletal remains because the juvenile skeleton changes drastically during growth and the consequent anatomical and morphological alterations are not possible to describe in a single chapter. The reader may consult the books given as suggested readings at the end of this chapter for resources on juvenile osteology as well as for additional information on the topics presented in the current chapter.

1.1 BONE FUNCTION

The human skeleton performs multiple functions. It supports the body and enables motion, while certain skeletal elements protect internal vital organs; for instance, cranial bones offer protection to the brain. In addition, the skeleton stores: (1) minerals, such as calcium and phosphorus; (2) blood-forming cells, as the red bone marrow produces red blood cells, white blood cells, and platelets via a process known as *hematopoiesis*; and (3) energy via the fat (lipids) stored in the yellow bone marrow.

1.2 BONE CLASSIFICATION

The adult skeleton (Fig. 1.2.1) typically consists of 206 bones, though this number may differ slightly among individuals owing to genetic factors. At birth, the skeleton has many more bones (over 270) but during adolescence many separate elements gradually fuse together.

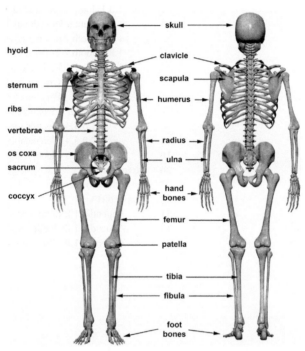

FIGURE 1.2.1 Three-dimensional model of the human skeleton. *Note:* The hyoid is not visible in this figure; the corresponding *arrow* denotes its location.

Based on their shape, human bones are divided into long, short, flat, and irregular bones. *Long bones* are elongated elements, as their name suggests, and consist of a tubular shaft terminating in an articular area at each end. Such bones are found in the upper and lower limbs (clavicle, humerus, radius, ulna—femur, tibia, fibula). Their main functions include supporting the weight of the body and enabling movement. Note that some authors place the metacarpals and metatarsals also in the long bone category on the grounds that their length is greater than their width. In *short bones* all dimensions are almost equal and their somewhat cubic shape provides them with compactness. Such bones are found mostly in the hands and feet (carpals, tarsals). *Flat bones* are flat, thin, and broad elements. As such, they provide extensive areas for muscle attachment and protect vital organs. This category includes most cranial bones (e.g., frontal, occipital, parietals), as well as the scapulae, os coxae, ribs, and sternum. Finally, as their name suggests, *irregular bones* have a complex morphology, which serves various functions. The elements of the spine (vertebrae, sacrum, coccyx) and certain cranial elements (e.g., sphenoid) belong in this category.

According to their location in the skeleton, bones are classified into axial and appendicular. The *axial skeleton* has 80 bones and includes the skull, hyoid, vertebrae, sacrum, coccyx, ribs, and sternum. The *appendicular skeleton* consists of 126 bones, which are the long bones of the arms and legs, patellae, hand and foot bones, clavicles, scapulae, and os coxae (Fig. 1.2.2).

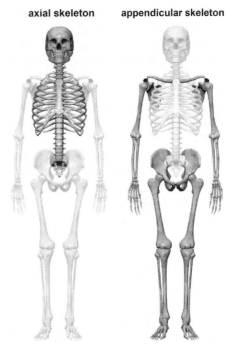

FIGURE 1.2.2 Axial and appendicular skeleton.

Two special categories of bones, which differ substantially in number between individuals, are sesamoid bones and sutural bones. *Sesamoid bones* are very small-sized and found within tendons. Their function is to protect tendons from excessive mechanical stress. *Sutural bones* are small-sized and found within the cranial sutures, that is, the joints that connect cranial bones.

Details on how to identify each bone and tooth are given in the following sections. Appendix 1.I presents a recording spreadsheet for the adult human skeleton and Appendix 1.II provides a recording spreadsheet for the permanent dentition. Finally, Appendix 1.III presents the bone and tooth inventories implemented in Osteoware, a free software program for the standardized recording of human skeletal remains, designed and provided by the Smithsonian Institution.

1.3 BONE STRUCTURE

1.3.1 Gross Anatomy

A typical long bone consists of (1) a *diaphysis*, the shaft of the bone; (2) two *epiphyses,* the extremities of the bone; and (3) two *metaphyses*, the areas that lie between the diaphysis and each of the epiphyses (Fig. 1.3.1). The epiphyses are initially

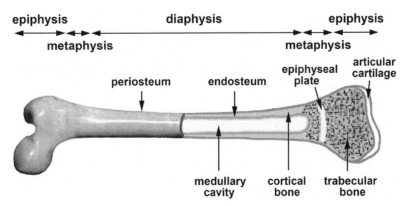

FIGURE 1.3.1 Long bone structure.

separated from the diaphysis, as the metaphyses contain a *growth plate* (or *epiphyseal plate*), consisting of hyaline cartilage, which allows longitudinal bone growth. Once an individual reaches adulthood and growth ceases, this cartilage is ossified and forms the *epiphyseal line*. The surface of the epiphyses that articulates with neighboring skeletal elements is covered with a thin layer of hyaline cartilage (*articular cartilage*) during life. The external bone surfaces that have no articular cartilage are covered by the *periosteum*. The periosteum enables bone growth in thickness, protects and nourishes the osseous tissues, facilitates fracture repair, and allows the attachment of ligaments and tendons. It attaches to the underlying osseous tissues by means of thick collagen fibers, called *Sharpey's fibers*. In the interior of the long bones lies the *medullary cavity*, which, during life, contains yellow bone marrow. The walls of this cavity are covered by the *endosteum*, a membrane that contains bone-forming cells.

Short, flat, and irregular bones have a rather simpler structure, consisting of trabecular bone covered by cortical bone (see Section 1.3.2 for definitions of the trabecular and cortical bone). The gross structure of a flat bone is shown schematically in Fig. 1.3.2.

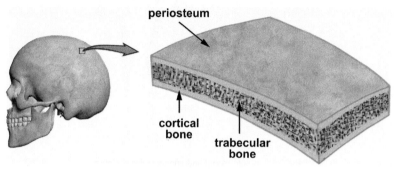

FIGURE 1.3.2 Flat bone structure.

1.3.2 Microscopic Anatomy

Histologically, bone tissue may be *woven* (immature) or *lamellar* (mature). During periods of skeletal growth or when certain pathological conditions have afflicted the skeleton, such as during fracture healing, the bone tissue produced consists of irregularly shaped collagen bundles with a random orientation. This type of bone is called *woven or primary bone*. Woven bone provides a means of responding rapidly to growth, disease, or mechanical loading; however, its disorganized structure makes it ineffective in offering long-term structural support. In contrast, *mature or lamellar bone* is formed in later childhood and during adulthood, and it consists of mineral crystals and collagen fibers that form layers called *lamellae*. Lamellar bone gradually replaces woven bone.

Lamellar bone has two structural types, cortical (or compact) bone and trabecular (or cancellous) bone. *Cortical bone* is dense and lies underneath the periosteum. Note that the cortical bone found in the joints is covered by cartilage during life and it is called *subchondral bone*. Its structural units are *osteons,* which consist of concentric layers of compact bone, *lamellae,* organized around a central canal, a *Haversian canal,* containing blood vessels and nerve fibers. *Trabecular bone* is found at the epiphyses of long bones and in the interior of all other bones. It consists of thin bony spicules, *trabeculae,* each of which is composed of a few layers of lamellae. The trabeculae are arranged irregularly, forming a honeycomb structure. Because of this structure, trabecular bone has minimal weight but at the same time provides great strength to the skeleton. During life, the spaces within the trabecular network contain hematopoietic red marrow.

1.4 BONE COMPOSITION AND CELLS

Bone tissue consists of inorganic ($\sim 70\%$) and organic ($\sim 30\%$) components. The principal inorganic component is *hydroxyapatite,* $Ca_{10}(PO_4)_6(OH)_2$, a mineral composed of calcium phosphate. *Collagen fibers* are the main organic component, along with noncollagenous proteins. The inorganic component makes the skeleton strong, whereas collagen offers elasticity.

As a living tissue, the human skeleton goes through a constant process of bone resorption (releasing of calcium and phosphate from mineralized bone) and deposition (use of calcium and phosphate to form new bone). This process is controlled by the main bone cells: osteogenic cells, osteoclasts, osteoblasts, osteocytes, and bone-lining cells. *Osteogenic* (or *osteoprogenitor*) *cells* derive from mesenchymal stem cells in bone marrow. These cells evolve into pre-osteoblasts, which subsequently give rise to mature osteoblasts. In the marrow of growing individuals, the number of osteogenic cells is high, but the number or potential of such cells to form mature osteoblasts declines with age. *Osteoclasts* are large, multinucleated cells, whose primary function is to resorb bone tissue by releasing lysosomal enzymes and acids. *Osteoblasts* facilitate new bone formation by secreting organic bone matrix, *osteoid*, and regulating its mineralization. They are mostly found under the periosteum and near the medullary cavity, where metabolic bone rates are higher. Once an osteoblast has completed bone formation it may (1) turn into a bone-lining cell (discussed later), (2) sustain apoptosis (programmed cell death), or (3) transform into an osteocyte. *Osteocytes* comprise 90% of all cells in mature bone and derive from osteoblasts that have become trapped in newly formed bone tissue. They facilitate cellular communication and maintain the daily functions of the skeleton by transporting nutrients and wastes. Finally, *bone-lining cells* derive from osteoblasts and cover bone surfaces. Their function is to release calcium when required, participate in the initiation of bone resorption and remodeling, and possibly maintain bone fluid balance.

1.5 BONE GROWTH AND DEVELOPMENT

Bone formation (*osteogenesis*) may occur through ossification within a connective tissue membrane (*intramembranous ossification*) or through ossification of cartilage precursors (*endochondral ossification*). Intramembranous ossification gives rise to the cranial vault and face, as well as partly to the clavicle and scapula. In contrast, long-bone epiphyses, short bones, vertebral bodies, and other elements largely consisting of trabecular bone grow by endochondral ossification.

Most bones are formed from at least two centers of ossification. The first center that appears is called the *primary ossification center*; its ossification usually begins in utero, and in long bones it corresponds to the diaphysis. Most *secondary ossification centers* appear after birth, and in long bones they correspond to the epiphyses. As mentioned in Section 1.3.1, between the diaphysis and the epiphyses lies a cartilaginous layer, the *growth plate*, which allows the bones to grow in length. During adolescence and early adulthood, the primary and secondary ossification centers fuse, giving rise to the complete bones.

As a bone develops, its form gradually alters to assume the final adult shape. This process is known as *modeling*. In contrast, *remodeling* is the replacement of mature bone during the repair of bone microdamage or as part of bone adaptation to mechanical loading (see Chapter 7).

1.6 PLANES OF REFERENCE AND DIRECTIONAL TERMS

This section presents brief definitions of the planes of reference and directional terms that are essential in the description of the human skeleton. All definitions provided here assume that the human skeleton is in *standard anatomical position*, that is, standing erect, looking forward, with the feet close and parallel to each other, the arms at the sides, and the palms facing forward (Fig. 1.6.1).

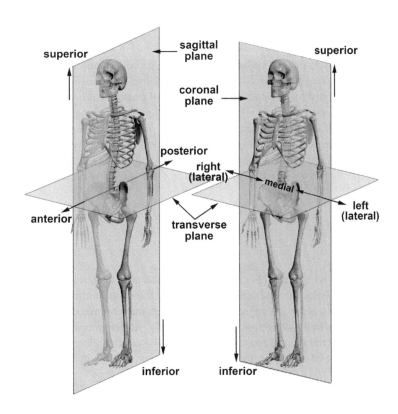

The main planes of reference for the human skeleton are used to divide the body into sections (Fig. 1.6.1). The *sagittal* (or *midsagittal*) *plane* separates the right half from the left half of the body, whereas the *coronal plane* is perpendicular to the sagittal and separates the anterior half from the posterior half of the body. Finally, the *transverse plane* is perpendicular to the sagittal and coronal planes and it may be located at different heights.

The main directions for parts of the body are superior, inferior, anterior, posterior, medial, and lateral, whereas the terms proximal and distal are more appropriate for the limbs (Figs. 1.6.1 and 1.6.2). *Superior* is toward the head, *inferior* toward the feet, *anterior* toward the front of the body, *posterior* toward the back of the body, *medial* toward the sagittal plane, and *lateral* away from the sagittal plane. For the limbs, *proximal* lies toward the trunk of the body, and *distal* lies away from the trunk. Terms that are often used for the hands and feet include *palmar,* which is the palm side of the hand; *plantar,* which is the sole side of the foot; and *dorsal*, that is, the top side of the foot or the back side of the hand. Note that when the terms *right* and *left* are used, they refer to the sides of the individual being studied and not to the sides of the observer.

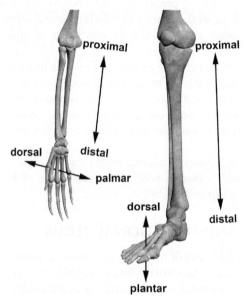

FIGURE 1.6.2   Directional terms for the upper and lower limbs.

1.7 BONE IDENTIFICATION

The identification of individual human skeletal remains may appear to be a daunting task; however, with experience it becomes straightforward. When the skeleton is well preserved, the figures provided in this section should offer sufficient information to allow the identification of each bone. In cases of partial preservation, the process of elimination should be followed. In this process, it is imperative to first determine if the elements under examination belong to an adult or a juvenile. Subsequently, we assess if the bone is long, short, flat, or irregular; though note that juvenile bones may be difficult to classify into these categories at certain stages of their development. Finally, we contrast the morphology of the bone under examination with that of the elements depicted in the following figures and find the most likely match. In the case of juvenile remains, we perform the earlier steps using as a guide one of the textbooks provided in the suggested reading list.

1.7.1 Axial Skeleton

1.7.1.1 Skull

At birth, the human skull consists of 45 elements but many of these gradually fuse, resulting in 28 bones in the adult skull. Fig. 1.7.1 shows the bones that are visible ectocranially on the lateral view of the adult skull. The bones of the skull may be divided into cranial bones and facial bones, though further divisions may be used. *Cranial bones* include the frontal, occipital, sphenoid, and ethmoid, as well as the right and left parietals and temporals. *Facial bones* include the right and left nasals, maxillae, zygomatics, lacrimals, palatines, and inferior nasal conchae, as well as the mandible and vomer. Six *auditory ossicles* (three on each side of the skull) form a separate category of skull bones.

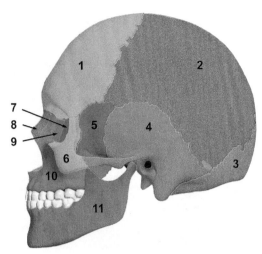

FIGURE 1.7.1   Skull bones: (1) frontal, (2) parietal (×2), (3) occipital, (4) temporal (×2), (5) sphenoid, (6) zygomatic (×2), (7) ethmoid, (8) nasal (×2), (9) lacrimal (×2), (10) maxilla (×2), (11) mandible. *Note 1:* In addition to these bones, the skull includes the vomer, palatine (×2), inferior nasal concha (×2), and three ear ossicles (malleus, incus, stapes) (×2). *Note 2:* The symbol ×2 indicates that the bone appears twice, once on each side of the skull.

It must be clarified that the term *skull* denotes all the bones of the head, including the mandible, whereas the *cranium* is the skull without the mandible. Cranial and facial bones articulate by means of interlocking fibrous joints called *sutures*. As will be discussed in Chapter 4, the sutures gradually ossify until they become completely obliterated. Because of this property, the degree of closure of the cranial sutures may be employed as an aging marker in adult skeletons.

When cranial and facial bones are intact, they are easy to identify because of the distinct morphology of each one of them. Figs. 1.7.2−1.7.5 show different views of an adult human cranium, whereas two endocranial views are given in Fig. 1.7.6. In addition, the cranial and facial bones that are most commonly individually retrieved are presented in Figs. 1.7.7−1.7.15, whereas smaller bones that are mostly found attached on larger and more diagnostic ones are simply described.

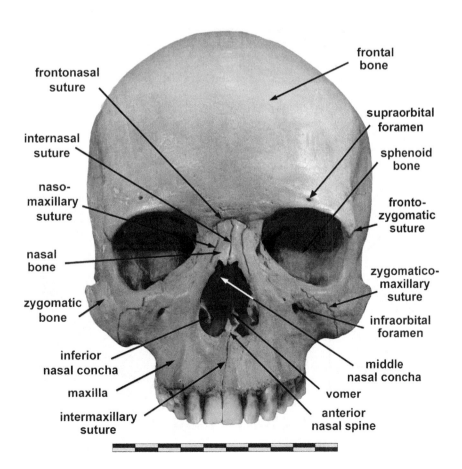

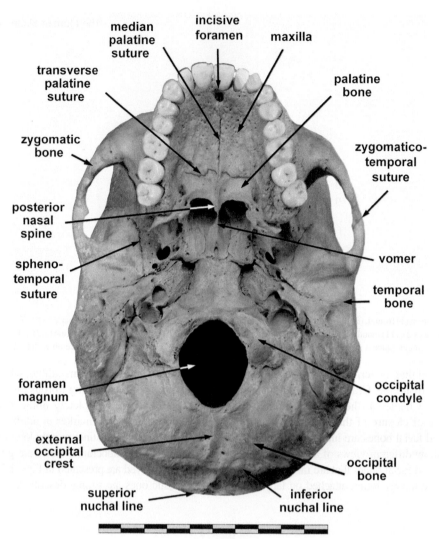

median palatine suture

incisive foramen

maxilla

transverse palatine suture

palatine bone

zygomatic bone

zygomatico-temporal suture

posterior nasal spine

spheno-temporal suture

vomer

temporal bone

foramen magnum

occipital condyle

external occipital crest

occipital bone

superior nuchal line

inferior nuchal line

FIGURE 1.7.3 Inferior view of the human cranium.

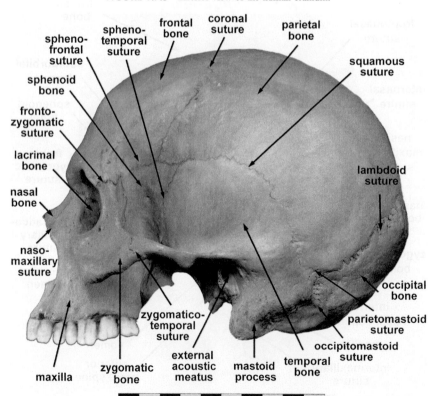

spheno-frontal suture

spheno-temporal suture

frontal bone

coronal suture

parietal bone

squamous suture

sphenoid bone

fronto-zygomatic suture

lambdoid suture

lacrimal bone

nasal bone

naso-maxillary suture

occipital bone

parietomastoid suture

zygomatico-temporal suture

external acoustic meatus

mastoid process

temporal bone

occipitomastoid suture

maxilla

zygomatic bone

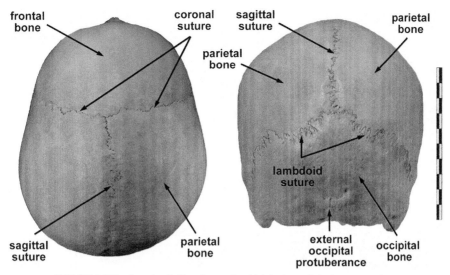

FIGURE 1.7.5   Superior (left) and posterior (right) views of the human cranium.

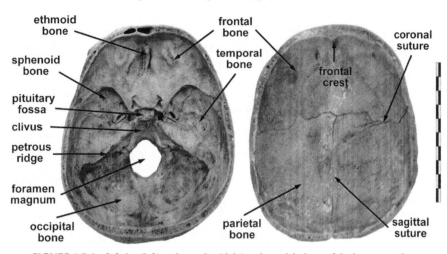

FIGURE 1.7.6   Inferior (left) and superior (right) endocranial views of the human cranium.

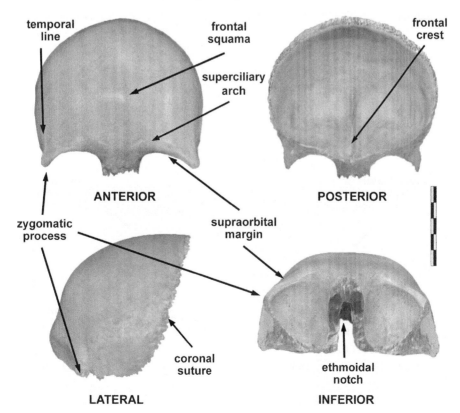

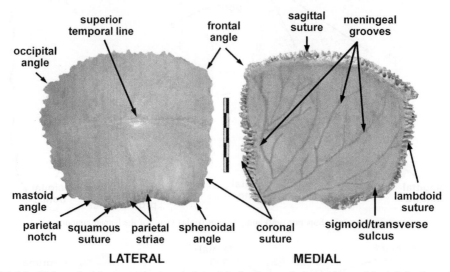

FIGURE 1.7.8 Right parietal bone; anterior is toward the right for the lateral view and toward the left for the medial view.

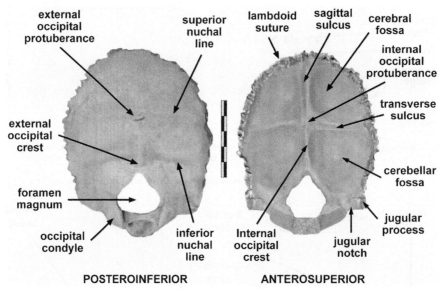

FIGURE 1.7.9 Occipital bone.

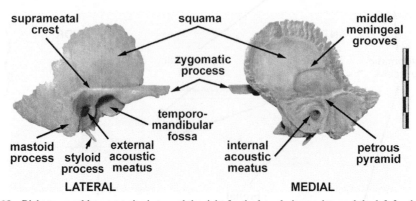

FIGURE 1.7.10 Right temporal bone; anterior is toward the right for the lateral view and toward the left for the medial view.

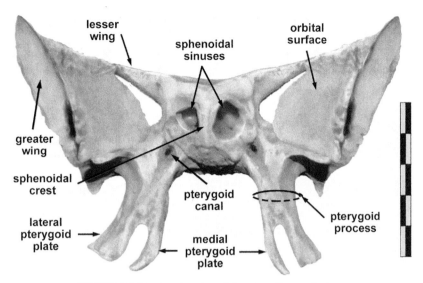

FIGURE 1.7.11   Anterior view of the sphenoid; superior is up.

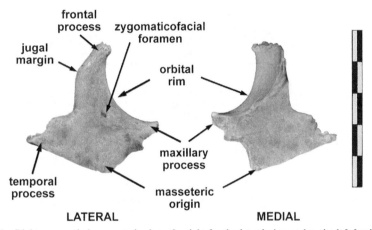

FIGURE 1.7.12   Right zygomatic bone; anterior is to the right for the lateral view and to the left for the medial view.

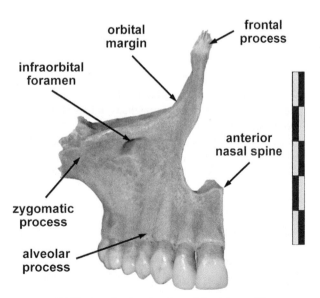

FIGURE 1.7.13   Anterior view of the right maxilla.

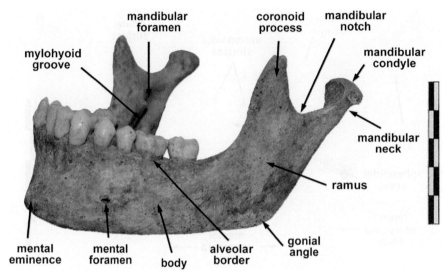

FIGURE 1.7.14 Anterolateral view of the mandible.

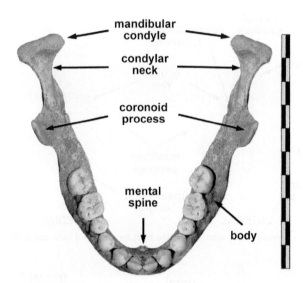

FIGURE 1.7.15 Superior view of the mandible.

Cranial Bones

The *frontal bone* (Boxes 1.7.1 and 1.7.2, Fig. 1.7.7) forms the forehead and the superior part of the orbits. It articulates with the parietals, sphenoid, ethmoid, lacrimals, zygomatics, maxillae, and nasals. At birth, it consists of two halves, which normally fuse by the end of the fourth year of life.

The *parietal bones* (Boxes 1.7.3 and 1.7.4, Fig. 1.7.8) form the roof and sides of the cranial vault. They articulate with each other, as well as with the frontal, occipital, sphenoid, and temporals.

BOX 1.7.1 Identification Tips—Frontal Bone

- Unique features: supraorbital margins, superciliary arches, and frontal crest
- Less pronounced meningeal grooves endocranially compared to the parietals
- Large sinus cavities (found only in the frontal, maxillae, and sphenoid)
- Temporal lines on the lateral ectocranial surface

BOX 1.7.2 Orientation Tips—Frontal Bone

- The coronal suture lies posteriorly and extends anterolaterally from the top of the cranium toward the face
- The frontal sinuses are anteromedial
- The supraorbital margins are anteroinferior
- The temporal lines become less prominent posteriorly

BOX 1.7.3 Identification Tips—Parietal Bones

- Pronounced meningeal grooves endocranially
- Striae ectocranially along the squamous suture
- Temporal line on the ectocranial surface
- More uniform thickness and regular endocranial surface compared to the occipital and frontal bones
- Parietal foramina often present on the posterior ectocranial surface near the sagittal suture

BOX 1.7.4 Siding Tips—Parietal Bones

- The meningeal grooves run posterosuperiorly from the sphenoidal angle; they have a vertical direction along the coronal suture and a horizontal one near the squamous suture; they become less prominent with distance from the coronal suture
- The frontal angle is nearly 90 degrees and lies anterosuperiorly
- The occipital and mastoid angles are thick
- The mastoid angle has an endocranial sulcus
- Striae are found ectocranially along the squamous suture and point posterosuperiorly
- When parietal foramina are present, they are found in the posterior third of the sagittal suture

The *occipital bone* (Box 1.7.5, Fig. 1.7.9) is situated in the posterior and inferior part of the cranium and it articulates with the parietals, temporals, sphenoid, and first cervical vertebra (atlas). The foramen magnum at the base of the occipital is the point through which the spinal cord enters the skull.

BOX 1.7.5 Identification Tips—Occipital Bone

- Unique features: foramen magnum and occipital condyles
- Highly variable cross-sectional thickness
- Marked ectocranial rugosity (external occipital protuberance, superior and inferior nuchal lines, external occipital crest)
- No meningeal grooves
- The endocranial surface is divided into four parts by two grooved ridges that cross each other at the internal occipital protuberance

The *temporal* bones (Boxes 1.7.6 and 1.7.7, Fig. 1.7.10) form part of the side and base of the cranium, and they contain the organs of hearing. They articulate with the occipital, parietals, mandible, zygomatics, and sphenoid. Each temporal has three main parts: squamous, mastoid, and petrous. Below each external auditory meatus lie the mastoid process and the styloid process. The mastoid process allows the attachment of various neck muscles, whereas the styloid process allows the attachment of muscles of the tongue and pharynx.

BOX 1.7.6 Identification Tips—Temporal Bones

- Unique features: mastoid process, styloid process, internal and external acoustic meatuses
- Meningeal grooves on the endocranial surface of the squamous part
- Squamous part is thinner than the parietals and frontal
- Zygomatic process of the temporals is less broad and flat than the temporal process of the zygomatic

---

BOX 1.7.7 Siding Tips—Temporal Bones

- The tips of the mastoid and styloid processes point anteroinferiorly
- The zygomatic process points anteriorly and its superior surface is sharper
- The petrous portion lies medially
- The mastoid process is posterior to the external auditory meatus
- Meningeal grooves have a posterior and rather superior orientation

---

The *ethmoid bone* (Fig. 1.7.6, left) is situated between the orbits, inferior to the frontal, in the midline of the skull. It participates in the formation of the floor of the anterior cranial fossa and nasal fossa, as well as the walls of the orbital fossa. It is virtually never found intact because of its fragility. It articulates with the frontal, sphenoid, nasals, lacrimals, maxillae, vomer, inferior nasal conchae, and palatines. Being roughly rectangular and consisting of multiple vertical layers of thin bone, even at a partially preserved state, fragments of the ethmoid are rather easy to identify.

The *sphenoid bone* (Box 1.7.8, Fig. 1.7.11) is an irregular element found at the anterior part of the cranium. It contributes to the formation of the floor and sides of the cranial vault and the posteroinferior surface of the eye orbits. It articulates with the occipital, parietals, frontal, ethmoid, temporals, palatines, vomer, zygomatics, and sometimes the maxillae. Because of its fragility, it is very rarely found intact in broken crania; rather it is usually retrieved in a fragmentary state attached to other cranial elements.

BOX 1.7.8 Identification Tips—Sphenoid Bone

- Characteristic features: large sinuses, sharp projections, many foramina
- Identification is facilitated by usually finding it attached to other cranial elements

---

Facial Bones

The *lacrimal bones* (Fig. 1.7.4) are thin, delicate bones situated in the anterior part of the medial wall of the orbits. They articulate with the ethmoid, maxillae, frontal, and inferior nasal conchae. In fragmentary crania, they are almost always found attached to other cranial elements with which they articulate.

The *nasal bones* (Figs. 1.7.2 and 1.7.4) are small, thin bones that form the roof of the bony nasal aperture. They are thick and narrow superiorly, but become increasingly thin and wide inferiorly. They articulate with each other as well as with the frontal, maxillae, and ethmoid. They can be identified and sided based on the nutrient foramina that are usually present on their ectocranial surface, the nasal suture that lies in between them, their nonarticulating inferior edge, and the fact that their outer surface is smooth, whereas the inner surface is rough.

The *vomer* (Figs. 1.7.2 and 1.7.3) is a thin, flat bone and is part of the posteroinferior portion of the nasal septum. It articulates with the ethmoid, sphenoid, palatines, and maxillae. It is hardly ever found unattached to other cranial elements and, because of its fragility, it is rarely retrieved in an intact state.

The *inferior nasal conchae* (Fig. 1.7.2) are slender, fragile bones attached to the lateral wall of the nasal cavity. They articulate with the maxillae, lacrimals, palatines, and ethmoid, whereas their inferior end is free. When in a fragmentary state, they may be confused with other cranial elements, but their corrugated surface makes them distinct.

The *zygomatic bones* (Boxes 1.7.9 and 1.7.10, Fig. 1.7.12) form the lateral part of the anterior face and the lateral–inferior part of the eye orbits. They articulate with the temporals, maxillae, frontal, and sphenoid.

BOX 1.7.9 Identification Tips—Zygomatic Bones

- Frontal process of the zygomatic is broader and flatter than the zygomatic process of the frontal
- Zygomatic process of the temporal is much thinner and longer than any process of the zygomatic

BOX 1.7.10 Siding Tips—Zygomatic Bones

- The masseter muscle attachment lies inferiorly
- The orbital margin lies anteriorly

The *maxillae* (Boxes 1.7.11 and 1.7.12, Fig. 1.7.13) are among the largest bones of the face, support the upper teeth, and contribute to the formation of the medial and inferior part of the orbits, the anterior part of the hard palate, and the lateral and inferior parts of the nasal aperture. The two maxillae articulate with each other as well as with the frontal, nasals, lacrimals, ethmoid, palatines, vomer, zygomatics, and inferior nasal conchae. In some cases, the maxillae may also articulate with the sphenoid.

BOX 1.7.11 Identification Tips—Maxillae

- Characteristic features: maxillary sinus, alveoli, infraorbital foramen, intermaxillary suture, and nasal aperture
- More prominent alveolar process compared to the mandible

BOX 1.7.12 Siding Tips—Maxillae

- The zygomatic process extends laterally; the frontal process is narrower than the zygomatic and lies superiorly
- The orbital margin lies superiorly
- The intermaxillary suture and nasal aperture lie medially
- The preservation of alveoli, with or without associated teeth, can assist in siding

The *palatine bones* (Fig. 1.7.3) are fragile, L-shaped bones, and form the posterior segment of the hard palate as well as part of the floor and lateral wall of the nasal cavity. They articulate with each other and with the maxillae, sphenoid, vomer, inferior nasal conchae, and ethmoid. They are very rarely found isolated; rather, they are retrieved fragmented and attached to other cranial elements.

The *mandible* (Boxes 1.7.13 and 1.7.14, Figs. 1.7.14 and 1.7.15) is the largest and strongest facial bone. It articulates with the two temporals and serves as an attachment site for the muscles of mastication and the tongue, and it also houses the lower dentition.

BOX 1.7.13 Identification Tips—Mandible

- Distinct overall anatomy (only very small fragments may be misidentified)
- No sinus (in contrast to the maxilla)
- Thicker cortical bone layer compared to the maxilla
- Distinct basal contour

BOX 1.7.14 Orientation Tips—Mandible

- The lingual surface is smoother than the buccal one
- If any teeth are preserved, they can help in orienting the mandible
- The mental foramen lies anterolaterally

Auditory Ossicles

The *auditory ossicles* are the malleus, incus, and stapes, and they are found within the petrous part of the temporal bone. The *malleus* is the largest auditory ossicle; it attaches to the tympanic membrane and articulates with the incus. The *incus* is situated between the malleus and the stapes, and the *stapes* is the innermost of the ear ossicles.

1.7.1.2 Hyoid and Spine

Hyoid Bone

The *hyoid bone* (Boxes 1.7.15 and 1.7.16, Fig. 1.7.16) is a U-shaped bone, lies in the anterior part of the neck, and does not articulate with any other bone. It offers support to the tongue and allows the attachment of numerous muscles used in speech.

BOX 1.7.15 Identification Tips—Hyoid Bone

- Much thinner body than any part of the vertebral arches
- Horns are longer and more delicate than vertebral spinous processes

---

BOX 1.7.16 Orientation Tips—Hyoid Bone

- The greater horns are wider anteriorly and gradually thin posteriorly
- The lesser horns lie superiorly

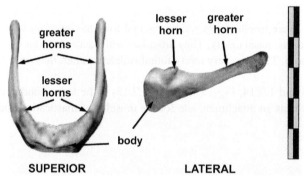

FIGURE 1.7.16 Hyoid; anterior is down for the superior view and toward the left for the lateral view.

Spine

The spine (Fig. 1.7.17) typically consists of 7 cervical (C1−C7), 12 thoracic (T1−T12), 5 lumbar (L1−L5), 5 sacral (S1−S5), and 3 to 5 coccygeal vertebrae, though deviations from this pattern can be observed. Note that the sacral and coccygeal vertebrae normally have fused by adulthood, forming the sacrum and coccyx, respectively.

The vertebral column protects the spinal cord, supports the head and the trunk of the body, and allows the attachment of muscles of the back and upper limbs. It is highly flexible, permitting a broad range of movements.

Four *curves* are visible in the spine, the *cervical*, *thoracic*, *lumbar*, and *sacral* (Fig. 1.7.17). These curves make the spine more resilient to mechanical stress and trauma, while they increase balance during bipedal walking. The thoracic and sacral curves are called *primary curves* because they start forming in utero, whereas the cervical and lumbar curves are called *secondary* because they appear after birth. Specifically, the cervical curve forms when a baby starts holding its head up, and the lumbar curve when a child starts walking.

Vertebrae vary in size and shape (Figs. 1.7.18−1.7.28), but they share some basic anatomical structures. A *typical vertebra* is composed of a body, vertebral arch, spinous process, transverse processes, and articular processes (Figs. 1.7.18,

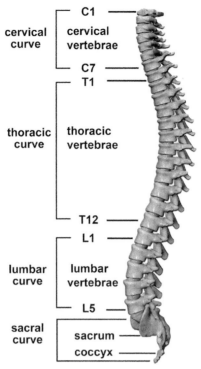

FIGURE 1.7.17   Three-dimensional model of the human spine.

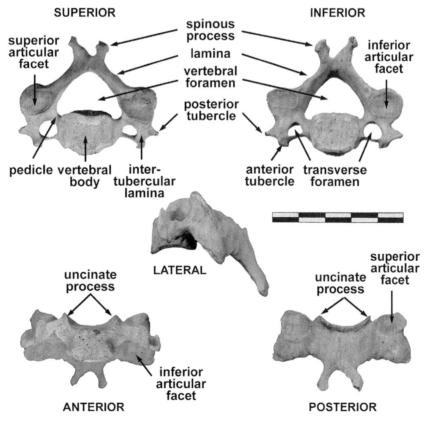

FIGURE 1.7.18   Typical cervical vertebra (C4).

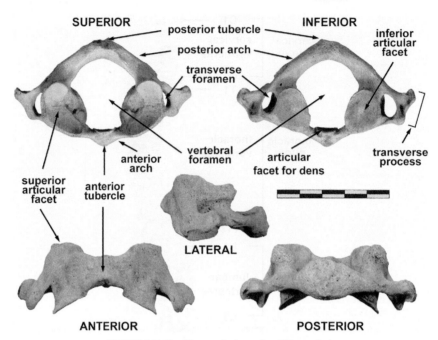

FIGURE 1.7.19   First cervical vertebra (C1, or atlas).

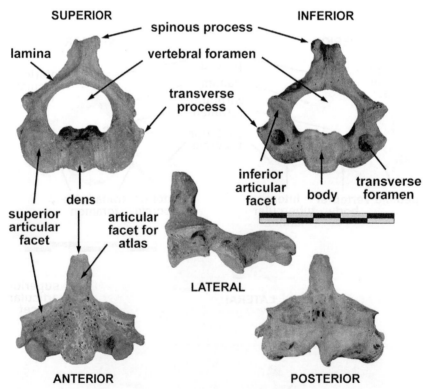

FIGURE 1.7.20   Second cervical vertebra (C2, or axis).

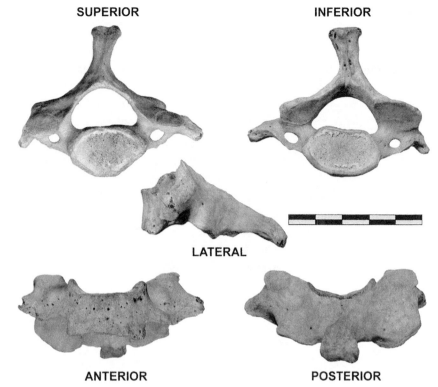

SUPERIOR   INFERIOR

LATERAL

ANTERIOR   POSTERIOR

FIGURE 1.7.21   Seventh cervical vertebra (C7).

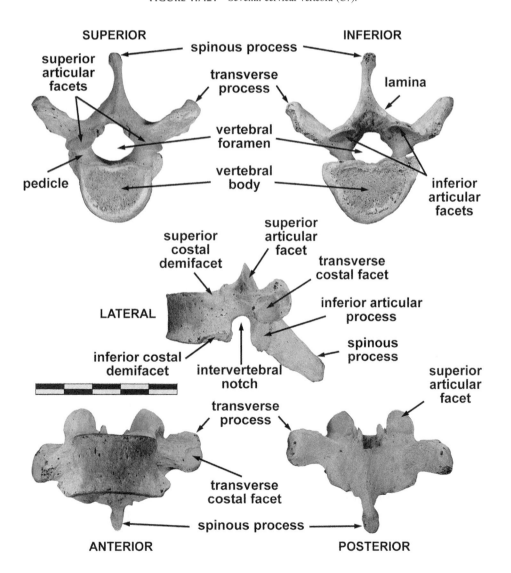

SUPERIOR   INFERIOR

spinous process

superior
articular   transverse
facets   process   lamina

vertebral
foramen

vertebral   inferior
pedicle   body   articular
                                                            facets

superior   superior
costal   articular
demifacet   facet
                              transverse
                              costal facet

LATERAL   inferior articular
                                              process

                                              spinous
inferior costal   process
demifacet   intervertebral
                 notch   superior
                                                             articular
transverse   facet
process

transverse
costal facet

spinous process

ANTERIOR   POSTERIOR

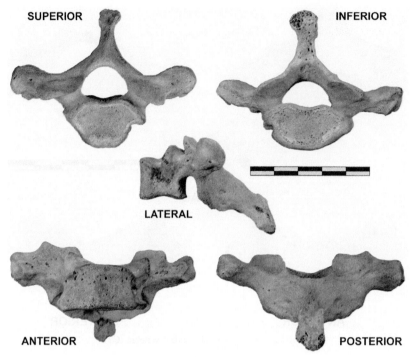

SUPERIOR

INFERIOR

LATERAL

ANTERIOR

POSTERIOR

FIGURE 1.7.23 First thoracic vertebra (T1).

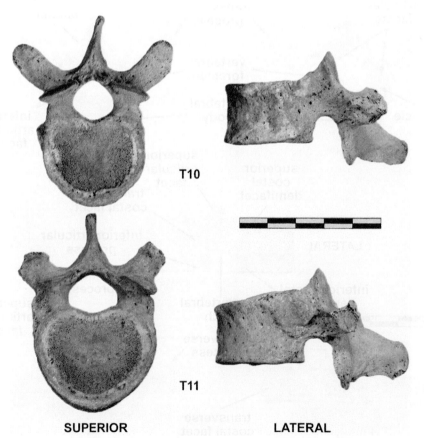

T10

T11

SUPERIOR

LATERAL

FIGURE 1.7.24 Tenth and eleventh thoracic vertebrae (T10, T11).

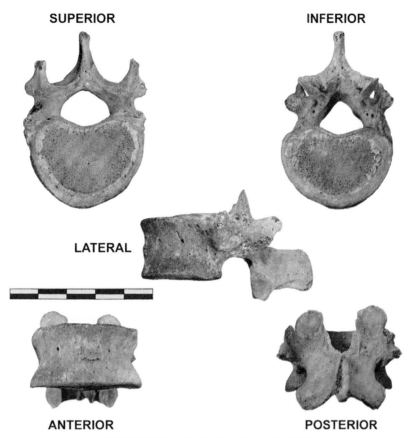

SUPERIOR   INFERIOR

LATERAL

ANTERIOR   POSTERIOR

FIGURE 1.7.25   Twelfth thoracic vertebra (T12).

1.7.22, and 1.7.26). The vertebral body lies anteriorly and it has a weight-bearing role. The spinous process lies posteriorly and the transverse processes are lateral. All processes allow the attachment of ligaments and muscles, thus permitting the movement of the vertebral column. Finally, the vertebral arch is the osseous ring that surrounds the spinal cord.

The various types of vertebrae (cervical, thoracic, lumbar) are easy to distinguish, as the aforementioned basic parts of all vertebrae have distinct characteristics in each vertebral type. Figs. 1.7.18–1.7.28 depict representative cervical, thoracic, and lumbar vertebrae, whereas Box 1.7.17 summarizes their distinct features.

Cervical Vertebrae

The cervical vertebrae are the smallest of the spine (without considering the sacral and coccygeal vertebrae, which are normally fused to one another) and characterized by great flexibility. Typical cervical vertebrae (C3–C6) have the morphology shown in Fig. 1.7.18, whereas vertebrae with atypical features are given in Figs. 1.7.19–1.7.21. The main anatomical characteristics of a typical cervical vertebra that separate it from other types of vertebrae are the small size, transverse foramina, saddle-shaped body, and bifid spinous process (Fig. 1.7.18). The atlas (C1) has no body or spinous process (Fig. 1.7.19), whereas the axis (C2) has a prominent superior process, the dens (odontoid process); lacks tubercles on the transverse processes; and has a robust spinous process (Fig. 1.7.20). The seventh cervical vertebra combines features of the cervical and thoracic vertebrae. In particular, it has transverse foramina, like all cervical vertebrae, but no tubercles. In addition, the anteroinferior margin of its body is flat instead of saddle shaped and the spinous process is rather horizontal and nonbifid (Fig. 1.7.21).

Thoracic Vertebrae

There are 12 thoracic vertebrae (T1–T12), among which eight are typical vertebrae, T2 to T9. Each of the typical vertebrae has a nonbifid spinous process, superior and inferior articulating facets, and articular demifacets on the lateral sides of the body, as well as articular facets on the transverse processes for the articulation of the ribs (Fig. 1.7.22).

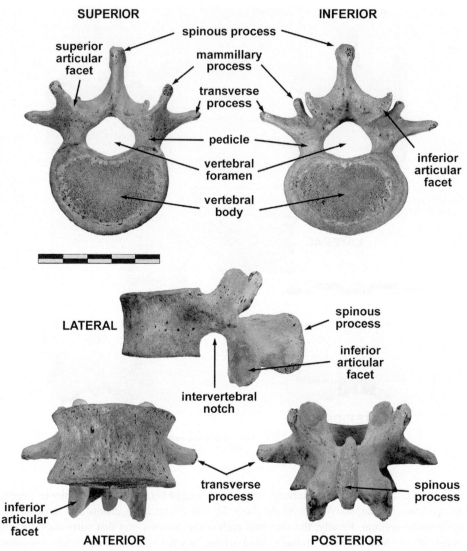

FIGURE 1.7.26 First lumbar vertebra (L1).

The atypical thoracic vertebrae are T1 and T10—T12. T1 has a complete superior costal facet instead of a demifacet; its body is flatter and the spinous process lies more horizontally than in the remaining thoracic vertebrae (Fig. 1.7.23). T10 also has a complete superior articular facet and it additionally lacks an inferior costal demifacet. Furthermore, its spinous process is horizontally oriented and rather short and thick (Fig. 1.7.24). Like T10, T11 lacks an inferior costal demifacet and it has a complete superior articular facet. In addition, it has no costal facets on the transverse processes, and its spinous process is also short, thick, and even more horizontally oriented (Fig. 1.7.24). Finally, T12 has a superior complete costal facet and no inferior demifacet, no articular facets on the transverse processes, and a horizontally oriented short and thick spinous process. Overall, this vertebra resembles the lumbar vertebrae (Fig. 1.7.25).

Lumbar Vertebrae

The lumbar vertebrae are differentiated from a typical thoracic vertebra as they exhibit: (1) large kidney-shaped bodies, (2) horizontally oriented transverse processes, (3) thick and stout spinous processes, (4) mammillary processes, (5) no articular facets on the bodies or transverse processes, and (6) U-shaped superior and inferior articular facets. Representative lumbar vertebrae are given in Figs. 1.7.26—1.7.28.

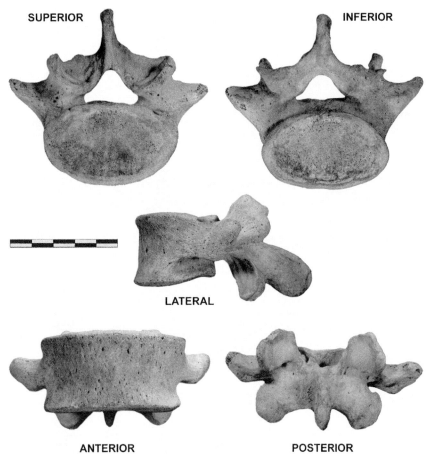

SUPERIOR   INFERIOR

LATERAL

ANTERIOR   POSTERIOR

FIGURE 1.7.27   Fifth lumbar vertebra (L5).

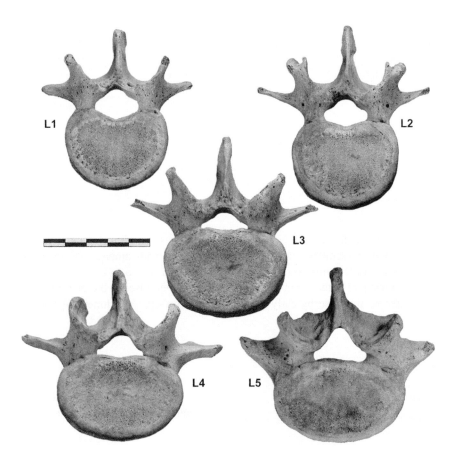

L1   L2

                  L3

L4   L5

BOX 1.7.17 Identification Tips—Typical Vertebrae

Characteristic	Cervical	Thoracic	Lumbar
Body size	Small	Medium	Large
Body shape	Saddle shaped	Rather triangular superiorly and circular inferiorly	Kidney shaped
Transverse foramina	Present	Absent	Absent
Articular facets/ demifacets on vertebral body	Absent	Present	Absent
Articular facets on transverse processes	Absent	Present	Absent
Transverse processes	Small tubercles	More prominent	Relatively smaller and thinner
Vertebral canal	Rather triangular and large	Rather circular and medium sized	Oval and small compared to the vertebral body
Spinous process	Short and bifid	Long, straight, pointing inferiorly, ending in a tubercle	Rather squared, large, blunt, horizontally oriented
Mammillary processes	Absent	Absent	Present
Superior/inferior articular facets	Flat	Flat	Curved

Sacrum—Coccyx

The *sacrum* is a large, curved, triangular-shaped bone at the base of the spine (Box 1.7.18, Figs. 1.7.29 and 1.7.30). It is initially composed of five separate sacral vertebrae (their number may vary among individuals), which fuse by early adulthood. It articulates with the fifth lumbar vertebra, the os coxae, and the coccyx.

The *coccyx* is the inferiormost part of the vertebral column and it is often fused to the sacrum (Fig. 1.7.31). It consists of three to five coccygeal vertebrae that fuse by early adulthood. It allows the attachment of various pelvic muscles and ligaments.

BOX 1.7.18 Identification Tips—Sacrum

- Unique features: alae, sacral foramina

- No bone surrounding the sacral auricular surface (in contrast to the iliac auricular surface)

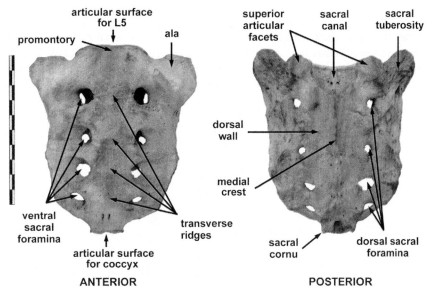

FIGURE 1.7.29   Anterior and posterior views of the sacrum.

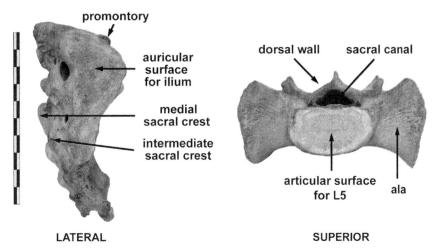

FIGURE 1.7.30   Lateral and superior views of the sacrum; anterior is toward the right for the lateral view and down for the superior view.

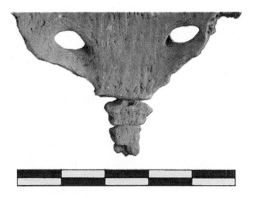

FIGURE 1.7.31   Anterior view of the coccyx.

1.7.1.3 Thoracic Cage

The term *thorax* describes the entire chest, whereas the *thoracic cage* is the skeletal part of the thorax and consists of the sternum, ribs, and thoracic vertebral bodies (Fig. 1.7.32). The thoracic cage gradually broadens from superior to inferior and flattens from anterior to posterior. It protects vital organs, such as the heart and lungs, and facilitates breathing and blood cell production. This section focuses on the sternum and ribs, because the thoracic vertebrae have already been presented.

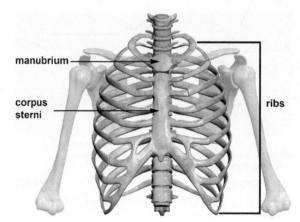

FIGURE 1.7.32   Three-dimensional model of the thoracic cage.

Sternum

The *sternum* (Box 1.7.19, Fig. 1.7.33) is a flat bone at the anterior part of the thoracic cage, which articulates with the clavicles and ribs. It has three parts: manubrium, corpus, and xiphoid process (Figs. 1.7.33 and 1.7.34). In young individuals it is

BOX 1.7.19 Identification Tips—Sternum

- Unique features: costal and clavicular notches
- Particularly light, consisting primarily of trabecular bone
- Rough and rather convex anterior surface, smooth and rather concave posterior surface

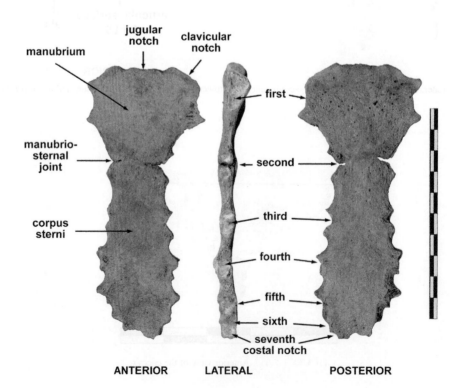

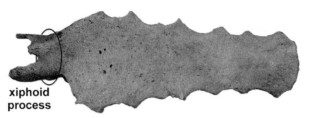

xiphoid process

FIGURE 1.7.34 Anterior view of the corpus sterni with xiphoid process.

composed of six segments. The first forms the manubrium, the second to fifth fuse and form the corpus, and the sixth forms the xiphoid process. The xiphoid process may take various shapes and allows the attachment of muscles of the abdomen.

Ribs

The human skeleton has 24 ribs (12 on each side), which form the *rib cage* (Boxes 1.7.20 and 1.7.21, Fig. 1.7.35). In some cases, there may be an extra pair of ribs or a pair of missing ribs, most often in the cervical or lumbar area. Each rib articulates posteriorly with the vertebrae, and the first 10 ribs articulate anteriorly with the sternum. Ribs 1−7 are called *true ribs* because they articulate directly with the sternum by means of cartilaginous attachments. Ribs 8−10 are known as *false ribs* because they articulate with the sternum indirectly, as their cartilage joins the cartilage of the seventh rib. Ribs 11 and 12 are called *floating ribs* because they do not articulate with the sternum at all. The anatomy of a typical rib (any rib from 3 to 9) is given in Fig. 1.7.36. Identification tips for the atypical ribs are given in Box 1.7.20.

BOX 1.7.20 Identification Tips—Atypical Ribs

- R1
  - Broad, short, and flat
  - Strongly curved
  - Small head with a single articular facet
  - Smooth inferior surface (no costal groove) and rough superior surface
- R2
  - Broad
  - Strongly curved
  - Roughened tuberosity in place of the tubercle
- R10
  - A single articular facet on the head

- R11
  - A single articular facet on the head
  - Less curved
  - Shallow costal groove
  - No neck or tubercle
  - Narrow sternal end
- R12
  - A single articular facet on the head
  - No neck, tubercle, angle, or costal groove
  - Particularly short

BOX 1.7.21 Siding Tips—Ribs

- The superior shaft surface is smooth and the inferior sharp. The opposite pattern is found in the first rib
- The head lies medially and the tubercle inferiorly, except for the first rib, on which the head points inferiorly

- The sternal end is flat with a U-shaped depression and lies anteriorly

---

1.7.2 Appendicular Skeleton

1.7.2.1 Shoulder Girdle

The *shoulder girdle* (*pectoral girdle*) consists of the clavicle and scapula (Fig. 1.7.37). It supports and facilitates the movement of the arms by providing sites for muscle attachment.

The clavicle and scapula (three-dimensional model in Fig. 1.7.37 and actual skeletal elements in Figs. 1.7.38—1.7.40) are rarely mistaken for other elements. Identification and siding tips are provided in Boxes 1.7.22—1.7.25. The clavicle has a distinct S shape, which renders it vulnerable to fractures. It articulates with the manubrium and the scapula, and

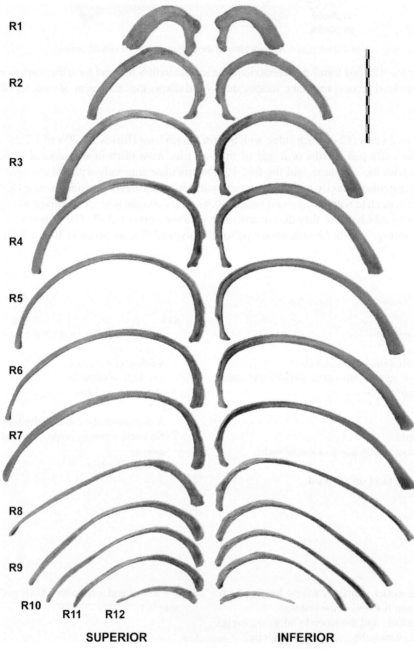

R1

R2

R3

R4

R5

R6

R7

R8

R9

R10

R11   R12

SUPERIOR   **INFERIOR**

FIGURE 1.7.35   Superior and inferior views of the right ribs.

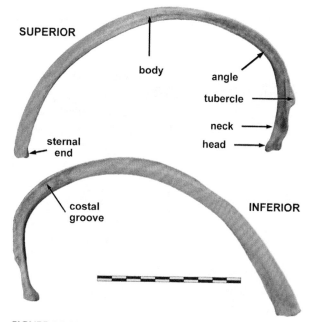

FIGURE 1.7.36 Superior and inferior views of the fourth right rib.

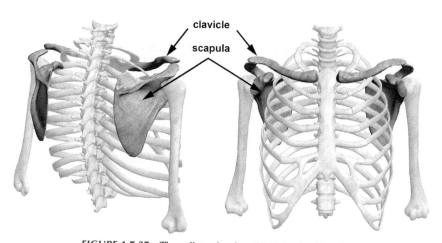

FIGURE 1.7.37 Three-dimensional model of the shoulder girdle.

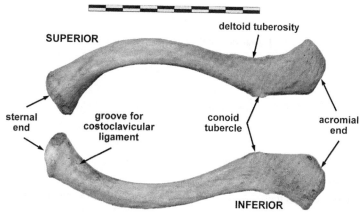

FIGURE 1.7.38 Superior and inferior views of the right clavicle; anterior is up for the superior view and down for the inferior view, lateral is toward the right for both views.

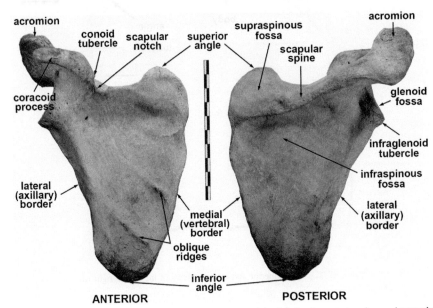

FIGURE 1.7.39 Anterior and posterior views of the right scapula; lateral is toward the left for the anterior view and toward the right for the posterior view.

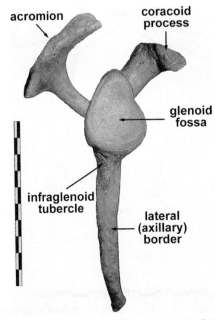

FIGURE 1.7.40 Lateral view of the right scapula; anterior is toward the right.

BOX 1.7.22 Identification Tip—Clavicle

- Distinctly S-shaped tubular shaft

BOX 1.7.23 Siding Tips—Clavicle

- The superior surface is smoother than the inferior surface
- The sternal end is bulbous, whereas the lateral end is flat

- The S shape of the bone is due to an anterior curvature toward the sternal end, a posterior curve in the midshaft, and another anterior curve toward the acromial end
- The conoid tubercle lies inferiorly and toward the acromial

BOX 1.7.24 Identification Tips—Scapula

- Overall distinct morphology
- Much thinner than the ilium (see Section 1.7.2.2)
- Glenoid fossa is smaller than the acetabulum (see Section 1.7.2.2)

- No articular facets on the coracoid process, in contrast to the transverse process of the thoracic vertebrae

BOX 1.7.25 Siding Tips—Scapula

- The scapular spine lies posteriorly
- The coracoid process lies anteriorly and points laterally
- The glenoid fossa is lateral; it is round inferiorly and rather pointy superiorly

- The vertebral border and the inferior angle are concave anteriorly and convex posteriorly
- The axillary border becomes thinner inferiorly
- The spine is thinner medially

contributes to the stabilization of the shoulder by allowing the attachment of muscles of the upper limbs, chest, and back. The scapula is a flat, triangular-shaped bone, which articulates with the humerus and clavicle and facilitates shoulder movement.

1.7.2.2 Pelvic Girdle

The pelvic girdle consists of the os coxae (Boxes 1.7.26 and 1.7.27, Figs. 1.7.41−1.7.43), sacrum, and coccyx. It largely supports the weight of the body, facilitates bipedal locomotion, and protects vital organs, such as the urinary bladder, part of the large intestine, and the internal reproductive organs.

BOX 1.7.26 Identification Tips—Os Coxae

- Overall distinct morphology
- Ilia much thicker than the scapulae, but lighter and not as uniformly thick as the cranial vault bones

- Bone surrounds the auricular surfaces, in contrast to the sacral auricular surfaces

BOX 1.7.27 Siding Tips—Os Coxae

- The pubic symphysis lies anteriorly and points medially
- The anterior surface of the pubic area is rougher than the posterior
- The superior ischiopubic ramus is rather thick and twisted, whereas the inferior is thinner and flat

- The ischial tuberosity lies inferiorly, posteriorly, and laterally
- The auricular surface lies posteromedially
- The acetabulum is lateral and the acetabular notch lies anteroinferiorly
- The greater and lesser sciatic notches lie posteriorly

The sacrum and coccyx have already been presented as parts of the spine, thus only the os coxae will be discussed here. The os coxae are irregularly shaped and exhibit morphological differences between males and females, which make them the primary skeletal elements examined for sex assessment (see Chapter 3). In subadults, each os coxa consists of three separate elements: the ilium, ischium, and pubis (Fig. 1.7.41), which gradually fuse. The os coxae articulate with each other, as well as with the sacrum and femur.

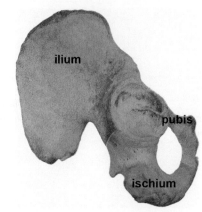

FIGURE 1.7.41 Parts of the os coxa.

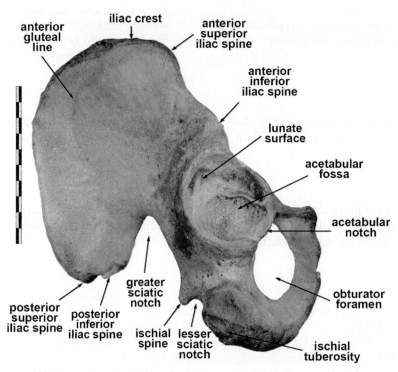

FIGURE 1.7.42 Lateral view of the right os coxa; anterior is toward the right.

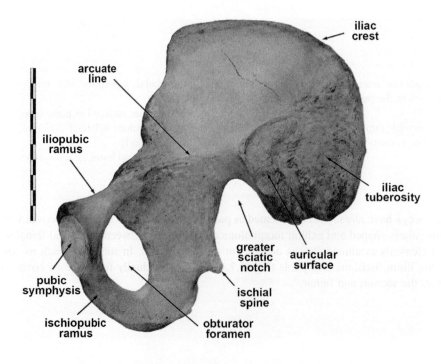

1.7.2.3 Arm and Leg Bones

The arm bones allow the attachment of muscles that enable upper limb movement. The *humerus* (Box 1.7.28, Figs. 1.7.44—1.7.46) is the largest arm bone and articulates with the scapula, radius, and ulna. The *radius* (Box 1.7.29, Figs. 1.7.47 and 1.7.48) is the lateral bone of the forearm and articulates with the humerus, ulna, lunate, and scaphoid. The *ulna* (Box 1.7.30, Figs. 1.7.49 and 1.7.50) is the medial bone of the forearm and articulates with the humerus and radius.

The leg bones support the weight of the body and enable motion. The *femur* (Box 1.7.31, Figs. 1.7.51—1.7.53) is the largest bone of the skeleton and articulates with the os coxa, tibia, and patella. The *patella* (Box 1.7.32, Fig. 1.7.54) is the

---

BOX 1.7.28 Siding Tips—Humerus

- The head points medially
- The lesser tubercle and intertubercular groove lie anteriorly
- The greater tubercle lies laterally and somewhat anteriorly
- The deltoid tuberosity lies laterally
- The capitulum is lateral

- The olecranon fossa is posterior
- The lateral epicondyle is smaller than the medial epicondyle
- The coronoid fossa is larger than the radial fossa and it is medial

---

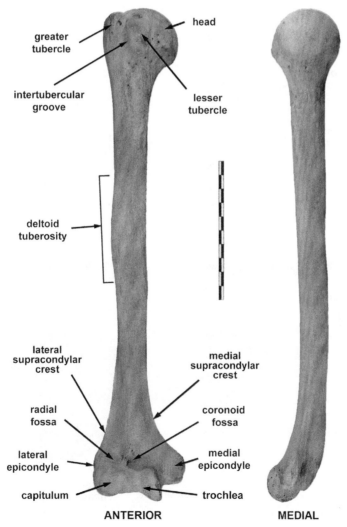

FIGURE 1.7.44   Anterior and medial views of the right humerus.

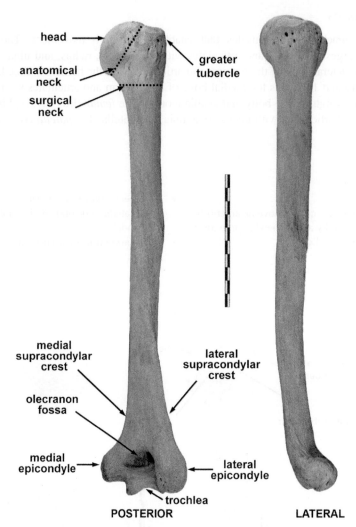

head

anatomical
neck

surgical
neck

greater
tubercle

medial
supracondylar
crest

lateral
supracondylar
crest

olecranon
fossa

medial
epicondyle

lateral
epicondyle

trochlea

POSTERIOR

LATERAL

FIGURE 1.7.45 Posterior and lateral views of the right humerus.

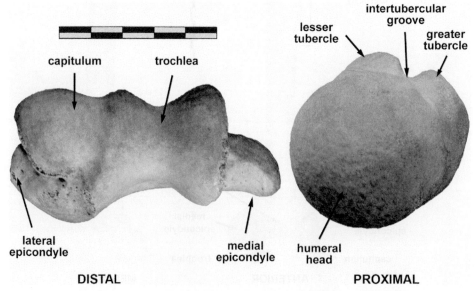

capitulum

trochlea

intertubercular
groove

lesser
tubercle

greater
tubercle

lateral
epicondyle

medial
epicondyle

humeral
head

DISTAL

PROXIMAL

FIGURE 1.7.46 Distal and proximal views of the right humerus; anterior is up.

BOX 1.7.29 Siding Tips—Radius

- The articular circumference of the head is wider medially
- The radial tuberosity lies medially and its posterior border protrudes more than the anterior
- The radial shaft anterior to the interosseous crest is rather concave, whereas the shaft posterior to the crest is slightly convex

- The styloid process is lateral
- The ulnar notch is medial
- The dorsal tubercle is posterior

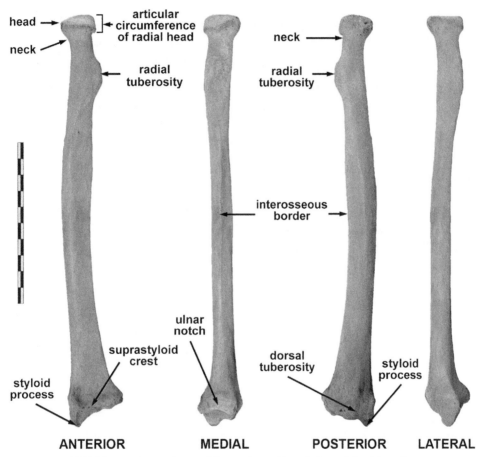

FIGURE 1.7.47   Anterior, medial, posterior, and lateral views of the right radius.

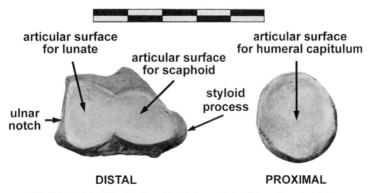

FIGURE 1.7.48   Distal and proximal views of the right radius; dorsal is up.

BOX 1.7.30 Siding Tips—Ulna

- The coronoid process is proximal and anterior
- The radial notch lies anterolaterally
- The interosseous border lies anterolaterally

- The styloid process is distal and posterior
- The groove for the extensor carpi ulnaris is lateral

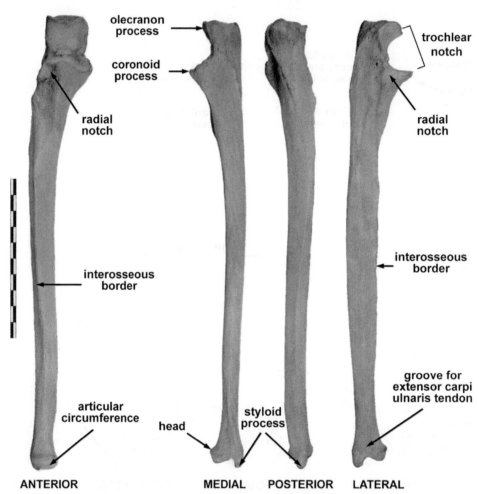

FIGURE 1.7.49   Anterior, medial, posterior, and lateral views of the right ulna.

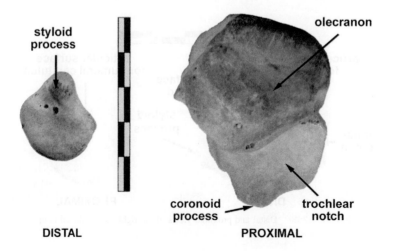

BOX 1.7.31 Siding Tips—Femur

- The head faces medially
- The *fovea capitis* lies slightly posteroinferiorly in relation to the center of the head
- The lesser trochanter is medial and the greater trochanter is lateral
- The shaft widens distally

- The *linea aspera* lies posteriorly and gradually becomes thinner from superior to inferior
- The medial supracondylar ridge is less pronounced than the lateral one
- The lateral part of the patellar surface expands more superiorly
- The lateral epicondyle is smaller than the medial one

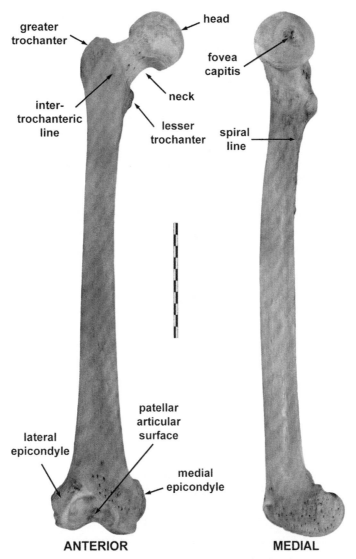

greater trochanter

head

fovea capitis

neck

inter-trochanteric line

lesser trochanter

spiral line

patellar articular surface

lateral epicondyle

medial epicondyle

ANTERIOR   **MEDIAL**

FIGURE 1.7.51 Anterior and medial views of the right femur.

largest sesamoid bone and articulates with the distal femur. It is found within the quadriceps tendon and its function is to protect the knee joint and enhance its function. The *tibia* (Box 1.7.33, Figs. 1.7.55−1.7.57) is the second largest bone of the skeleton; it lies medially and articulates with the femur, fibula, and talus. Finally, the *fibula* (Box 1.7.34, Figs. 1.7.58 and 1.7.59) is the lateral bone in the leg and it is not weight-bearing. It articulates with the tibia and talus.

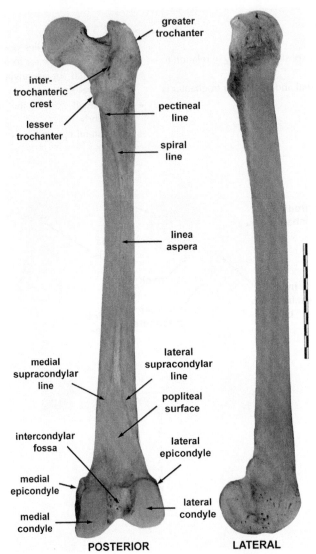

POSTERIOR   **LATERAL**

FIGURE 1.7.52 Posterior and lateral views of the right femur.

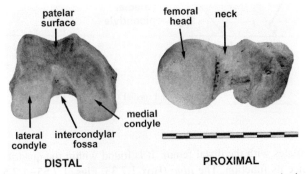

DISTAL   **PROXIMAL**

FIGURE 1.7.53 Distal and proximal views of the right femur; anterior is up.

- The apex is distal
- The medial articular facet is smaller than the lateral

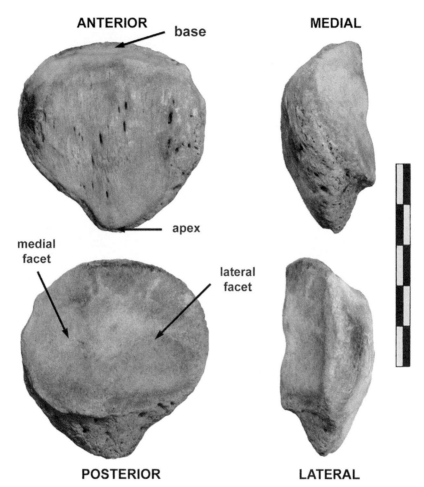

ANTERIOR

base

apex

medial facet

lateral facet

MEDIAL

POSTERIOR

LATERAL

FIGURE 1.7.54   Anterior, medial, posterior, and lateral views of the right patella.

- The medial articular surface of the proximal epiphysis is larger and more oval shaped than the lateral one
- The fibular articular surface is posterolateral
- The tibial tuberosity and anterior crest are anterior
- The soleal line has a superolateral to inferomedial direction
- The proximal diaphysis has a triangular cross section, whereas the distal is rectangular
- The interosseous crest lies laterally
- The malleolus is medial and its most prominent projection points anteriorly

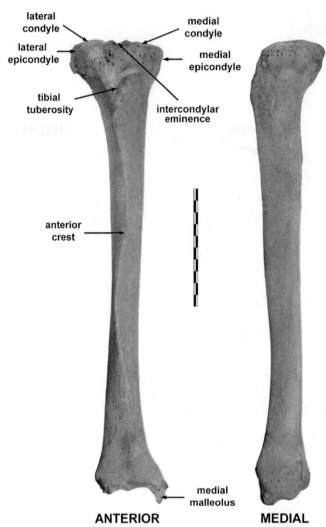

lateral
condyle

medial
condyle

lateral
epicondyle

medial
epicondyle

tibial
tuberosity

intercondylar
eminence

anterior
crest

medial
malleolus

ANTERIOR   **MEDIAL**

FIGURE 1.7.55 Anterior and medial views of the right tibia.

Arm and leg bones have morphological similarities that may inhibit proper identification in cases of partially preserved remains. Box 1.7.35 presents the main distinctive traits to be used for anatomical areas most commonly confused.

1.7.2.4 Hand and Foot Bones

Each hand consists of 8 carpals, 5 metacarpals, and 14 phalanges arranged in three rows (proximal, intermediate, distal) (Fig. 1.7.60). It must be noted that the thumb has no middle phalanx. Similarly, each foot consists of 7 tarsals, 5 metatarsals, and 14 phalanges, also arranged in three rows, and the hallux is also lacking a middle phalanx (Fig. 1.7.61).

The *carpal bones* are arranged in two rows, a proximal and a distal. In anatomical position, the carpals in the proximal row (lateral to medial) are the scaphoid, lunate, triquetral, and pisiform, and the carpals in the distal row (lateral to medial) are the trapezium, trapezoid, capitate, and hamate. The *scaphoid* (Fig. 1.7.62) articulates with the lunate and the distal radius, as well as with the capitate, trapezium, and trapezoid. The *lunate* (Fig. 1.7.63) articulates with the distal radius, scaphoid, capitate, and triquetral and indirectly with the ulna. The *triquetral* (Fig. 1.7.64) articulates with the lunate, hamate, pisiform, and distal ulna. The *pisiform* (Fig. 1.7.65) articulates only with the triquetral. The *trapezium* (Fig. 1.7.66) articulates with the scaphoid, trapezoid, and first metacarpal. The *trapezoid* (Fig. 1.7.67) articulates with the trapezium, scaphoid, capitate, and second metacarpal. The *capitate* (Fig. 1.7.68) is the largest carpal bone and articulates with the trapezoid, scaphoid, lunate, hamate, and second, third, and fourth metacarpals. Finally, the *hamate* (Fig. 1.7.69) articulates with the triquetral, capitate, lunate, and fourth and fifth metacarpals.

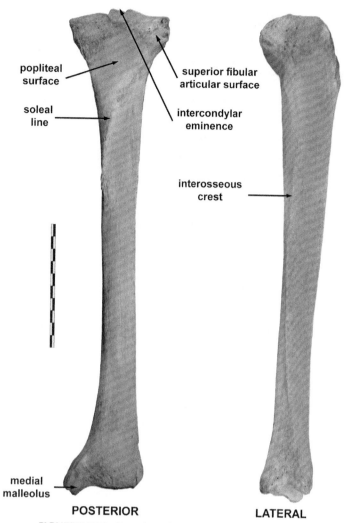

popliteal
surface

soleal
line

superior fibular
articular surface

intercondylar
eminence

interosseous
crest

medial
malleolus

POSTERIOR

LATERAL

FIGURE 1.7.56 Posterior and lateral views of the right tibia.

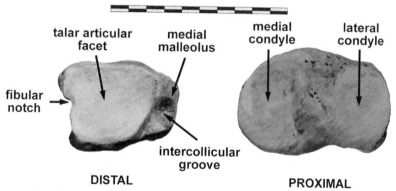

talar articular
facet

medial
malleolus

medial
condyle

lateral
condyle

fibular
notch

intercollicular
groove

DISTAL

PROXIMAL

FIGURE 1.7.57 Distal and proximal views of the right tibia; anterior is up.

BOX 1.7.34 Siding Tips—Fibula

- The head is rather bulbous, whereas the base is flat
- The styloid process is lateral and posterior, whereas the proximal articular facet is medial
- The malleolar fossa is posterior and the distal articular surface faces medially

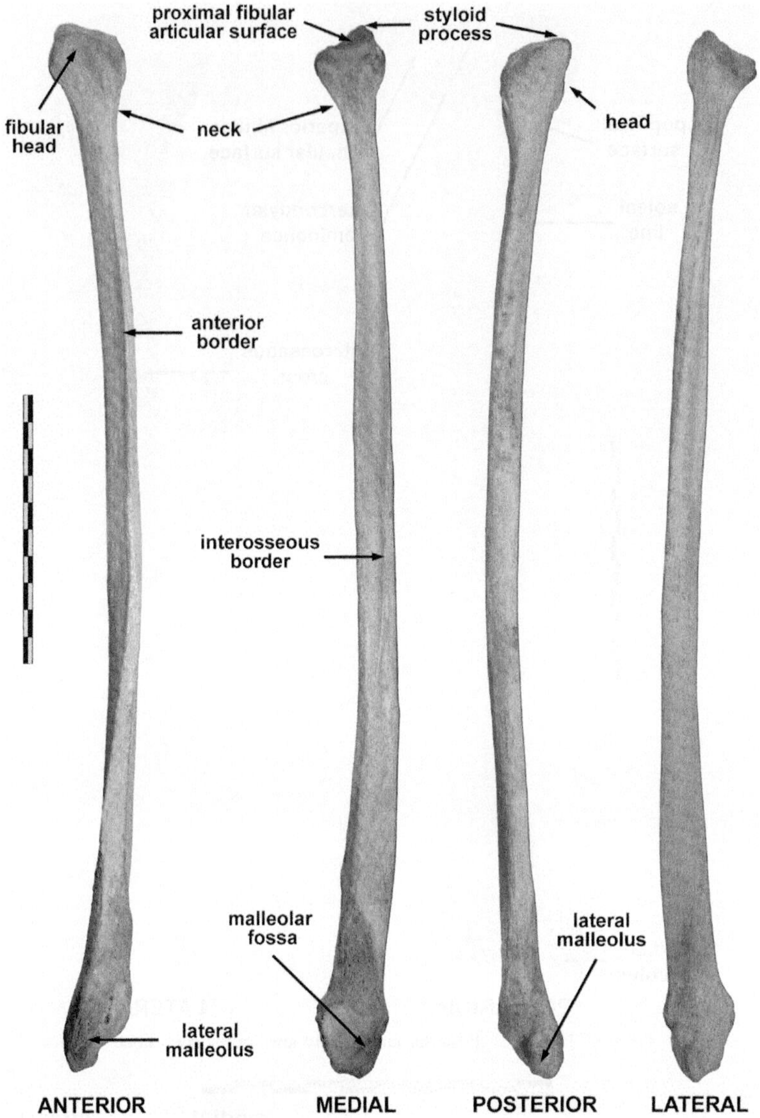

proximal fibular
articular surface

styloid
process

fibular
head

neck

head

anterior
border

interosseous
border

malleolar
fossa

lateral
malleolus

lateral
malleolus

lateral
malleolus

ANTERIOR   **MEDIAL**   **POSTERIOR**   **LATERAL**

FIGURE 1.7.58   Anterior, medial, posterior, and lateral views of the right fibula.

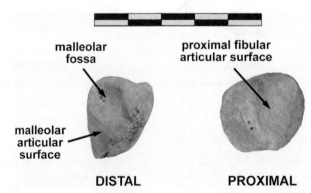

malleolar
fossa

proximal fibular
articular surface

malleolar
articular
surface

DISTAL   **PROXIMAL**

FIGURE 1.7.59   Distal and proximal views of the right fibula; anterior is down.

BOX 1.7.35 Identification Tips—Arm and Leg Bones

- Head
  - Hemispherical humeral head compared to spherical femoral head
  - *Fovea capitis* in femoral head (absent in the humerus)
  - Larger and flatter radial head compared to ulnar distal end (plus no styloid process)
- Diaphysis
  - Humeral diaphysis is larger and more circular in cross section than the radial, ulnar, or fibular diaphyses; smaller and more irregular than the femoral diaphysis; and less triangular than the tibial diaphysis

- Ulnar diaphysis is rather triangular in cross section, with interosseous crest, and decreases in circumference from proximal to distal, in contrast to the radius or fibula
- Radial diaphysis has characteristic teardrop cross section
- Femoral diaphysis is larger and more circular in cross section than all other elements
- Tibial diaphysis is much larger than the ulnar and radial diaphyses, with triangular cross section
- Fibular diaphysis is thin and irregular in cross section

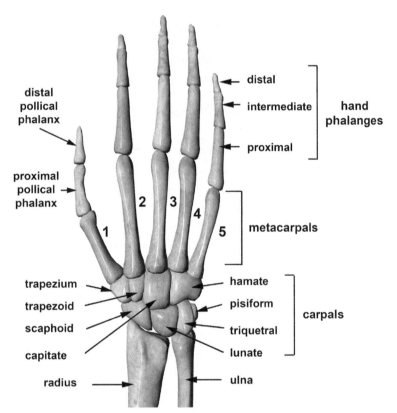

FIGURE 1.7.60 Three-dimensional model of right hand bones.

The *metacarpals* (MCs) (Box 1.7.36, Figs. 1.7.70−1.7.73) are tube-shaped bones, each with a single rounded distal articular surface (head) and a proximal square base. The *first MC* (MC 1) articulates with the trapezium and first proximal phalanx; the *second MC* (MC 2) articulates with the trapezoid, capitate, trapezium, MC 3, and second proximal phalanx; the *third MC* (MC 3) articulates with the capitate, MC 2, MC 4, and third proximal phalanx; the *fourth MC* (MC 4) articulates with the hamate, MC 3, MC 5, fourth proximal phalanx, and sometimes the capitate; the *fifth MC* (MC 5) articulates with the hamate, MC 4, and fifth proximal phalanx.

The hand has 14 phalanges (Box 1.7.37, Figs. 1.7.60 and 1.7.74). Each finger has a proximal, middle, and distal phalanx except for the thumb, which has only a proximal and a distal phalanx, as mentioned above.

The *tarsals* lie in the posterior part of the foot. The *calcaneus* (Figs. 1.7.75 and 1.7.76) is the largest tarsal and articulates with the talus and cuboid. The *talus* (Figs. 1.7.77 and 1.7.78) is the second largest tarsal bone and articulates with

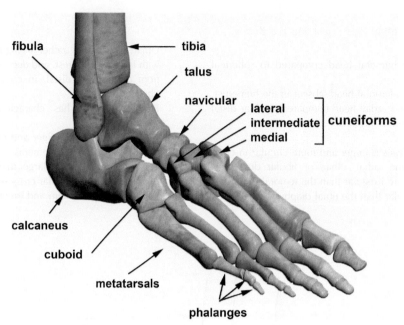

FIGURE 1.7.61   Three-dimensional model of right foot bones.

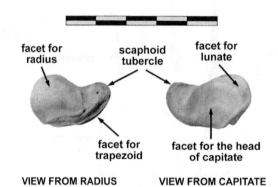

FIGURE 1.7.62   Right scaphoid: views from the radius and capitate; palmar is up.

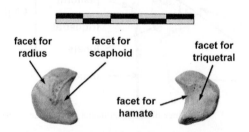

FIGURE 1.7.63   Right lunate: views from the scaphoid and triquetral; palmar is up.

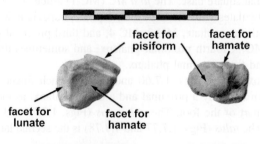

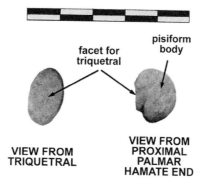

FIGURE 1.7.65 Right pisiform: views from the triquetral and proximal palmar hamate end; distal is down.

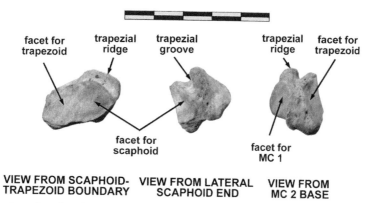

FIGURE 1.7.66 Right trapezium: views from the scaphoid—trapezoid boundary, lateral scaphoid end, and metacarpal (MC) 2 base; palmar is up.

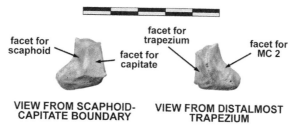

FIGURE 1.7.67 Right trapezoid: views from the scaphoid—capitate boundary and distalmost trapezium; palmar is up. *MC*, metacarpal.

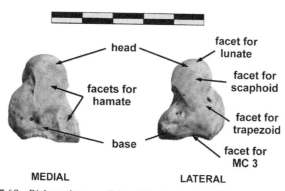

FIGURE 1.7.68 Right capitate: medial and lateral views; proximal is up. *MC*, metacarpal.

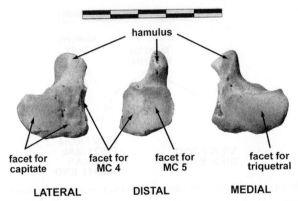

FIGURE 1.7.69 Right hamate: lateral, distal, and medial views; palmar is up. *MC*, metacarpal.

BOX 1.7.36 Siding Tips—Metacarpals

- General: The palmar shaft surface is slightly concave and the dorsal slightly convex
- MC 1: The maximum projection on the palmar surface of the base lies medially
- MC 2: The proximalmost part of the base has a medial wedge for articulation with MC 3

- MC 3: The styloid process is lateral
- MC 4: The proximal medial facet has a single articular surface
- MC 5: The nonarticular facet of the base lies medially

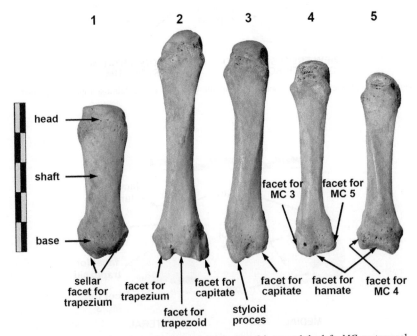

FIGURE 1.7.70 Dorsal view of right metacarpals; lateral is toward the left. *MC*, metacarpal.

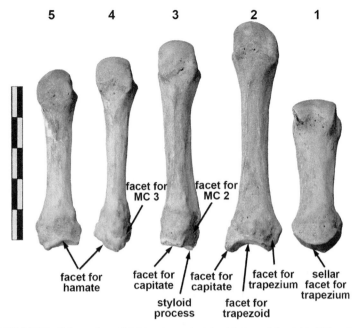

FIGURE 1.7.71 Palmar view of right metacarpals; lateral is toward the right. *MC*, metacarpal.

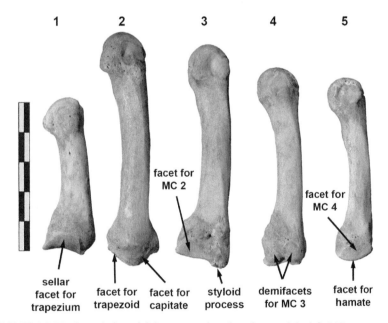

FIGURE 1.7.72 Lateral view of right metacarpals; palmar is toward the left. *MC*, metacarpal.

the tibia, fibula, calcaneus, and navicular. The *navicular* (Fig. 1.7.79) articulates with the talus, cuboid, and medial, intermediate, and lateral cuneiforms. The *cuboid* (Fig. 1.7.80) articulates with the calcaneus, navicular, lateral cuneiform, and fourth and fifth metatarsals. The *medial (first) cuneiform* (Fig. 1.7.81) is the largest cuneiform and articulates with the navicular, first and second metatarsals, and intermediate (second) cuneiform. The *intermediate (second) cuneiform* (Fig. 1.7.82) is the smallest cuneiform and articulates with the navicular, second metatarsal, and medial and lateral cuneiforms. Finally, the *lateral (third) cuneiform* (Fig. 1.7.83) articulates with the navicular, second and third metatarsals, intermediate cuneiform, and cuboid.

The *metatarsals* (MTs) (Box 1.7.38, Figs. 1.7.84−1.7.87) are found between the tarsals and the phalanges. The *first MT* (MT 1) is the shortest and thickest and articulates with the first proximal phalanx, medial (first) cuneiform, and second MT;

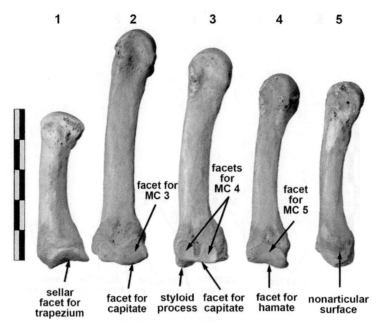

FIGURE 1.7.73 Medial view of right metacarpals; palmar is toward the right. *MC*, metacarpal.

BOX 1.7.37 Identification Tips—Manual Phalanges

- Proximal phalanges
  - Single proximal articular facet
  - Smooth, round distal articular facet, bearing a groove
- Intermediate phalanges
  - Double proximal articular facet
  - Smooth, round distal articular facet, bearing a slight "crest" in the midline

- Distal phalanges
  - Double proximal articular facet
  - No distal articular facet

Note: Right and left manual phalanges are extremely difficult to differentiate.

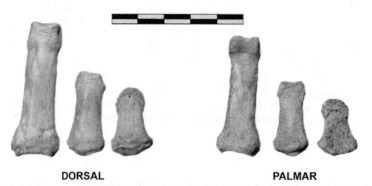

DORSAL   **PALMAR**

FIGURE 1.7.74 Dorsal and palmar views of representative proximal (left), intermediate (middle), and distal (right) manual phalanges.

the *second MT* (MT 2) articulates with the second proximal phalanx, intermediate cuneiform, and first and third MTs; the *third MT* (MT 3) articulates with the lateral cuneiform, third proximal phalanx, and second and fourth MTs; the *fourth MT* (MT 4) articulates with the cuboid, fourth proximal phalanx, and third and fifth MTs; the *fifth MT* (MT 5) articulates with the cuboid, fifth proximal phalanx, and MT 4.

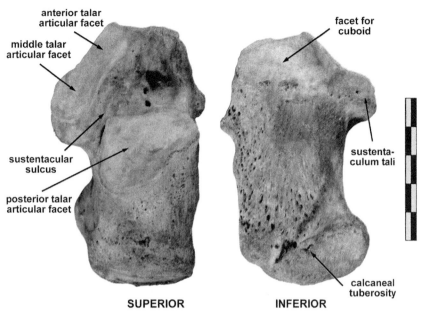

FIGURE 1.7.75   Right calcaneus: superior and inferior views; distal is up.

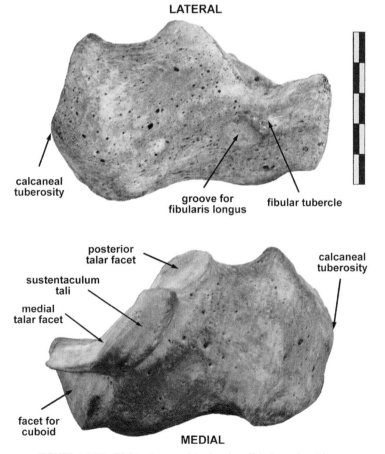

FIGURE 1.7.76   Right calcaneus: lateral and medial views; dorsal is up.

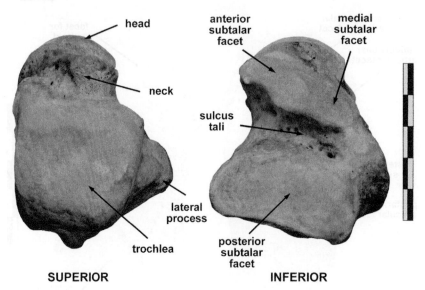

FIGURE 1.7.77 Right talus: superior and inferior views; distal is up.

As with the hand, the foot has 14 *phalanges* (Box 1.7.39, Figs. 1.7.61 and 1.7.88). Each toe has a proximal, middle, and distal phalanx except for the great toe, which has only a proximal and a distal phalanx, as noted above.

Hand and foot bones are usually separated during collection from the field. However, in cases of commingled remains, the criteria outlined in Box 1.7.40 may be used to differentiate the elements most commonly misidentified.

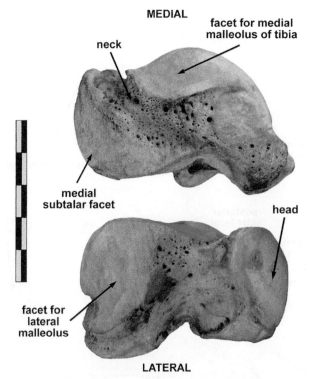

FIGURE 1.7.78 Right talus: medial and lateral views; dorsal is up.

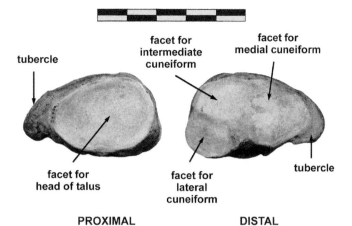

tubercle

facet for
intermediate
cuneiform

facet for
medial cuneiform

facet for
head of talus

facet for
lateral
cuneiform

tubercle

PROXIMAL

DISTAL

FIGURE 1.7.79 Right navicular: proximal and distal views; dorsal is up.

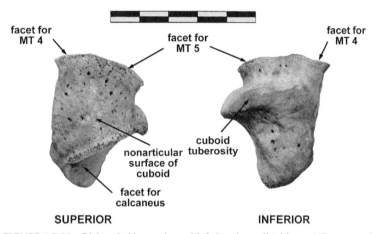

facet for
MT 4

facet for
MT 5

facet for
MT 4

nonarticular
surface of
cuboid

cuboid
tuberosity

facet for
calcaneus

SUPERIOR

INFERIOR

FIGURE 1.7.80 Right cuboid: superior and inferior views; distal is up. *MT*, metatarsal.

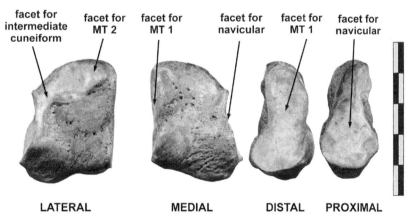

facet for
intermediate
cuneiform

facet for
MT 2

facet for
MT 1

facet for
navicular

facet for
MT 1

facet for
navicular

LATERAL

MEDIAL

DISTAL

PROXIMAL

FIGURE 1.7.81 Right medial cuneiform: lateral, medial, distal, and proximal views; dorsal is up. *MT*, metatarsal.

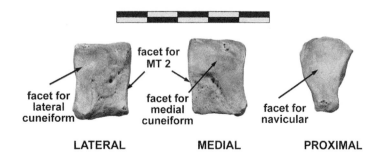

facet for
MT 2

facet for
lateral
cuneiform

facet for
medial
cuneiform

facet for
navicular

LATERAL

MEDIAL

PROXIMAL

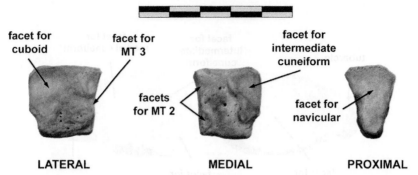

FIGURE 1.7.83 Right lateral cuneiform: lateral, medial, and proximal views; dorsal is up. *MT*, metatarsal.

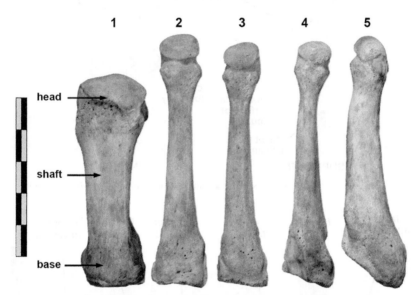

FIGURE 1.7.84 Dorsal view of right metatarsals; lateral is toward the right.

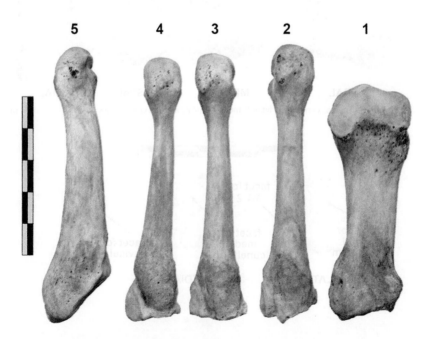

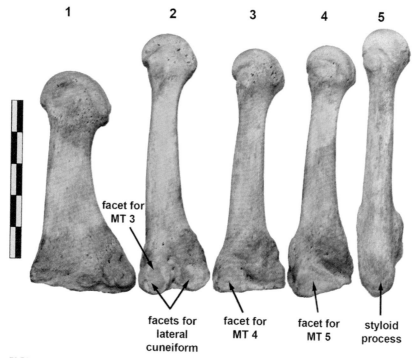

FIGURE 1.7.86 Lateral view of right metatarsals; plantar is toward the right. *MT*, metatarsal.

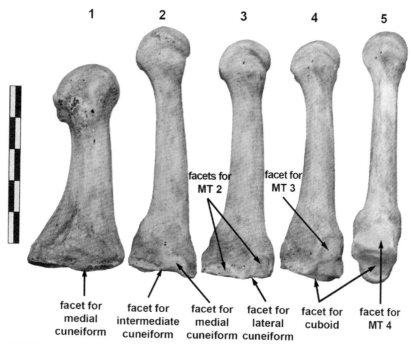

FIGURE 1.7.87 Medial view of right metatarsals; plantar is toward the left. *MT*, metatarsal.

BOX 1.7.39 Identification Tips—Pedal Phalanges

- Proximal phalanges
  - Narrow shaft, large base and head
  - Single proximal articular facet
  - Slight groove in the midline of the head
- Intermediate phalanges
  - Small and cubic shaped
  - Double proximal articular facet

- Symmetrical and round distal articular facet
- Distal phalanges
  - Very small and stout
  - No articulation at distal end
  - Double proximal articular facet

Note: Right and left pedal phalanges are extremely difficult to differentiate.

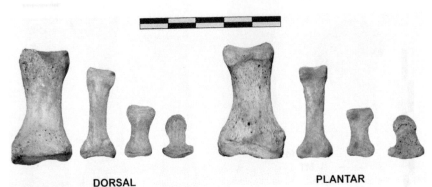

FIGURE 1.7.88 Dorsal and plantar views of representative right pedal phalanges (from left to right: first proximal phalanx, second proximal phalanx, second intermediate phalanx, second distal phalanx).

BOX 1.7.40 Identification Tips—Hand and Foot Bones

- MC diaphyses are less slender than MT diaphyses
- MC heads are round; MT heads are mediolaterally compressed

- Manual phalanges have flat palmar surfaces; the diaphyses of pedal phalanges are circular in cross section
- Pedal phalanges are constricted at the midshaft, in contrast to manual phalanges

1.8 TEETH

Teeth are usually the best preserved skeletal elements. This section focuses on the permanent dentition and only representative deciduous teeth are given, in the context of facilitating the discrimination between permanent and deciduous tooth types. For a thorough presentation of the deciduous dentition, the reader may consult the books on juvenile osteology provided as suggested readings at the end of the chapter.

1.8.1 Tooth Types and Dental Numbering Systems

The human dentition is divided into four quadrants: upper left, upper right, lower left, and lower right. Humans are *heterodontic*, that is, within each quadrant there are teeth with different forms and functions: incisors, canines, premolars, and molars (Fig. 1.8.1). To express the number of teeth of each type in each quadrant, a *dental formula* is used. In humans, the permanent dentition consists of 32 teeth in total, with the dental formula 2.1.2.3/2.1.2.3 indicating two incisors, one canine, two premolars, and three molars in each quadrant. In contrast, the deciduous teeth are 20, with five teeth per quadrant: two incisors, one canine, and two molars (dental formula 2.1.0.2/2.1.0.2).

Several methods have been devised for the coding of various tooth types in the maxilla and mandible. The most descriptive way is shown in Fig. 1.8.2. The capital letters I (incisor), C (canine), P (premolar), and M (molar) denote the type of permanent

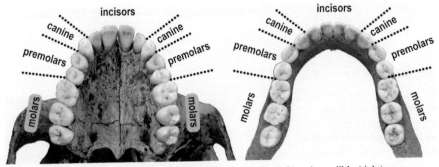

FIGURE 1.8.1 Permanent dentition of the maxilla (left) and mandible (right).

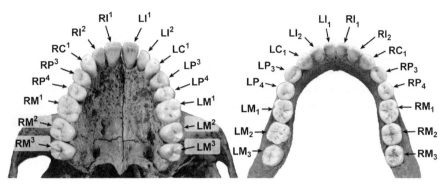

FIGURE 1.8.2 Descriptive coding scheme for the permanent dentition of the maxilla (left) and mandible (right). *C,* canine; *I,* incisor; *L,* left; *M,* molar; *P,* premolar; *R,* right.

tooth. The side of the tooth, that is, right or left, is denoted by R and L, respectively. Finally, incisors are numbered as either 1 or 2, for central and lateral teeth, respectively; the canines are all 1's; the two premolars are denoted as 3 or 4; and the molars can be 1, 2, or 3. Note that these numbers are given as either superscripts or subscripts. Superscripts are used for maxillary and subscripts for mandibular teeth. Thus, for example, the maxillary right permanent central incisor is denoted by RI^1.

For the deciduous dentition the symbols used are the same but lowercase. Thus, i, c, and m are used to denote the incisors, canines, and molars (there are no premolars), and the letter d precedes the tooth type. For example, the maxillary right deciduous central incisor is denoted by Rdi^1.

At this point a nomenclature issue should be clarified. The mammalian dentition generally consists of three incisors, one canine, four premolars, and three molars per quadrant. The numbering of the teeth follows the aforementioned general formula even in genera that have lost certain teeth during the course of evolution, such as humans. Specifically, humans have lost their first and second premolars; therefore, the remaining two premolars are numbered as P3 and P4 instead of P1 and P2, as they correspond to the third and fourth premolars of the mammalian dentition.

Two other broadly used dental coding schemes are the Universal Numbering System (UNS) and the Fédération Dentaire Internationale (FDI) system. The UNS is adopted primarily in the United States and assigns a number from 1 to 32 to each tooth, as seen in Fig. 1.8.3. The FDI system is used worldwide and provides a two-digit number for each tooth, whereby the first number expresses the quadrant and the second number the tooth (Fig. 1.8.4).

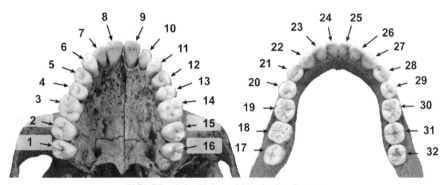

FIGURE 1.8.3 Universal Numbering System.

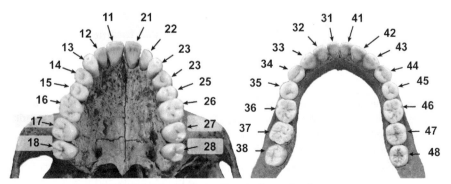

FIGURE 1.8.4 Fédération Dentaire Internationale system.

1.8.2 Dental Directional Terms

For the human dentition, the principal directional terms are shown in Fig. 1.8.5. As can be seen, *mesial* means toward the midline of the dental arch, and *distal* is the opposite of mesial. *Lingual* means toward the tongue, *labial* toward the lips, and *buccal* toward the cheek. Note that labial is used for incisors and canines, and buccal for premolars and molars. In addition, *interproximal* is the area where adjacent teeth are in contact; the *occlusal* surface is the chewing surface of premolars and molars, *incisal* is the biting surface of the incisors and canines, and *apical* means toward the tip of the root.

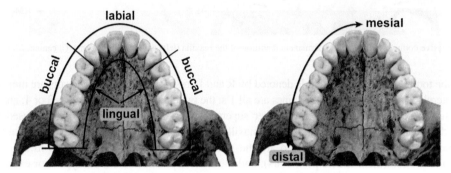

FIGURE 1.8.5 Directional terms for the human dentition.

1.8.3 Tooth Anatomy and Composition

Teeth have two major parts (Fig. 1.8.6): the *crown* (above the gumline) and the *root* (below the gumline). The point where the crown and the root meet is called the *cervix* or *neck*, whereas the *cementoenamel* junction encircles the cervix.

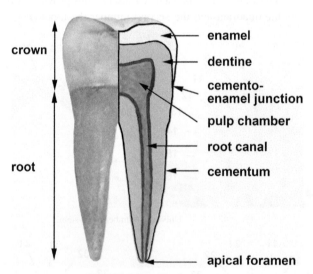

FIGURE 1.8.6 Tooth structure.

The most important anatomical features of the various tooth types are the following (Fig. 1.8.7): A *cusp* is a conical eminence on the occlusal surface of the crown. The main cusps on premolars and molars have specific names, as shown in Fig. 1.8.8. A *fissure* is a cleft between cusps, and a *groove* is a large fissure. Finally, a *fovea* is a small depression, and a *tuberculum* is a bulge on the lower part of the lingual surface of the anterior teeth.

Teeth are made of three tissue types: enamel, cementum, and dentine (Fig. 1.8.6). The *enamel* covers the crowns; it is extremely hard, and once it is formed, it cannot remodel as it has no blood supply and it consists of almost 95% inorganic

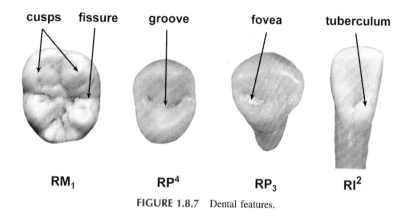

FIGURE 1.8.7 Dental features.

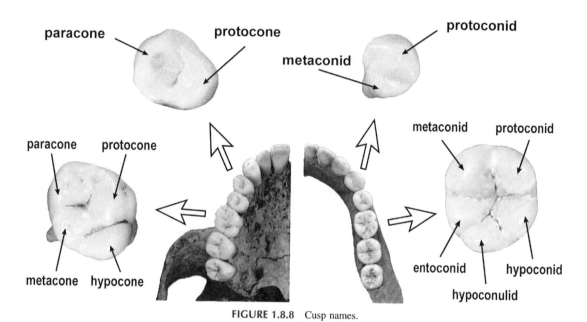

FIGURE 1.8.8 Cusp names.

components (hydroxyapatite), 4% water, and 1% organic material. The tissue beneath the enamel in the crown and forming most of the root is called *dentine* and consists of about 70% hydroxyapatite, 20% organic materials (mainly collagen), and 10% water. Within the dentine is the *pulp cavity*, which extends from the crown into the roots and contains nerves and blood vessels. The *cementum* covers the dentine at the root and consists of approximately 45% hydroxyapatite, 33% proteins (mainly collagen), and 22% water.

1.8.4 Tooth Formation and Development

Teeth develop inside the jaws in spaces called *crypts* through a process known as *odontogenesis*. Humans first develop the *deciduous dentition* (or *primary dentition*), which is subsequently replaced by the *permanent dentition* (or *secondary dentition*). The rate of dental formation and eruption, as well as the rate of replacement of the deciduous teeth by permanent ones, is largely controlled genetically and constitutes one of the most accurate aging methods for juveniles (see Chapter 4).

Dentine is the first dental tissue that starts to form through a process called *dentinogenesis*. Cells called *odontoblasts* secrete an organic matrix, which subsequently mineralizes and forms dentine in layers, starting from the crown and progressing toward the tip of the root. The cells responsible for enamel formation are called *ameloblasts* and also start to form the enamel in layers from the tip of the crown toward the cervix. *Amelogenesis* is also based on the initial formation of an organic matrix that subsequently mineralizes; however, in this process there is also a *maturation phase* during which the enamel loses almost its entire organic component. Finally, cementum is also formed by the secretion of an organic matrix and its subsequent mineralization. It continues to be formed throughout life; thus it increases in thickness with age.

1.8.5 Tooth Identification

Teeth are not difficult to identify when they are retrieved embedded in the maxillary or mandibular alveoli, but the identification of loose teeth may be challenging. The criteria presented in this section should facilitate the process of discriminating human dental remains. However, as it will become clear, some of the standards employed are based on the size and shape of teeth relative to one another. As a result, certain standards are difficult to implement in commingled remains, in which it is often impossible to determine which teeth belong to each one of the individuals.

In each case, the steps to be followed are:

1. determine if the tooth is deciduous or permanent;
2. determine the tooth type (incisor, canine, premolar, molar);
3. determine if the tooth is maxillary or mandibular;
4. determine whether the tooth belongs to the right or left side; and
5. for the incisors, premolars, and molars, determine if the tooth is first, second, etc.

1.8.5.1 Discrimination Between Deciduous and Permanent Teeth (Box 1.8.1, Figs. 1.8.9 and 1.8.10)

> **BOX 1.8.1 Deciduous Versus Permanent Teeth**
> - Deciduous teeth are smaller than corresponding permanent teeth
> - Deciduous crowns are more bulbous than permanent crowns (deciduous molar crowns may be oddly shaped)
>
> - Deciduous roots are thinner and shorter than permanent roots and, in the case of molars, more divergent; deciduous roots are partly resorbed during the replacement of deciduous teeth by permanent ones

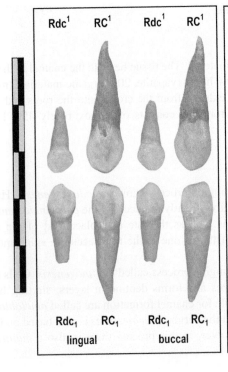
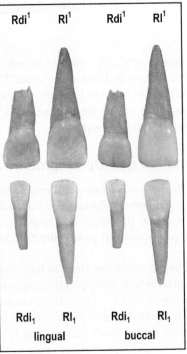

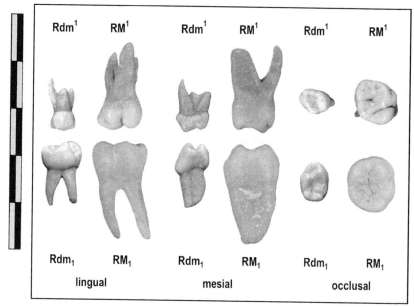

| Rdm¹ | RM¹ | Rdm¹ | RM¹ | Rdm¹ | RM¹ |

| Rdm₁ | RM₁ | Rdm₁ | RM₁ | Rdm₁ | RM₁ |
| lingual | | mesial | | occlusal | |

FIGURE 1.8.10 Comparison between deciduous and permanent molars.

1.8.5.2 Identification of Incisors (Boxes 1.8.2–1.8.6, Fig. 1.8.11)

BOX 1.8.2 Maxillary Versus Mandibular Incisors

- Maxillary incisor crowns are larger than mandibular crowns (maxillary central incisors are the largest)
- The mesiodistal diameter of maxillary incisors is greater than their buccolingual diameter; it is the opposite pattern in mandibular incisors

- There is more lingual relief in maxillary incisors (tuberculum, marginal ridges)
- Maxillary crowns are more asymmetrical than mandibular crowns
- Maxillary roots have rounded triangular cross section; mandibular roots are mesiodistally compressed

BOX 1.8.3 Right Versus Left Maxillary Incisors

- Rather upright mesial margin and bulging distal margin
- Incisal surface is sloping from mesial to distal

- Root apex is pointing distally

BOX 1.8.4 Right Versus Left Mandibular Incisors

- Mesioincisal corner is less rounded than distoincisal corner (especially in lateral incisors)

- Root apex is pointing distally

BOX 1.8.5 Central (First) Versus Lateral (Second) Maxillary Incisors

- First incisor crown is larger but less asymmetrical than the second incisor crown

- Second incisor root is longer than the first incisor root

BOX 1.8.6 Central (First) Versus Lateral (Second) Mandibular Incisors

- First incisor crown is a bit smaller than the second incisor crown

- Second incisor root is a bit longer and more distally curved than the first incisor root

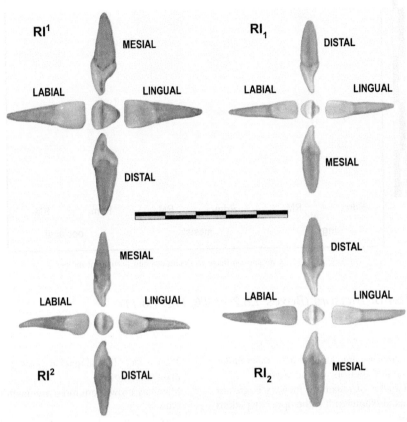

FIGURE 1.8.11 Incisors.

1.8.5.3 Identification of Canines (Boxes 1.8.7 and 1.8.8, Fig. 1.8.12)

BOX 1.8.7 Maxillary Versus Mandibular Canines

- Maxillary canines are broader and more robust than mandibular canines, but mandibular crowns are longer
- Maxillary crowns bulge mesially and distally more markedly than mandibular crowns
- There is more lingual relief in maxillary canines (cingulum, marginal ridges)
- Occlusal wear is mostly lingual in maxillary canines and labial in mandibular canines
- Mandibular roots are shorter and more compressed in cross section than maxillary roots

BOX 1.8.8 Right Versus Left Canines (Maxillary and Mandibular)

- Wear facets are more pronounced distally
- Root apex is pointing distally

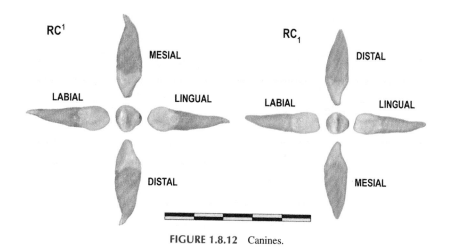

FIGURE 1.8.12 Canines.

1.8.5.4 Identification of Premolars (Boxes 1.8.9–1.8.13, Fig. 1.8.13)

BOX 1.8.9 Maxillary Versus Mandibular Premolars

- Two almost equally sized cusps in maxillary crowns; one buccal cusp and one or two smaller lingual cusps in mandibular crowns

- Deeper occlusal grooves in maxillary crowns

BOX 1.8.10 Right Versus Left Maxillary Premolars

- Lingual cusp tip is pointing mesially
- Root apex is pointing distally

- Buccal cusp tip is set distally compared to lingual cusp tip

---

BOX 1.8.11 Right Versus Left Mandibular Premolars

- Buccal cusp is much larger than lingual cusp(s)
- Mesiolingual cusp is usually larger than the distolingual when two lingual cusps are present

- Buccal and lingual cusp tips are pointing mesially
- Root apex is pointing distally

BOX 1.8.12 Third Versus Fourth Maxillary Premolars

- Fourth premolars are slightly smaller than third premolars
- Buccal cusp is much larger than lingual cusps in third premolars; cusp size difference is not as marked in fourth premolars
- Lingual cusp is more markedly mesially oriented in third premolars
- There are more marked central groove and fossae in third premolars
- There are more prominent marginal ridges in fourth premolars
- Third premolars are usually two-rooted; fourth premolars are usually single-rooted

BOX 1.8.13 Third Versus Fourth Mandibular Premolars

- Fourth premolars are somewhat larger than third premolars
- Third premolar crown is usually two-cusped; fourth premolar crown is usually three-cusped
- Third premolar crown has a circular occlusal outline; fourth premolar crown has a square occlusal outline
- Buccal cusp is much larger than the lingual cusps in third premolars (cusp size difference not as marked in fourth premolars)
- Double roots are rather common in third premolars (not in fourth premolars)

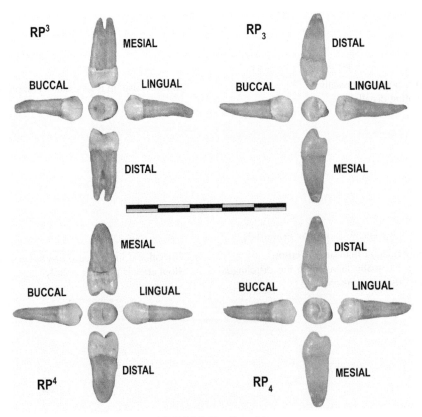

FIGURE 1.8.13 Premolars.

1.8.5.5 Identification of Molars (Boxes 1.8.14—1.8.18, Fig. 1.8.14)

BOX 1.8.14 Maxillary Versus Mandibular Molars

- Maxillary molars are usually three- or four-cusped; mandibular molars are usually four- or five-cusped
- Maxillary molar occlusal outline is rhomboidal; mandibular molar occlusal outline is square, rectangular, or oblong
- Mandibular molar cusps are symmetrically arranged relative to the mesiodistal axis; maxillary molar cusps are asymmetrically arranged
- Maxillary molars are three-rooted; mandibular molars are two-rooted
- Mesiolingual cusp is larger than distolingual cusp in maxillary molars; lingual cusps in mandibular molars are equally sized

BOX 1.8.15 Right Versus Left Maxillary Molars

- Occlusal wear facets slope lingually
- Mesial cusps are larger and more occlusally protruding than distal cusps
- Lingual root is clearly separated from buccal root

BOX 1.8.16 Right Versus Left Mandibular Molars

- Buccal crown surface is more bulging, with lower cervical margin and heavier wear
- Mesial root is larger and more grooved than distal root
- Roots are mesiodistally compressed and pointing distally

BOX 1.8.17 First Versus Second Versus Third Maxillary Molars

- First molar crowns are the largest and third molar crowns are the smallest
- Occlusal outline of the first molar crowns is trapezoidal, second molar crowns are rather square, and third molar crowns triangular
- Mesiobuccal and distobuccal cusps are of roughly equal size in first molars; mesiobuccal cusp is larger than the distobuccal on second molars
- Distolingual cusp size decreases from the first molar to the third, where it may be absent
- Mesial and distal interproximal wear facets in first and second molars; only mesial wear facets in third molars
- Root divergence decreases from the first molar to the third, where roots may be fused

BOX 1.8.18 First Versus Second Versus Third Mandibular Molars

- First molars are usually five-cusped, second molars usually four-cusped, and third molars variable with five, four, or three cusps
- Mesial and distal interproximal wear facets in first and second molars; only mesial wear facets in third molars
- Root divergence decreases from the first molar to the third, where roots may be fused

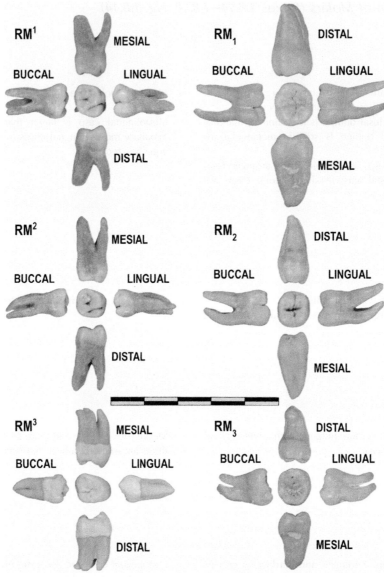

FIGURE 1.8.14 Molars.

REFERENCES

Buikstra JE, Ubelaker DH, editors. Standards for data collection from human skeletal remains. Fayetteville, Arkansas: Arkansas Archaeological Survey Report Number 44; 1994.

Moorrees CFA, Fanning EA, Hunt Jr EE. Formation and resorption of three deciduous teeth in children. American Journal of Physical Anthropology 1963;21:205−13.

Smith BH. Patterns of molar wear in hunter-gatherers and agriculturalists. American Journal of Physical Anthropology 1984;63:39−56.

SUGGESTED READINGS

This chapter does not provide in-text references because the information presented here can largely be found in any human anatomy textbook. The reader is advised to consult the following books for further information:

Bone Structure and Composition

Bilezikian JP, Raisz LG, Martin TJ. Principles of bone biology. 3rd ed. San Diego: Elsevier; 2008.
McKinley M, O'Loughlin V. Human anatomy. 4th ed. New York: McGraw-Hill; 2014.
Sevitt S. Bone repair and fracture healing in man. Edinburgh: Churchill Livingstone; 1981.
Shier D, Butler J, Lewis R. Hole's human anatomy and physiology. 14th ed. New York: McGraw-Hill; 2015.
Tortora GJ, Derrickson BH. Principles of anatomy and physiology. 14th ed. New York: Wiley; 2014.

Skeletal Development and Morphology

Bass WM. Human osteology: a laboratory and field manual. 5th ed. Columbia: Missouri Archaeological Society; 2005.
Bronner F, Farach-Carson MC, editors. Bone formation. London: Springer-Verlag; 2004.
Hall BK. Bones and cartilage: developmental and evolutionary skeletal biology. 2nd ed. San Diego: Elsevier; 2015.
Massaro EJ, Rogers JM, editors. The skeleton. biochemical, genetic, and molecular interactions in development and homeostasis. New Jersey: Humana Press; 2004.
Matshes E, Burbridge B, Sher B, Mohamed A, Juurlink B. Human osteology and skeletal radiology. An Atlas and guide. Boca Raton: CRC Press; 2004.
Sampson HW, Montgomery JL, Henryson GL. Atlas of the human skull. 2nd ed. College Station: Texas A&M University Press; 1991.
Steele DG, Bramblett CA. The anatomy and biology of the human skeleton. 4th ed. College Station: Texas A&M University Press; 1994.
White TD, Black MT, Folkens PA. Human osteology. 3rd ed. San Diego: Elsevier; 2011.

Dental Anatomy and Morphology

Fuller JL, Denehy GE, Schulein TM. Concise dental anatomy and morphology. 4th ed. Iowa: University of Iowa Publications Department; 2001.
Hillson S. Dental anthropology. Cambridge: Cambridge University Press; 1996.
Hillson S. Teeth. 2nd ed. Cambridge: Cambridge University Press; 2005.
Türp JC, Alt KW. Anatomy and morphology of human teeth. In: Alt KW, Rösing FW, Teschler-Nicola M, editors. Dental anthropology: fundamentals, limits and prospects. New York: Springer; 1998. p. 71–94.

Juvenile Osteology

Baker BJ, Dupras TL, Tocheri MW. The osteology of infants and children. College Station: Texas A&M University Press; 2005.
Fazekas IG, Kósa F. Forensic fetal osteology. Budapest: Akadémiai Kiadó; 1978.
Schaefer M, Black S, Scheuer L. Juvenile osteology. A laboratory and field manual. San Diego: Elsevier; 2008.
Scheuer L, Black S. Developmental Juvenile osteology. San Diego: Elsevier; 2000.

Discrimination Between Human and Nonhuman Bones

France DL. Human and nonhuman bone identification. Boca Raton: CRC Press; 2008.

Osteoware

Dudar JC. Inventories, adding individuals, and tracking skeletal elements. In: Wilczak CA, Dudar JC, editors. Osteoware™ software manual, volume I. Washington: Smithsonian Institution; 2011. p. 10–8.
Dudar JC, Ousley SD, Wilczak CA. Introduction to the Osteoware program. In: Wilczak CA, Dudar JC, editors. Osteoware™ software manual, volume I. Washington: Smithsonian Institution; 2011. p. 2–9.

APPENDICES

Appendix 1.I: Bone Inventory

This appendix provides diagrammatic and tabular inventories for recording the completeness of human skeletons.

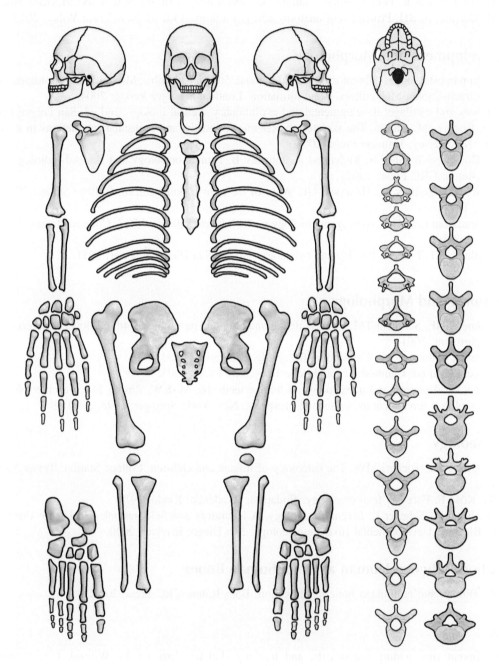

Note: The skeletal elements in the earlier figure are not given in correct scale; instead they are size adjusted so that they can all be visible and recorded.

TABLE 1.I.1 Bone Inventory—Skull

Single Bones	Paired Bones	R	L
Frontal	Parietal		
Occipital	Maxilla		
Ethmoid	Zygomatic		
Sphenoid	Temporal		
Mandible	Palatine		
Vomer	Lacrimal		
	Nasal		
	Inferior nasal concha		

TABLE 1.I.2 Bone Inventory—Shoulder and Pelvic Girdles

Single Bones	Paired Bones	R	L
Sacrum	Clavicle		
Coccyx	Scapula		
	Os coxa		

TABLE 1.I.3 Bone Inventory—Arm/Hand Bones and Leg/Foot Bones

Arm/Hand	R	L	Leg/Foot	R	L
Humerus			Femur		
Radius			Patella		
Ulna			Tibia		
Hamate			Fibula		
Scaphoid			Talus		
Capitate			Calcaneus		
Triquetral			Navicular		
Trapezium			First cuneiform		
Trapezoid			Second cuneiform		
Lunate			Third cuneiform		
Pisiform			Cuboid		
Metacarpal 1			Metatarsal 1		
Metacarpal 2			Metatarsal 2		
Metacarpal 3			Metatarsal 3		
Metacarpal 4			Metatarsal 4		
Metacarpal 5			Metatarsal 5		
No. of phalanges			No. of phalanges		

TABLE 1.1.4 Bone Inventory—Vertebrae

Cervical		Thoracic		Lumbar	
Atlas		T1		L1	
Axis		T2		L2	
C3		T3		L3	
C4		T4		L4	
C5		T5		L5	
C6		T6			
C7		T7		**Extra**	
		T8			
		T9			
		T10			
		T11			
		T12			

TABLE 1.1.5 Bone Inventory—Thorax

Single Bone		Paired Bones	R	L
Sternum		Rib 1		
		Rib 2		
		Rib 3		
		Rib 4		
		Rib 5		
		Rib 6		
		Rib 7		
		Rib 8		
		Rib 9		
		Rib 10		
		Rib 11		
		Rib 12		

Note 1: This inventory is designed for single skeletons. In cases of commingled remains and/or isolated bones, make a list of the element(s) preserved and specify the segments of these elements and the corresponding anatomical structures that are present (see also Appendix 2.I).

Note 2: The above recording scheme may be used for a simple presence/absence recording of each element, but it is advisable to record more specific information. For example, in the case of vertebrae, the preservation of vertebral bodies and neural arches may be recorded separately, whereas the long bones may be divided into the diaphysis and epiphyses, and so on.

Appendix 1.II: Tooth Inventory

Fill in the boxes of the following graph using the categories described in Table 1.II.1.

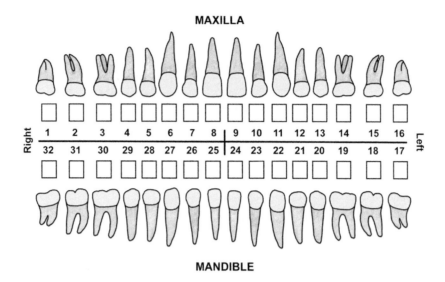

TABLE 1.II.1 Dental Recording Scheme

Category	Description
1	Present—unerupted
2	Present—erupting
3	Present—in occlusion
4	Missing—antemortem loss
5	Missing—postmortem loss
6	Missing—unclear time of loss

For a more detailed scheme see Buikstra and Ubelaker (1994).

Appendix 1.III: Bone and Tooth Inventory Using Osteoware

The Osteoware Program

Osteoware is a freely available software for recording qualitative and quantitative human skeletal data. It was developed by the Repatriation Osteology Lab at the Smithsonian Institution. The program, an installation guide, and a two-volume manual are available for download from the Osteoware website: http://osteoware.si.edu/.

When the program is running, the Osteoware interface appears (Fig. 1.III.1). As can be seen, Osteoware provides a series of modules for data recording, whereas the Catkey (Catalog Key) window can be used to search for a certain record in a data set.

In the top left corner of the Osteoware interface there is the *Data Subset* window, which presents the databases entered in the program. At this stage you cannot enter your own data directly via the Osteoware interface. A simple method to

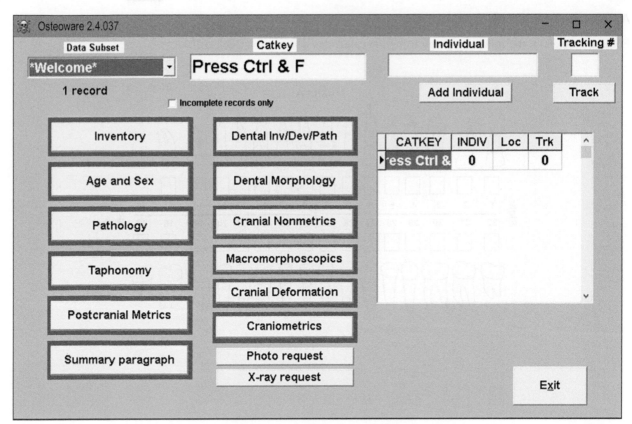

FIGURE 1.III.1   Osteoware home screen.

create and organize your own database is via the program *Advantage Data Architect*, which may be downloaded from the Osteoware website: http://osteoware.si.edu/content/software-downloads.

Once you install the Advantage Data Architect program (versions 9−11), open it and click on "Connection → New Connection Wizard" from the menu bar. In the dialog box that appears, select "Create a connection to a directory of existing tables" and click on the "Next" button. In the field DatabaseName type in "Osteoware," click on "ConnectionPath," select "Browse for Directory" from the drop-down list, and navigate to the *C:\Osteoware/ProtData* folder (Fig. 1.III.2).

On the left side of the Advantage Data Architect window and in the *Connection Repository* panel you can now observe the database *Osteoware* and the tables connected to it (Fig. 1.III.3). Double click on "CaseListProtInvt.ADT." The *CaseListProtInvt* table appears, which includes the list of the test Catkey numbers appearing in the Osteoware interface. *CaseListProtInvt* is the master database table, which is used to enter the ID numbers of the skeletal material of a certain site as follows.

Consider that in the site CRETE-MO we have found the skeletal remains of five individuals coded as CMO-01 to CMO-05. To enter these data in *CaseListProtInvt*, click on the "+" button, ▸▸ ▸| + − ▴, at the bottom of the *CaseListProtInvt* table (Fig. 1.III.4), so that an empty row is added to the database. In this row type in the first code number, CMO-01, in the empty *CATKEY* field; type in "0" (zero) in the *INDIV* column and "0" (zero) in the *TRACKNO* column; in the Prefix column type in "P;" under the RepatSeries column type in the code of the site, "CRETE-MO," and, finally, in the *Catkey Active* column enter a "Y." Repeat this procedure for all five records and refresh the table by clicking on the curved arrow button, ✓ ✗ ↻ (Fig. 1.III.5). The Osteoware home screen showing the new dataset CRETE-MO is depicted in Fig. 1.III.6.

Bone Inventory

To input the elements preserved per skeleton in a specific assemblage, Osteoware uses the *Inventory* module. This module has four tabs labeled *Cranium, Axial Skeleton, Appendicular Skeleton,* and *Hands and Feet* (Figs. 1.III.7 and 1.III.8). In

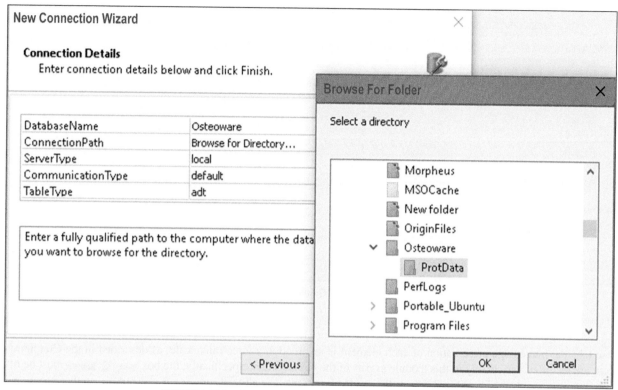

FIGURE 1.III.2   Connecting *Advantage Data Architect* to Osteoware.

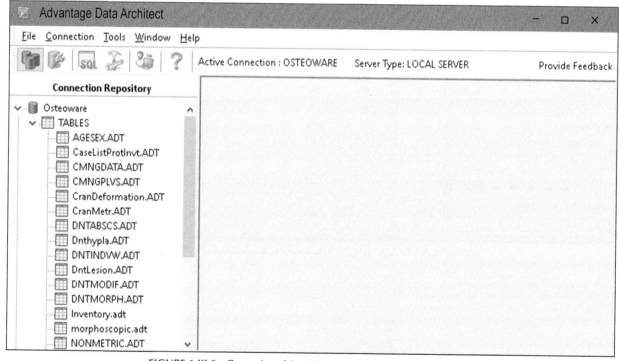

FIGURE 1.III.3   Connection of the *Advantage Data Architect* to Osteoware.

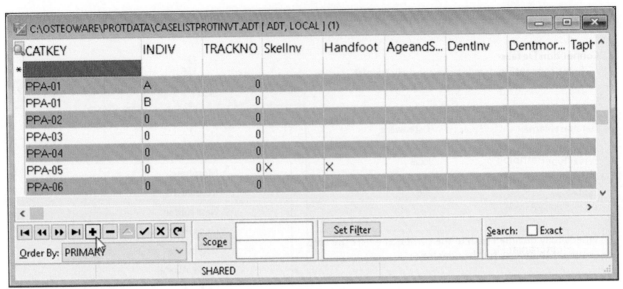

FIGURE 1.III.4   Creation of an empty row.

these tabs the percentage preservation of each element is recorded in a three-rank scale, as described in the Cranium tab. Teeth are recorded very briefly in this module as part of the *Cranium* tab. Specifically, the box Teeth Required must be filled in by entering an integer from 0 to 3, where 0 is no teeth present, 1 is all teeth present, 2 is >50% of teeth present, and 3 is <50% of teeth present.

FIGURE 1.III.5   Refreshment of the database.

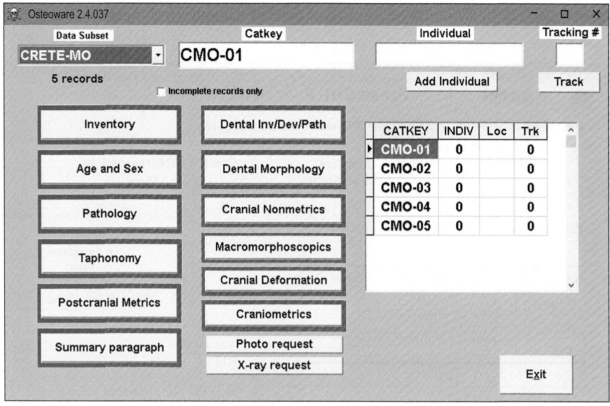

FIGURE 1.III.6 Osteoware home screen showing the data set CRETE-MO.

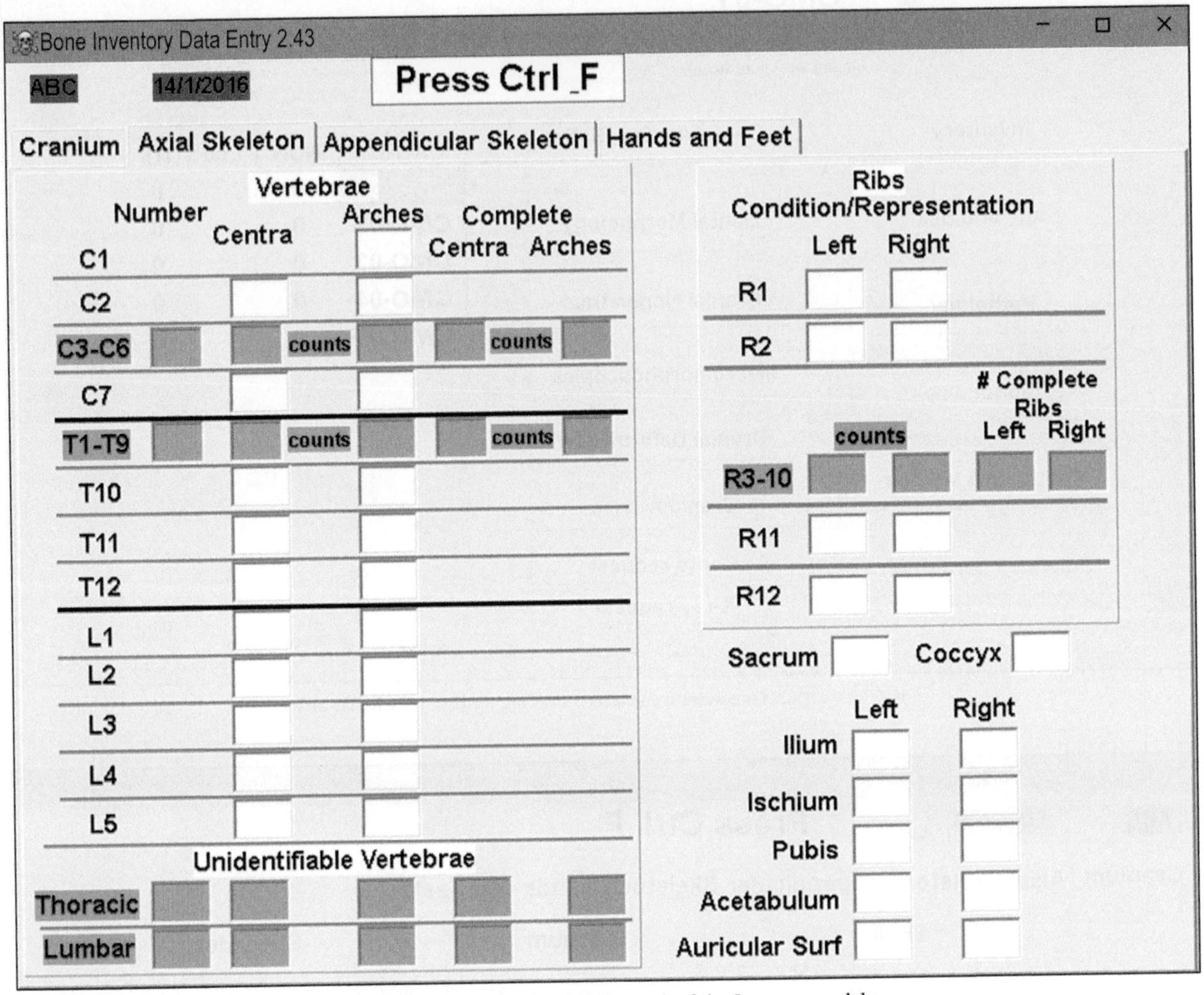

FIGURE 1.III.8 The *Axial Skeleton* tab of the *Inventory* module.

In the *Axial Skeleton* as well as in the *Hands and Feet* tab, the white boxes are filled in with preservation scores, whereas the turquoise boxes are used for inputting counts of each element. In the turquoise boxes labeled "# Complete" only elements preserved at more than 75% should be included in the counts (Fig. 1.III.8). Finally, in the *Appendicular Skeleton* tab each long bone is divided into five segments, which are scored independently.

Tooth Inventory

For a more detailed dental inventory, use the *Dental Inv/Dev/Path* module (Fig. 1.III.9). This module allows the recording of the preservation of each tooth. In addition, the number of supernumerary teeth, if any are present, may be input along with any relevant information. The *Dental Inv/Dev/Path* module may also be used for recording the stages of tooth formation, dental wear, and dental pathology. The inventory codes are shown in the inventory tab, whereas those used for dental development and wear appear by clicking on the "Help" button. Note that the scores used for dental development arise from the stages of tooth formation suggested by Moorrees et al. (1963) (Section 4.2.4), whereas the dental wear recording scheme proposed by Smith (1984) (Appendix 7.III) is used to score dental wear. The recording of dental age, dental wear, and dental pathology in Osteoware is discussed in more detail in Chapters 4, 7, and 8, respectively.

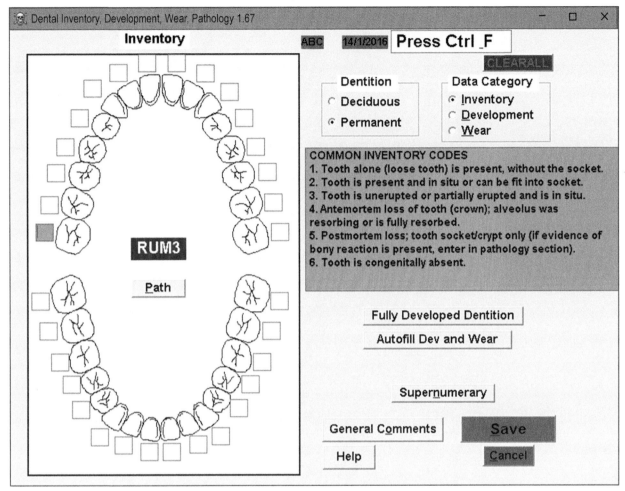

FIGURE 1.III.9   The Dental Inventory, Development, Wear, and Pathology module.

Chapter 2

Taphonomy

Chapter Outline

Chapter Objectives

By the end of this chapter, the reader will be able to:

- appreciate the factors that may affect the state of human skeletal remains from the time of death of the individual to the moment of laboratory examination;
- identify the most common taphonomic factors in a given skeletonized assemblage;
- determine if specific modifications have been caused by human or nonhuman agents and subsequently draw conclusions regarding the peri- and postmortem treatment of the deceased; and
- calculate the minimum and most likely numbers of individuals in commingled assemblages.

This chapter outlines the main factors that determine the state of preservation of human bone assemblages recovered from archaeological and forensic contexts. These factors may be natural (e.g., soil composition, temperature, animal activity) or cultural (e.g., mortuary practices, excavation strategy). The focus of this chapter is on natural forces because cultural parameters are too numerous and variable across time and space to present here. As a general introduction to cultural parameters determining the postmortem fate of human skeletal remains, the reader may consult Duday (2009). Population-specific publications on funerary practices are many and the reader should look into the literature pertaining to his or her study area for relevant information.

2.1 TAPHONOMY IN ARCHAEOLOGICAL AND FORENSIC CONTEXTS

Taphonomy etymologically derives from the Greek words *taphos* (=burial) and *nomos* (=law). It is a term originally used by Efremov (1940, p. 85) to refer to "the study of the transition of organic remains from the biosphere into the lithosphere." Nowadays, taphonomy covers the study of the physical and chemical processes that act upon an organism after death until the moment of examination, and it has become an integral part of archaeological and forensic studies. The reader may consult Lyman (1994), Haglund and Sorg (1996, 2001a), and Pokines and Symes (2013) as invaluable resources regarding taphonomy.

In archaeological contexts taphonomic methods aim primarily at interpreting postmortem processes that have modified the skeletal remains, to assess whether the material under study is representative of the original population. In addition, human-induced taphonomic modifications can offer information regarding past mortuary practices (Fig. 2.1.1). The methods adopted originate largely in zooarchaeology, where extensive studies have been performed regarding weathering and fragmentation patterns, animal scavenging activity, and fire- and tool-induced bone alterations (Lyman, 1994).

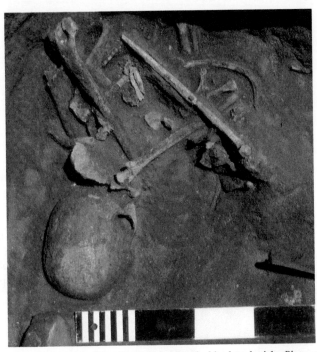

FIGURE 2.1.1 Disarticulated skeleton from a Roman burial at Leptiminus, disturbed by later burials. *Photo courtesy of Professor David Mattingly, University of Leicester, UK.*

Forensic taphonomy also examines the postmortem fate of skeletal remains, but its aims are largely different from those of archaeological taphonomy. Following the definition of Haglund and Sorg (1996, p. 13), forensic taphonomy focuses on the "study of postmortem processes which affect (1) the preservation, observation, or recovery of dead organisms, (2) the reconstruction of their biology or ecology, or (3) the reconstruction of the circumstances of their death." The study of these factors aims principally at determining the time since death (postmortem interval), differentiating antemortem, perimortem, and postmortem events (such as trauma), and assessing human manipulation of the remains at the scene, e.g., selective transportation of elements (Christensen et al., 2014; Komar and Buikstra, 2007).

Given this definition, forensic taphonomy is similar to archaeological taphonomy in the sense that it tries to identify the natural and cultural factors that acted upon the remains postmortem and resulted in the observed patterns of preservation of the material. However, its strong focus on determining time since death and the overall circumstances of death differentiates it from archaeological approaches, in which the nature and antiquity of the material render such research questions rather marginal.

As the factors that may affect the preservation of human remains are particularly diverse, human taphonomy is interdisciplinary and combines site formation processes, cultural factors relating to the management of the deceased, chemical degradation (diagenesis), animal and plant activity, and many other agents that may affect the remains at the ante-, peri-, or postdepositional stage. Therefore, taphonomic research involves the collaboration of archaeologists, geologists, biological anthropologists, zoologists, botanists, and other specialists.

This chapter focuses on the taphonomic processes that take place after skeletonization. Representative steps in taphonomic analysis of skeletonized remains are given in Box 2.1.1. Appendix 2.I presents a suggested protocol for the degree of completeness of the skeleton, and Appendices 2.II and 2.III give examples of recording protocols for taphonomic alterations.

BOX 2.1.1 Steps in Taphonomic Analysis

1. Document the context of the skeletal remains.
2. Record skeletal alterations resulting from handling the remains during the recovery and postrecovery stages.
3. Inventory all skeletal elements.
4. Record the state of preservation of all elements.
5. Conjoin fractured elements.
6. Assess whether commingling has occurred (identify articulating elements, pair bilateral elements).

7. Record any bone modifications due to taphonomic agents that affected the remains prior to recovery.

Adapted from Marden K, Sorg MH, Haglund WD. Taphonomy. In: DiGangi EA, Moore MK, editors. Research methods in human skeletal biology. San Diego: Elsevier; 2012. p. 241–62.

2.2 DECOMPOSITION PROCESS

Decomposition includes the self-destruction of cells by their own enzymes (*autolysis*) as well as the breakdown of cells by the activity of bacteria and other microorganisms (*putrefaction*) (Komar and Buikstra, 2007). The stage of decomposition of the remains can offer valuable information regarding the postmortem interval and postburial interval, which are pivotal in forensic taphonomic studies (Komar and Buikstra, 2007). Nevertheless, calculation of these intervals is based primarily on soft tissue modifications; thus such calculations are not part of osteological studies. For this reason, the decomposition process prior to skeletonization is only briefly outlined here (Table 2.2.1).

TABLE 2.2.1 Decomposition Stages and Corresponding Body Changes

Decomposition Stage	Body Changes
Fresh	Rigor mortis; marbled skin; fly eggs in orifices; possibly fluids around the oral and nasal cavities
Primary bloat	Gases within the body; loose hair and epidermis; strong odor
Secondary bloat	Bloating; limb disarticulation; purging; strong odor
Active decay	Deflation; desiccation; limb and head disarticulation; strong odor; early bone exposure
Advanced decay	Collapse of abdomen and thoracic cage; decayed soft tissues though skin, fat, and cartilage still present; adipocere formation
Skeletonization	Complete decay of all soft tissues except for some adipocere and ligaments; possible bone weathering

Adapted from Bass WM. Outdoor decomposition rates in Tennessee. In: Haglund WD, Sorg MH, editors. Forensic taphonomy: the postmortem fate of human remains. Boca Raton: CRC Press; 1996. p. 181–6 and Bristow J, Simms Z, Randolph-Quinney P. Taphonomy. In: Black S, Ferguson E, editors. Forensic anthropology 2000 to 2010. Boca Raton: CRC Press; 2011. p. 279–318.

It must be remembered that although the sequence of decomposition is fixed, the rate at which a skeleton may reach each decomposition stage is highly variable, as it depends upon many intrinsic and extrinsic factors. As a result, it is difficult to calculate time since death directly from the stage of decomposition of a body (Komar and Buikstra, 2007; Lyman, 2001). For example, when a body is exposed to animal activity, decay is rapid compared to when it is buried in a deep grave, making it inaccessible to scavengers (Haglund et al., 1989; Janaway, 1996). Similarly, high temperatures and humidity increase the rate of decomposition (Pinheiro, 2006). Indeed, it has been found that in warm and humid environments skeletonization may be complete within 1–2 weeks (Mann et al., 1990), whereas putrefaction is severely retarded under freezing conditions (below 4°C) (Micozzi, 1996).

Once the remains reach the skeletonization stage, a number of factors affect the preservation of the material. The organic and inorganic bone components initially protect one another against decay (Trueman and Martill, 2002), but eventually physical and chemical alterations occur (Nielsen-Marsh and Hedges, 2000). Among the primary post-depositional alterations found on bones is *weathering*. Weathering manifests as bleaching, exfoliation, and cracking (Fig. 2.2.1), and results from exposure to sunlight, fluctuating temperatures, humidity, and other factors (Behrensmeyer, 1978; Junod and Pokines, 2013). Specifically, when bones are exposed to sunlight and heat, they dehydrate, and their organic and inorganic components are separated through diagenesis, eventually destroying the bone completely (Dupras and Schultz, 2013; Lyman and Fox, 1996). The rate of diagenesis depends upon numerous factors, such as the size and porosity of the bone, duration of the burial, soil acidity, presence of bacteria, underground water, temperature, and others (Hollund et al., 2012). In general, the rate of bone weathering decreases in cold climates and under reduced sunlight exposure (Andrews and Cook, 1985), whereas it increases in warm climates, with temperature fluctuations and direct sunlight exposure (Tappen, 1995; Western and Behrensmeyer, 2009; but see Andrews and Whybrow, 2005). Table 2.2.2 presents representative stages of bone weathering, whereas the taphonomic factors that produce weathering and other bone modifications are presented in more detail in the following sections.

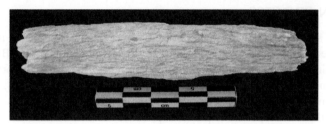

FIGURE 2.2.1   Fragment of weathered tibial diaphysis.

TABLE 2.2.2 Weathering Stages

WS	Bone Condition
0	No evidence of cracking or flaking on the bone surface
1	Cracking on the bone surface and mosaic cracking on the articular surfaces
2	Flaking and cracking of the outermost cortical bone layers, resulting in the complete destruction of most of the outer cortical bone layer at the end of this stage
3	Areas of weathered cortical bone gradually covering the entire bone surface; weathering as deep as 1.0−1.5 mm
4	Fibrous and rough bone surface with splinters; weathering deeper than 1.5 mm
5	Disintegrated bone; original shape difficult to identify

WS, weathering stage.
Adapted from Behrensmeyer AK. Taphonomic and ecologic information from bone weathering. Paleobiology 1978;4:150−62.

2.3 SCAVENGERS

Scavengers may have a significant impact on the preservation of skeletal remains by causing various bone modifications, as well as by actively participating in the dispersal and disarticulation of the remains.

2.3.1 Insects

Insects are usually the first scavengers to attack a dead body. The study of insects can offer useful information on the estimated time since death, season of death, potential relocation of the remains, and other important forensic questions (Anderson and Cervenka, 2001). For this reason, forensic entomology constitutes a major part of forensic taphonomy. Despite its importance, entomological evidence exceeds the purpose of this chapter, as insects affect almost exclusively the soft tissues (but see, for example, Huchet et al., 2011, for termite impact on human bones).

2.3.2 Carnivores

When carnivores consume large carcasses, they tend to proceed from the most easily accessible parts of the body to the anatomical areas with the lowest nutrient availability (Blumenschine, 1988). As such, they usually start with the internal organs that require limited bone crushing to access (e.g., heart, lungs, liver). Then they consume the large muscles of the hinter limbs, followed by the muscles of the thorax and the front limbs. The disarticulation of the skeletal elements that results from muscle consumption minimizes competition over the carcass and facilitates feeding the cubs (Kerbis Peterhans, 1990; Pokines and Kerbis Peterhans, 2007). It must be stressed that this pattern is generally seen when large mammals are consumed; however, in the case of humans, Haglund et al. (1989) found that the first part of the body attacked is usually the throat, possibly because clothes restrict scavenger access to other body parts normally consumed earlier.

Damage to the skeleton follows the same general pattern of first attacking the easiest parts and gradually proceeding to better-protected areas. The elements of the thoracic cage are usually among the first to be destroyed. Small elements, such as the hand and foot bones, may be consumed whole rather than being crushed. The long bones usually exhibit the clearest evidence of carnivore activity. Consumption of the long bones starts from the epiphyses, which are easier to crush. If one epiphysis is more robust than the other, scavengers often gnaw exclusively at the more fragile end. Subsequently, gnawing proceeds to the diaphysis to access the medullary cavity (Pokines and Kerbis Peterhans, 2007). The cranium is usually too large to be gnawed; however, it may be transported for long distances for later consumption (Horwitz and Smith, 1988). Box 2.3.1 presents the general impact carnivores may have on skeletal remains, and Box 2.3.2 outlines the carnivore tooth marks that may be identified on bones.

BOX 2.3.1 Impact of Large Carnivores on Skeletal Remains

- Preference for fresh bone
- Destruction of elements rich in trabecular bone (e.g., ribs, long-bone epiphyses)
- Tooth marks (pits and scores) near bone edges (Fig. 2.3.1)
- Furrowing of trabecular bone

- Extensive bone scattering and possible bone accumulation in a feeding spot

Adapted from Pokines JT. Faunal dispersal, reconcentration, and gnawing damage to bone in terrestrial environments. In: Pokines JT, Symes SA, editors. Manual of forensic taphonomy. Boca Raton: CRC Press; 2013. p. 201–48.

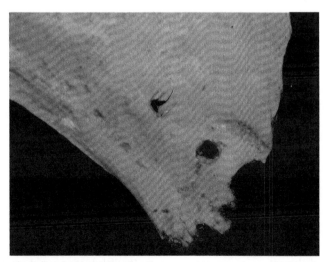

FIGURE 2.3.1   Carnivore punctures on a scapula. *Original photo in Christensen AM, Passalacqua NV, Bartelink EJ. Forensic anthropology. Current methods and practice. San Diego: Elsevier; 2014, reprinted with permission.*

Despite numerous attempts, identifying the carnivore that produced the observed tooth marks in each case is difficult. Domínguez-Rodrigo and Piqueras (2003) concluded that tooth marks can distinguish only between large and small carnivores, whereas no distinction of specific taxa can be made. This conclusion was supported by Murmann et al. (2006), who found substantial overlap between the marks produced by many common carnivores.

BOX 2.3.2 Types of Carnivore Tooth Marks

- Pits
  - Small oval or irregular indentations on the cortical bone
  - No penetration to the interior of the bone
  - Maximum length up to three times the maximum width
- Punctures
  - Shape similar to that of pits
  - Penetration to the interior of the bone
- Scores (or striations)
  - Long scratches (length longer than three times the maximum width)
  - No penetration to the interior of the bone

- Furrows
  - Long marks (length longer than three times the maximum width)
  - Penetration to the interior of the bone
  - Usually found in already exposed trabecular bone

Adapted from Pobiner BL. Hominin-carnivore interactions: evidence from modern carnivore bone modification and early Pleistocene archaeofaunas (Koobi Fora, Kenya; Olduvai Gorge, Tanzania). [Ph.D. dissertation], Department of Anthropology, Rutgers University; 2007; Pokines JT. Faunal dispersal, reconcentration, and gnawing damage to bone in terrestrial environments. In: Pokines JT, Symes SA, editors. Manual of forensic taphonomy. Boca Raton: CRC Press; 2013. p. 201—48 and references therein.

A final important modification of the skeletal remains due to carnivore activity is *gastric corrosion*. When large carnivores consume a carcass, they ingest masticated bone fragments as well as small intact elements (e.g., carpals, phalanges). Ingested bone undergoes gastric corrosion, whereby gastric acid and digestive enzymes produce thinning of the bone edges and corrugation of the bone surfaces to the point where small holes appear (*windowing*) (Pokines and Kerbis Peterhans, 2007).

2.3.3 Rodents

Rodent damage on the bones is generally less extensive than that produced by carnivores (Boxes 2.3.3 and 2.3.4). One of the main reasons rodents gnaw on bone is to wear down their maxillary and mandibular incisors, which are constantly growing. Moreover, certain rodents obtain nutrients, such as fat and minerals, from bones (Klippel and Synstelien, 2007). Various skeletal areas are targeted, depending on the purpose of the gnawing activity. Klippel and Synstelien (2007) found that brown rats preferred cancellous bone, as their aim was to acquire nutrients (fat), whereas gray squirrels targeted cortical bone to access mineral components. When the aim is to sharpen the anterior dentition, rodents focus on projecting surfaces, such as the orbital margins (Fig. 2.3.2) and the iliac crest (Haglund, 1996).

BOX 2.3.3 Impact of Large Rodents on Skeletal Remains

- Preference for dry bone
- Accumulation of larger bones to a den (seen in certain species)
- Parallel striations, gradually becoming obliterated through repeated gnawing

Adapted from Pokines JT. Faunal dispersal, reconcentration, and gnawing damage to bone in terrestrial environments. In: Pokines JT, Symes SA, editors. Manual of forensic taphonomy. Boca Raton: CRC Press; 2013. p. 201—48.

BOX 2.3.4 Impact of Small Rodents on Skeletal Remains

Fresh or dry bones
- No dispersal of large skeletal elements
- Uniform damage to bone margins

Fresh bones
- Modification of anatomical areas that are easy to fracture (e.g., nasals, epiphyses)
- Production of pedestaled trabecular bone areas

Dry/weathered bones
- Parallel striations on sharp bone margins

Adapted from Pokines JT. Faunal dispersal, reconcentration, and gnawing damage to bone in terrestrial environments. In: Pokines JT, Symes SA, editors. Manual of forensic taphonomy. Boca Raton: CRC Press; 2013. p. 201—48.

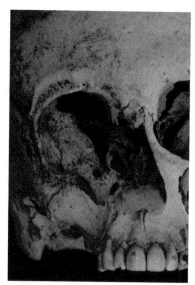

FIGURE 2.3.2 Parallel striations on orbital margin produced by rodent gnawing. *Original photo in Christensen AM, Passalacqua NV, Bartelink EJ. Forensic anthropology. Current methods and practice. San Diego: Elsevier; 2014, reprinted with permission.*

2.3.4 Pigs

Pig tooth marks appear as long, and often multiple, parallel lesions resulting from turning the bone against their teeth or dragging their teeth across cortical bone (Berryman, 2001). Experimental studies suggest that during the consumption of a carcass, pigs tend to destroy weaker elements (e.g., vertebrae) and modify long-bone epiphyses (Domínguez-Solera and Domínguez-Rodrigo, 2009).

2.3.5 Marine Predators

Large marine predators may produce gastric corrosion or leave traces of tooth marks on bones (Lentz et al., 2010). Shark teeth usually cause linear superficial striations on the cortical bone layer, deeper punctures with or without associated fractures, as well as incised gouges (Allaire et al., 2012; Byard et al., 2000; Ihama et al., 2009).

2.3.6 Avian Predators

Scavenging birds may produce characteristic osseous alterations while consuming the soft tissues (review in Pokines and Baker, 2013). Reeves (2009) found two types of markings produced by vulture feeding on pig and goat carcasses: shallow, irregular linear scratches, primarily found on the skull and secondarily on the scapulae, vertebrae, ribs, and long bones, and shallow scratches mostly visible as surface discoloration, which may become gradually obliterated. Similarly, Domínguez-Solera and Domínguez-Rodrigo (2011) identified punctures on the crania and scapulae of deer carcasses, along with shallow scores and striae on long-bone diaphyses.

Other large raptors produce marks similar to those of vultures. Such marks are mostly found on surfaces covered by a thin layer of cortical bone, for example, on the facial bones and scapulae. They typically manifest as scratches and punctures around and through the orbits to access the eyes, scratches on the cranial vault to remove the scalp, and fracturing of the zygomatics and maxillae to access the tongue. Occasionally the occipital bone is also broken to access the brain (McGraw et al., 2006). In addition, large raptors may scatter human remains because of the large number of birds that feed simultaneously and the competition between them (Pokines and Baker, 2013).

2.4 HUMAN AGENTS

Human activity generates three major types of modification to human remains: (1) tool marks, (2) fractures, and (3) thermal alteration. The principal aims of taphonomy in human-modified assemblages are to distinguish: (1) violent acts resulting in trauma and death, (2) perimortem or postmortem body processing as part of the mortuary ritual, and (3) cannibalism (Stodder, 2008). In this section we will not deal with fractures because these, along with their distinction into perimortem and postmortem trauma, are discussed in Chapter 8.

2.4.1 Tool Marks

Tool marks found on human skeletal remains are mainly due to dismemberment and cannibalism (Box 2.4.1). The most common reasons to dismember a body are: (1) to prevent identification by removing the head, fingers, and other diagnostic anatomical parts; (2) to fit the body into a container; and (3) cultural practices (Reichs, 1998). The number, size, type, and anatomical location of the tool marks are important in determining the etiology of this type of bone modification (Stodder, 2008).

BOX 2.4.1 Long-Bone Modifications Indicative of Cannibalism (Turner and Turner, 1999; Villa and Mahieu, 1991; White, 1992)

- Cut marks at muscle attachment sites (defleshing)
- Cut marks near articulations (dismemberment)

- Percussion marks (accessing the bone marrow)
- Pot polish on bone ends (cooking and burning)

The main tool mark categories identified on skeletal remains are cut, chop, scrape, and percussion marks. Various experimental studies have attempted to establish criteria for the identification and differentiation of these marks and representative results are given in Box 2.4.2.

BOX 2.4.2 Tool Mark Identification Criteria (Lewis, 2008; White et al., 2011)

Cut marks
- Produced by a sharp tool that impacts the bone surface perpendicularly
- Narrow and V-shaped cross section
  Sword marks (Fig. 2.4.1, left)
- Longer, wider, and deeper than knife marks
- Extensive damage to the sides of the cut mark in cross section
- One curved wall and one straight wall
  Knife marks (Fig. 2.4.1, right)
- Shallow and narrow

- Limited damage to the sides of the cut mark
- V-shaped cross section

Chop marks
- Produced by forceful impact of the tool on the bone
- Shorter and broader than cut marks
- V-shaped cross section

Scrape marks
- Shallow
- Consisting of many parallel and subparallel striations

Percussion marks
- Combination of pits, grooves, or striae

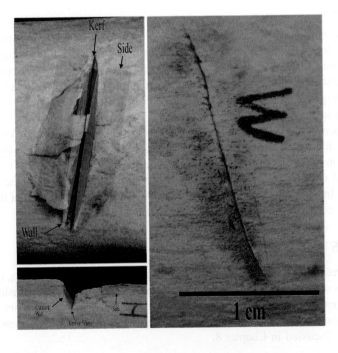

2.4.2 Fire

Heat can cause extensive modifications to skeletal remains; however, total destruction of osseous elements through fire is exceptionally rare or even impossible (Bass, 1984; Komar and Buikstra, 2007). Excellent books on cremated remains (*cremains*) in forensic contexts include Fairgrieve (2007) and Schmidt and Symes (2008).

2.4.2.1 Fire-Induced Bone Alterations

When exposed to high temperatures, bone dehydrates; subsequently, its organic components decompose and, finally, microstructural changes to the inorganic matrix occur. Heat-induced alterations to the skeleton have been formally divided into four stages: dehydration, decomposition, inversion, and fusion (Shipman et al., 1984). Table 2.4.1 gives a brief outline of the alterations occurring at each stage and the corresponding temperatures. It must be stressed that in addition to temperature, a number of other factors also contribute to heat-induced bone changes. In particular, the rate of bone destruction is dependent on the fire temperature and duration, as well as the nature of heating (direct contact, boiling, etc.), the position of the body in the fire, the size of the body, the extent of soft tissue coverage, the degree of articulation of the remains, whether the bones were fresh or dry and whether they consist mostly of cortical or trabecular bone, and other parameters (Buikstra and Swegle, 1989; DeHaan, 2012; Symes et al., 2008).

TABLE 2.4.1 Stages of Heat-Induced Bone Transformation

Stage	Heat-Induced Change	Bone Alteration	Temperature Range (°C)
Dehydration	Water loss	Fragmentation and weight loss	100–600
Decomposition	Organic component loss	Color and porosity alteration, weight loss, and reduced resistance to mechanical loading	300–800
Inversion	Carbonate loss	Crystal size increase	500–1100
Fusion	Crystals melting	Increased resistance to mechanical loading, increased crystal size, porosity changes, and size reduction	700 and greater

Adapted from Mayne Correia P. Fire modification of bone: a review of the literature. In: Haglund WD, Sorg MH, editors. Forensic taphonomy: the postmortem fate of human remains. Boca Raton: CRC Press; 1996. p. 275–94; Thompson TJU. Recent advances in the study of burned bone and their implications for forensic anthropology. Forensic Science International 2004;146:S203–5.

The macroscopic changes occurring on bones exposed to fire include discoloration, shrinkage, warping, and fragmentation (Fairgrieve, 2007). In particular, when organic material is subjected to intense heat, it undergoes *carbonization* due to its high content in carbon atoms. The color of carbonized (charred/smoked) bone is black, as this is the natural color of carbon (Symes et al., 2008). At this stage the affected bones exhibit shrinkage and deformation (Thompson, 2004). If additional thermal stress is applied on carbonized bone, *calcination* occurs. During this stage, the carbon that has been released from the organic components of bone combines with oxygen and forms carbon dioxide or carbon monoxide. Because the only bone component remaining at this stage is hydroxyapatite, which is naturally white in color, the color of calcined bones turns from black to white (Mayne Correia, 1996; Thompson, 2004). Calcined bones are particularly fragile and often preserved in a fractured and distorted state (Hiller et al., 2003). However, these bones may actually be more resistant to subsequent diagenetic changes in the soil (Gilchrist and Mytum, 1986).

The bone modifications occurring during exposure to fire are described in more detail in the following sections. When examining the burning patterns of the human body, it should be kept in mind that when the body burns, it tends to assume the *pugilistic posture* because flexor muscles contract when they dehydrate (Fairgrieve, 2007; Symes et al., 2008) (Figs. 2.4.2–2.4.4).

Color Changes

Color changes on thermally altered bone express the disintegration and chemical alteration of the organic and inorganic bone components and they can provide information regarding fire intensity and duration. However, factors such as

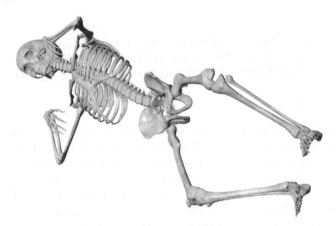

FIGURE 2.4.2 The pugilistic posture.

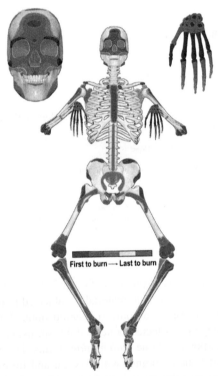

FIGURE 2.4.3 Order of burning of the human skeleton in pugilistic posture; anterior view. *Top left and right*: Magnified views of burn patterns on anterior skull and dorsal hand. *Adapted from Symes SA, Rainwater CW, Chapman EN, Gipson DR, Piper AL. Patterned thermal destruction of human remains in a forensic setting. In: Schmidt CW, Symes SA, editors. The analysis of burned human remains. San Diego: Elsevier; 2008. p. 15—54.*

whether the bones were fresh or dry when exposed to fire, oxygen availability, and others should also be taken into account before firm conclusions are drawn (Devlin and Herrmann, 2008; Walker and Miller, 2005).

Shipman et al. (1984) identified five broad color stages resulting from exposure to increasing temperatures. In bones exposed to temperatures below 285°C the main colors were neutral white, pale yellow, and yellow. In temperatures from 285 to 525°C bones were reddish brown, very dark gray-brown, neutral dark gray, and reddish yellow. In temperatures up to 645°C bones were neutral black, medium blue, and reddish yellow, whereas in temperatures of up to 940°C neutral white prevailed, with occasional light blue-gray and light gray present. Finally, in temperatures over 940°C neutral white and medium gray dominated, because the bones had entered the calcination stage. However, as mentioned earlier, in

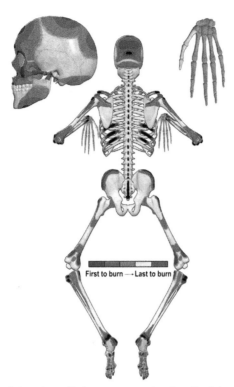

FIGURE 2.4.4 Order of burning of the human skeleton in pugilistic posture; posterior view. *Top left and right*: Magnified views of burn patterns on the lateral skull and palmar hand. *Adapted from Symes SA, Rainwater CW, Chapman EN, Gipson DR, Piper AL. Patterned thermal destruction of human remains in a forensic setting. In: Schmidt CW, Symes SA, editors. The analysis of burned human remains. San Diego: Elsevier; 2008. p. 15−54.*

addition to the temperature to which the bones are exposed, many other parameters affect heat-induced bone discoloration and overall modification (Walker et al., 2008).

Structural Breakdown

Increased exposure to fire produces structural breakdown of bone. In particular, the dehydration process involves the combustion of organic materials and the subsequent recrystallization of the mineral matrix. The end result is shrinkage and warping, and the subsequent cooling of the bone results in fracturing (Fairgrieve, 2007).

There are several types of heat-induced fractures on the long bones (Box 2.4.3). Because bone fractures result from dehydration, the concentration of water in the bone before burning is an important parameter in the study of fracture patterns (Shipman et al., 1984). Baby (1954) was the first to note that dry bone exhibits patina and longitudinal

---

BOX 2.4.3 Thermal Fractures (Symes et al., 2008)

Longitudinal
- Along the longitudinal axis of a long bone (Fig. 2.4.5)

Step
- From the margin of a longitudinal fracture, transversing the bone shaft, and intersecting another longitudinal fracture (Fig. 2.4.5)

Transverse
- Perpendicular to the longitudinal axis of a long bone

Patina
- Superficial and less destructive mesh of uniform cracks

- Mostly found on flat postcranial and cranial bones and long-bone epiphyses

Splintering and delamination
- Pealing of cortical bone layers
- Separation of endocranial and ectocranial bone tissues
- Exposure of epiphyseal trabecular bone

Burn line fractures
- Along the borders of the burnt bone surface

Curved transverse
- Rarely manifesting as "concentric rings"

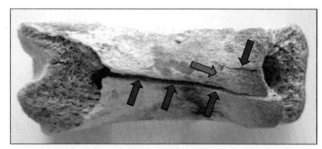

FIGURE 2.4.5 Longitudinal fractures (*red arrows*) and a step fracture (*yellow arrow*). *Original photo in Keough N, L'Abbé EN, Steyn M, Pretorius S. Assessment of skeletal changes after post-mortem exposure to fire as an indicator of decomposition stage. Forensic Science International 2015;246:17−24, reprinted with permission.*

fractures, as well as transverse splintering, but no warping, in contrast to fresh bone. Similarly, Binford (1963) found that dry bones develop straight transverse cracking, in contrast to the curved transverse cracking seen in green bones. Buikstra and Swegle (1989) observed that dry bones exhibit shallow longitudinal fissures and transverse cracks, whereas in green bones the cracks and fissures run deep. More recently, DeHaan and Nurbakhsh (2001) also noted that the presence of blood, marrow, moisture, and fat in bones under firing conditions affects the pattern of alteration of the remains. However, it must be stressed that these general differences in the heat-induced changes occurring in dry and fresh/green bones are representative, and on certain occasions, patterns typical of one bone category may be seen in another. For example, Gonçalves et al. (2011) identified bone warping and curved transverse fractures (thumbnail fractures) in a small number of dry bones that were submitted to thermal stress, even though these deformities are considered typical of fresh bone.

Cranial fractures due to heat stress are produced by the same mechanisms as in the postcranial skeleton but they are additionally caused by increased intracranial pressure (Bohnert et al., 1997). Most cranial fractures are found along the sutures, except for when the cranial vault has been broken by trauma. In such cases, the traumatic lesion would allow the escape of increased intracranial pressure (Rhine, 1998).

Bone shrinkage due to heat stress affects skeletal dimensions. Herrmann (1976, 1977) proposed associations between the percentage of shrinkage and the temperatures that could have generated it. However, temperature alone is not an accurate predictor of the amount of shrinkage, as the duration of exposure to heat as well as the bone composition are also highly influential (Thompson, 2005).

2.4.2.2 Fire-Induced Dental Alterations

Thermal changes in teeth are similar overall to those observed in bone (see review in Schmidt, 2008). When tooth exposure to heat is advanced, the dental tissues dehydrate and lose their organic component. The greater concentration of organic components in dentine compared to the enamel results in the earlier affliction of this dental tissue by fire. As a result, the dentine is affected by shrinkage to a greater degree than the enamel and the latter may fall off a tooth almost intact (Hughes and White, 2009). An interesting point to note is that if the temperature rises above 800°C, the inorganic crystals fuse to one another, preventing further shrinkage and fracturing (Shipman et al., 1984). Table 2.4.2 summarizes the color changes seen in each dental tissue under various temperatures.

TABLE 2.4.2 Dental Color Alterations After 1-h Heat Exposure at Various Temperatures

Temperature (°C)	Enamel	Dentine	Cementum
300	Dark grayish brown	Light grayish brown	Dark grayish brown
500	Gray	Dark grayish black	Light brownish gray
700	Light grayish white	Pale gray	Light grayish white
900	Almost white	Almost white	Almost white
1000−1300	Porcelain white	Porcelain white	Porcelain white

Adapted from Fairgrieve SI. Forensic cremation: recovery and analysis. Boca Raton: CRC Press; 2007, and drawn from Harsányi L. Scanning electron microscopic investigation of thermal damage of the teeth. Acta Morphologica Academiae Scientiarium Hungaricae 1975;23:271−281.

Alveolar bone can protect unerupted deciduous and permanent teeth by reducing direct exposure to fire. This applies particularly to the mandibular teeth and posterior maxillary teeth because of the increased density of the alveolar bone in these regions. However, the protection offered by the jaws is limited under intense heat stress (Schmidt, 2008).

2.4.3 Mortuary Practices

As mentioned in the introduction of this chapter, funerary practices are varied worldwide and their detailed discussion exceeds the purposes of this book. However, some general observations on the impact of broadly used mortuary practices are made here because the treatment of the deceased affects greatly the preservation of their skeletal remains.

Mortuary practices that pertain to the treatment of the body are considered taphonomic processes as they affect its postmortem fate (Ubelaker, 2000). In a mortuary context, one or more individuals may be buried together, whereas a group burial may represent a single episode or successive burial events (Stodder, 2008). Furthermore, bodies may be well arranged, placed in a random position in the tomb, or well arranged at first and subsequently disturbed as part of the secondary treatment of the deceased. In any case, it must be stressed that the position of the skeleton in the tomb does not necessarily represent its original arrangement, because factors such as soft tissue decomposition, underground water, gravity, soil pressure, micromammal activity, and others tend to relocate the skeletal elements (Roksandic, 2001).

Burial depth plays an important role in the rate of decomposition of a body because shallow graves are characterized by temperature fluctuations and are more likely to experience insect and other scavenger invasions, accelerating the decomposition rate (Weitzel, 2005). Furthermore, in deep burials there is limited oxygen availability; thus the chemical reactions required to break down the body tissues are slowed down (Mann et al., 1990).

When the body is clothed or wrapped in a shroud, or when organic matter, such as straw, is present in the burial site, decay is faster (Lieverse et al., 2006). However, certain objects occasionally accompanying the deceased may partially protect the bones and associated soft tissues from extrinsic agents. A typical example is leather footwear or gloves, which protect the feet and hands from contact with the soil, plant roots, and micromammal activity (Pokines, 2008; Pokines and Baker, 2013).

Coffins initially protect the body from decay as they limit contact with the soil, plant roots, microorganisms, micromammals, and other taphonomic agents. However, as the coffin gradually decomposes, the aforementioned factors access the body (Schultz et al., 2003). Special mention must be made of iron coffins, which are more durable compared to wooden ones, thus offering better protection against taphonomic factors (Owsley and Compton, 1996). In addition, iron coffins facilitate the formation of anaerobic conditions, further promoting the long-term preservation of organic remains (Breuning-Madsen et al., 2001). Note that the remains inside iron coffins are often stained dark or even black, possibly due to iron oxides leaching from the coffin (Schultz et al., 2003).

2.5 NATURAL ENVIRONMENT

2.5.1 Plant Activity

Plants may produce taphonomic alterations to human bones by causing fractures and root etching. Bones contain nutrients that are important to plants, especially nitrogen and phosphorus. The porous structure of trabecular bone facilitates the release of these nutrients to the soil, and it also increases the amount of absorbed water, promoting the growth of plant roots. Plant roots may grow around buried bone or penetrate it through foramina and the medullary cavity. As the roots grow thicker with time, they often fracture the bones (Pokines and Baker, 2013).

In addition to fracturing, plant roots produce bone destruction by means of their acidic exudates that dissolve the mineral content of the bone. The end result of this process is called *root etching* and it creates a branching pattern on the bone surface (Bais et al., 2006; Lyman, 1994; Rudrappa et al., 2008).

2.5.2 Soil

The soil at the burial site is very important in bone preservation. Acidic soils produce more extensive damage, expressed as thinning of the cortical bone or even windowing, because the dissolution of minerals is faster. Alkaline soils facilitate microbial attack (or microbial damage is easier to identify because of enhanced mineral preservation), resulting in histological damage, loss of the organic components, and biomolecular degradation. In contrast, in burial sites with neutral or slightly basic pH, bone is usually well preserved (Casallas and Moore, 2012; Nielsen-Marsh et al., 2007).

Another important impact that soil may have on the preservation of skeletal remains pertains to deformations produced by soil pressure. This phenomenon is more pronounced in subadult bones, which are not fully mineralized yet (Buikstra and Ubelaker, 1994). Soil pressure may also have a dramatic effect on the commingling of human remains, especially in the case of mass burials (Pokines and Baker, 2013).

2.5.3 Aquatic Environments

Aquatic environments exhibit varied characteristics with regard to chemistry, water currents, and temperature depending on their type (lake, river, ocean), the region, the season, and other parameters (Sorg et al., 1996). As a result, different aquatic environments reflect different taphonomic conditions (for a review see Evans, 2013 for fluvial environments, and Higgs and Pokines, 2013 for marine environments).

Bodies in aquatic environments may float or sink, be buried under sediments, be transported for long distances by currents, or be washed up on the shore. Furthermore, depending on the taphonomic agents acting upon them, they may disarticulate, be consumed by scavengers, or decompose (Haglund and Sorg, 2001b). Although the rate at which tissue decomposition occurs in water depends upon many factors, the remains generally decompose more slowly in water than in terrestrial environments (Anderson and Bell, 2010; Sorg et al., 1996). This slower decomposition rate is due to the limited exposure of the body to fly maggots (Westling, 2012), combined with low water temperatures (Heaton et al., 2010). Even though the decomposition rate of remains in water is rather slow, once a body is submerged in water, invertebrates produce tissue breakdown (Vanin and Zancaner, 2011), whereas body parts exposed above water are affected by terrestrial invertebrates (Barrios and Wolff, 2011).

When the skeletonization stage has been reached, water environments can modify bones through a number of factors which are given briefly in Table 2.5.1. In addition to the taphonomic forces that act upon the bones within aquatic environments, bone cracking and warping can occur if the skeletal material is removed from the water (Evans, 2013).

2.6 INTRINSIC PRESERVATION FACTORS

The main intrinsic factors that affect postmortem bone preservation include the density, shape, and size of the bones; the age and sex of the individual; and certain pathological conditions. Bone density is the primary intrinsic factor

TABLE 2.5.1 Taphonomic Modifications of Bones in Aquatic Environments

Modification	Effects
Abrasion	Thinning of the bone surface by means of smoothing, polishing, scratching, pitting, chipping, or grooving; the end result is windowing (small openings that gradually enlarge) (Fernández-Jalvo and Andrews, 2003; Shipman and Rose, 1983)
Encrustation	Produced by marine organisms, such as coralline algae, serpulid worms, barnacles, certain mollusks, and others (Parsons and Brett, 1991); indicates that the bones had been exposed above the sediment–water interface (Haglung and Sorg, 2001b)
Bioerosion	Removal of bone by living organisms, which tunnel into the bone for shelter or nutrients or mark the bone surface while consuming soft tissues or other adhering organisms (Belaústegui et al., 2012 and references therein)
Dissolution	Corrosion of skeletal surfaces occurring in aquatic environments with high salinity, low temperature, or bioturbation (Sorg et al., 1996)
Erosion	Rounding of broken bone edges due to dissolution or abrasion (Haglung and Sorg, 2001b)
Decomposition	Occuring in the presence of oxygen; attracting scavengers and facilitating soft tissue loss (Haglung and Sorg, 2001b)
Disarticulation	Affecting principally flexible joints (hands, skull, limbs); depending on whether the body is floating or submerged, indicates the presence of trauma, scavengers, clothing, and other factors; produces further taphonomic alterations by facilitating long-distance transportation of skeletal elements (Christensen et al., 2014)
Scavenging	Promoting dispersal and fragmentation (Haglung and Sorg, 2001b)

determining the postmortem fate of skeletal remains, as bones with high density are generally better preserved (Bello and Andrews, 2009; Willey et al., 1997). This is why appendicular elements, which consist largely of cortical bone tissue, tend to be better preserved than axial ones, which have a higher concentration of trabecular bone. In particular, trabecular bone has a larger surface area, facilitating chemical exchange between the bone and the soil, thus accelerating decomposition (Grupe, 1988), and it provides ample fat and nutrients to scavengers, making it one of their primary targets (Blumenschine and Marean, 1993).

The size and shape of specific bones may also affect their degree of survival because small bones are more easily lost during excavation or during the secondary treatment of the deceased as part of mortuary practices, and they may also be more easily dispersed by scavengers (Bello and Andrews, 2009; Henderson, 1988).

The age of the individual may also be important because the bones of younger individuals are smaller, have low density, and have high organic content; thus they decay faster than those of adults (Guy et al., 1997). Similarly, the bones of older individuals, especially females, may exhibit osteoporosis, which also accelerates the decay process (Bello and Andrews, 2009; Henderson, 1988). The sex of the deceased is also potentially influential in taphonomy because many societies treat females and males in different ways as part of the funerary ritual and this differential treatment may affect the rate of bone decay (Bello and Andrews, 2009; Henderson, 1988).

Finally, pathological conditions can accelerate the rate of decomposition of skeletal remains. Injured or otherwise pathological bone is more easily accessed by microorganisms, whereas metabolic and other disorders result in reduced bone mineralization and increased porosity, which facilitates bone decomposition (Breitmeier et al., 2005; Henderson, 1988; Lewis, 2010).

2.7 COMMINGLING

Commingling is the mixing of the skeletal remains of different individuals (Fig. 2.7.1); it is not a taphonomic factor but rather the outcome of many different taphonomic processes. Excellent edited volumes that discuss various approaches to the study of commingled remains have been published by Osterholtz et al. (2014) and Adams and Byrd (2008).

The study of commingled assemblages is a primary issue for paleontologists and archaeozoologists; thus most of the relevant methodology has been developed in the context of these disciplines (e.g., Allen and Guy, 1984; Bökönyi, 1970; Chase and Hagaman, 1987; Fieller and Turner, 1982; Grayson, 1984; Krantz, 1968; Lyman, 1987; Nichol and Creak, 1979; Wild and Nichol, 1983; Winder, 1991).

The first step in the study of human commingled remains is to create a list of all the bones present in the assemblage by type and side. The presence of more than one bone of the same type and side (e.g., two right humeri) suggests that commingling has occurred. During the sorting of commingled remains, it is helpful to take into account the age at death (e.g., fused or unfused epiphyses), bone size, and other potentially useful aspects of morphological variation (Ubelaker, 2001). It must be noted that despite efforts to employ metric methods in sorting commingled remains, these are of limited use when the individuals that comprise the assemblage do not differ substantially in overall size (Byrd and Adams, 2003).

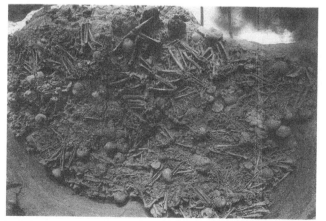

FIGURE 2.7.1 Commingled skeletal remains in a collective burial from Sarrians (Vaucluse, Southern France). *Original photo in Villa P, Mahieu E. Breakage patterns of human long bones. Journal of Human Evolution 1991;21:27–48, reprinted with permission.*

The next step is to estimate the number of individuals that formed the commingled assemblage. Two approaches are usually adopted for this estimation. The first approach calculates the minimum number of individuals (MNI), whereas the second computes the most likely number of individuals (MLNI).

The MNI was introduced into zooarchaeological studies by White (1953). According to White, the number of preserved bones of the most abundant element is equal to the MNI. For instance, consider a sample that includes 12 right and 8 left femora, 7 right and 11 left clavicles, and 10 right and 9 left humeri. Based on White's definition, the MNI is 12, given that the most abundant element is the right femora. It is evident that the MNI approximates the number of individuals originally present in the assemblage satisfactorily only when a high percentage of the original material is present in the sample (Adams and Konigsberg, 2008).

An alternative but equivalent formulation of the MNI takes into account the number of pairs formed between bilateral elements. Consider that P_i pairs between R_i right and L_i left bones of type i are identified in the assemblage. Then the MNI may be calculated from the following (Chaplin, 1971):

$$N = \max(R_i + L_i - P_i) \tag{2.7.1}$$

where max denotes the maximum value of $(R_i + L_i - P_i)$ among the various skeletal elements. In this expression, the presence of *altered* elements, i.e., bones that have been damaged postdepositionally so that it is still possible to determine if they are right or left but it is not feasible to pair them, should be excluded from the calculations.

A straightforward extension of Eq. (2.7.1) to include altered elements is:

$$N = \max(R_i + L_i - P_i, R_i + AR_i, L_i + AL_i) \tag{2.7.2}$$

where AR_i and AL_i are the number of right and left altered bones, whereas R_i and L_i indicate the number of right and left bones, respectively, which are not altered. This expression is expected to give better estimations than Eq. (2.7.1) but, again, the accuracy of the calculated N is acceptable only if bone loss is relatively low. A hypothetical example demonstrating the application of the earlier equations is given in Box 2.7.1.

As mentioned, MNI estimators produce satisfactory results of the original number of individuals in an assemblage only when the preservation of the material under study is very good, with very few elements lost postdepositionally. For this reason, estimators of the MLNI are preferred. MLNI estimators assess the initial number of individuals that comprised the assemblage under study based on the fact that the probability of identifying P pairs between R right and L left bones from N initial individuals follows the hypergeometric distribution (Adams and Konigsberg, 2004).

For the estimation of the MLNI the most frequently used equation is the so-called *Lincoln's index* (Adams and Konigsberg, 2004):

$$N = \frac{RL}{P} \tag{2.7.3}$$

BOX 2.7.1 Calculation of the Minimum Number of Individuals

Consider the following assemblage of human skeletal elements:

    Femora: $R = 12$, $L = 8$, $AR = 3$, $AL = 1$, $P = 5$;

    Tibiae: $R = 9$, $L = 11$, $AR = 2$, $AL = 0$, $P = 8$;

    Humeri: $R = 13$, $L = 8$, $AR = 4$, $AL = 1$, $P = 7$;

where R is the number of intact right elements, L is the number of intact left elements, AR is the number of altered right elements, AL is the number of altered left elements, and P is the number of pairs.

According to White (1953), the MNI is equal to the most abundant element in the assemblage, which in this example is the right humerus: $N = R + AR = 13 + 4 = 17$. Therefore, the assemblage includes at least 17 individuals.

Using Chaplin's (1971) formula, we have:

$N_{femora} = 12 + 8 - 5 = 15$;

$N_{tibiae} = 9 + 11 - 8 = 12$;

$N_{humeri} = 13 + 8 - 7 = 14$.

By definition, the MNI is the maximum of the obtained values per element, thus the assemblage under study included at least 15 individuals. We observe that this value is lower than the one calculated using White's (1953) approach. The reason is that altered elements have not been included in the calculations based on Chaplin's formula, resulting in an underestimation of the number of individuals. To amend this, we use Eq. (2.7.2):

$N_{femora} = \max(12 + 8 - 5,\ 12 + 3,\ 8 + 1) = \max(15,\ 15,\ 9) = 15$;

$N_{tibiae} = \max(9 + 11 - 8,\ 9 + 2,\ 11 + 0) = \max(12,\ 11,\ 11) = 12$;

$N_{humeri} = \max(13 + 8 - 7,\ 13 + 4,\ 8 + 1) = \max(14,\ 17,\ 9) = 17$.

Once again, we take into account the maximum of the obtained values per element; thus the assemblage had at least 17 individuals. This value is the same as White's (1953).

For example, in the hypothetical data set described in Box 2.7.1, five pairs have been identified between 12 left and 8 right femora. Therefore, the MLNI in the sample is (12 × 8)/5 = 19. We observe that this estimate is slightly different from the MNI but this should be expected because the two methods estimate different things.

A main precondition of MLNI estimators is that all pairs between the right and the left elements have been accurately identified. However, this is not always feasible, particularly in cases of very large sample sizes or when bone preservation is poor. In such cases the misidentification of the number of pairs between the existing bilateral elements may produce a high error in the MLNI value. This problem may be addressed through the use of proper computer algorithms. Such an algorithm that produces a number of potential pairs between bilateral elements is discussed by Nikita and Lahr (2011), whereas the macro Pairing, which can be used for this purpose, is provided in the companion website in the Excel file Pairing in the folder ExcelMacros.

The accuracy of MLNI estimators is expected to improve when multiple skeletal elements are taken into account simultaneously instead of using only the most abundant bone. For this reason, the following equations have been proposed (Nikita, 2014):

$$N = \frac{R_1 L_1 + R_2 L_2 + \ldots + R_n L_n}{P} \tag{2.7.4}$$

$$N = \frac{(R_1 + R_2 + \ldots + R_n + L_1 + L_2 + \ldots + L_n)^2}{4nP} \tag{2.7.5}$$

$$N = \frac{(R_1 + L_1)^2 + (R_2 + L_2)^2 + \ldots + (R_n + L_n)^2}{4P} \tag{2.7.6}$$

$$N = \frac{(R_1 + 1)(L_1 + 1) + (R_2 + 1)(L_2 + 1) + \ldots + (R_n + 1)(L_n + 1)}{P + n} - 1 \tag{2.7.7}$$

In these equations n is the number of the various types of bones, subscripts 1, 2, …, n denote each skeletal element under study (e.g., 1, femora; 2, tibiae; etc.), and P is the sum of all pairs. An application of various MLNI estimators in a hypothetical assemblage is given in Box 2.7.2.

Once N is calculated in a commingled assemblage, using the aforementioned methods, we may proceed to calculate the probabilities $Pr(Loss)$ and $Pr(Alteration)$, which express the probability of a bone of a certain type $i = 1, 2, \ldots, n$ to be lost or altered postdepositionally. On average, if bone alteration does not occur, the number of bones of a certain type that will be lost is equal to $2NPr(Loss)$, because initially there are $2N$ bones in the assemblage (e.g., 5 individuals have 10 femora). Therefore, the number of bones of a certain type that will remain in the sample is equal to $2N[1 - Pr(Loss)]$. From these bones some will be altered and the rest will remain intact. If $Pr(Alteration)$ is the probability of alteration, the number of

---

BOX 2.7.2 Calculation of the Most Likely Number of Individuals

Consider the following assemblage of human skeletal elements:

Femora: $R = 9$, $L = 9$, $P = 6$;
Tibiae: $R = 7$, $L = 7$, $P = 4$;
Humeri: $R = 7$, $L = 9$, $P = 2$.

Lincoln's expression, Eq. (2.7.3), gives the following estimates:

$N_{femora} = (9 \times 9)/6 = 13.5$, thus 14 individuals;
$N_{tibiae} = (7 \times 7)/4 = 12.25$, thus 12 individuals;
$N_{humeri} = (7 \times 9)/2 = 31.5$, thus 32 individuals.

The discrepancy of the values obtained from different elements is due to the differential preservation of these elements and, in our case, it is attributed to the small number of pairs identified between right and left humeri. In contrast, the values obtained from equations employing multiple elements simultaneously are:

$N = [(9 \times 9) + (7 \times 7) + (7 \times 9)]/(6 + 4 + 2) =$ 193/ 12 = 16.1;
$N = (9 + 7 + 7 + 9 + 7 + 9)^2/[4 \times 3 \times (6 + 4 + 2)] =$ 2304/144 = 16;
$N = [(9 + 9)^2 + (7 + 7)^2 + (7 + 9)^2]/[4 \times (6 + 4 + 2)] =$ 776/48 = 16.2;
$N = \{[(9 + 1) \times (9 + 1)] + [(7 + 1) \times (7 + 1)] + [(7 + 1)$ $\times (9 + 1)]\}/[(6 + 4 + 2) + 3] - 1 = 244/15 - 1 = 15.3$.

It is seen that the first three equations employing multiple elements yield the same result, $N = 16$, and this may be adopted as the MLNI for the assemblage under consideration.

bones that will be altered is $2N[1 - Pr(Loss)]Pr(Alteration)$ and the number of bones that will remain intact is equal to $2N[1 - Pr(Loss)][1 - Pr(Alteration)]$. Therefore, we have the relationships:

$$2N[1 - Pr(Loss)]Pr(Alteration) = AR + AL \tag{2.7.8}$$

$$2N[1 - Pr(Loss)][1 - Pr(Alteration)] = R + L \tag{2.7.9}$$

If there are no altered elements, then $Pr(Alteration) = 0$ and $Pr(Loss)$ can be estimated from Eq. (2.7.9), which yields:

$$Pr(Loss) = \frac{2N - R - L}{2N} \tag{2.7.10}$$

If $Pr(Alteration) \neq 0$, we divide Eqs. (2.7.8) and (2.7.9), solve the resulting expression with respect to $Pr(Alteration)$, and obtain:

$$Pr(Alteration) = \frac{AR + AL}{AR + AL + R + L} \tag{2.7.11}$$

which allows the calculation of $Pr(Alteration)$. If Eq. (2.7.8) is solved with respect to $Pr(Loss)$, we obtain:

$$Pr(Loss) = \frac{2N \, Pr(Alteration) - AR - AL}{2N \, Pr(Alteration)} \tag{2.7.12}$$

which, in combination with Eq. (2.7.11), can be used for the calculation of $Pr(Loss)$ when $Pr(Alteration) \neq 0$.

Note that the probabilities $Pr(Loss)$ of the various bone types are interrelated through the following equation:

$$Pr(Loss_i) = 1 - [1 - Pr(Loss_1)] \times Robusticity(i) \tag{2.7.13}$$

where $Pr(Loss_1)$ is the probability of the loss of a reference bone, say a femur, and the relative $Robusticity(i)$ is calculated from the ratio $(R_i + L_i)/(R_1 + L_1)$, i.e.,

$$Robusticity(i) = \frac{R_i + L_i}{R_1 + L_1} \tag{2.7.14}$$

Eq. (2.7.13) arises from Eq. (2.7.10), which can be rewritten as $1 - Pr(Loss) = (R + L)/(2N)$. This relationship yields $1 - Pr(Loss_i) = (R_i + L_i)/(2N)$ and $1 - Pr(Loss_1) = (R_1 + L_1)/(2N)$, which readily results in Eq. (2.7.13).

The earlier relationships can play an important role in the evaluation of the accuracy of the calculated N values from Eqs. (2.7.4)–(2.7.7). Fig. 2.7.2 depicts the relationship between N(estimated) and $Pr(Loss)$, as well as the corresponding standard deviations of N. For the creation of this figure, artificial data were used (Nikita, 2015). From this figure as well as from similar simulations, the following observations may be made:

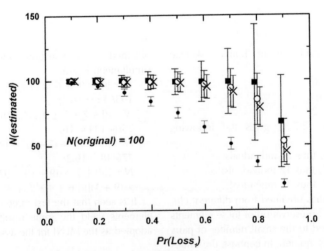

FIGURE 2.7.2 Relationship between N(estimated) and $Pr(Loss_1)$. Corresponding standard deviations are also depicted. N(estimated) were averaged over 1000 iterations calculated from Eq. (2.7.1) with $n = 5$ (●) and Eq. (2.7.7) with $n = 1$ (■), 3 (○), and 5 (×) using N(original) = 100, $Pr(Alteration) = 0$, and Robusticity = 1, 0.75, 0.75, 0.6, and 0.5 per element.

1. The estimation of N based on MNI is valid only when less than 10% of the original elements are missing [$Pr(Loss) \leq$ 0.1] and no altered elements are included in the calculations. For $Pr(Loss)$ values over 0.1, the higher these are, the greater the underestimation of N becomes.
2. Eqs. (2.7.4)–(2.7.7) give in general convergent results and estimations based on them overall perform well even when the percentage of lost elements reaches 50% [$Pr(Loss) \leq 0.5$]. Note that the mean estimated N values are accurate even for $Pr(Loss)$ around 0.7 or 0.8. However, in practice, with archaeological (nonsimulated) material we cannot calculate the mean values of N, and the great variances for $Pr(Loss) \geq 0.6$ make any prediction for N ambiguous.
3. With respect to the number of skeletal elements (n) that should be incorporated in the MLNI functions, by increasing n, the dispersal of the N values decreases; therefore it is preferable to incorporate multiple elements instead of using a single one. However, we should be careful not to incorporate elements with a high degree of alteration, which can affect pairing, i.e., the accurate estimation of P, and subsequently the validity of the estimated N values. As a general rule, the use of the three most robust long bones (femur, tibia, humerus) should be preferred over the use of a single element.

Fig. 2.7.2 highlights that to determine how accurate the estimated N values are, it is important to calculate the standard deviations of these estimates. This can be achieved by means of the macros provided in the companion website (spreadsheet MLNI). This spreadsheet uses Eqs. (2.7.1) and (2.7.2) denoted by MNI and MNIC; Eqs. (2.7.4)–(2.7.7) denoted by MLNI1, MLNI2, MLNI3, MLNI4; and the Hypergeometric Estimator (JHE) as presented by Konigsberg (konig.la.utk.edu/MLNI.html). All these equations (estimators) have also been written in Excel VBA to facilitate the calculations required for each estimator. In addition, the macro MLNI_Stdev can be used for the computation of the standard deviation of N. The functions and the macro are provided in the companion website in the Excel files MLNI and OSTEO. For the application of this macro, an average N value is calculated using the various MLNI functions. In addition, the probabilities $Pr(Loss)$ and $Pr(Alteration)$ are computed from Eqs. (2.7.11) and (2.7.12) or Eq. (2.7.10) when $Pr(Alteration) = 0$. Using these data, the macro MLNI_Stdev is run and the averaged values of N for each estimator as well as the standard deviations of these values are obtained.

As an example of the application of the aforementioned method, the skeletal assemblage presented in Fig. 2.7.3 is examined. This is an archaeological assemblage consisting of 25 individuals buried together. The direct application of all estimators to these data is also shown in Fig. 2.7.3.

It is seen that because of the great number of altered elements, the MNI estimator underestimates the initial number of individuals, whereas the MNIC estimator gives rather satisfactory results. In general, the use of just one type of bone ($n = 1$, femur) yields an underestimation of N. The prediction of N is improved if we include all three types of bones. It is seen that estimators MLNI1 to MLNI3 give N ranging from 23 to 25 when three elements are used, whereas estimators MLNI4 and JHE give N of 22.

To compute the standard deviation of the estimated N values, the probabilities $Pr(Loss)$ and $Pr(Alteration)$ are calculated from Eqs. (2.7.11) and (2.7.12). We obtain $Pr(Loss) = 0.16$, 0.4, and 0.22, and $Pr(Alteration) = 0.476$, 0.367, and 0.692 for the femur, humerus, and tibia, respectively. For the application of the macro MLNI_Stdev, we may use as an initial value $N = 24$, which is the average value of N estimated from Eqs. (2.7.4)–(2.7.6) using all three elements. The averaged N values and their standard deviations are depicted in Fig. 2.7.4. Eqs. (2.7.4)–(2.7.6) yield on average $N = 25 \pm 7$ when $n = 3$, and $N = 27 \pm 11$ when $n = 1$.

	A	B	C	D
1	**Estimators using 1 and 3 types of bones**			
2	Data from Boeotian cemetery			
3	Bone =	Femur	Humerus	Tibia
4	R =	11	9	6
5	L =	11	10	6
6	P =	6	3	1
7	Altered_R =	10	6	13
8	Altered_L =	10	5	14
9				
10	**Estimators:**	n=1		n=3
11	MNI :	16		16
12	MNIC :	21		21
13	MLNI1 :	20		25
14	MLNI2 :	20		23
15	MLNI3 :	20		25
16	MLNI4 :	20		22
17	JHE :	19		22

	A	B	C	D	E
1	**Averaged estimations of the original number of individuals**				
2					
3	Iterations=	10000			
4	N =	24			
5	Pr(loss) =	0.16	0.4	0.22	
6	Pr(alteration) =	0.4762	0.3667	0.6923	
7					
8					
9	n =	3			
10					
11					
12	**Averaged estimations:**				
13					
14		n=1		n=3	
15		AVERAGE	STDEV	AVERAGE	STDEV
16	MNI :	16	2.3	17	1.9
17	MNIC :	21	1.4	21	1.2
18					
19	MLNI1 :	27	10.5	25	6.5
20	MLNI2 :	27	11.0	24	6.6
21	MLNI3 :	27	11.0	26	6.9
22	MLNI4 :	24	7.2	22	3.8
23	JHE :	23	6.3	22	3.5

FIGURE 2.7.4   Results from the MLNI_Stdev macro when altered elements are included in the treatment.

It is seen that although Eqs. (2.7.4)−(2.7.7) estimate very satisfactorily the original number of individuals in the assemblage ($N = 25$), the computed standard deviations are rather large, indicating a high uncertainty in the estimated N values. This example shows how important it is to calculate the standard deviation of N as a means of determining the accuracy of the obtained results.

REFERENCES

Adams BJ, Konigsberg LW. Estimation of the most likely number of individuals from commingled human skeletal remains. American Journal of Physical Anthropology 2004;125:138−51.

Adams BJ, Konigsberg LW. How many people? Determining the number of individuals represented by commingled human remains. In: Adams BJ, Byrd JE, editors. Recovery, analysis and identification of commingled human remains. New York: Springer; 2008. p. 241−56.

Adams BJ, Byrd JE, editors. Recovery, analysis, and identification of commingled human remains. New York: Springer; 2008.

Allaire MT, Manheim MH, Burgess GH. Shark-inflicted trauma: a case study of unidentified remains recovered from the Gulf of Mexico. Journal of Forensic Sciences 2012;57:1675−8.

Allen J, Guy JBM. Optimal estimations of individuals in archaeological faunal assemblages: how minimal is the MNI? Archaeology in Oceania 1984;19:41−7.

Anderson GS, Cervenka VJ. Insects associated with the body: their use and analysis. In: Haglund WD, Sorg MH, editors. Advances in forensic taphonomy: method, theory, and archaeological perspectives. Boca Raton: CRC Press; 2001. p. 173−200.

Anderson G, Bell LS. Deep coastal marine taphonomy: interim results from an ongoing experimental investigation of decomposition in the Saanich Inlet, British Columbia. Proceedings of the American Academy of Forensic Sciences 2010;16:381−2.

Andrews P, Cook J. Natural modifications to bones in a temperate setting. Man 1985;20:675−91.

Andrews P, Whybrow P. Taphonomic observations on a camel skeleton in a desert environment in Abu Dhabi. Palaeontologia Electronica 2005;8:23A.

Baby R. Hopewell cremation practices. Papers in Archaeology 1. Columbus, OH: The Ohio Historical Society; 1954. p. 1−7.

Bais HP, Weir TL, Perry LG, Gilroy S, Vivanco JM. The role of root exudates in rhizosphere interactions with plants and other organisms. Annual Review of Plant Biology 2006;57:233−66.

Barrios M, Wolff M. Initial study of arthropods succession and pig carrion decomposition in two freshwater ecosystems in the Colombian Andes. Forensic Science International 2011;212:164−72.

Bass WM. Time interval since death. In: Rathbun TA, Buikstra JE, editors. Human identification: case studies in forensic anthropology. Springfield, IL: Charles C. Thomas; 1984. p. 136−47.

Bass WM. Outdoor decomposition rates in Tennessee. In: Haglund WD, Sorg MH, editors. Forensic taphonomy: the postmortem fate of human remains. Boca Raton: CRC Press; 1996. p. 181−6.

Behrensmeyer AK. Taphonomic and ecologic information from bone weathering. Paleobiology 1978;4:150—62.

Belaústegui Z, de Gibert JM, Domènech R, Muñiz F, Martinell J. Clavate borings in a Miocene cetacean skeleton from Tarragona (NE Spain) and the fossil record of marine bone bioerosion. Palaeogeography, Palaeoclimatology, Palaeoecology 2012;323—325:68—74.

Bello S, Andrews P. The intrinsic pattern of preservation of human skeletons and its influence on the interpretation of funerary behaviours. In: Gowland R, Knüsel C, editors. Social archaeology of funerary remains. Oxford: Oxbow Books; 2009. p. 1—13.

Bello S, Signoli M, Thomann A, Lalys L, Dutour O. Nouvelle méthode de quantification de l'état de conservation des surfaces corticales et son application dans les études paléopathologiques et paléoépidémiologiques. Bulletin et Mémoires de la Société d'Anthropologie de Paris 2003;15:7—8.

Bello S, Thomann A, Signoli M, Dutour O, Andrews P. Age and sex bias in the reconstruction of past population structures. American Journal of Physical Anthropology 2006;129:24—38.

Berryman HE. Disarticulation pattern and tooth mark artifacts associated with pig scavenging of human remains: a case study. In: Haglund WD, Sorg MH, editors. Advances in forensic taphonomy. Method, theory, and archaeological perspectives. Boca Raton: CRC Press; 2001. p. 495—7.

Binford LR. An analysis of cremations from three Michigan sites. Wisconsin Archaeologist 1963;44:98—110.

Blumenschine RJ. An experimental model of the timing of hominid and carnivore influence on archaeological bone assemblages. Journal of Archaeological Science 1988;15:483—502.

Blumenschine R, Marean C. A carnivore's view of archaeological bone assemblages. In: Hudson J, editor. From bones to behaviour: ethnoarchaeological and experimental contributions to the interpretation of faunal remains. Carbonale: Center for Archaeological Investigations, Southern Illinois University; 1993. p. 273—300.

Bohnert M, Rost T, Faller-Marquardt M, Ropohl D, Pollak S. Fractures of the base of the skull in charred bodies — post-mortem heat injuries or signs of mechanical traumatisation? Forensic Science International 1997;87:55—62.

Bökönyi S. A new method for the determination of the number of individuals in animal bone material. American Journal of Archaeology 1970;74:291—2.

Breitmeier D, Graefee-Kircl U, Albrecht K, Weber M, Tröger HD, Kleemann WJ. Evaluation of the correlation between time corpses spent in in-ground graves and findings at exhumation. Forensic Science International 2005;154:218—23.

Breuning-Madsen H, Holst MK, Rasmussen M. The chemical environment in a burial mound shortly after construction—an archaeological-pedological experiment. Journal of Archaeological Science 2001;28:691—7.

Bristow J, Simms Z, Randolph-Quinney P. Taphonomy. In: Black S, Ferguson E, editors. Forensic anthropology 2000 to 2010. Boca Raton: CRC Press; 2011. p. 279—318.

Buikstra JE, Swegle M. Bone modification due to burning: experimental evidence. In: Bonnichsen R, Sorg M, editors. Bone modification. Orono: Maine center for the study of the first Americans; 1989. p. 247—58.

Buikstra JE, Ubelaker DH, editors. Standards for data collection from human skeletal remains. Fayetteville: Arkansas Archaeological Survey Research Series No. 44; 1994.

Byard RW, Gilbert JD, Brown K. Pathologic features of fatal shark attacks. The American Journal of Forensic Medicine and Pathology 2000;21:225—9.

Byrd JE, Adams BJ. Osteometric sorting of commingled human remains. Journal of Forensic Sciences 2003;48:717—24.

Casallas DA, Moore MK. High soil acidity associated with near complete mineral dissolution of recently buried human remains. Proceedings of the American Academy of Forensic Sciences 2012;18:400—1.

Chaplin RE. The study of animal bones from archaeological sites. London: Seminar Press; 1971.

Chase PG, Hagaman RM. Minimum number of individuals and its alternatives: a probability theory perspective. OSSA 1987;13:75—86.

Christensen AM, Passalacqua NV, Bartelink EJ. Forensic anthropology. Current methods and practice. San Diego: Elsevier; 2014.

DeHaan JD. Sustained combustion of bodies: some observations. Journal of Forensic Sciences 2012;57:1578—84.

DeHaan J, Nurbakhsh S. Sustained combustion of an animal carcass and its implications for the consumption of human bodies in fires. Journal of Forensic Sciences 2001;46:1076—81.

Devlin JB, Herrmann NP. Bone color as an interpretive tool of the depositional history of archaeological cremains. In: Schmidt CW, Symes SA, editors. The analysis of burned human remains. San Diego: Elsevier; 2008. p. 109—28.

Dobney K, Rielly K. A method for recording archaeological animal bones: the use of diagnostic zones. Circaea 1988;5:79—96.

Dodson P, Wexlar D. Taphonomic investigations of owl pellets. Paleobiology 1979;5:279—84.

Domínguez-Rodrigo M, Piqueras A. The use of tooth pits to identify carnivore taxa in tooth-marked archaeofaunas and their relevance to reconstruct hominid carcass processing behaviors. Journal of Archaeological Sciences 2003;30:1385—91.

Domínguez-Solera SD, Domínguez-Rodrigo M. A taphonomic study of bone modification and of tooth-mark patterns on long limb bone portions by suids. International Journal of Osteoarchaeology 2009;19:345—63.

Domínguez-Solera S, Domínguez-Rodrigo M. A taphonomic study of a carcass consumed by griffon vultures (*Gyps fulvus*) and its relevance for the interpretation of bone surface modifications. Archaeological and Anthropological Sciences 2011;3:385—92.

Duday H. The archaeology of the dead. Lectures in archaeothanatology. Oxford: Oxbow Books; 2009.

Dupras TL, Schultz JJ. Taphonomic bone staining and color changes in forensic contexts. In: Pokines JT, Symes SA, editors. Manual of forensic taphonomy. Boca Raton: CRC Press; 2013. p. 315—40.

Efremov IA. Taphonomy: a new branch of paleontology. Pan-American Geologist 1940;74:81—93.

Evans T. Fluvial taphonomy. In: Pokines JT, Symes SA, editors. Manual of forensic taphonomy. Boca Raton: CRC Press; 2013. p. 115—42.

Fairgrieve SI. Forensic cremation: recovery and analysis. Boca Raton: CRC Press; 2007.

Fernández-Jalvo Y, Andrews P. Experimental effects of water abrasion on bone fragments. Journal of Taphonomy 2003;1:147—63.

Fieller NRJ, Turner A. Number estimation in vertebrate samples. Journal of Archaeological Science 1982;9:49—62.

Gilchrist M, Mytum H. Experimental archaeology and burnt animal bone from archaeological sites. Circaea 1986;4:29–38.

Gonçalves D, Thompson TJU, Cunha E. Implications of heat-induced changes in bone on the interpretation of funerary behaviour and practice. Journal of Archaeological Science 2011;38:1308–13.

Grayson DK. Quantitative zooarchaeology: topics in the analysis of archaeological Faunas. New York: Academic Press; 1984.

Grupe G. Impact of the choice of bone samples on trace element data in excavated human skeletons. Journal of Archaeological Science 1988;15:123–9.

Guy H, Masset C, Baud CA. Infant taphonomy. International Journal of Osteoarchaeology 1997;7:221–9.

Haglund WD. Rodents and human remains. In: Haglund WD, Sorg MH, editors. Forensic taphonomy: the postmortem fate of human remains. Boca Raton: CRC Press; 1996. p. 405–14.

Haglund WD, Sorg MH, editors. Forensic taphonomy: the postmortem fate of human remains. Boca Raton: CRC Press; 1996.

Advances in forensic taphonomy. In: Haglund WD, Sorg MH, editors. Method, theory, and archaeological perspectives. Boca Raton: CRC Press; 2001a.

Haglund WD, Sorg MH. Human remains in water environments. In: Haglund WD, Sorg MH, editors. Advances in forensic taphonomy. Method, theory, and archaeological perspectives. Boca Raton: CRC Press; 2001b. p. 202–18.

Haglund WD, Reay DT, Swindler DR. Canid scavenging/disarticulation sequence of human remains in the Pacific northwest. Journal of Forensic Sciences 1989;34:587–606.

Harsányi L. Scanning electron microscopic investigation of thermal damage of the teeth. Acta Morphologica Academiae Scientiarium Hungaricae 1975;23:271–81.

Heaton VG, Lagden A, Moffatt C, Simmons T. Predicting the postmortem submersion interval for human remains recovered from U.K. waterways. Journal of Forensic Sciences 2010;55:302–7.

Henderson J. Factors determining the state of preservation of human remains. In: Boddington A, Garland AN, Janaway RC, editors. Death, decay and reconstruction. Approaches to archaeology and forensic science. Manchester: Manchester University Press; 1988. p. 43–54.

Herrmann B. Experimentelle und theoretische beiträge zur leichenbrand unter schung. HOMO-Journal of Comparative Human Biology 1976;27:114–8.

Herrmann B. On histological investigations of cremated human remains. Journal of Human Evolution 1977;6:101–3.

Higgs ND, Pokines JT. Marine environmental alterations to bone. In: Pokines JT, Symes SA, editors. Manual of forensic taphonomy. Boca Raton: CRC Press; 2013. p. 143–80.

Hiller JT, Thompson JU, Evison MP, Chamberlain AT, Weiss TJ. Bone mineral change during experimental heating: an X-ray scattering investigation. Biomaterials 2003;24:5091–7.

Hollund HI, Jans MME, Collins MJ, Kars H, Joosten I, Kars SM. What happened here? Bone histology as a tool in decoding the post-mortem histories of archaeological bone from Castricum, The Netherlands. International Journal of Osteoarchaeology 2012;22:537–48.

Horwitz L, Smith P. The effects of striped hyaena activity on human remains. Journal of Archaeological Science 1988;15:471–81.

Huchet J-B, Deverly D, Gutierrez B, Chauchat C. Taphonomic evidence of a human skeleton gnawed by termites in a Moche-civilisation grave at Huaca de la Luna, Peru. International Journal of Osteoarchaeology 2011;21:92–102.

Hughes CE, White CA. Crack propagation in teeth: a comparison of perimortem and postmortem behavior of dental materials and cracks. Journal of Forensic Sciences 2009;54:263–6.

Ihama Y, Ninomiya K, Noguchi M, Fuke C, Miyazaki T. Characteristic features of injuries due to shark attacks: a review of 12 cases. Legal Medicine 2009;11:219–25.

Janaway RC. The decay of buried human remains and their associated materials. In: Hunter J, Roberts C, Martin A, editors. Studies in crime: an introduction to forensic archaeology. London: Routledge; 1996. p. 58–85.

Junod CA, Pokines JT. Subaerial weathering. In: Pokines JT, Symes SA, editors. Manual of forensic taphonomy. Boca Raton: CRC Press; 2013. p. 287–314.

Keough N, L'Abbé EN, Steyn M, Pretorius S. Assessment of skeletal changes after post-mortem exposure to fire as an indicator of decomposition stage. Forensic Science International 2015;246:17–24.

Kerbis Peterhans JC. The roles of porcupines, leopards, and hyenas in ungulate carcass dispersal: implications for paleoanthropology [Ph.D. dissertation]. Chicago, IL: Department of Anthropology, University of Chicago; 1990.

Klippel WE, Synstelien JA. Rodents as taphonomic agents: bone gnawing by brown rats and gray squirrels. Journal of Forensic Sciences 2007;53:765–73.

Knüsel CJ, Outram AK. Fragmentation: the zonation method applied to fragmented human remains from archaeological and forensic contexts. Environmental Archaeology 2004;9:85–97.

Komar DA, Buikstra JE. Forensic anthropology: contemporary theory and practice. New York: Oxford University Press; 2007.

Krantz GS. A new method of counting mammal bones. American Journal of Archaeology 1968;72:286–8.

Lentz AK, Burgess GH, Perrin K, Brown JA, Mozingo DW, Lottenberg L. Mortality and management of 96 shark attacks and development of a shark bite severity scoring system. The American Surgeon 2010;76:101–6.

Lewis JE. Identifying sword marks on bone: criteria for distinguishing between cut marks made by different classes of bladed weapons. Journal of Archaeological Science 2008;35:2001–8.

Lewis ME. Life and death in a civitas capital: metabolic disease and trauma in the children from late Roman Dorchester, Dorset. American Journal of Physical Anthropology 2010;142:405–16.

Lieverse AR, Weber AW, Goriunova OI. Human taphonomy at Khuzhir-Nuge Xiv, Siberia: a new method for documenting skeletal condition. Journal of Archaeological Science 2006;33:1141–51.

Lyman RL. Zooarchaeology and taphonomy: a general consideration. Journal of Ethnobiology 1987;7:93–117.

Lyman RL. Vertebrate taphonomy. Cambridge: Cambridge University Press; 1994.

Lyman RL. Foreword from paleontology. In: Haglund WD, Sorg MH, editors. Advances in forensic taphonomy: method, theory, and archaeological perspectives. Boca Raton: CRC Press, p. xix−xxi; 2001.

Lyman RL, Fox GL. A critical evaluation of bone weathering as an indication of bone assemblage formation. In: Haglund WD, Sorg MH, editors. Forensic taphonomy: the postmortem fate of human remains. Boca Raton: CRC Press; 1996. p. 223−47.

Mann RW, Bass WM, Meadows L. Time since death and decomposition of the human body: variables and observations in case and experimental field studies. Journal of Forensic Sciences 1990;35:103−11.

Marden K, Sorg MH, Haglund WD. Taphonomy. In: DiGangi EA, Moore MK, editors. Research methods in human skeletal biology. San Diego: Elsevier; 2012. p. 241−62.

Mayne Correia P. Fire modification of bone: a review of the literature. In: Haglund WD, Sorg MH, editors. Forensic taphonomy: the postmortem fate of human remains. Boca Raton: CRC Press; 1996. p. 275−94.

McGraw WS, Cooke C, Shultz S. Primate remains from African crowned eagle (*Stephanoaetus coronatus*) nests in Ivory Coast's Tai Forest: implications for primate predation and early hominid taphonomy in South Africa. American Journal of Physical Anthropology 2006;131:151−65.

Micozzi M. Frozen environments and soft tissue preservation. In: Haglund WD, Sorg MH, editors. The postmortem fate of human remains. Boca Raton: CRC Press; 1996. p. 171−80.

Murmann DC, Brumit PC, Schrader BA, Senn DR. A comparison of animal jaws and bite mark patterns. Journal of Forensic Sciences 2006;51:846−60.

Nichol RK, Creak GA. Matched paired elements among archaeological bone remains: a computer procedure and some practical limitations. Newsletter of Computer Archaeology 1979;14:6−16.

Nielsen-Marsh CM, Hedges REM. Patterns of diagenesis in bone I: the effects of site environments. Journal of Archaeological Science 2000;27:1139−50.

Nielsen-Marsh CM, Smith CI, Jans MME, Nord A, Kars H, Collins MJ. Bone diagenesis in the European Holocene II: taphonomic and environmental considerations. Journal of Archaeological Science 2007;34:1523−31.

Nikita E. Estimation of the original number of individuals using multiple skeletal elements. International Journal of Osteoarchaeology 2014;24:660−4.

Nikita E. Dust to dust and what is left? The impact of partial preservation in the calculation of the number of individuals from commingled assemblages. In: Oral presentation at the 116th annual meeting of the archaeological institute of America, 8th−11th January 2015; 2015. New Orleans, LA.

Nikita E, Lahr MM. Simple algorithms for the estimation of the initial number of individuals in commingled skeletal remains. American Journal of Physical Anthropology 2011;146:629−36.

Osterholtz AJ, Baustian KM, Martin DL, editors. Commingled and disarticulated human remains. Working toward improved theory, method, and data. New York: Springer; 2014.

Owsley DW, Compton BE. Preservation in late 19th century iron coffin burials. In: Haglund WD, Sorg MH, editors. Forensic taphonomy: the postmortem fate of human remains. Boca Raton: CRC Press; 1996. p. 511−26.

Parsons KM, Brett CE. Taphonomic processes and biases in modern marine environments: an actualistic perspective of fossil assemblage preservation. In: Donovan SK, editor. The processes of fossilization. New York: Columbia University Press; 1991. p. 22−65.

Pinheiro J. Introduction to forensic medicine and pathology. In: Schmitt A, Cunha E, Pinheiro J, editors. Forensic anthropology and medicine: complementary sciences from recovery to cause of death. New York: Springer; 2006. p. 13−38.

Pobiner BL. Hominin-carnivore interactions: evidence from modern carnivore bone modification and early Pleistocene archaeofaunas (Koobi Fora, Kenya; Olduvai Gorge, Tanzania) [Ph.D. dissertation]. Department of Anthropology, Rutgers University; 2007.

Pokines JT. Forensic recoveries of U.S. war dead and the effects of taphonomy and other site-altering processes. In: Steadman DW, editor. Hard evidence: case studies in forensic anthropology. 2nd ed. Upper Saddle River: Routledge; 2008. p. 141−54.

Pokines JT. Faunal dispersal, reconcentration, and gnawing damage to bone in terrestrial environments. In: Pokines JT, Symes SA, editors. Manual of forensic taphonomy. Boca Raton: CRC Press; 2013. p. 201−48.

Pokines JT, Kerbis Peterhans JC. Spotted hyena (*Crocuta crocuta*) den use and taphonomy in the Masai Mara National Reserve, Kenya. Journal of Archaeological Science 2007;34:1914−31.

Pokines JT, Baker JE. Effects of burial environment on osseous remains. In: Pokines JT, Symes SA, editors. Manual of forensic taphonomy. Boca Raton: CRC Press; 2013. p. 73−114.

Pokines JT, Symes SA, editors. Manual of forensic taphonomy. Boca Raton: CRC Press; 2013.

Reeves NM. Taphonomic effects of vulture scavenging. Journal of Forensic Sciences 2009;54:523−8.

Reichs K. Postmortem dismemberment: recovery, analysis and interpretation. In: Reichs KJ, editor. Forensic osteology: advances in the identification of human remains. 2nd ed. Springfield: Charles C. Thomas; 1998. p. 353−88.

Rhine S. Bone voyage: a journey in forensic anthropology. Albuquerque: University of New Mexico Press; 1998.

Roksandic M. Position of skeletal remains as a key to understanding mortuary behavior. In: Haglund WD, Sorg MH, editors. Advances in forensic taphonomy. Method, theory, and archaeological perspectives. Boca Raton: CRC Press; 2001. p. 99−117.

Rudrappa T, Czymmek KJ, Paré PW, Bais HP. Root-secreted malic acid recruits beneficial soil bacteria. Plant Physiology 2008;148:1547−56.

Schmidt CW. The recovery and study of burned human teeth. In: Schmidt CW, Symes SA, editors. The analysis of burned human remains. San Diego: Elsevier; 2008. p. 55−74.

Schmidt CW, Symes SA, editors. The analysis of burned human remains. San Diego: Elsevier; 2008.

Schultz J, Williamson M, Nawrocki SP, Falsetti A, Warren M. A taphonomic profile to aid in the recognition of human remains from historic and/or cemetery contexts. Florida Anthropologist 2003;56:141−7.

Shipman P, Rose JJ. Early hominid hunting, butchering, and carcass processing behaviors: approaches to the fossil record. Journal of Anthropological Archaeology 1983;2:57−98.

Shipman P, Foster G, Schoeninger M. Burnt bones and teeth: an experimental study of color, morphology, crystal structure and shrinkage. Journal of Archaeological Science 1984;2:307−25.

Sorg MH, Dearborn JH, Monahan EI, Ryan HF, Kristin G, Sweeney KG, et al. Forensic taphonomy in marine contexts. In: Haglund WD, Sorg MH, editors. Forensic taphonomy: the postmortem fate of human remains. Boca Raton: CRC Press; 1996. p. 1−9.

Stodder ALW. Taphonomy and the nature of archaeological assemblages. In: Katzenberg MA, Saunders SR, editors. Biological anthropology of the human skeleton. 2nd ed. New York: Wiley-Liss; 2008. p. 71−114.

Symes SA, Rainwater CW, Chapman EN, Gipson DR, Piper AL. Patterned thermal destruction of human remains in a forensic setting. In: Schmidt CW, Symes SA, editors. The analysis of burned human remains. San Diego: Elsevier; 2008. p. 15−54.

Tappen M. Savanna ecology and natural bone deposition: implications for early hominid site formation, hunting, and scavenging. Current Anthropology 1995;36:223−60.

Thompson TJU. Recent advances in the study of burned bone and their implications for forensic anthropology. Forensic Science International 2004;146:S203−5.

Thompson TJU. Heat-induced dimensional changes in bone and their consequences for forensic anthropology. Journal of Forensic Sciences 2005;50:1008−15.

Trueman CN, Martill DM. The long-term survival of bone: the role of bioerosion. Archaeometry 2002;44:371−82.

Turner II CG, Turner JA. Man corn: cannibalism and violence in the prehistoric American southwest. Salt Lake City: The University of Utah Press; 1999.

Ubelaker DH. A history of Smithsonian-FBI collaboration in forensic anthropology, especially in regard to facial imagery. Forensic Science Communications 2000;2.

Ubelaker DH. Approaches to the study of commingling in human skeletal biology. In: Haglund WD, Sorg MH, editors. Advances in forensic taphonomy. Method, theory, and archaeological perspectives. Boca Raton: CRC Press; 2001. p. 331−52.

Vanin S, Zancaner S. Post-mortal lesions in freshwater environment. Forensic Science International 2011;212:e18−20.

Villa P, Mahieu E. Breakage patterns of human long bones. Journal of Human Evolution 1991;21:27−48.

Walker PL, Miller KP. Time, temperature, and oxygen availability: an experimental study of the effects of environmental conditions on the color and organic content of cremated bone. In: Poster presented at the 104th annual meeting of the American association of physical anthropologists, 8th April 2005, Milwaukee, WI; 2005.

Walker PL, Miller KWP, Richman R. Time, temperature, and oxygen availability: an experimental study of the effects of environmental conditions on the color and organic content of cremated bones. In: Schmidt CW, Symes SA, editors. The analysis of burned human remains. San Diego: Elsevier; 2008. p. 129−35.

Weitzel MA. Human taphonomy: Khuzhir-Nuge XIV, Siberia and Edmonton, Alberta [Ph.D. dissertation]. Alberta: University of Alberta; 2005.

Western D, Behrensmeyer AK. Bone assemblages track animal community structure over 40 years in an African savanna ecosystem. Science 2009;324:1061−4.

Westling L. Underwater decomposition: an examination of factors surrounding freshwater decomposition in Eastern Massachusetts [M.Sc. thesis]. Boston University; 2012.

White TE. A method of calculating the dietary percentage of various food animals utilized by aboriginal people. American Antiquity 1953;18:396−8.

White TD. Prehistoric cannibalism at Mancos 5MTUMR-2346. Princeton: Princeton University Press; 1992.

White TD, Black MT, Folkens PA. Human osteology. 3rd ed. San Diego: Elsevier; 2011.

Wild L, Nichol R. Estimation of the original number of individuals using estimators of the Krantz type. Journal of Field Archeology 1983;10:337−44.

Willey P, Galloway A, Snyder L. Bone mineral density and survival of elements and element portions in the bones of the Crow Creek massacre victims. American Journal of Physical Anthropology 1997;104:513−28.

Winder NP. How many bones make five? The art and science of guesstimation in archaeozoology. International Journal of Osteoarchaeology 1991;1:111−26.

APPENDICES

Appendix 2.I: Assessment of the Degree of Preservation of the Skeleton

- Use the recording sheets provided in Appendices 1.I and 1.II.
- Express the identified elements as a percentage of the number of elements expected to be found if every skeleton under study had been intact.
- Express the overall degree of completeness of the skeleton using the following categories:
  1. Particularly poor preservation: <20%
  2. Poor preservation: 20−40%
  3. Moderate preservation: 40−50%
  4. Fair preservation: 50−70%
  5. Good preservation: 70−90%
  6. Excellent preservation: >90%

Note 1: The percentages of completeness that correspond to each category may be modified depending on the overall preservation of the skeletal elements.

Note 2: This process can be performed separately for males and females, as well as for each age group, to explore sex- or age-related biases in preservation.

Note 3: Bello et al. (2006) proposed the use of three indexes: the *anatomical preservation index* (API), the *bone representation index* (BRI), and the *qualitative bone index* (QBI), to express different aspects of bone preservation.

The API expresses the percentage of preserved bones of the total number of bones per skeleton. Based on this index, the percentage of bone preservation falls into one of the following classes:

Class 1: 0%
Class 2: 1−24%
Class 3: 25−49%
Class 4: 50−74%
Class 5: 75−99%
Class 6: 100%

The BRI was originally proposed by Dodson and Wexlar (1979) and is the ratio between the number of retrieved bones and the total number of skeletal elements that should have been present if no bones had been lost postmortem.

The QBI is the ratio between the well-preserved cortical bone surface and the damaged cortical surface of each skeletal element (Bello et al., 2003). According to this ratio, the percentage of undamaged cortical bone surface falls into the same classes as for the API.

Note 4. For the standardized recording of fragmentation patterns on skeletal elements, an adaptation of the zonation method, originally proposed by Dobney and Rielly (1988) for animal remains, may be adopted. Such an adaptation has been proposed by Knüsel and Outram (2004) and separates bones into areas (zones) based on common fracturing patterns occurring because of the architecture of each element. The bones of representative elements are given schematically in Figs. 2.I.1−2.I.4 and the reader may consult the original publication for a description of these zones.

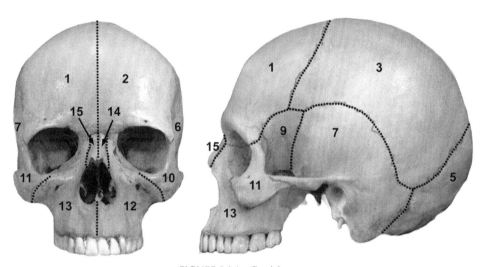

FIGURE 2.I.1   Cranial zones.

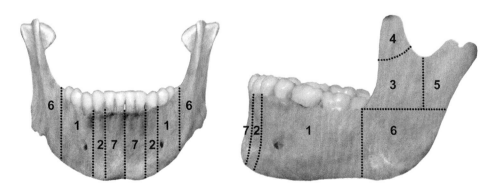

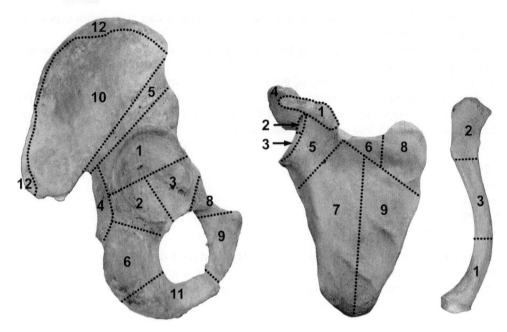

FIGURE 2.1.3   Os coxal scapular, and clavicular zones.

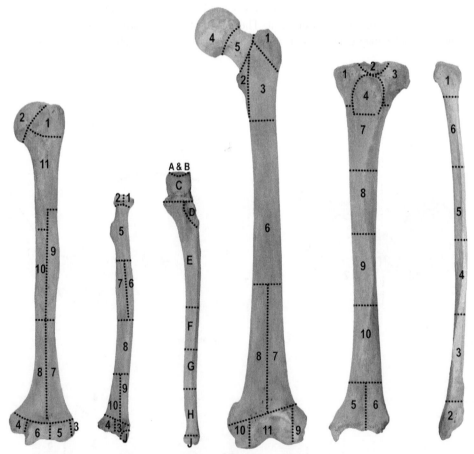

FIGURE 2.1.4   Long-bone zones.

Appendix 2.II: Recording Taphonomic Alterations

Weathering level (based on Behrensmeyer, 1978): 0 1 2 3 4 5

- Tooth marks

Skeletal Element Affected	Animal	Type of Mark

- Thermal modifications

Skeletal Element Affected	Discoloration	Shrinkage (%)	Fracture	Deformation/Warping

Note 1: For discoloration, record the color of the remains as white, gray, etc., but also provide a Munsell color chart value. If more than one color appears on a single bone, list all appropriate colors.
Note 2: Record thermal fractures as longitudinal, step, transverse, patina, splintering/delamination, burn line, curved transverse, or unidentified.

- Tool marks

Skeletal Element Affected	Type of Mark	Location	Orientation

• Miscellaneous modifications

Skeletal Element Affected	Type of Modification	Possible Causative Agent

Appendix 2.III: Recording Taphonomic Alterations Using Osteoware

Taphonomic data can be recorded in Osteoware using the Taphonomy module. The properties that are recorded include the bone color, adherent materials and staining, possible cultural and curation modifications, surface damage, and overall condition of the bone (Fig. 2.III.1). The last is coded using a six-rank scale, the stages of which are described by clicking on the "Help" button.

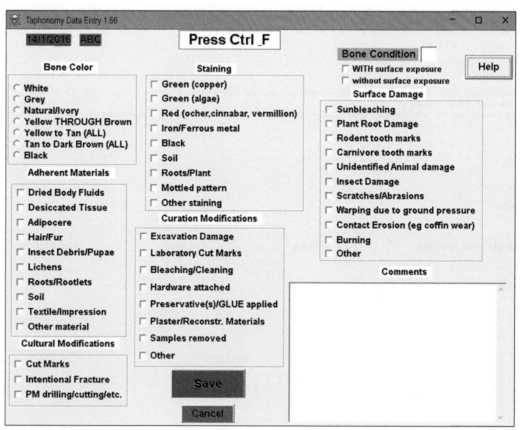

FIGURE 2.III.1 The Taphonomy module.

Chapter 3

Sex and Ancestry Assessment

Chapter Outline

Chapter Objectives

By the end of this chapter, the reader will be able to:

- understand the mechanisms that produce sexual dimorphism in various skeletal structures;
- assess sex based on cranial and postcranial elements, using morphological and metric methods;
- recognize the limitations and prospects of assessing sex from juvenile skeletal remains;
- understand the concept of ancestry and its importance in forensic contexts;
- assess the ancestry of an individual based on skeletal markers; and
- understand the conceptual and methodological limitations of the approaches used in ancestry studies.

This chapter presents the main morphological and metric methods for the assessment of the sex and ancestry of individuals based on skeletal remains. Sex assessment is one of the first steps in any osteological study, whether on archaeological or forensic material. In archaeological contexts such information can provide insights into the demographic profile of past communities and allows the exploration of associations between sex and cultural traits (e.g., grave goods), as well as between sex and other skeletal traits (e.g., specific pathologies or activity markers). In forensic contexts sex is among the primary variables used in the identification of the unknown individual.

Ancestry assessment is primarily relevant in forensic studies, in which the ancestral background of the individual under study can also contribute to his or her identification. In osteoarchaeological studies, a more appropriate means of exploring biological affinity is biodistance analysis, which is discussed in detail in Chapter 5. An important difference between ancestry assessment and biodistance estimation is that the former focuses primarily on the individual, whereas the latter explores broader patterns at the level of the population.

3.1 SEX ASSESSMENT

Sexual dimorphism expresses the morphological and physiological differences between males and females. The degree of sexual dimorphism in humans is small, with adult males generally being larger and more robust than females, but with substantial overlap between male and female dimensions. Despite this limitation, various morphological and metric methods have been developed for assessing sex from skeletal remains, as will be described in the following sections. Suggested recording protocols for various sex markers are provided in Appendix 3.I

Sex, not gender!

Sex refers to all biological traits that differentiate males from females. In contrast, the term *gender* expresses the social dimensions of being male or female in a specific community.

3.1.1 Morphological Methods

3.1.1.1 Pelvis

Sexual dimorphism in the human pelvis has traditionally been attributed to the fact that the female pelvis is adapted for both effective locomotion and parturition, whereas the male pelvis is adapted only for efficient bipedalism. This mechanism underlying pelvic sexual dimorphism has been questioned. For example, Warrener et al. (2015) showed that sexual dimorphism in pelvic shape does not affect energy expenditure during locomotion. However, a study by Huseynov et al. (2016) has found that the female pelvic developmental trajectory changes from puberty until menopause, whereas prepubertal and postmenopausal women exhibit pelvises largely similar to those of males. This finding suggests that pelvic shape indeed changes during the fertile years in a woman's life to accommodate both parturition and locomotion.

Irrespective of the underlying factors that generate sexual dimorphism in the pelvic girdle, the female pelvis is broader than the male one, with a round pelvic inlet. In contrast, the male pelvis is narrower and has a heart-shaped inlet (Chamberlain, 2006). The increased female pelvic inlet is achieved by the mediolateral elongation of the pubic bone, which creates a wide U-shaped subpubic angle, in contrast to the narrow V-shaped angle found in male pelvises (Klepinger, 2006). Table 3.1.1 presents a summary of sexually dimorphic pelvic traits, the most important of which are described in more detail in the following paragraphs.

TABLE 3.1.1 Sexually Dimorphic Pelvic Traits

Trait	Female	Male
Pelvic inlet	Oval	Heart shaped
Ilium	Low and wide	High and vertical
Iliac auricular surface	Elevated from surrounding bone	Not elevated
Greater sciatic notch	Wide and shallow	Narrow and deep
Preauricular sulcus	Present	Absent or very small and shallow
Subpubic concavity	Present	Absent
Subpubic arch	Broad U shaped	V shaped
Ventral arc	Present	Absent
Medial ischiopubic ramus	Narrow and sharp, often a ridge is present	Wide and dull
Obturator foramen	Triangular	Ovoid
Acetabulum	Small, laterally directed	Large, forwardly directed
Sacral shape	Short, wide, and less curved	Long, narrow, and curved

Phenice (1969) developed the most widely used method for sexing human remains based on the pelvis. Specifically, he observed three sexually dimorphic traits: the ventral arc, subpubic concavity, and medial aspect of the ischiopubic ramus (Fig. 3.1.1). The *ventral arc* is a bony ridge on the ventral (anterior) surface of the pubic bone that extends from the pubic crest posteroinferiorly toward the most lateral extension of the subpubic concavity and then it merges with the medial border of the ischiopubic ramus (Fig. 3.1.2). This trait is present only in females. Note that a bony ridge may occasionally be seen on the

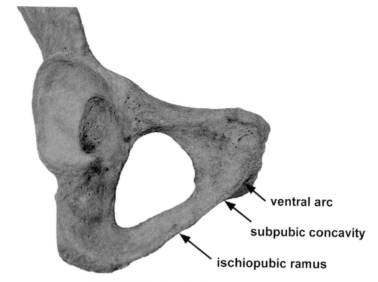

FIGURE 3.1.1 Sexually dimorphic pelvic traits.

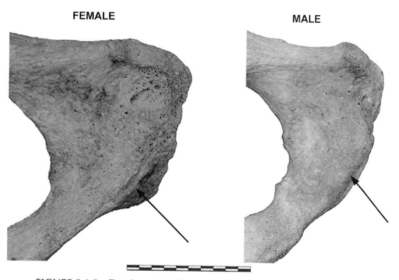

FIGURE 3.1.2 Female–male difference in the expression of the ventral arc.

ventral side of a male pubis, but in this case the ridge does not arc posteroinferiorly, as happens with a true ventral arc; rather it extends parallel to the face of the pubic symphysis (Anderson, 1990). The *subpubic concavity* manifests as a concavity on the ischiopubic ramus, below the pubic symphysis (Fig. 3.1.3). This concavity is absent or very shallow in males. To record this

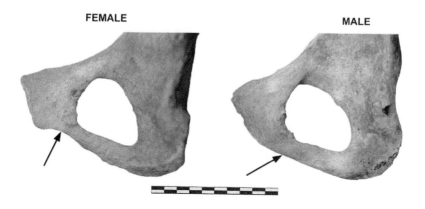

trait, the pubic bone must be viewed dorsally. Finally, the *medial aspect of the ischiopubic ramus*, below the pubic symphysis, is broad and flat in males but narrow and bearing a crestlike ridge in females (Fig. 3.1.4).

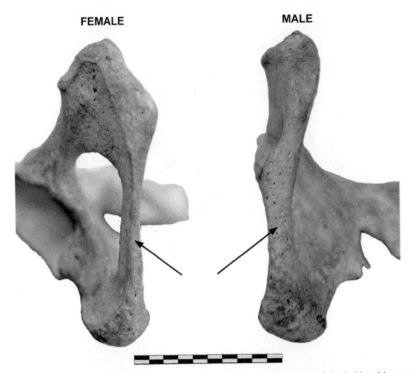

FEMALE   MALE

FIGURE 3.1.4 Female—male difference in the shape of the medial aspect of the ischiopubic ramus.

Phenice suggested that when one or two of these traits give ambiguous results, the remaining ones should be used. It is generally held that the ventral arc offers the most reliable results and the ischiopubic ramus ridge the least reliable ones, as noted by Phenice (1969); however, this may differ between samples. Tests of this method have generally found that it performs well (Lovell, 1989; Sutherland and Suchey, 1991; Ubelaker and Volk, 2002).

A 2012 study (Klales et al., 2012) refined the Phenice method by developing five grades of expression for each of the three traits proposed by Phenice (Fig. 3.1.5). The ordinal scores were subsequently statistically analyzed using logistic regression (see Chapter 9) and the following equation was proposed to assess if an individual was male or female:

$$y = 16.312 - 2.726 \times V - 1.214 \times M - 1.073 \times S \quad (98/74) \qquad (3.1.1)$$

Here, V is the ventral arc, M is the medial aspect of the ischiopubic ramus, and S is the subpubic concavity, while the numbers in parentheses indicate the percentage accuracy for female and male classification. Based on y, the probabilities of an individual being female (p_f) or male (p_m) can be calculated using the following equations:

$$p_f = 1/(1 + e^{-y}) \text{ and } p_m = 1 - p_f \qquad (3.1.2)$$

These equations, as well as additional unpublished functions used for sex assessment, are provided in the Excel spreadsheet Klales_Phenice_Characteristics_Innominate1.3, which can be downloaded from http://math.mercyhurst.edu/~sousley/Software/. The unpublished functions extracted from this spreadsheet are the following:

$$y = 17.470 - 1.952 \times M - 3.711 \times V \quad (92/97) \qquad (3.1.3)$$

$$y = 19.093 - 1.361 \times S - 1.807 \times M - 3.308 \times V \quad (89/98) \qquad (3.1.4)$$

$$y = 16.444 - 2.560 \times S - 3.145 \times V \quad (88/98) \qquad (3.1.5)$$

$$y = 10.460 - 1.028 \times M - 2.862 \times S \quad (87/96) \qquad (3.1.6)$$

Note that the accuracy of the originally published Eq. (3.1.1) is rather low for males (74%), whereas Eqs. (3.1.3)−(3.1.6) appear to provide a more balanced sex assessment. These functions, as well as Eq. (3.1.1), are also used to assess sex in the

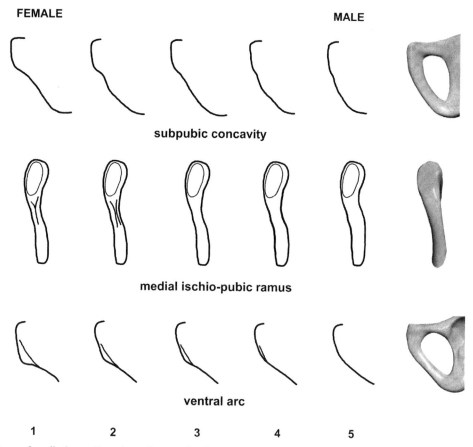

FIGURE 3.1.5 Five-grade ordinal recording scheme for sexually dimorphic pelvic traits. *Adapted from Klales AR, Ousley SD, Vollner JM. A revised method of sexing the human innominate using Phenice's nonmetric traits and statistical methods. American Journal of Physical Anthropology 2012;149:104–14, reproduced with permission.*

macro SexAssessment provided in Software/ExcelMacros/SexAssessment in the companion website of this book. An application of this macro is described in Appendix 3.II.

The shape and breadth of the greater sciatic notch are also sexually dimorphic, with females exhibiting broader and shallower greater sciatic notches (Figs. 3.1.6 and 3.1.7). Note that when examining the shape of the greater sciatic notch, it

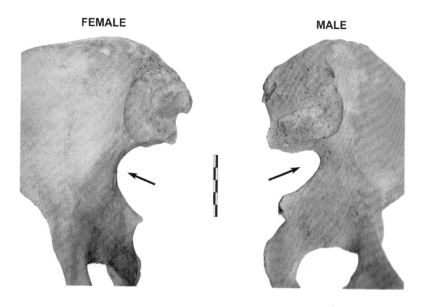

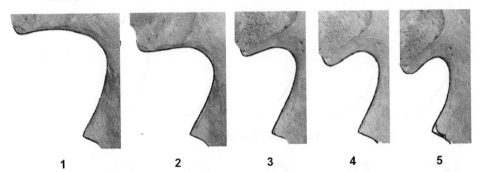

1   **2**   **3**   **4**   **5**

FIGURE 3.1.7   Ordinal scale for recording the shape of the greater sciatic notch. *Adapted from Walker in Buikstra JE, Ubelaker DH, editors. Standards for data collection from human skeletal remains. Fayetteville, Arkansas: Arkansas Archaeological Survey Report Number 44; 1994.*

is advisable not to take into account any exostoses near the preauricular sulcus and the inferior posterior iliac spine (Buikstra and Ubelaker, 1994). This trait is a potentially good sex indicator; however, age at death should be taken into account because young individuals tend to have wider sciatic notches, whereas significant interpopulation variation also exists (Patriquin et al., 2003; Steyn et al., 2004; Walker, 2005).

The presence of a preauricular sulcus, a groove between the auricular surface and the greater sciatic notch, is another potentially useful sex marker, because such a sulcus is present in female skeletons but absent altogether or particularly small and shallow in male ones (Buikstra and Ubelaker, 1994) (Fig. 3.1.8).

FEMALE   **MALE**

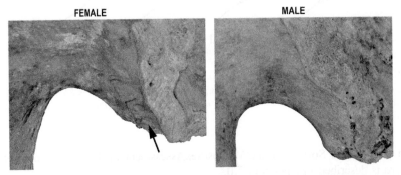

FIGURE 3.1.8   Presence of preauricular sulcus in female os coxa and absence from male os coxa.

Bruzek (2002) proposed a method that combines multiple pelvic sex markers, namely the preauricular sulcus, greater sciatic notch, composite arch, inferior pelvis, and ischiopubic proportion. Each marker is defined by one or three conditions, and each condition provides a male or female classification depending on its skeletal manifestation, as shown in Table 3.1.2. Specifically, at first each marker is examined separately and each condition is classified as f_i (feminine), m_i (masculine), or intermediate. Subsequently, the sex of the individual is assessed for each marker based on whether the majority of the conditions are f_i or m_i. Therefore, for each marker, we end up with an overall female, intermediate, or male classification. The sex of the individual will be female if the majority of markers support a female classification and vice versa, unless the majority of markers provide an intermediate classification. Figs. 3.1.9–3.1.11 visualize the expression of some of these markers on female and male os coxae. Bruzek reported a correct sex classification in 95% of his samples. The method may be implemented using the spreadsheet Bruzek in the Excel file SexAssessment, provided in the companion website in the folder ExcelMacros.

3.1.1.2 Cranium and Mandible

Most differences between the male and the female cranium and mandible can be attributed to the fact that males are generally more muscular than females. Because robusticity is strongly related to occupational factors, cranial sexual dimorphism may differ among populations (Buikstra and Ubelaker, 1994).

Male crania are overall larger and more robust compared to female ones, which tend to be smaller and more gracile. The increased robusticity of male crania manifests primarily in specific structures, with males having larger mastoid

TABLE 3.1.2 Bruzek Method for Sex Assessment Based on Five Pelvic Markers

Marker	Conditions and Sexual Dimorphism[a]
Preauricular surface	f_1: Pronounced depression
	m_1: No or slight depression
	f_2: Well-defined grooves or pits
	m_2: Diffuse grooves or pits
	f_3: No tubercle
	m_3: Tubercle or protuberance
Greater sciatic notch (Fig. 3.1.10)	f_1: Posterior sciatic notch chord longer than or equal to anterior chord
	m_1: Posterior sciatic notch chord shorter than anterior chord
	f_2: Symmetric notch contour relative to depth
	m_2: Asymmetric notch contour relative to depth
	f_3: Contour of posterior chord does not cross line A–P
	m_3: Contour of posterior chord crosses line A–P
Composite arch (Fig. 3.1.9)	f_1: Sciatic notch outline and auricular surface outline form a double curve
	m_1: Sciatic notch outline and auricular surface outline form a single curve
Inferior pelvis	f_1: External eversion of margo inferior ossis coxae
	m_1: No eversion of margo inferior ossis coxae
	f_2: Phallic ridge absent or small
	m_2: Phallic ridge present
	f_3: Gracile ischiopubic ramus
	m_3: Robust ischiopubic ramus
Ischiopubic proportion (Fig. 3.1.11)	f_1: Pubis longer than ischium
	m_1: Ischium longer than pubis

A–P, see Fig. 3.1.10 for definition.
[a]*If the skeletal manifestation of a marker does not fall in the f_i or m_i category, it is classified as intermediate.*
Adapted from Bruzek J. A method for visual determination of sex, using the human hip bone. American Journal of Physical Anthropology 2002;117:157–168.

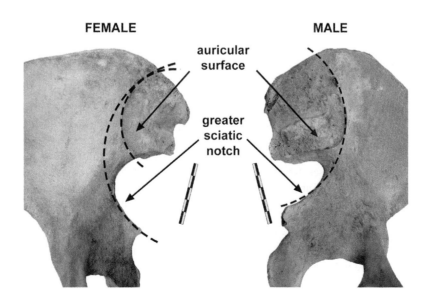

FEMALE   MALE

auricular
surface

greater
sciatic
notch

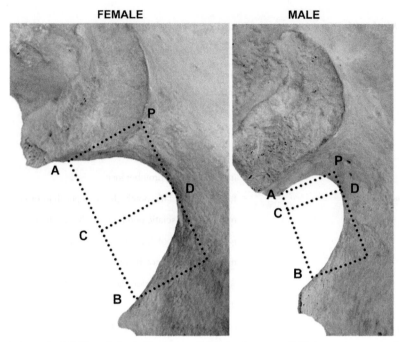

FIGURE 3.1.10 Greater sciatic notch, definition of chords. Female: posterior chord segment (AC) longer than or equal to the anterior chord (CB), symmetry of notch contour, contour of posterior chord does not cross line A−P. Male: AC shorter than CB, asymmetry of notch contour, contour of posterior chord crosses line A−P.

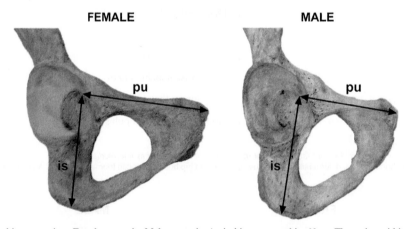

FIGURE 3.1.11 Ischiopubic proportion. Female: pu > is. Male: pu < is. *is*, ischium; *pu*, pubis. *Note*: The point within the acetabulum marks the intersection of the ilium, pubis, and ischium (Schultz 1930; Washburn 1948)

processes, supraorbital ridges, and glabella, as well as a larger and more protruding nuchal crest. In addition, the supraorbital margins tend to be rounded in males, whereas they are sharp in females, and the frontal bone is more vertical in females than in males. Finally, male mandibles have squarer chins and show gonial eversion, as a consequence of having larger masseter muscles, whereas female mandibles are more gracile with round chins (Hu et al., 2006; Novotný et al., 1993; Williams and Rogers, 2006; but see Kemkes-Grottenthaler et al., 2002 for a critique of gonial eversion as a sex marker). These traits are summarized in Table 3.1.3 and the most important ones are visualized in Figs. 3.1.12−3.1.14.

In addition to examining the earlier traits independently and drawing qualitative conclusions regarding the sex of the individual, certain authors proposed ways to quantitatively combine multiple cranial traits in sex assessment. A notable study in this direction was performed by Walker (2008), who used morphological criteria for a logistic regression analysis based on visually assessed traits recorded on a five-degree ordinal scale. The traits included and their recording scheme are given in Fig. 3.1.15. When all five traits were used in sex assessment, Walker obtained a correct classification rate of up to

TABLE 3.1.3 Sexually Dimorphic Cranial Traits

Trait	Female	Male
Overall size	Smaller	Larger
Robusticity	Less robust	More robust
Supraorbital margin	Sharp	Blunt
Supraorbital ridges/glabella	Less pronounced	More pronounced
Frontals and parietals	More bossed	Less bossed
Mastoid process	Small	Large
External occipital protuberance	Small	Well developed
Nuchal lines	Less pronounced	More pronounced
Chin shape	Round	Square
Mental eminence	Less pronounced	More pronounced
Mandibular ramus	No or very slight flexure	Flexure
Gonial eversion	Minimal	Pronounced

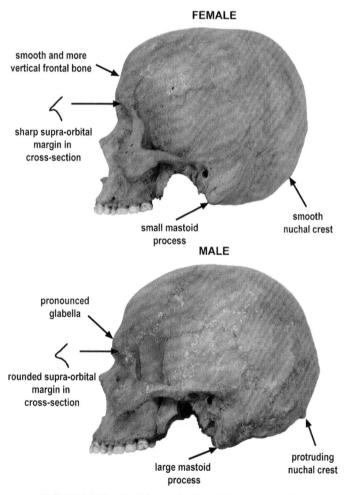

FEMALE

smooth and more vertical frontal bone

sharp supra-orbital margin in cross-section

small mastoid process

smooth nuchal crest

MALE

pronounced glabella

rounded supra-orbital margin in cross-section

large mastoid process

protruding nuchal crest

FIGURE 3.1.12   Cranial sexually dimorphic traits—overview.

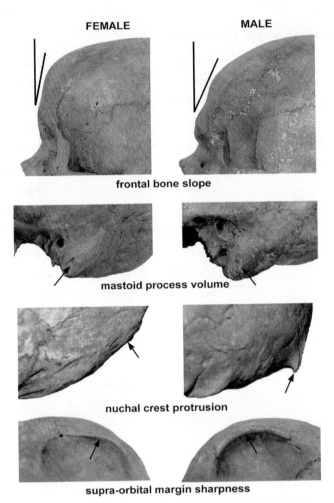

FIGURE 3.1.13   Cranial sexually dimorphic traits.

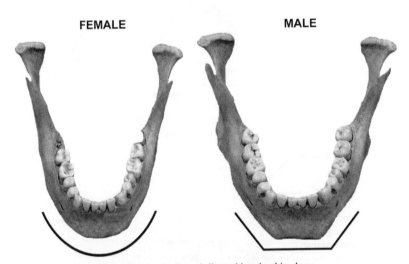

FIGURE 3.1.14   Sexual dimorphism in chin shape.

88%. As the author adopted logistic regression in his analysis, he produced a series of equations that may be used for sexing skeletal remains employing different sets of cranial variables. These discriminant functions are provided in Table 3.1.4, whereas the probability of being female (p_f) or male (p_m) can be calculated using Eq. (3.1.2).

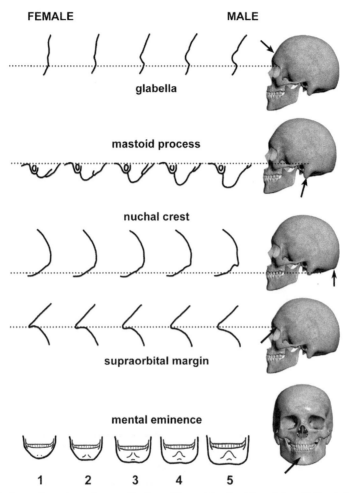

FIGURE 3.1.15 Five-grade ordinal recording scheme for sexually dimorphic cranial traits. *Adapted from Walker in Buikstra JE, Ubelaker DH, editors. Standards for data collection from human skeletal remains. Fayetteville, Arkansas: Arkansas Archaeological Survey Report Number 44; 1994, reproduced with permission.*

TABLE 3.1.4 Logistic Regression Equations for Predicting Sex From Cranial Trait Scores for American/English and Native American Samples

Discriminant Functions	% Classified Correctly (Males/Females)
American/English	
$y = 9.128 - 1.375 \times GL - 1.185 \times MA - 1.151 \times ME$	88.4/86.4
$y = 7.434 - 1.568 \times GL - 1.459 \times MA$	85.4/82.9
$y = 7.372 - 1.525 \times GL - 1.485 \times ME$	86.6/82.1
$y = 7.382 - 1.415 \times MA - 1.629 \times ME$	79.9/83.6
$y = 6.018 - 1.007 \times ORB - 1.850 \times ME$	78.1/77.9
$y = 5.329 - 0.700 \times NU - 1.559 \times MA$	76.8/82.9
Native American	
$y = 3.414 - 0.499 \times ORB - 0.606 \times ME$	78.1/77.9
$y = 4.765 - 1.136 \times MA - 0.576 \times ME$	74.1/72.7
$y = 5.025 - 0.797 \times GL - 1.085 \times MA$	69.5/82.9

GL, glabella; *MA*, mastoid process; *ME*, mental eminence; *NU*, nuchal crest; *ORB*, supraorbital margin.
From Walker PL. Sexing skulls using discriminant function analysis of visually assessed traits. American Journal of Physical

The Walker method for sex assessment is implemented in the Excel spreadsheet Walker_Cranial_SexingWithImages10, downloadable from http://math.mercyhurst.edu/~sousley/Software/. In addition, this method is implemented in the macro SexAssessment, an application of which is presented in Appendix 3.II.

A mandibular trait that may function as a useful sex marker is mandibular ramus flexure. Loth and Henneberg (1996) noted that the posterior border of the mandibular ramus in adult male mandibles has an angulation at the level of the molar occlusal surface. In females there is no mandibular ramus flexure, or it is very slight and occurs close to the condylar neck (Fig. 3.1.16). The authors reported a sexing accuracy rate of over 90% using this trait. However, blind tests yielded results with much lower accuracy (e.g., Kemkes-Grottenthaler et al., 2002). More recently, Balci et al. (2005) reexamined the validity of mandibular ramus flexure and found that if mandibles missing more than two molars are excluded from the analysis, the correct classification rate was 90.6% (95.6% in males, 70.6% in females). Furthermore, they noted that if they focused only on mandibles that exhibited either bilateral flexure or bilateral nonflexure, correct classification was 100% for both sexes. However, it should be stressed that the female sample that conformed to the authors' criteria was particularly small, so further validation of these results is required.

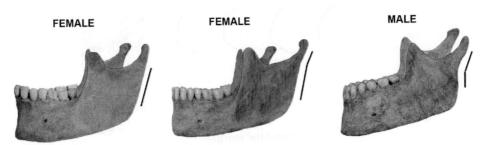

FIGURE 3.1.16 Sexual dimorphism in mandibular ramus flexure.

The use of cranial traits as sex markers may be complicated by the fact that, owing to the progressive deposition of new bone tissue with increasing age, the skull tends to appear increasingly masculine in older individuals, even among females. Thus, an old female skull may be mistaken for a young male one (Meindl et al., 1985). To that end, Nikita (2014) digitized crania of individuals of known sex and age at death and examined whether differences in shape and size with increasing age are statistically significant in the two sexes. The results of her study showed that the shape of the cranium indeed changes over time but this alteration is not statistically significant in either sex. In contrast, the size of the cranium changes slightly in females, but significantly so in males, with increasing age. Another potential limitation pertains to the secular changes that occur in the cranial skeleton, primarily as a result of changes in the life quality of individuals over time (Jantz and Jantz, 2000).

3.1.1.3 Long Bones

Clavicular and humeral morphological traits have been employed for sex assessment, though not frequently. Sexual dimorphism on the clavicle manifests primarily in the rhomboid fossa, a depression on the inferior medial clavicle. According to Rogers et al. (2000), when this trait is present, it almost certainly denotes a male individual; however, the lack of a fossa is not necessarily suggestive of a female, because males also may not exhibit a fossa. Therefore, this technique is useful only if fossae can be detected. Prado et al. (2009) verified the general lack of fossae among female skeletons and their rather frequent presence in males.

Regarding the humerus, Rogers (1999) reported that females generally have a more oval-shaped olecranon fossa, an angled medial epicondyle, and a symmetrical and rather constricted trochlea compared to males. Falys et al. (2005) evaluated this technique and found that a combination of all these traits provided a correct classification in 79.1% of the cases examined, whereas the olecranon fossa shape alone correctly classified 84.6% of the individuals in their sample. More recently, Vance et al. (2011) managed to correctly identify the sex of 75.5% of individuals using morphological traits of the distal humerus.

3.1.2 Metric Methods

Metric methods involve taking measurements so that size and shape differences between the sexes can be quantitatively assessed by means of univariate or multivariate statistical tests (most notably discriminant function analysis—see Chapter 9).

Traditionally, metric analyses use linear measurements and are based on the property that males are generally larger than females; thus, they focus on capturing size differences between sexes.

More recently, research has shifted toward geometric morphometrics, that is, shape-based analysis. Geometric morphometrics are discussed in detail in Chapter 5. At this point it is worth mentioning that geometric morphometric techniques analyze landmark coordinates. In this way they offer the option to control for the effect of size on the data by translating, rotating, and, most importantly in this respect, scaling the subjects under study, thus facilitating the discrimination of males and females based on skeletal shape (González et al., 2009, 2011).

As levels of sexual dimorphism differ among populations, it is important to adopt discriminant functions produced from the same population as the one under study or from populations with close biological affinity. Literature concerning worldwide studies on metric sex assessment is provided in the companion website in the file Studies_on_sex_stature_BM. In contrast to the trend of producing population-specific equations, Albanese (2013) proposed equations from a population-diverse study, employing long-bone and cranial measurements. These equations are used to assess sex in the Excel file SexAssessment provided as online material in the folder ExcelMacros.

The main advantage of metric methods is that they are more objective than morphological ones and usually result in lower intra- and interobserver errors. In addition, the continuous data produced can be subjected to a wider range of statistical analyses, facilitating within- and between-population comparisons. On the other hand, metric analyses typically require well-preserved skeletal elements, and the appropriate population-specific equations should generally be adopted.

3.1.3 Sex Assessment in Juveniles

The assessment of sex in juveniles is of particular importance in osteoarchaeological and forensic studies. Nevertheless, sex assessment based on the immature skeleton is difficult, or even impossible, because levels of testosterone, the hormone largely responsible for the development of male physical characteristics, are very low in males before puberty. Testosterone levels start to rise in the male fetus at about 8 weeks in utero and remain high until birth. Just before birth testosterone levels drop and stay low until puberty. Thus, although slight sexual dimorphism can be observed in perinatal skeletal remains, skeletal differences between males and females are minimal prior to adolescence (Berg, 2012; Wilson et al., 1981).

Despite the difficulty in assigning sex to nonadult remains, there have been a number of papers that explored sexual dimorphism in specific skeletal structures at different ages. These studies have focused primarily on the os coxae and the mandible, and their findings are briefly presented below.

3.1.3.1 Sexual Dimorphism in the Juvenile Pelvis

Among the early studies exploring sex differences in pelvic morphology, Reynolds (1945, 1947) identified sexual dimorphism with regard to various pelvic dimensions, whereas Boucher (1955, 1957) found sex differences in the subpubic angle and greater sciatic notch. Fazekas and Kósa (1978) noted that the relation between the depth of the curvature of the sciatic notch to the length of the ilium and length of the femur is rather constant in males, in contrast to females. The authors also observed a higher correlation between the length and depth of the sciatic notch in male fetuses compared to female ones. Schutkowski (1987) produced discriminant functions using iliac and femoral measurements based on data from Fazekas and Kósa (1978). Weaver (1980) found that the iliac auricular surface may be useful in assessing the sex of fetuses and infants because an elevated surface is more commonly observed in females than in males. Mittler and Sheridan (1992) obtained good results when testing this method for males but not for females, whereas Hunt (1990) did not find it successful.

Schutkowski (1993) identified the following dimorphic features in juvenile pelvic morphology (Fig. 3.1.17): (1) the greater sciatic notch angle is approximately 90 degrees in males and greater than 90 degrees in females; (2) the greater sciatic notch is rather shallow in females and deep in males; (3) the superoposterior extension of the vertical side of the sciatic notch crosses the auricular surface in females, but is adjacent to the lateral rim of the auricular surface in males; and (4) the iliac crest forms a more pronounced S shape in males. Sutter (2003) found the first three criteria to provide an accuracy of approximately 80%, but Vlak et al. (2008) found limited sexual dimorphism when using the first two criteria.

Holcomb and Konigsberg (1995) also examined the fetal greater sciatic notch and identified significant dimorphism in its shape, especially with respect to the location of the maximum depth of the notch when viewed anteroposteriorly. However, the authors concluded that the greater sciatic notch cannot be used for reliable sex assessment in juveniles because of the great overlap between male and female values. Rissech et al. (2003) reported significant differences in the

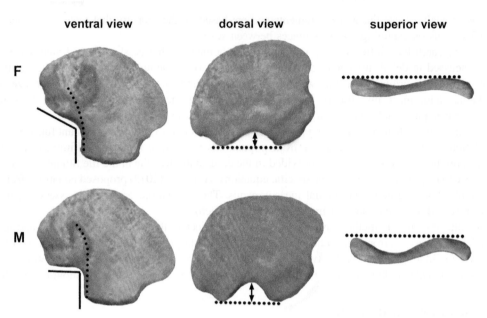

FIGURE 3.1.17 Sexually dimorphic pelvic traits in juveniles. Ventral (anterior) view: greater sciatic notch angle and superoposterior extension of the vertical side of the sciatic notch. Dorsal (posterior) view: greater sciatic notch depth. Superior view: iliac crest curvature. *Adapted from Schutkowski H. Sex determination of infant and juvenile skeletons: I. Morphognostic features. American Journal of Physical Anthropology 1993;90:199–205.*

ratio of the vertical to the horizontal ischial acetabular surface diameter in males and females of ages between 5 and 9 years and possibly even earlier at 0–4 years.

Wilson et al. (2008, 2011) examined variation in the juvenile ilium employing geometric morphometric methods; they found marked sexual dimorphism in this area, but recommended the use of population-specific discriminant functions. More recently, Mokrane et al. (2013) also explored the shape of the fetal ilium using geometric morphometric methods but failed to find any difference between males and females. Finally, Bilfeld et al. (2015) used geometric morphometric analysis to explore sexual dimorphism in the shape of the pubis and found that sexual dimorphism in this anatomical area is evident from the age of 13 years, though certain shape differences can be traced earlier, from the age of 9 years.

3.1.3.2 Sexual Dimorphism in the Juvenile Skull

The mandible is a potentially useful element for sex assessment in juveniles because a number of endocrine, functional, and anatomical factors affect its development. Schutkowski (1993) found that males tend to have more angular chins, wide anterior dental arcades, and gonial eversion, whereas females exhibit smooth nonprominent chins, round anterior dental arcades, and no eversion. However, these traits appeared to be effective only in identifying males. Similarly, Loth and Henneberg (2001) noticed that the transition from the symphyseal region to the lateral mandibular body is sharply angled in males and the chin is pointy or squared. In contrast, the female mandibular body curves gradually and the chin is rounded. However, when Scheuer (2002) tested this method, she achieved an accuracy of merely 64%. Geometric morphometric analysis of the mandible has supported that sex discrimination based on this element is problematic. The multivariate regressions of Franklin et al. (2007) found no significant sexual dimorphism in the sample under study, with a cross-validated classification accuracy of only 59%. A more recent study by Coquerelle et al. (2011) found that sexual dimorphism in the mandible is evident before the age of 4 years and after 14 years, whereas it is almost completely absent between 4 and 14 years of age.

Regarding the cranium, Gonzalez (2012) analyzed a series of craniofacial measurements using discriminant function analysis in a sample of individuals aged 5–16 years and obtained a correct sex classification in 78–89% of the cases. The cranial base has also been explored as a potentially sexually dimorphic area in juveniles. Veroni et al. (2010) analyzed the dimensions of the foramen magnum and the occipital condyles by means of discriminant function analysis and achieved a correct classification of 75.8%.

Dental dimensions have also been used in sexing subadult remains. Black (1978) developed discriminant functions for deciduous teeth, achieving correct classification rates of up to 75%, but he noted that sexual dimorphism is less marked in deciduous teeth compared to permanent ones. Similarly, De Vito and Saunders (1990) produced discriminant functions to assess sex based on deciduous teeth and reported even higher accuracies (76−90%). More recently, Cardoso (2008) proposed a series of approaches for developing sample-specific sex-assessment methods for juveniles employing permanent tooth dimensions. The author supported that the canine is the most sexually dimorphic tooth, producing sexing accuracies ranging from 58.8% to 100%. However, as the author pointed out, the sample sizes employed in this study were small; thus further validation in different assemblages is required. Similarly, Hassett (2011) found that canine dimensions are sufficiently dimorphic to correctly identify the sex in 65−88% (cross-validated classifications) of the juveniles in an English sample. Similar results were obtained in a much larger sample by Viciano et al. (2013), who achieved correct sex classifications in over 78% of the cases using the dimensions of deciduous and permanent teeth.

3.1.3.3 Other Elements and Approaches

Rogers (2009) used the same distal humeral traits she had examined among adults and found an accuracy of 81% in individuals aged 11−20 years. Metric methods have also been proposed, with Choi and Trotter (1970) using factor analysis and discriminant analysis to determine fetal sex using measurements of weight and length from postcranial elements of the axial and appendicular skeleton. More recently, Stull and Godde (2013) produced a series of discriminant functions for sex assessment of individuals between birth and 1 year employing humeral and femoral measurements. Finally, an interesting approach was proposed by Hunt and Gleiser (1955), who suggested sexing juveniles using the correlation between dental and skeletal age, based on the principle that the rate of dental development is similar between sexes but skeletal development is delayed in males compared to females.

3.2 ANCESTRY

Ancestry expresses an individual's geographic region of origin and it may be assessed from skeletal remains by means of morphological and metric methods (The Scientific Working Group for Forensic Anthropology). Ancestry assessments are often treated with skepticism given the typological nature of early studies, which supported that different groups of people belong to different races, often with some of them perceived as "superior" to others. Genetic studies have now proven that genetic variation at the intrapopulation level is greater than at the interpopulation one (e.g., Long et al., 2009; Rosenberg et al., 2002). However, the fact that distinct human races do not exist does not mean that there is not some form of temporal and geographical patterning in human morphology, generated by evolutionary forces such as natural selection and genetic drift, which can be explored by means of ancestry studies (Box 3.2.1). The discussion on the issue of races is an extensive one and beyond the scope of this chapter. The reader may consult the special volume of the *American Journal of Physical Anthropology* ("Race Reconciled: How Biological Anthropologists View Human Variation," vol. 139, issue 1, 2009) for a compilation of papers on the issue of race and its place in modern biological anthropology, as well as Ta'ala (2015) for a brief outline of the history of ancestry studies and the race concept in anthropology.

BOX 3.2.1 Ancestry Groups

By convention, there are four broad ancestry groups into which an individual may be classified: the sub-Saharan African group ("Negroid"), the European group ("Caucasoid"), the Central Asian group ("Mongoloid"), and the Australasian group ("Australoid") (Ferguson et al., 2011). It must be stressed that other scholars identify different ancestry groups, largely dependent upon the specific geographic area they examine and its population history. As such, for North America, Byers (2010) suggests the use of the categories "white," "black," "Asian," "Native American," and "Hispanic." This variability in the recording schemes of ancestry groups reflects the main limitation of ancestry studies, that is, although groups living under different conditions exhibit skeletal variation, this variation cannot be classified into strict racial categories.

3.2.1 Morphological Methods

A number of morphological traits have been employed in ancestry assessment and these are often called *macromorphoscopic* (Ousley and Hefner, 2005) or more simply *morphoscopic* (Hefner, 2009) traits. Such traits have focused primarily on the overall cranial shape or the shape of specific bones, with an emphasis on facial anatomy, as well as the morphology of the sutures and the dentition (e.g., Gill, 1998). They have traditionally been organized in lists ("trait lists") that were thought to correspond to particular ancestral groups. Among the most widely cited studies is the one by Rhine (1990), who described 45 characteristics and examined their expression in whites, blacks, Hispanics, and Amerindians. Rhine identified some ancestry-related variation, but his sample sizes were very small and many traits did not appear in their expected ancestry groups.

Morphoscopic traits versus nonmetric traits

Morphoscopic traits are morphological variants observable in all skeletons, whereas nonmetric traits (discussed in Chapter 5) are morphological characters that may be present or absent.

The trait list approach has been criticized on the grounds that (1) it does not adopt a scientific approach for weighing the character states of different traits, (2) the association between specific traits and ancestry groups has been based on samples of small size, and (3) some of the character states are not found in the expected ancestry groups (e.g., Clark et al., 2016; Maddux et al., 2015; Sholts and Wärmländer, 2012; and discussion in Hefner, 2009; but see also Hughes et al., 2011 for a support of the trait list approach). To render morphoscopic traits more useful in ancestry assessment, Hefner (2009) proposed a systematic scoring system for a series of cranial traits and divided these traits into five categories: (1) assessing bone shape, (2) assessing bony feature morphology, (3) assessing suture shape, (4) presence/absence data, and (5) assessing feature prominence (for examples see Figs. 3.2.1—3.2.6). In addition, Hefner et al. suggested specific statistical tests for the more effective analysis of these traits (Hefner, 2009; Hefner and Ousley, 2006, 2014; Hefner et al., 2012; Ousley and Hefner, 2005). Klales and Kenyhercz (2015) tested the utility of the traits defined by Hefner (2009) in ancestry assessment and found them to perform well when males and females were pooled (73.3—86.6% correct classification), but not so well when each sex was examined separately (46.7—64.3% correct classification).

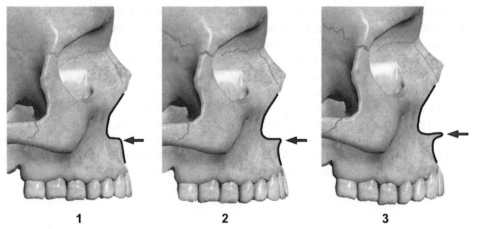

FIGURE 3.2.1 Character states for the anterior nasal spine. *Adapted from Hefner JT. Cranial nonmetric variation and estimating ancestry. Journal of Forensic Sciences 2009;54:985—95.*

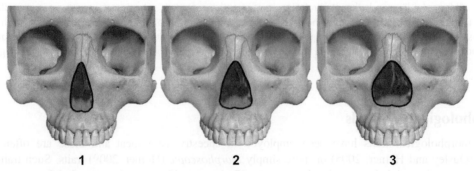

FIGURE 3.2.2 Character states for the nasal aperture width. *Adapted from Hefner JT. Cranial nonmetric variation and estimating ancestry. Journal of Forensic Sciences 2009;54:985—95.*

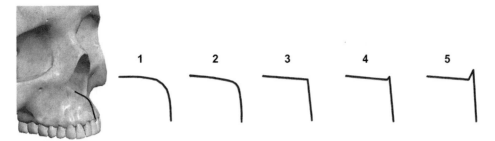

FIGURE 3.2.3   Character states for the inferior nasal aperture. *Adapted from Hefner JT. Cranial nonmetric variation and estimating ancestry. Journal of Forensic Sciences 2009;54:985—95.*

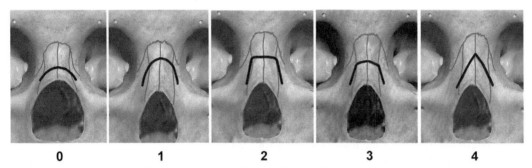

FIGURE 3.2.4   Character states for the nasal bone contour. *Adapted from Hefner JT. Cranial nonmetric variation and estimating ancestry. Journal of Forensic Sciences 2009;54:985—95.*

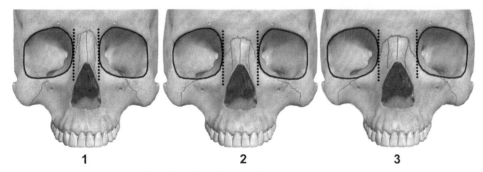

FIGURE 3.2.5   Character states for the interorbital breadth. *Adapted from Hefner JT. Cranial nonmetric variation and estimating ancestry. Journal of Forensic Sciences 2009;54:985—95.*

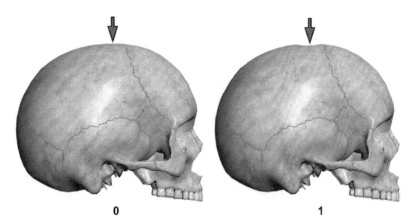

FIGURE 3.2.6   Character states for the postbregmatic depression. *Adapted from Hefner JT. Cranial nonmetric variation and estimating ancestry. Journal of Forensic Sciences 2009;54:985—95.*

Among the most recent methods for ancestry assessment is *optimized summed scored attributes* (OSSA; for a description see Hefner and Ousley, 2014). This method classifies individuals as black or white based on the traits presented in Figs. 3.2.1−3.2.6. According to this method, the anterior nasal spine, nasal aperture width, inferior nasal aperture, nasal bone contour, interorbital breadth, and postbregmatic depression are recorded ordinally as shown in the aforementioned figures (Hefner, 2009). Subsequently, these scores are transformed into "OSSA scores," 0 and 1, following Table 3.2.1. To assess if an individual is black or white, all OSSA scores are summed. If the sum is greater than 3, the individual is white, otherwise he or she is black. Appendix 3.III gives a simple recording protocol based on this method, and Appendix 3.IV presents the recording of several morphoscopic traits suggested by Hefner (2009) in Osteoware. This appendix also presents the recording of sex markers in Osteoware.

TABLE 3.2.1 Transformation of Ordinal Scores to OSSA Scores

Score	ANS		NAW		INA		NBC		IOB		PBD	
Ordinal	1	2−3	1−2	3	1−3	4−5	0−1	2−4	1−2	3	0	1
OSSA	0	1	1	0	0	1	0	1	1	0	1	0

ANS, anterior nasal spine; *INA*, inferior nasal aperture; *IOB*, interorbital breadth; *NAW*, nasal aperture width; *NBC*, nasal bone contour; *OSSA*, optimized summed scored attributes; *PBD*, postbregmatic depression.

The spreadsheet HefnerNonMetricAncestry-OSSA2.1 performs all the aforementioned calculations and can be downloaded from http://math.mercyhurst.edu/∼sousley/Software/. Alternatively, the spreadsheet AncestryAssessment, provided in the companion website in the folder ExcelMacros, can be used.

More recently, Hefner (2015) produced a series of discriminant function equations for the classification of blacks, Hispanics, and whites using combinations of the morphoscopic traits given in Figs. 3.2.1−3.2.6, plus one more, the *nasal overgrowth*, which refers to an inferiorly directed projection of the nasal bones. These equations correctly classified 63.1−85.4% of the individuals under study.

The use of dental morphological characters has recently also started being explored in ancestry studies (for example, Edgar, 2015; Irish, 2015) even though dental nonmetric traits have a long history in biodistance studies (see Chapter 5). Finally, a few papers have explored the potential of postcranial elements in ancestry assessment. Indicative of this direction is the work of Bidmos (2006), who attempted to discriminate South Africans of European descent from indigenous South Africans using the number of calcaneal articular facets.

3.2.2 Metric Methods

As briefly mentioned in the previous section, the cranium has been among the primary anatomical areas examined in ancestry studies. As such, attempts have been made to quantify the cranial size and shape differences identified among various ancestral groups by means of linear measurements and geometric morphometrics (see Chapter 5 for a discussion on genetic versus environmental control over cranial morphology). Giles and Elliot (1962) were pioneers in developing a series of equations using discriminant analysis to classify individuals as white, black, or Amerindian. Since then, a number of scholars have tested the accuracy of the obtained ancestry classifications using the Giles and Elliot equations in different samples (e.g., Ayers et al., 1990; Birkby, 1966), and attempts have been made to develop new functions (e.g., Burris and Harris, 1998; İşcan and Steyn, 1999; Stull et al., 2014; also see Berg, 2015 for discriminant functions based on mandibular measurements, and Pilloud et al., 2014, and Harris and Foster, 2015, for discriminant functions based on tooth dimensions).

Metric methods for ancestry assessment are not restricted to cranial measurements. Liebenberg et al. (2015) examined the effectiveness of measurements obtained from 11 postcranial elements in assessing the ancestry of South African groups and achieved accuracies higher than 85% when measurements of diverse elements were combined. Similarly, Okrutny (2010) used measurements of various postcranial elements to differentiate between Koreans, Africans, and Europeans. The discriminant functions she produced correctly classified at least 80% of the Koreans and 77% of the Africans/Europeans, with higher classifications obtained from the upper limbs. When Africans and Europeans were compared to one another, over 70% of the former and 72% of the latter were correctly classified, but this time measurements of the lower limbs and pelvis were more informative. In addition, Spradley (2015) achieved correct classification in American black, American white, and Hispanic males, ranging from 72% to 85% when combining multiple postcranial measurements in stepwise discriminant function analysis.

The pelvis has been a rather favored area in ancestry assessment, with İşcan (1983) reporting accuracies up to 88% when classifying American blacks and American whites from the Terry Collection, and Patriquin et al. (2002) also reaching up to 88% classification accuracy for males and 85% for females in South African blacks and whites. DiBennardo and Taylor (1983) achieved accuracies as high as 97% when combining pelvic and femoral measurements in the Terry Collection, and high accuracies were also retrieved in the same collection by İşcan and Cotton (1990) when they combined pelvic, femoral, and tibial measurements. In contrast to the promising results obtained by these studies, Igbigbi and Nanono-Igbigbi (2003) achieved merely 63% correct ancestry classification for a sample of indigenous Ugandans using the subpubic angle.

The femur alone has been used in several studies, although its morphology is largely controlled by activity patterns and environmental conditions, potentially limiting its utility as an ancestry marker. Specifically, anterior femoral curvature has been found to be less pronounced in blacks compared to Asian/Amerindians, with Caucasians falling in between (Stewart, 1962). Anteroposterior flattening below the lesser trochanter appears to be more pronounced in American Indians than in American blacks or whites (Gilbert and Gill, 1990), as well as in Thai groups compared to American whites (Tallman and Winburn, 2015), and in Native Americans and Polynesians compared to American blacks and whites (Wescott, 2005). The intercondylar shelf angle has been found to be more acute in American blacks compared to whites (Craig, 1995), whereas the intercondylar notch tends to be higher in American blacks compared to American whites (Baker et al., 1990). In contrast, the femoral neck axis length has been found not to discriminate satisfactorily American black, American white, and Native American groups (Meeusen et al., 2015; but see Christensen et al., 2014). In a study that combined computed tomography scans with statistical bone atlases, Shirley et al. (2015) found that male American black femora are longer, straighter, and distally narrower than those of American whites, whereas they exhibit less anteroposterior neck torsion and are more circular in cross section. The same study also found that American blacks have longer and more robust tibiae and longer lateral tibial condyles.

Hand and foot bones have also been used for ancestry assessment. McFadden and Bracht (2009) found that the metacarpals of American blacks tend to be larger and more similar in length to one another than those of American whites. Furthermore, the study by Bidmos (2006) explored the potential of calcaneal measurements (in addition to the number of articular facets mentioned earlier) in separating South Africans of European descent from indigenous South Africans.

Finally, Kindschuh et al. (2012) used hyoid measurements to assess the ancestry of Europeans versus Africans from the Terry Anatomical Collection, achieving accuracies of 73% and 77%.

Metric ancestry assessment using cranial and postcranial measurements has been greatly facilitated through the software FORDISC, presented in Box 3.2.2 (Ousley and Jantz, 2012). In addition to FORDISC, CRANID (downloadable from www.box.net/shared/h0674knjzl) can also perform linear discriminant and nearest-neighbor analysis using metric cranial data. Its data bank includes more than 3000 skulls with a global distribution (Wright, 2008).

BOX 3.2.2 FORDISC

FORDISC allows the user to input numerous postcranial and cranial metrics of an unknown skeleton into a worksheet. Subsequently, the program performs discriminant function analysis to classify the remains into ancestral groups according to reference samples available in the software database.

The reference samples used in FORDISC have been largely obtained from identified forensic cases, which form part of the Forensic Data Bank (Box 3.2.3), as well as other recent North American individuals. In addition, samples from Japan, China, Vietnam, and Latin America, as well as archaeological specimens from museums worldwide (Howells, 1973, 1989), are included.

FORDISC has the advantage that it simplifies calculations and offers cross-validated results, as well as posterior and typicality probabilities, which are helpful in determining the degree of confidence in the classifications provided. A limitation of FORDISC is that the classification requires that the ancestry of the individual under study falls under one of the available reference samples. The accuracy of the classification results of FORDISC has been questioned (for example, L'Abbé et al., 2013; Ubelaker et al., 2002; Williams et al., 2005), but its developers have attributed the poor results occasionally obtained to the incorrect use of the program or the misinterpretation of the obtained classifications (Freid et al., 2005).

BOX 3.2.3 Forensic Anthropology Data Bank

The Forensic Data Bank (FDB) was established in 1986 to accumulate data from contemporary skeletons (Jantz and Moore-Jansen, 1988). Today, it has information on more than 3400 individuals. Specifically, it includes cranial measurements and nonmetric traits, postcranial measurements, congenital traits, trauma data, and dental information. In certain cases, additional information such as age at death, sex, ancestry, height, weight, and occupation are also available (Ousley and Jantz, 1998). A copy of the FDB may be downloaded from http://www.icpsr.umich.edu/icpsrweb/ICPSR/ by searching for "forensic anthropology."

3.2.3 Ancestry Assessment in Juveniles

Assessing ancestry in juveniles is difficult because most ancestry-related differences develop fully in adulthood. However, a number of scholars have worked in this direction. Steyn and Henneberg (1997) found that children of black South African descent exhibit narrower and longer heads compared to children of European origin from approximately age 5 onward. However, their sample size was small, and the effect of sexual dimorphism was not controlled for. Weinberg et al. (2005) found that white infants exhibit narrow occipital squamae, pronounced vomers and anterior nasal spines, "deep" subnasal margins, and semicircular temporal squamae more often than black infants. In addition, Buck and Strand Vidarsdottir (2004) found differences in the mandibular morphology of subadult African Americans, Native Americans, Caucasians, Inuit, and Pacific Islanders, though sexual dimorphism was not included as a possible variable.

Metric and morphological traits of the deciduous and permanent dentition have also been used for subadult ancestry assessment. Harris et al. (2001) found greater deciduous molar dimensions in American blacks than whites, whereas Lease and Sciulli (2005) combined metric and morphological deciduous dental characters in distinguishing European American from African American children and achieved correct classification rates of over 90%.

A 2015 publication (Wood, 2015) examined the expression of cranial traits often employed in adult ancestry studies in subadults aged 4 months in utero to approximately 20 years. The author found that growth and development affect the expression of these traits and different traits become stable at different time periods. However, she also noted that interpopulation variation in the expression of these traits is evident even before they become stable. Therefore, it seems that ancestry studies in juveniles are promising and research should focus more in this direction.

REFERENCES

Albanese J. A method for estimating sex using the clavicle, humerus, radius, and ulna. Journal of Forensic Sciences 2013;58:1413−9.

Anderson BE. Ventral arc of the os pubis: anatomical and developmental considerations. American Journal of Physical Anthropology 1990;83:449−58.

Ayers HG, Jantz RL, Moore-Jansen PH. Giles and Elliot race discriminant functions revisited: a test using recent forensic cases. In: Gill GW, Rhine S, editors. Skeletal attribution of race: methods for forensic anthropology. Albuquerque: Maxwell Museum of Anthropology; 1990. p. 65−71.

Baker SJ, Gill GW, Kieffer DH. Race and sex determination from the intercondylar notch of the distal femur. In: Gill GW, Rhine S, editors. Skeletal attribution of race: methods for forensic anthropology. Albuquerque: Maxwell Museum of Anthropology; 1990. p. 91−5.

Balci Y, Yavuz MF, Cağdir S. Predictive accuracy of sexing the mandible by ramus flexure. HOMO - Journal of Comparative Human Biology 2005;55:229−37.

Berg GE. Determining the sex of unknown human skeletal remains. In: Tersigni-Tarrant MT, Shirley NR, editors. Forensic anthropology: an introduction. Boca Raton: CRC Press; 2012. p. 139−60.

Berg GE. Biological affinity and sex from the mandible utilizing multiple world populations. In: Berg GE, Ta'ala SC, editors. Biological affinity in forensic identification of human skeletal remains. Beyond black and white. Boca Raton: CRC Press; 2015. p. 43−82.

Bidmos M. Metrical and non-metrical assessment of population affinity from the calcaneus. Forensic Science International 2006;159:6−13.

Bilfeld MF, Dedouit F, Sans N, Rousseau H, Rougé D, Telmon N. Ontogeny of size and shape sexual dimorphism in the pubis: a multislice computed tomography study by geometric morphometry. Journal of Forensic Sciences 2015;60:1121−8.

Birkby WH. An evaluation of race and sex identification from cranial measurements. American Journal of Physical Anthropology 1966;24:21−8.

Black III TK. Sexual dimorphism in the tooth-crown diameters of the deciduous teeth. American Journal of Physical Anthropology 1978;48:77−82.

Boucher B. Sex differences in the foetal sciatic notch. Journal of Forensic Medicine 1955;2:51−4.

Boucher BJ. Sex differences in the foetal pelvis. American Journal of Physical Anthropology 1957;15:581−600.

Bruzek J. A method for visual determination of sex, using the human hip bone. American Journal of Physical Anthropology 2002;117:157−68.

Buck TJ, Strand Vidarsdottir U. A proposed method for the identification of race in sub-adult skeletons: a geometric morphometric analysis of mandibular morphology. Journal of Forensic Sciences 2004;49:1159−64.

Buikstra JE, Ubelaker DH, editors. Standards for data collection from human skeletal remains. Fayetteville, Arkansas: Arkansas Archaeological Survey Report Number 44; 1994.

Burris BG, Harris EF. Identification of race and sex from palate dimensions. Journal of Forensic Sciences 1998;43:959−63.

Byers SN. Introduction to forensic anthropology. fourth ed. New York: Prentice Hall; 2010.

Cardoso HFV. Sample-specific (universal) approaches for determining the sex of immature human skeletal remains using permanent tooth dimensions. Journal of Archaeological Science 2008;35:158−68.

Chamberlain AT. Demography in archaeology. Cambridge: Cambridge University Press; 2006.

Choi SC, Trotter M. A statistical study of the multivariate structure and race-sex differences of American white and Negro fetal skeletons. American Journal of Physical Anthropology 1970;33:307−12.

Christensen AM, Leslie WD, Baim S. Ancestral differences in femoral neck axis length: possible implications for forensic anthropological analyses. Forensic Science International 2014;236. 193.e1−193.e4.

Clark MA, Guatelli-Steinberg D, Hubbe M, Stout S. Quantification of maxillary dental arcade curvature and the estimation of biological ancestry in forensic anthropology. Journal of Forensic Sciences 2016;61:141−6.

Coquerelle M, Bookstein FL, Braga J, Halazonetis DJ, Weber GW, Mitteroecker P. Sexual dimorphism of the human mandible and its association with dental development. American Journal of Physical Anthropology 2011;145:192−202.

Craig EA. Intercondylar shelf angle: a new method to determine race from the distal femur. Journal of Forensic Sciences 1995;40:777−82.

De Vito C, Saunders SR. A discriminant function analysis of deciduous teeth to determine sex. Journal of Forensic Sciences 1990;35:845−58.

DiBennardo R, Taylor JV. Multiple discriminant function analysis of sex and race in the postcranial skeleton. American Journal of Physical Anthropology 1983;61:305−14.

Edgar HJH. Dental morphological estimation of ancestry in forensic contexts. In: Berg GE, Ta'ala SC, editors. Biological affinity in forensic identification of human skeletal remains. Beyond black and white. Boca Raton: CRC Press; 2015. p. 191−207.

Falys CG, Schutkowski H, Weston DA. The distal humerus − a blind test of Rogers' sexing technique using a documented skeletal collection. Journal of Forensic Sciences 2005;50:1−5.

Fazekas G, Kósa F. Forensic fetal osteology. Budapest: Akadémiai Kiadó; 1978.

Ferguson E, Kerr N, Rynn C. Race and ancestry. In: Black S, Ferguson E, editors. Forensic anthropology 2000−2010. Boca Raton: CRC Press; 2011. p. 119−54.

Franklin D, Cardini A, O'Higgins P, Oxnard CE, Dadour I. Sexual dimorphism in the subadult mandible: quantification using geometric morphometrics. Journal of Forensic Science 2007;52:6−10.

Freid DL, Jantz RL, Ousley SD. The truth is out there: how NOT to use FORDISC. In: Poster presented at the 74th annual meeting of the American Association of Physical Anthropologists, Milwaukee, WI, April 6−9; 2005.

Gilbert R, Gill GW. A metric technique for identifying American Indian femora. In: Gill GW, Rhine S, editors. Skeletal attribution of race: methods for forensic anthropology. Albuquerque: Maxwell Museum of Anthropology; 1990. p. 97−9.

Giles E, Elliot O. Race identification from cranial measurements. Journal of Forensic Sciences 1962;7:147−57.

Gill GW. Craniofacial criteria in the skeletal attribution of race. In: Reichs KJ, editor. Forensic osteology: advances in the identification of human remains. second ed. Springfield: Charles C. Thomas; 1998. p. 293−318.

González PN, Bernal V, Perez SI. Geometric morphometric approach to sex estimation of human pelvis. Forensic Science International 2009;189:68−74.

González PN, Bernal V, Perez SI. Analysis of sexual dimorphism of craniofacial traits using geometric morphometric techniques. International Journal of Osteoarchaeology 2011;21:89−91.

Gonzalez RA. Determination of sex from juvenile crania by means of discriminant function analysis. Journal of Forensic Sciences 2012;57:24−34.

Harris EF, Foster CL. Size matters: discrimination between American blacks and whites, males and females, using tooth crown dimensions. In: Berg GE, Ta'ala SC, editors. Biological affinity in forensic identification of human skeletal remains. Beyond black and white. Boca Raton: CRC Press; 2015. p. 209−38.

Harris EF, Hicks JD, Barcroft BD. Tissue contributions to sex and race: differences in tooth crown size of deciduous molars. American Journal of Physical Anthropology 2001;115:223−37.

Hassett B. Technical note: estimating sex using cervical canine odontometrics: a test using a known sex sample. American Journal of Physical Anthropology 2011;146:486−9.

Hefner JT, Ousley SD. Morphoscopic traits and the statistical determination of ancestry II. In: Proceedings of the 58th annual meeting of the American Academy of Forensic Science, Seattle, WA; 2006.

Hefner JT, Ousley SD. Statistical classification methods for estimating ancestry using morphoscopic traits. Journal of Forensic Sciences 2014;59:883−90.

Hefner JT, Ousley SD, Dirkmaat DC. Morphoscopic traits and the assessment of ancestry. In: Dirkmaat DC, editor. A companion to forensic anthropology. Oxford: Wiley-Blackwell Publishing; 2012. p. 287−310.

Hefner JT. Cranial nonmetric variation and estimating ancestry. Journal of Forensic Sciences 2009;54:985−95.

Hefner JT. Macromorphoscopics. In: Wilczak CA, Dudar CJ, editors. Osteoware™ software manual, vol. I. Washington: Smithsonian Institution; 2011. p. 66−78.

Hefner JT. Cranial morphoscopic traits and the assessment of American black, American white, and Hispanic ancestry. In: Berg GE, Ta'ala SC, editors. Biological affinity in forensic identification of human skeletal remains. Beyond black and white. Boca Raton: CRC Press; 2015. p. 27−42.

Holcomb SMC, Konigsberg LW. A statistical study of sexual dimorphism in the human fetal sciatic notch. American Journal of Physical Anthropology 1995;97:113−25.

Howells WW. Cranial variation in man. A study by multivariate analysis of patterns of difference among recent human populations. Cambridge, MA: Harvard University Press; 1973. Papers of the Peabody Museum of Archaeology and Ethnology 67.

Howells WW. Skull shapes and the map. Craniometric analyses in the dispersion of modern Homo. Cambridge, MA: Harvard University Press; 1989. Papers of the Peabody Museum of Archaeology and Ethnology 79.

Hu K-S, Koh K-S, Han S-H, Shin K-J, Kim H-J. Sex determination using nonmetric characteristics of the mandible in Koreans. Journal of Forensic Sciences 2006;51:1376−82.

Hughes CE, Juarez CA, Hughes TL, Galloway A, Fowler G, Chacon S. A simulation for exploring the effects of the "trait list" method's subjectivity on consistency and accuracy of ancestry estimations. Journal of Forensic Sciences 2011;56:1094−106.

Hunt EE, Gleiser I. The estimation of age and sex of preadolescent children from bones and teeth. American Journal of Physical Anthropology 1955;13:479−87.

Hunt DR. Sex determination in the subadult ilia: an indirect test of Weaver's nonmetric sexing method. Journal of Forensic Sciences 1990;35:881−5.

Huseynov A, Zollikofer CPE, Coudyzer W, Gascho D, Kellenberger C, Hinzpeter R, et al. Developmental evidence for obstetric adaptation of the human female pelvis. Proceedings of the National Academy of Sciences of the United States of America 2016;113:5227−32.

Igbigbi PS, Nanono-Igbigbi AM. Determination of sex and race from the subpubic angle in Ugandan subjects. American Journal of Medical Pathology

Irish JD. Dental nonmetric variation around the world: using key traits in populations to estimate ancestry in individuals. In: Berg GE, Ta'ala SC, editors. Biological affinity in forensic identification of human skeletal remains. Beyond black and white. Boca Raton: CRC Press; 2015. p. 165—90.

İşcan MY, Cotton TS. Osteometric assessment of racial affinity from multiple sites in the postcranial skeleton. In: Gill GW, Rhine S, editors. Skeletal attribution of race. Albuquerque: Maxwell Museum of Anthropology; 1990. p. 83—91.

İşcan MY, Steyn M. Craniometric determination of population affinity in South Africans. International Journal of Legal Medicine 1999;112:91—7.

İşcan MY. Assessment of race from the pelvis. American Journal of Physical Anthropology 1983;62:205—8.

Jantz RL, Jantz LM. Secular change in craniofacial morphology. American Journal of Human Biology 2000;12:327—38.

Jantz RL, Moore-Jansen PH. A database for forensic anthropology: structure, content and analysis. Tennessee, Knoxville: University of Tennessee, Department of Anthropology; 1988. Report of Investigations No. 47.

Kemkes-Grottenthaler A, Löbig K, Stock F. Mandibular ramus flexure and gonial eversion as morphologic indicator of sex. HOMO - Journal of Comparative Human Biology 2002;53:97—111.

Kindschuh SC, Dupras TL, Cowgill LW. Exploring ancestral variation of the hyoid. Journal of Forensic Sciences 2012;57:41—6.

Klales AR, Kenyhercz MW. Morphological assessment of ancestry using cranial macromorphoscopics. Journal of Forensic Sciences 2015;60:13—20.

Klales AR, Ousley SD, Vollner JM. A revised method of sexing the human innominate using Phenice's nonmetric traits and statistical methods. American Journal of Physical Anthropology 2012;149:104—14.

Klepinger LL. Fundamentals of forensic anthropology. Hoboken: Wiley-Liss; 2006.

L'Abbé EN, Kenyhercz M, Stull KE, Keough N, Nawrocki S. Application of Fordisc 3.0 to explore differences among crania of North American and South African blacks and whites. Journal of Forensic Sciences 2013;58:1579—83.

Lease LR, Sciulli PW. Brief communication: discrimination between European-American and African-American children based on deciduous dental metrics and morphology. American Journal of Physical Anthropology 2005;126:56—60.

Liebenberg L, L'Abbé EN, Stull KE. Population differences in the postcrania of modern South Africans and the implications for ancestry estimation. Forensic Science International 2015;257:522—9.

Long JC, Li J, Healy ME. Human DNA sequences: more variation and less race. American Journal of Physical Anthropology 2009;139:23—34.

Loth SR, Henneberg M. Mandibular ramus flexure: a new morphologic indicator of sexual dimorphism in the human skeleton. American Journal of Physical Anthropology 1996;99:473—85.

Loth SR, Henneberg M. Sexually dimorphic mandibular morphology in the first few years of life. American Journal of Physical Anthropology 2001;115:179—86.

Lovell NC. Test of Phenice's technique for determining sex from the os pubis. American Journal of Physical Anthropology 1989;79:117—20.

Maddux SD, Sporleder AN, Burns CE. Geographic variation in zygomaxillary suture morphology and its use in ancestry estimation. Journal of Forensic Sciences 2015;60:966—73.

McFadden D, Bracht MS. Sex and race differences in the relative lengths of metacarpals and metatarsals in human skeletons. Early Human Development 2009;85:117—24.

Meeusen RA, Christensen AM, Hefner JT. The use of femoral neck axis length to estimate sex and ancestry. Journal of Forensic Sciences 2015;60:1300—4.

Meindl RS, Lovejoy C, Mensforth RP, Don Carlos L. Accuracy and direction of error in sexing of the skeleton: implications for paleodemography. American Journal of Physical Anthropology 1985;68:79—85.

Mittler DM, Sheridan SG. Sex determination in subadults using auricular surface morphology: a forensic science perspective. Journal of Forensic Sciences 1992;37:1068—75.

Mokrane F-Z, Dedouit F, Gellée S, Sans N, Rousseau H, Rougé D, et al. Sexual dimorphism of the fetal ilium: a 3D geometric morphometric approach with multislice computed tomography. Journal of Forensic Sciences 2013;58:851—8.

Nikita E. Age-associated variation and sexual dimorphism in adult cranial morphology: implications in anthropological studies. International Journal of Osteoarchaeology 2014;24:557—69.

Novotny V, İşcan MY, Loth SR. Morphological and osteometric assessment of age, sex and race from the skull. In: İşcan MY, Helmer RP, editors. Forensic analysis of the skull. New York: Wiley-Liss; 1993. p. 71—88.

Okrutny EC-J. Postcranial osteometric assessment of Korean ancestry [Master's thesis]. Orlando, Florida: University of Central Florida; 2010.

Ousley SD, Hefner JT. The statistical determination of ancestry. In: Proceedings of the 56th annual meeting of the American Academy of forensic Sciences, Seattle, WA; 2005.

Ousley SD, Jantz RL. The Forensic Data Bank: documenting skeletal trends in the United States. In: Reichs KJ, editor. Forensic osteology: advances in the identification of human remains. second ed. Springfield: Charles C. Thomas; 1998. p. 441—58.

Ousley SD, Jantz RL. Fordisc 3 and statistical methods for estimating sex and ancestry. In: Dirkmaat DC, editor. A companion to forensic anthropology. Oxford: Wiley-Blackwell Publishing; 2012. p. 400—12.

Patriquin ML, Steyn M, Loth SR. Metric assessment of race from the pelvis in South Africans. Forensic Science International 2002;127:104—13.

Patriquin M, Loth SR, Steyn M. Sexually dimorphic pelvic morphology in South African whites and blacks. HOMO - Journal of Comparative Human Biology 2003;53:255—62.

Phenice TW. A newly developed visual method of sexing the os pubis. American Journal of Physical Anthropology 1969;30:297—302.

Pilloud MA, Hefner JT, Hanihara T, Hayashi A. The use of tooth crown measurements in the assessment of ancestry. Journal of Forenic Sciences 2014;59:1493—501.

Prado FB, De Mollos Santos LS, Caria PHF, Kawaguchi JT, Preza ADOG, Daruge E, et al. Incidence of clavicular rhomboid fossa (impression of costoclavicular ligament) in the Brazilian population: forensic application. Journal of Forensic Odonto-Stomatology 2009;27:12—6.

Reynolds EL. The bony pelvic girdle in early infancy. A roentgenometric study. American Journal of Physical Anthropology 1945;3:321 54.

Reynolds EL. The bony pelvis in pre-pubertal childhood. American Journal of Physical Anthropology 1947;5:165—200.

Rhine S. Nonmetric skull racing. In: Gill GW, Rhine S, editors. Skeletal attribution of race: methods for forensic anthropology. Albuquerque: Maxwell Museum of Anthropology; 1990. p. 9—20.

Rissech C, Garcia M, Malgosa A. Sex and age diagnosis by ischium morphometric analysis. Forensic Science International 2003;135:188—96.

Rogers TL, Flournoy LE, McCormick WF. The rhomboid fossa of the clavicle as a sex and age estimator. Journal of Forensic Sciences 2000;39:1047—56.

Rogers TL. A visual method of determining the sex of skeletal remains using the distal humerus. Journal of Forensic Sciences 1999;44:57—60.

Rogers TL. Sex determination of adolescent skeletons using the distal humerus. American Journal of Physical Anthropology 2009;140:143—8.

Rosenberg NA, Pritchard JK, Weber JL, Cann HM, Kidd KK, Zhivotovsky LA, et al. Genetic structure of human populations. Science 2002;298:2381—5.

Scheuer L. Brief communication: a blind test of mandibular morphology for sexing mandibles in the first few years of life. American Journal of Physical Anthropology 2002;119:189—91.

Schultz AH. The skeleton of the trunk and limbs of higher primates. Human Biology 1930;2:303—456.

Schutkowski H. Sex determination of fetal and neonate skeletons by means of discriminant analysis. International Journal of Anthropology 1987;2:347—52.

Schutkowski H. Sex determination of infant and juvenile skeletons: I. Morphognostic features. American Journal of Physical Anthropology 1993;90:199—205.

Shirley NR, Fatah EEA, Mahfouz M. Beyond the cranium: ancestry estimation from the lower limb. In: Berg GE, Ta'ala SC, editors. Biological affinity in forensic identification of human skeletal remains. Beyond black and white. Boca Raton: CRC Press; 2015. p. 133—54.

Sholts SB, Wärmländer SK. Zygomaticomaxillary suture shape analyzed with digital morphometrics: reassessing patterns of variation in American Indian and European populations. Forensic Science International 2012;217. 234.e1—234.e6.

Spradley K. Metric ancestry estimation from the postcranial skeleton. In: Berg GE, Ta'ala SC, editors. Biological affinity in forensic identification of human skeletal remains. Beyond black and white. Boca Raton: CRC Press; 2015. p. 83—94.

Stewart TD. Anterior femoral curvature: its utility for race identification. Human Biology 1962;34:49—62.

Steyn M, Henneberg M. Cranial growth in the prehistoric sample from K2 at Mapungubwe (South Africa) is population specific. HOMO - Journal of Comparative Human Biology 1997;48:62—71.

Steyn M, Pretorius E, Hutten L. Geometric morphometric analysis of the greater sciatic notch in South Africans. HOMO - Journal of Comparative Human Biology 2004;54:197—206.

Stull KE, Godde K. Sex estimation of infants between birth and one year through discriminant analysis of the humerus and femur. Journal of Forensic Sciences 2013;58:13—20.

Stull KE, Kenyhercz MW, L'Abbé EN. Ancestry estimation in South Africa using craniometrics and geometric morphometrics. Forensic Science International 2014;245. 206.e1—206.e7.

Sutherland LD, Suchey JM. Use of the ventral arc in pubic sex determination. Journal of Forensic Sciences 1991;36:501—11.

Sutter RC. Nonmetric subadult skeletal sexing traits: I. A blind test of the accuracy of eight previously proposed methods using prehistoric known-sex mummies from northern Chile. Journal of Forensic Sciences 2003;48:927—35.

Ta'ala SC. A brief history of the race concept in physical anthropology. In: Berg GE, Ta'ala SC, editors. Biological affinity in forensic identification of human skeletal remains. Beyond black and white. Boca Raton: CRC Press; 2015. p. 1—16.

Tallman SD, Winburn AP. Forensic applicability of femur subtrochanteric shape to ancestry assessment in Thai and White American males. Journal of Forensic Sciences 2015;60:1283—9.

Ubelaker DH, Volk CG. A test of the Phenice method for the estimation of sex. Journal of Forensic Sciences 2002;47:19—24.

Ubelaker DH, Ross AH, Graver SM. Application of forensic discriminant functions to a Spanish cranial sample. Forensic Science Communications 2002;4(3).

Vance VL, Steyn M, L'Abbé EN. Non-metric sex determination from the distal and posterior humerus in black and white South Africans. Journal of Forensic Sciences 2011;56:710—4.

Veroni A, Nikitovic D, Schillaci MA. Brief communication: sexual dimorphism of the juvenile basicranium. American Journal of Physical Anthropology 2010;141:147—51.

Viciano J, López-Lázaro S, Alemán I. Sex estimation based on deciduous and permanent dentition in a contemporary Spanish population. American Journal of Physical Anthropology 2013;152:31—43.

Vlak D, Roksandic M, Schillaci MA. Greater sciatic notch as a sex indicator in juveniles. American Journal of Physical Anthropology 2008;137:309—15.

Walker PL. Greater sciatic notch morphology: sex, age, and population differences. American Journal of Physical Anthropology 2005;127:385—91.

Walker PL. Sexing skulls using discriminant function analysis of visually assessed traits. American Journal of Physical Anthropology 2008;136:39—50.

Warrener AG, Lewton KL, Pontzer H, Lieberman DE. A wider pelvis does not increase locomotor cost in humans, with implications for the evolution of childbirth. PLoS One 2015;10(3):e0118903.

Washburn SL. Sex differences in the pubic bone. American Journal of Physical Anthropology 1948;6:199—207.

Weaver DS. Sex differences in the ilia of a known sex and age sample of fetal and infant skeletons. American Journal of Physical Anthropology 1980;52:191—5.

Weinberg SM, Putz DA, Mooney MP, Siegel MI. Evaluation of non-metric variation in the crania of black and white perinates. Forensic Science International 2005;151:177—85.

Wescott D. Population variation in femur subtrochanteric shape. Journal of Forensic Science 2005;50:1—8.

Williams BA, Rogers T. Evaluating the accuracy and precision of cranial morphological traits for sex determination. Journal of Forensic Sciences 2006;51:729 35.

Williams FL, Belcher RL, Armelagos GJ. Forensic misclassification of Ancient Nubian crania: implications for assumptions about human variation. Current Anthropology 2005;46:340−6.

Wilson J, George F, Griffin J. The hormonal control of sexual development. Science 1981;211:1278−84.

Wilson LA, MacLeod N, Humphrey LT. Morphometric criteria for sexing juvenile human skeletons using the ilium. Journal of Forensic Sciences 2008;53:269−78.

Wilson LAB, Cardoso HFV, Humphrey LT. On the reliability of a geometric morphometric approach to sex determination: a blind test of six criteria of the juvenile ilium. Forensic Science International 2011;206:35−42.

Wood C. The age-related emergence of cranial morphological variation. Forensic Science International 2015;251(220):e1−20.

Wright R. Detection of likely ancestry using CRANID. In: Oxenham M, editor. Forensic approaches to death, disaster and abuse. Brisbane: Australian Academic Press; 2008. p. 111−22.

APPENDICES

Appendix 3.I: Sex Assessment Recording Protocol

TABLE 3.I.1 Sex Assessment Using Pelvic Morphological Traits

Trait/Method	Subcharacter	Score	Sex
Overall pelvic shape	—	—	
Overall sacral shape	—	—	
Iliac auricular surface elevation	—	—	
Greater sciatic notch depth/breadth	—		
Preauricular sulcus	—	—	
Obturator foramen size and shape	—	—	
Acetabular size and direction	—	—	
Phenice (1969) method	Ventral arc	—	
	Subpubic concavity	—	
	Medial ischiopubic ramus	—	
	Overall sex	—	
Klales et al. (2012) method	Ventral arc		—
	Subpubic concavity		—
	Medial ischiopubic ramus		—
	Discriminant equation score		—
	Probability male		—
	Probability female		—
	Overall sex	—	
Bruzek (2002) method	Preauricular surface—first condition		
	Preauricular surface—second condition		
	Preauricular surface—third condition		
	Greater sciatic notch—first condition		
	Greater sciatic notch—second condition		
	Greater sciatic notch—third condition		
	Composite arch		

TABLE 3.I.1 Sex Assessment Using Pelvic Morphological Traits—cont'd

Trait/Method	Subcharacter	Score	Sex
	Inferior pelvis—first condition		
	Inferior pelvis—second condition		
	Inferior pelvis—third condition		
	Ischiopubic proportion		
	Overall sex	–	

TABLE 3.I.2 Sex Assessment Using Cranial Morphological Traits

Cranial Trait	Subcharacter	Score	Sex
Overall size	–	–	
Overall robusticity	–	–	
External occipital protuberance	–	–	
Nuchal lines	–	–	
Mastoid process	–	–	
Supraorbital margin	–	–	
Supraorbital ridges/glabella	–	–	
Frontal/parietal bossing	–	–	
Mental eminence	–	–	
Chin shape	–	–	
Mandibular ramus flexure	–	–	
Gonial eversion	–	–	
Walker (2008) method	Supraorbital ridges/glabella		–
	Mastoid process		–
	Nuchal crest		–
	Supraorbital margin		–
	Mental eminence		–
	Discriminant equation score		–
	Probability male		–
	Probability female		–
	Overall sex	–	

TABLE 3.I.3 Sex Assessment Using Other Morphological Traits

Method	Sex

TABLE 3.I.4 Sex Assessment Using Metric Analysis

Method (Publication/Skeletal Element/Equation)	Result	Sex

Appendix 3.II: Case Study for Sex Assessment

Figs. 3.II.1 and 3.II.2 depict aspects of the cranial and pelvic morphology of a 27-year-old male from the Athens Collection (WLH 72). Assume that the sex of the individual is unknown and assess it based on the provided information.

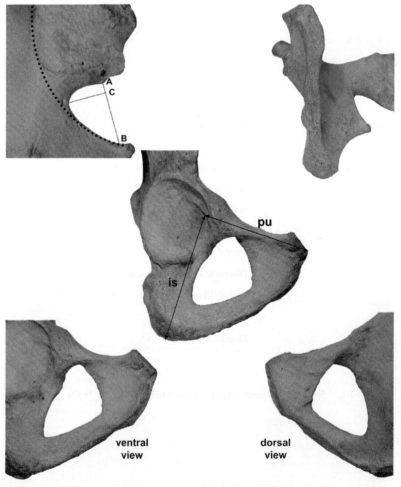

FIGURE 3.II.1   Pelvic morphological traits. *is*, ischium; *pu*, pubis.

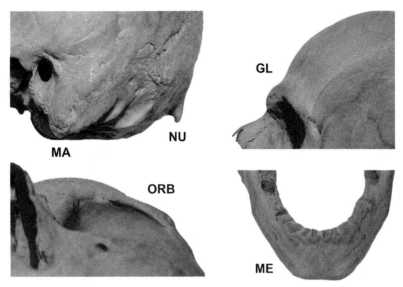

FIGURE 3.II.2 Cranial and mandibular morphological traits. *GL*, glabella; *MA*, mastoid process; *ME*, mental eminence; *NU*, nuchal crest; *ORB*, supraorbital margin.

If we examine the morphological characteristics of the pelvis (Fig. 3.II.1), we observe that the subpubic concavity is only slightly present, there is minimal manifestation of a ventral arc, and the medial aspect of the ischiopubic ramus is broad. Moreover, the ischiopubic proportion is typical of a male individual (pu < is), whereas the greater sciatic notch is narrow, there is no composite arch, the notch contour is asymmetric, and the posterior chord segment, AC, is shorter than the anterior chord, CB. Therefore, the pelvic traits support a male sex.

The cranium of the individual (Fig. 3.II.2) is also typically male. The glabella is pronounced, the frontal bone has a clear slope, the nuchal crest protrudes, the chin is squared, the supraorbital margin is blunt, and the mastoid process is large.

Employing the method by Klales et al. (2012), we can assign the following scores to each pelvic trait: ventral arc (V) = 3, medial aspect of the ischiopubic ramus (M) = 4, and subpubic concavity (S) = 4. If these values are inserted into the logistic regression Eq. (3.1.1), we obtain:

$$y = -1.014, \; p_f = 1/(1 + e^{-y}) = 0.266, \text{ and } p_m = 1 - p_f = 0.734$$

From Eqs. (3.1.3)−(3.1.6) we similarly obtain $y = -1.471, -3.503, -3.231,$ and -5.1, respectively, which result in p_m values greater than 0.81.

In addition, assigning the following scores to each cranial trait, glabella (GL) = 5, supraorbital margin (ORB) = 3, mental eminence (ME) = 4, nuchal crest (NU) = 5, and mastoid process (MA) = 4, and applying Walker's equations for American/English populations (Table 3.1.4), we obtain $y = -7.09, -6.242, -6.193, -4.794, -4.403,$ and $-4.407,$ which yield p_m values greater than 0.988.

It is seen that the logistic regressions based on pelvic and cranial traits support the original observation that the individual is male, as is indeed the case.

All the aforementioned computations can be easily performed using either the OSTEO software and the menu Add-Ins → OSTEO → Estimation → SexAssessment or directly the macro SexAssessment from the homonymous Excel file, provided in the companion website. For the application of the macro, the traits should be arranged in a single row in the following order:

GL, ORB, ME, NU, MA, S, M, V

If some scores are missing, the corresponding cells should be left vacant. For example, if cranial data are not available, the first five cells (GL, ORB, ME, NU, MA) should be empty. When running the macro, select the entire range of the scores (GL, ORB, ME, NU, MA, S, M, V), and subsequently select the output cell. Fig. 3.II.3 presents the results obtained from the application of the macro SexAssessment. As expected, they are identical to the aforementioned.

Sex estimation using cranial or/and pelvic morphological traits								
Vars:	glabella	supraorbital margin	mental eminence	nuchal crest	mastoid process	subpubic concavity	medial Ischio-pubic	ventral arc
Abbreviation:	**GL**	**ORB**	**ME**	**NU**	**MA**	**S**	**M**	**V**
Scores:	5	3	4	5	4	4	4	3

Estimation from cranial data - Accuracy % for male and female classification

American/English

vars	P(Female)	P(Male)	sex	accuracy
GL-MA-ME	0.001	0.999	MALE	88/86
GL-MA	0.002	0.998	MALE	85/83
GL-ME	0.002	0.998	MALE	87/82
ME-MA	0.008	0.992	MALE	80/84
ORB-ME	0.012	0.988	MALE	78/78
NU-MA	0.012	0.988	MALE	77/83

NativeAmerican

vars	P(Female)	P(Male)	sex	accuracy
ORB-ME	0.376	0.624	MALE	78/78
ME-MA	0.111	0.889	MALE	74/73
GL-MA	0.036	0.964	MALE	70/83

Estimation from Phenice method using linear discriminant functions
Accuracy % for male and female classification

vars	P(Female)	P(Male)	sex	accuracy
S-M-V	0.029	0.971	MALE	98/89
M-V	0.187	0.813	MALE	97/92
S-V	0.038	0.962	MALE	98/88
S-M	0.006	0.994	MALE	96/87

Estimation from Phenice method using logistic regression equation

vars	P(Female)	P(Male)	sex	accuracy
S-M-V	0.266	0.734	MALE	74/98

FIGURE 3.II.3 Sex assessment results from the OSTEO software.

Appendix 3.III: Ancestry Assessment Recording Protocol

Morphoscopic Trait	Score	OSSA score
Anterior nasal spine	(1—3)	
Inferior nasal aperture	(1—5)	
Interorbital breadth	(1—3)	
Nasal aperture width	(1—3)	
Nasal bone contour	(0—4)	
Postbregmatic depression	(0—1)	
OSSA sum =		
Ancestry		

OSSA, optimized summed scored attributes.

Appendix 3.IV: Recording Sex and Ancestry Markers in Osteoware

Osteoware allows the recording of pelvic and cranial sex markers in the Age and Sex module using the Morphology tab (Fig. 3.IV.1). Note that the same tab also includes certain age indicators, which will be discussed in Chapter 4. The pelvic sexually dimorphic traits that may be recorded include the ventral arc, subpubic concavity, ischiopubic ramus ridge, auricular surface elevation, greater sciatic notch width, sacral curvature, and preauricular sulcus. Most of these traits are scored as male (M), female (F), or indeterminate (?); however, for the greater sciatic notch and the preauricular sulcus more detailed recordings are provided, as seen in Fig. 3.IV.1. Cranial sexually dimorphic traits include the nuchal crest, mastoid process, supraorbital sharpness, supraorbital ridge size, glabellar prominence, and mental eminence, for which a five-point recording is proposed following Walker (in Buikstra and Ubelaker, 1994).

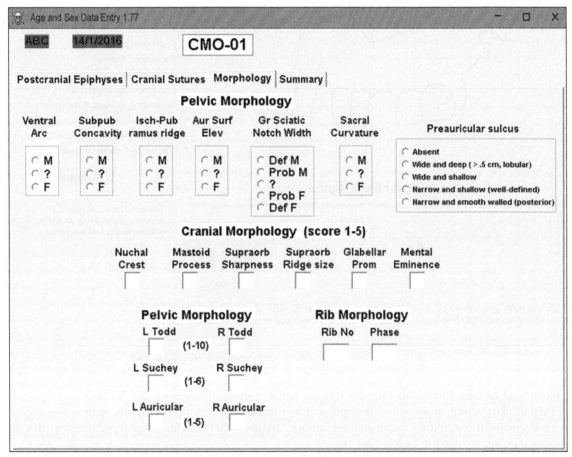

FIGURE 3.IV.1   The Morphology tab of the Age and Sex module.

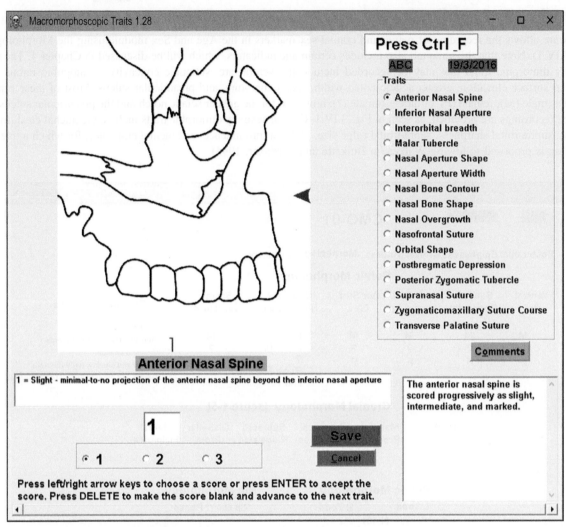

FIGURE 3.IV.2 Osteoware data entry screen for macromorphoscopic traits.

For ancestry, Osteoware allows data entry for 16 traits in the Macromorphoscopics tab. The definition for each trait is given in the data entry screen, along with a description of its various character states, as can be seen in Fig. 3.IV.2 for the anterior nasal spine. All descriptions and definitions are from Hefner (2009). Additional photographs depicting each trait and character state are provided in Hefner (2011).

Chapter 4

Age Estimation

Chapter Objectives

By the end of this chapter, the reader will be able to:

- understand the mechanisms that produce age-related changes in juvenile and adult skeletal remains;
- estimate the age at death of an individual using different methods; and
- understand the limitations of each method.

This chapter presents the main macroscopic methods for the estimation of the age at death of individuals based on skeletal remains. Age estimation is important to both osteoarchaeologists and forensic anthropologists. In archaeological material age is a significant parameter in paleodemographic profiles and an essential factor to consider when examining activity, pathology, and other aspects of past life. In forensic contexts, age is important in identifying the unknown individual(s) represented by the skeletal remains.

4.1 AGE ESTIMATION

Age at death estimation in osteological studies is based on the biological changes that occur on the skeleton with time and activity (*biological age*). However, this is not the same as *chronological age*, that is, how much time has passed since the birth of the individual. Chronological and biological age are interrelated; thus one can be used to estimate the other, but this relationship is not perfect. Whereas chronological age progresses steadily, biological age is affected by multiple factors such as activity, diet, and disease. As a result, chronological and biological age become increasingly divergent from each other, making the estimation of chronological age from biological age problematic. This is why age estimation for adults is less precise than for juveniles (Nawrocki, 2010). An additional reason for the higher precision of juvenile age estimation is that in juveniles this is based on anatomical changes that occur because of the gradual development of the body, whereas in adults age estimation is based on skeletal degenerative changes that do not strictly reflect biological age.

Owing to the inherent inaccuracies in age at death estimation, age classes are used to classify individuals, rather than assigning a strict age to each skeleton. These classes become increasingly broad as the individual grows older. Such classes may be *fetus* (before birth), *infant* (0−3 years old), *child* (3−12 years old), *adolescent* (12−20 years old), *young adult* (20−34 years old), *middle adult* (35−49 years old), and *old adult* (50+ years old) (Buikstra and Ubelaker, 1994). However, each sample can be divided into different age groups, with smaller or larger ranges, depending on the level of preservation and research questions. For instance, if a study focuses on juvenile remains, one may wish to follow the more detailed age groups provided by Scheuer and Black (2000).

The age at death of an individual may be estimated based on morphological and metric methods, which are presented in the following sections. Suggested recording protocols for aging juveniles and adults are given in Appendices 4.I to 4.III.

4.2 JUVENILES

Excellent sources on skeletal growth and development are Fazekas and Kósa (1978), Scheuer and Black (2000), Schaefer et al. (2008), and Baker et al. (2005). Of these, Schaefer et al. is the most updated and complete manual as of this writing, providing a compilation of metric and morphological developmental standards for the estimation of the age of infants to young adults. The work of Fazekas and Kósa may be rather old but it is still an essential source regarding fetal developmental standards.

4.2.1 Appearance and Union of Ossification Centers

Ossification of the skeleton starts from specific centers, which gradually fuse together. In the fetus there are originally 806 ossification centers; at birth these have been reduced to 450, and eventually these turn to the 206 bones of the adult skeleton. Most centers commence ossification during the embryonic or fetal period of life, but it is only once they have grown sufficiently to be recognized that they may be used in aging. This differs per element; for example, most parts of the cranium can be recognized from the midfetal stage, whereas the carpals become identifiable in later childhood (Scheuer and Black, 2000).

The next stage of bone development is characterized by the fusion of the primary centers or between a primary and a secondary center (Scheuer and Black, 2000). Indeed, most bones derive from a primary ossification center and several (usually at least two) secondary ossification centers. The fusion of the primary and secondary ossification centers is known as *epiphyseal union*. Epiphyseal union occurs gradually (Figs. 4.2.1 and 4.2.2); thus, when recording it, it is important to use a scale that expresses the degree of the union of the ossification centers, such as "open," "partial union," or "complete union" (Buikstra and Ubelaker, 1994).

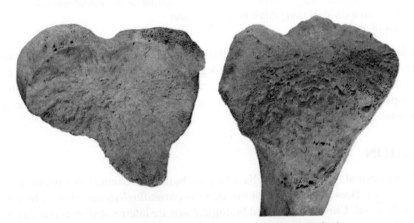

FIGURE 4.2.1 Unfused proximal tibial epiphysis and diaphysis.

The exact age of fusion of the ossification centers differs among individuals and populations but some general patterns for the primary ossification centers most often used for age at death estimation are provided in Table 4.2.1. The fusion of the sphenooccipital synchondrosis is a special case and it is described in Box 4.2.1. Finally, representative ages of fusion of the primary and secondary ossification centers for elements of the axial and appendicular skeleton are given in Figs. 4.2.3−4.2.8. Note that, because of interpopulation variation in the timing of development, it is advisable to use the data presented in this section only if population-specific standards are not available.

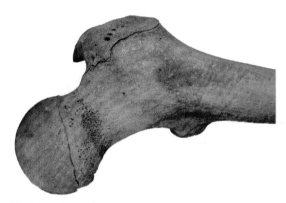

FIGURE 4.2.2   Fusing proximal femoral epiphyses and diaphysis.

TABLE 4.2.1 Age of Fusion of Primary Ossification Centers

Skeletal Element	Anatomical Parts	Age of Fusion
Frontal bone	Metopic suture	By end of 4th year
Occipital bone	Squamous part—lateral parts	1st–3rd year
	Basilar part—lateral parts	5th–7th year
Mandible	Mandibular symphysis	By end of 1st year
Os coxa	Ischium—pubis	3rd–8th year
	Ilium—ischium and pubis	10th–17th year
Vertebrae	Two halves of the neural arches (cervical)	By early 2nd year
	Two halves of the neural arches (lower thoracic and upper lumbar)	1st year
	Two halves of the neural arches (lower lumbar)	By early 6th year
	Neural arch—vertebral centrum	3rd–7th year

From Schaefer M, Black S, Scheuer L. Juvenile Osteology: A Laboratory and Field Manual. San Diego: Academic Press; 2008.

BOX 4.2.1 Fusion of the Sphenooccipital Synchondrosis

The occipital bone and the sphenoid are joined at the sphenooccipital synchondrosis. This is gradually ossified and the two bones unite in the cranial base. Traditionally this fusion was believed to take place between the ages of 17 and 20–25 years. However, more recent research supports that this fusion actually occurs earlier (between 11 and 16 years of age in females and between 13 and 18 years in males) (see Scheuer and Black, 2000 for a review).

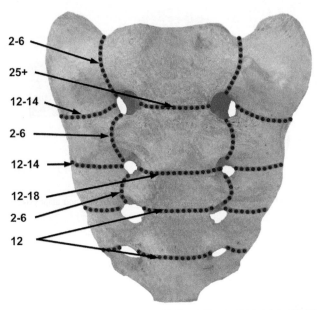

FIGURE 4.2.3 Age of fusion (in years) of ossification centers in the sacrum. *Adapted from Schaefer M, Black S, Scheuer L. Juvenile Osteology: A Laboratory and Field Manual. San Diego: Academic Press; 2008.*

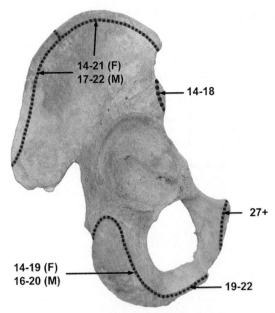

FIGURE 4.2.4 Age of fusion (in years) of primary and secondary ossification centers in the os coxa. *F*, female; *M*, male. *Adapted from Schaefer M, Black S, Scheuer L. Juvenile Osteology: A Laboratory and Field Manual. San Diego: Academic Press; 2008.*

A factor that should be taken into consideration when using ossification center union as an age marker is that many centers start fusing earlier in females than in males, as can be seen in Figs. 4.2.3–4.2.8. Therefore, ideally the sex of the individual should be assessed prior to age estimation. However, as mentioned in Chapter 3, assessing the sex of juveniles is particularly tenuous. The safest option is to use both criteria for males and females and estimate age with the appropriate margin of error. In addition, there are interpopulation differences in the rate of epiphyseal union; thus the patterns depicted

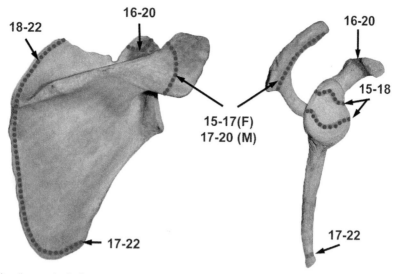

FIGURE 4.2.5 Age of fusion (in years) of primary and secondary ossification centers in the scapula. *F*, female; *M*, male. *Adapted from Schaefer M, Black S, Scheuer L. Juvenile Osteology: A Laboratory and Field Manual. San Diego: Academic Press; 2008.*

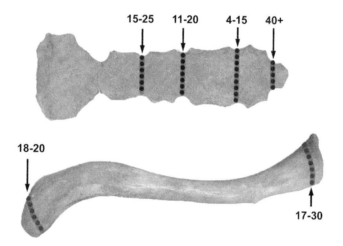

FIGURE 4.2.6 Age of fusion (in years) of primary and secondary ossification centers in the sternum and clavicle. *Adapted from Schaefer M, Black S, Scheuer L. Juvenile Osteology: A Laboratory and Field Manual. San Diego: Academic Press; 2008.*

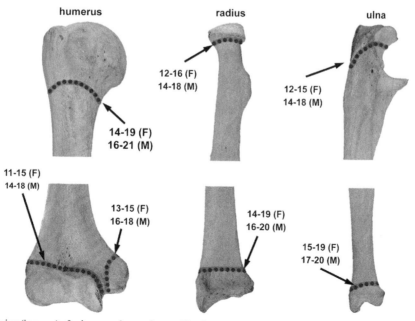

FIGURE 4.2.7 Age of fusion (in years) of primary and secondary ossification centers in the humerus, radius, and ulna. *F*, female; *M*, male. *Adapted from*

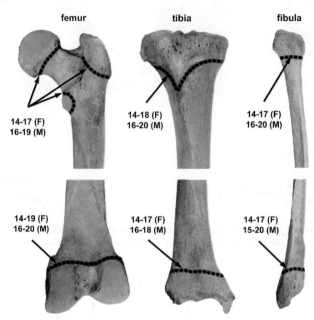

femur　　　　tibia　　　　fibula

14-17 (F)
16-19 (M)

14-18 (F)
16-20 (M)

14-17 (F)
16-20 (M)

14-19 (F)
16-20 (M)

14-17 (F)
16-18 (M)

14-17 (F)
15-20 (M)

FIGURE 4.2.8　Age of fusion (in years) of primary and secondary ossification centers in the femur, tibia, and fibula. *F*, female; *M*, male. *Adapted from Schaefer M, Black S, Scheuer L. Juvenile Osteology: A Laboratory and Field Manual. San Diego: Academic Press; 2008.*

in these figures may vary among groups. It should also be kept in mind that the association between the stage of union of the ossification centers and the chronological age has been based on modern data, but it is unclear to what extent the same standards apply to earlier populations because of secular changes.

4.2.2 Long-Bone Length

There is a strong linear relationship between long-bone length and age, which makes the length of long bones a potentially useful age marker (Fazekas and Kósa, 1978). This is particularly so for fetuses because the development of fetal bones appears to be minimally influenced by extrinsic factors, such as poor nutrition (Lewis, 2009). For this reason, regression equations have been produced using modern data to predict the age of an individual based on diaphyseal length. Regression equations for estimating fetal age of 3 to 9 months from long-bone diaphyseal length are given in Table 4.2.2. These have been obtained from data published by Fazekas and Kósa (1978). Note that although Fazekas and Kósa (1978) is a principal source that correlated gestational age to bone size, there are some serious issues. An important problem is that the skeletal material examined by the authors was largely of unknown age; fetuses were seriated

TABLE 4.2.2 Regression Equations for Estimating Fetal Age of 3 to 9 months From Long-Bone Length (in mm)

Regression Equation	Standard Error of Estimate
Age $= 0.00145 \times$ (humeral length)$^2 + 0.033 \times$ (humeral length) $+ 2.71$	0.14
Age $= 0.00245 \times$ (radial length)$^2 + 0.0256 \times$ (radial length) $+ 2.82$	0.12
Age $= 0.00183 \times$ (ulnar length)$^2 + 0.0284 \times$ (ulnar length) $+ 2.79$	0.12
Age $= 0.00068 \times$ (femoral length)$^2 + 0.063 \times$ (femoral length) $+ 2.45$	0.18
Age $= 0.00113 \times$ (tibial length)$^2 + 0.0538 \times$ (tibial length) $+ 2.69$	0.14
Age $= 0.00135 \times$ (fibular length)$^2 + 0.05 \times$ (fibular length) $+ 2.74$	0.13

Based on data published by Fazekas G, Kósa F. Forensic fetal osteology. Budapest: Akadémiai Kiadó; 1978.

according to crown–heel length and subsequently assigned an age. An additional issue is that some of the fetuses examined had been naturally aborted; therefore, they may have suffered from developmental defects (Scheuer and Black, 2000). More recently, various aging standards for fetal remains based on diaphyseal lengths have been published by Scheuer and Black (2000) and Schaefer et al. (2008), and a number of population-specific studies can be found in the literature.

Long-bone length can also be used for age estimation after birth (see Schaefer et al., 2008 for a compilation of the results of numerous studies on the subject). Table 4.2.3 presents regression equations for estimating age in individuals of 0.125 to 12 years from long-bone diaphyseal length (in mm). These equations were derived from data given in Maresh (1970). Note that the regression equations for females are different from those for males, so in cases in which the sex of the individual is unknown, the estimates from the two sexes should be combined.

TABLE 4.2.3 Regression Equations for Estimating Age in Individuals of 0.125 to 12 years From Long-Bone Diaphyseal Length (x in mm)

Bone	Regression Equation
Females	
Humerus	$\text{Age} = (-7.588 \times 10^{-7})x^3 + (5.550 \times 10^{-4})x^2 - (5.391 \times 10^{-2})x + 1.435$
Ulna	$\text{Age} = (-2.230 \times 10^{-6})x^3 + (1.187 \times 10^{-3})x^2 - (1.104 \times 10^{-1})x + 2.947$
Radius	$\text{Age} = (-2.401 \times 10^{-6})x^3 + (1.193 \times 10^{-3})x^2 - (8.979 \times 10^{-2})x + 1.813$
Femur	$\text{Age} = (-1.823 \times 10^{-7})x^3 + (1.955 \times 10^{-4})x^2 - (1.822 \times 10^{-2})x + 0.336$
Tibia	$\text{Age} = (-4.264 \times 10^{-7})x^3 + (3.368 \times 10^{-4})x^2 - (2.820 \times 10^{-2})x + 0.602$
Fibula	$\text{Age} = (-3.323 \times 10^{-7})x^3 + (2.947 \times 10^{-4})x^2 - (2.219 \times 10^{-2})x + 0.414$
Males	
Humerus	$\text{Age} = (-6.144 \times 10^{-7})x^3 + (5.008 \times 10^{-4})x^2 - (4.840 \times 10^{-2})x + 1.239$
Ulna	$\text{Age} = (-1.573 \times 10^{-6})x^3 + (9.604 \times 10^{-4})x^2 - (8.776 \times 10^{-2})x + 2.159$
Radius	$\text{Age} = (-1.636 \times 10^{-6})x^3 + (9.563 \times 10^{-4})x^2 - (7.065 \times 10^{-2})x + 1.254$
Femur	$\text{Age} = (-1.440 \times 10^{-7})x^3 + (1.724 \times 10^{-4})x^2 - (1.430 \times 10^{-2})x + 0.124$
Tibia	$\text{Age} = (-3.290 \times 10^{-7})x^3 + (2.926 \times 10^{-4})x^2 - (2.265 \times 10^{-2})x + 0.361$
Fibula	$\text{Age} = (-2.613 \times 10^{-7})x^3 + (2.638 \times 10^{-4})x^2 - (1.873 \times 10^{-2})x + 0.261$

Based on data published by Maresh MM. Measurements from roentgenograms. In: McCammon RW, editor. Human growth and development. Springfield, IL: Charles C. Thomas; 1970. p. 157–200.

The regression equations of both Tables 4.2.2 and 4.2.3 can be easily applied using the macro AgeEstimation either directly from the homonymous Excel file or from the OSTEO software via the menu OSTEO → Estimation → Age estimation provided in the companion website.

When adopting published standards, it is important to keep in mind that the regression equations for age estimation based on long-bone length were formed using measurements obtained from radiographs of modern individuals. However, in archaeological material it is the dried bones that are directly measured, so a certain degree of error exists. Additional limitations arise from the fact that although extrinsic factors appear to have a minimal impact on fetal and neonatal bone dimensions, they do exert some influence, especially after birth, which cannot always be controlled for (Hauspie et al., 1994). Finally, children in the past were probably smaller than modern children because of secular changes (Humphrey, 2000).

4.2.3 Other Bone Dimensions

In addition to the use of long-bone diaphyses in regression equations for age estimation, certain studies have focused on the dimensions of other skeletal elements. Scheuer and MacLaughlin-Black (1994) found that if the width of the pars basilaris of the occipital bone is less than the sagittal length, then the individual is likely to be younger than 28 weeks in utero, whereas if the width is greater than the maximum length, then the individual is likely to be older than 5 months of age postpartum. Tocheri and Molto (2002) showed that in 87% of the individuals from their sample, age estimates based on the pars basilaris, femoral diaphyseal length, and dental development (see following section) agreed, supporting the value of occipital bone dimensions as an age at death marker. Finally, some studies have explored the potential of vertebral dimensions for age estimation (Kósa and Castellana, 2005).

4.2.4 Dentition

The estimation of age at death based on the dentition is particularly accurate for juveniles because teeth follow a well-defined developmental pattern from the fetal stage until the end of the second decade (Whittaker, 2000). Moreover, dental development appears to be under stronger genetic control than skeletal development and minimally affected by extrinsic factors (but see Gaur and Kumar, 2012 for evidence of delayed deciduous tooth emergence in cases of under-nourishment in modern populations and Pechníková et al., 2014 for a significant divergence in the timing of dental development even between monozygotic twins).

Dental development includes both the formation and the eruption of teeth. Deciduous tooth formation begins in utero, and most deciduous teeth erupt in the mouth during the second year after birth, with the second molars being the last to erupt. Permanent teeth begin to form during the first year of life, with the third molar being the last to form and emerge (Scheuer and Black, 2000; Whittaker, 2000).

The easiest method to estimate age based on dental development is an atlas, that is, a reference drawing depicting the stage of dental development at different ages. The atlas most commonly used in the literature is that devised by Ubelaker (1989), which was based on the work of Schour and Massler (1941). In Ubelaker's atlas (Fig. 4.2.9) data regarding tooth eruption were based on Native Americans and other "nonwhite" groups, as well as white North Americans, whereas information on tooth formation was derived primarily from white North American groups.

More recently, AlQahtani et al. (2010) produced the London Atlas, freely available at www.atlas.dentistry.qmul.ac.uk. This atlas is designed for individuals aged 28 weeks in utero to 23 years, and it is based on material of known age at death from collections at the Royal College of Surgeons of England and the Natural History Museum (London, UK), as well as from dental radiographs of living individuals. Note that a test of the Ubelaker (1989), Schour and Massler (1941), and London Atlas methods by AlQahtani et al. (2014) on individuals of known age with a broad geographic distribution found the London Atlas to provide the most accurate results. Nevertheless, it would be advisable to use population-specific standards of dental development, if such standards are available for the assemblage under study.

Another approach, alternative to atlases, focuses on the determination of the developmental stage of each available tooth by reference to relevant illustrations. Subsequently, the skeletal age to which this developmental stage corresponds is found based on graphs or tables generated from modern samples. The most commonly employed methods using this approach are those of Moorrees et al. (1963), Demirjian et al. (1973), and Liversidge and Molleson (2004).

At this point we should stress the following. According to Smith (1991), the *age of attainment* of a certain developmental stage is not the same as the *predicted age* of an individual. This is because when a tooth belongs to a certain developmental stage, it actually reached this stage at some point in the past. Therefore, when using the developmental stage per se, age is underestimated. A correction suggested by Smith (1991) is to predict age using the midpoint between the stage at which tooth formation falls and the subsequent stage. Liversidge (1994) retrieved better results when using predicted age than with age of attainment, whereas Saunders et al. (1993) found no significant difference between the two approaches. For a comprehensive discussion on this issue see Hoppa and FitzGerald (2005).

Whereas calculating the mean predicted age from the age of attainment is straightforward following Smith's (1991) approach, for the estimation of the corresponding standard deviation, we may work as follows: If $m_1 \pm s_1$ and $m_2 \pm s_2$ are the mean ages of attainment plus or minus the standard deviations of two successive stages, with $m_1 < m_2$, then the predicted age from stage 1 may be calculated from:

$$m = \frac{m_1 + m_2}{2} \tag{4.2.1}$$

In this case the standard deviation of the predicted age may be estimated using the expression:

$$\sigma = \sqrt{\frac{s_1^2 + m_1^2 + s_2^2 + m_2^2}{2} - \frac{(m_1 + m_2)^2}{4}} \tag{4.2.2}$$

which arises from the fact that the variance of a random variable X is given by:

$$\sigma^2 = \overline{X^2} - \left(\overline{X}\right)^2 \tag{4.2.3}$$

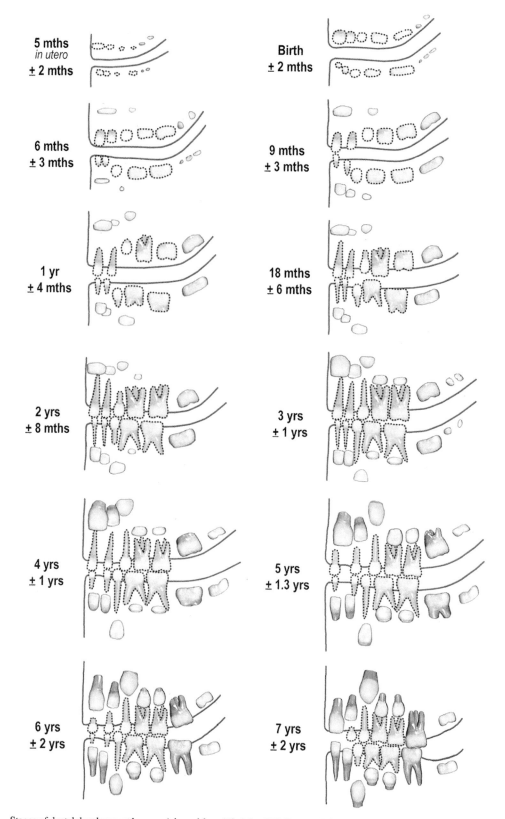

FIGURE 4.2.9   Stages of dental development by age. *Adapted from Ubelaker DH. Human skeletal remains: excavation, analysis, interpretation. 2nd ed. Washington: Taraxacum; 1989.*

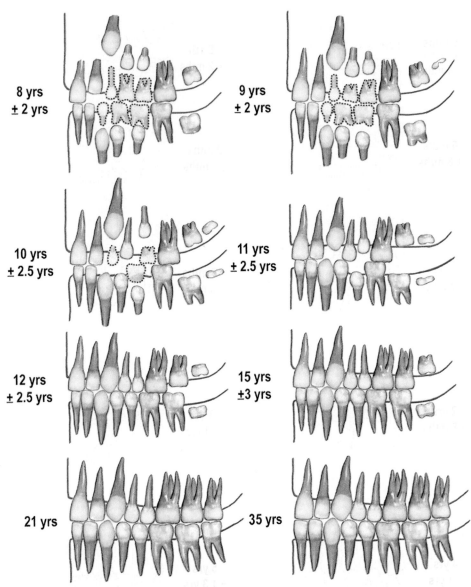

FIGURE 4.2.9 Continued.

where $\overline{X^2}$ and $\overline{X}$ are the mean values of X^2 and X, respectively, whereas when X follows the normal distribution with mean value m and standard deviation s, then:

$$\overline{X^2} = s^2 + m^2 \qquad (4.2.4)$$

As mentioned earlier, the most commonly used method employing dental developmental stages is that of Moorrees et al. (1963). This method is based on radiographs of Americans of European ancestry. Table 4.2.4 presents mandibular tooth formation stages, along with the corresponding age of attainment, predicted age, and standard deviations. The ages of attainment and their standard deviations were obtained from the charts provided in the original paper, whereas the predicted ages and standard deviations were calculated using the aforementioned equations. Tables 4.2.5 and 4.2.6 present the same information for root resorption.

Demirjian et al. (1973) also proposed dental developmental standards for individuals aged 3–17 years based on radiographs of permanent mandibular teeth (see also updated version in Demirjian and Goldstein, 1976). Once each tooth is allocated to a developmental stage, tables of maturity scores correlated with stages of tooth formation for males and females are used, and subsequently all maturity scores are added for each individual. Dental ages can be

TABLE 4.2.4 Definition of Tooth Formation Stage, Age of Attainment, and Predicted Age, According to Moorrees et al. (1963)

Symbol	Schematic Image	Stage, AOA, and PA (mean ± SD in years)
C_{oc}		*Cusp outline complete*
		AOA (M): dc = 0.2 ± 0.1; dm$_2$ = 0.2 ± 0.1
		AOA (F): dc = 0.2 ± 0.1
		PA (M): dc = 0.2 ± 0.1; dm$_2$ = 0.2 ± 0.1
		PA (F): dc = 0.2 ± 0.1
$Cr_{1/2}$		*Crown half complete*
		AOA (M): dc = 0.3 ± 0.1; dm$_1$ = 0.2 ± 0.1; dm$_2$ = 0.3 ± 0.1
		AOA (F): dc = 0.3 ± 0.1; dm$_1$ = 0.2 ± 0.1; dm$_2$ = 0.2 ± 0.1
		PA (M): dc = 0.4 ± 0.2; dm$_1$ = 0.2 ± 0.1; dm$_2$ = 0.4 ± 0.2
		PA (F): dc = 0.4 ± 0.1; dm$_1$ = 0.2 ± 0.1; dm$_2$ = 0.3 ± 0.2
$Cr_{3/4}$		*Crown three-quarters complete*
		AOA (M): dc = 0.5 ± 0.1; dm$_1$ = 0.3 ± 0.1; dm$_2$ = 0.5 ± 0.1
		AOA (F): dc = 0.5 ± 0.1; dm$_1$ = 0.2 ± 0.1; dm$_2$ = 0.5 ± 0.1
		PA (M): dc = 0.6 ± 0.2; dm$_1$ = 0.4 ± 0.1; dm$_2$ = 0.6 ± 0.2
		PA (F): dc = 0.6 ± 0.2; dm$_1$ = 0.3 ± 0.1; dm$_2$ = 0.6 ± 0.2
Cr_c		*Crown complete*
		AOA (M): dc = 0.7 ± 0.1; dm$_1$ = 0.5 ± 0.1; dm$_2$ = 0.7 ± 0.2
		AOA (F): dc = 0.7 ± 0.1; dm$_1$ = 0.3 ± 0.1; dm$_2$ = 0.7 ± 0.1
		PA (M): dc = 0.7 ± 0.2; dm$_1$ = 0.5 ± 0.1; dm$_2$ = 0.8 ± 0.2
		PA (F): dc = 0.8 ± 0.2; dm$_1$ = 0.4 ± 0.2; dm$_2$ = 0.8 ± 0.2
R_i		*Initial root formation*
		AOA (M): dc = 0.8 ± 0.2; dm$_1$ = 0.6 ± 0.1; dm$_2$ = 0.9 ± 0.2
		AOA (F): dc = 0.9 ± 0.2; dm$_1$ = 0.6 ± 0.1; dm$_2$ = 0.9 ± 0.2
		PA (M): dc = 0.9 ± 0.2; dm$_1$ = 0.6 ± 0.1; dm$_2$ = 0.9 ± 0.2
		PA (F): dc = 1.0 ± 0.2; dm$_1$ = 0.6 ± 0.1; dm$_2$ = 0.9 ± 0.2
Cl_i		*Initial cleft formation*
		AOA (M): dm$_1$ = 0.7 ± 0.1; dm$_2$ = 1.0 ± 0.2
		AOA (F): dm$_1$ = 0.6 ± 0.1; dm$_2$ = 1.0 ± 0.2
		PA (M): dm$_1$ = 0.7 ± 0.1; dm$_2$ = 1.2 ± 0.2
		PA (F): dm$_1$ = 0.6 ± 0.1; dm$_2$ = 1.1 ± 0.2
$R_{1/4}$		*Root length one-quarter*
		AOA (M): dc = 1.0 ± 0.2; dm$_1$ = 0.8 ± 0.2; dm$_2$ = 1.3 ± 0.2
		AOA (F): dc = 1.1 ± 0.2; dm$_1$ = 0.7 ± 0.1; dm$_2$ = 1.3 ± 0.2
		PA (M): dc = 1.1 ± 0.2; dm$_1$ = 0.8 ± 0.2; dm$_2$ = 1.4 ± 0.2
		PA (F): dc = 1.2 ± 0.2; dm$_1$ = 0.8 ± 0.1; dm$_2$ = 1.4 ± 0.3

Continued

TABLE 4.2.4 Definition of Tooth Formation Stage, Age of Attainment, and Predicted Age, According to Moorrees et al. (1963)—cont'd

Symbol	Schematic Image	Stage, AOA, and PA (mean ± SD in years)
$R_{1/2}$		*Root length half*
		AOA (M): dc = 1.3 ± 0.2; dm_1 = 0.9 ± 0.2; dm_2 = 1.6 ± 0.2
		AOA (F): dc = 1.3 ± 0.2; dm_1 = 0.9 ± 0.1; dm_2 = 1.5 ± 0.3
		PA (M): dc = 1.6 ± 0.4; dm_1 = 1.1 ± 0.2; dm_2 = 1.7 ± 0.3
		PA (F): dc = 1.5 ± 0.3; dm_1 = 1.0 ± 0.2; dm_2 = 1.7 ± 0.3
$R_{3/4}$		*Root length three-quarters*
		AOA (M): dc = 1.8 ± 0.3; dm_1 = 1.2 ± 0.2; dm_2 = 1.9 ± 0.3
		AOA (F): dc = 1.8 ± 0.3; dm_1 = 1.1 ± 0.2; dm_2 = 1.9 ± 0.3
		PA (M): dc = 1.9 ± 0.3; dm_1 = 1.3 ± 0.2; dm_2 = 1.9 ± 0.3
		PA (F): dc = 1.9 ± 0.3; dm_1 = 1.2 ± 0.2; dm_2 = 1.9 ± 0.3
R_c		*Root length complete*
		AOA (M): dc = 1.9 ± 0.3; dm_1 = 1.3 ± 0.2; dm_2 = 2.0 ± 0.3
		AOA (F): dc = 2.1 ± 0.3; dm_1 = 1.3 ± 0.2; dm_2 = 2.0 ± 0.3
		PA (M): dc = 2.2 ± 0.4; dm_1 = 1.5 ± 0.3; dm_2 = 2.2 ± 0.4
		PA (F): dc = 2.3 ± 0.4; dm_1 = 1.4 ± 0.2; dm_2 = 2.2 ± 0.4
$A_{1/2}$		*Apex half closed*
		AOA (M): dc = 2.5 ± 0.3; dm_1 = 1.7 ± 0.2; dm_2 = 2.4 ± 0.3
		AOA (F): dc = 2.5 ± 0.3; dm_1 = 1.5 ± 0.2; dm_2 = 2.4 ± 0.3
		PA (M): dc = 2.8 ± 0.5; dm_1 = 1.8 ± 0.3; dm_2 = 2.7 ± 0.5
		PA (F): dc = 2.7 ± 0.4; dm_1 = 1.6 ± 0.3; dm_2 = 2.6 ± 0.4
A_c		*Apical closure complete*
		AOA (M): dc = 3.1 ± 0.4; dm_1 = 1.9 ± 0.3; dm_2 = 3.0 ± 0.4
		AOA (F): dc = 3.0 ± 0.4; dm_1 = 1.8 ± 0.3; dm_2 = 2.8 ± 0.4

AOA, age of attainment; *F*, females; *M*, males; *PA*, predicted age.

calculated by matching the total sum of the maturity scores to the age curves provided in the original study. Note that when the Demirjian method was tested in different samples, it was found to miscalculate age (e.g., Różyło-Kalinowska et al., 2008; Urzel and Bruzek, 2013), yet population-specific aging techniques have been proposed based on this method (e.g., Lee et al., 2008).

More recently, Liversidge and Molleson (2004) proposed new developmental stages for deciduous teeth following the Demirjian et al. (1973) approach, using data from observations of isolated teeth and radiographs. The stages of crown and root formation along with the corresponding ages of attainment and predicted ages are shown in Table 4.2.7. Note that, whereas in the original publication separate age standards are provided for maxillary and mandibular teeth, Table 4.2.7 presents pooled data. In addition, ages of attainment and predicted ages for tooth eruption stages are given in Table 4.2.8, along with their corresponding standard deviations.

TABLE 4.2.5 Definition of Root Resorption Stages According to Moorrees et al. (1963)

Symbol	Schematic Image	Definition
Res.1/4		Root resorbed ¼
Res.1/2		Root resorbed ½
Res.3/4		Root resorbed ¾
Exf.		Exfoliation

TABLE 4.2.6 Age of Attainment and Predicted Age Based on Root Resorption, According to Moorrees et al. (1963)

	dc	$dm_1(m)$	$dm_1(d)$	$dm_2(m)$	$dm_2(d)$
Males					
Res.1/4	6.1 ± 0.4	5.4 ± 0.6	6.4 ± 0.7	6.7 ± 0.8	7.5 ± 0.8
	7.2 ± 1.4	**6.5 ± 1.3**	**7.4 ± 1.3**	**7.6 ± 1.3**	**8.5 ± 1.4**
Res.1/2	8.4 ± 1.0	7.6 ± 0.9	8.3 ± 1.0	8.6 ± 0.9	9.5 ± 1.1
	9.1 ± 1.3	**8.5 ± 1.3**	**9.2 ± 1.4**	**9.5 ± 1.4**	**10.3 ± 1.4**
Res.3/4	9.8 ± 1.1	9.4 ± 1.1	10.0 ± 1.1	10.4 ± 1.2	11.1 ± 1.2
	10.2 ± 1.2	**10.1 ± 1.3**	**10.4 ± 1.2**	**11.0 ± 1.4**	**11.4 ± 1.3**
Exf.	10.7 ± 1.1	10.8 ± 1.1	10.8 ± 1.1	11.7 ± 1.3	11.7 ± 1.3
Females					
Res.1/4	4.9 ± 0.6	4.9 ± 0.6	5.2 ± 0.6	6.0 ± 0.7	7.0 ± 0.7
	6.1 ± 1.3	**6.1 ± 1.4**	**6.4 ± 1.4**	**7.2 ± 1.4**	**7.8 ± 1.2**
Res.1/2	7.2 ± 0.9	7.3 ± 0.8	7.7 ± 0.9	8.3 ± 0.9	8.6 ± 1.0
	7.9 ± 1.2	**8.1 ± 1.2**	**8.5 ± 1.3**	**9.1 ± 1.4**	**9.3 ± 1.2**
Res.3/4	8.7 ± 1.0	8.8 ± 0.9	9.4 ± 1.0	10.0 ± 1.2	9.9 ± 1.1
	9.1 ± 1.1	**9.5 ± 1.2**	**9.7 ± 1.1**	**10.6 ± 1.3**	**10.5 ± 1.3**
Exf.	9.5 ± 1.1	10.1 ± 1.2	10.1 ± 1.2	11.1 ± 1.3	11.1 ± 1.3

TABLE 4.2.7 Description of Crown and Root Formation Stage, Age of Attainment, and Predicted Age

Stage	Schematic Image	Stage Description, AOA, and PA
C		*Completion of enamel formation on incisal/occlusal surface* AOA: dc $= 0.4 \pm 0.2$, dm1 $= 0.2 \pm 0.3$, dm2 $= 0.3 \pm 0.2$ PA: dc $= 0.6 \pm 0.3$, dm1 $= 0.3 \pm 0.3$, dm2 $= 0.6 \pm 0.4$
D		*Enamel formation down to the cementoenamel junction; beginning of root formation* AOA: di1 $= 0.1 \pm 0.2$, di2 $= 0.3 \pm 0.2$, dc $= 0.8 \pm 0.3$, dm1 $= 0.4 \pm 0.2$, dm2 $= 0.9 \pm 0.3$ PA: di1 $= 0.2 \pm 0.3$, di2 $= 0.4 \pm 0.2$, dc $= 0.9 \pm 0.3$, dm1 $= 0.6 \pm 0.3$, dm2 $= 1.1 \pm 0.3$
E		*Root length less than crown height* AOA: di1 $= 0.4 \pm 0.3$, di2 $= 0.5 \pm 0.2$, dc $= 1.0 \pm 0.3$, dm1 $= 0.7 \pm 0.3$, dm2 $= 1.3 \pm 0.3$ PA: di1 $= 0.6 \pm 0.4$, di2 $= 0.7 \pm 0.4$, dc $= 1.4 \pm 0.5$, dm1 $= 1.0 \pm 0.3$, dm2 $= 1.8 \pm 0.7$
F		*Root length equal to or greater than crown height* AOA: di1 $= 0.9 \pm 0.3$, di2 $= 1.0 \pm 0.3$, dc $= 1.8 \pm 0.2$, dm1 $= 1.3 \pm 0.1$, dm2 $= 2.3 \pm 0.5$ PA: di1 $= 1.1 \pm 0.4$, di2 $= 1.3 \pm 0.4$, dc $= 2.1 \pm 0.4$, dm1 $= 1.8 \pm 0.7$, dm2 $= 2.6 \pm 0.5$
G		*Almost complete root length* AOA: di1 $= 1.3 \pm 0.4$, di2 $= 1.5 \pm 0.3$, dc $= 2.4 \pm 0.4$, dm1 $= 2.4 \pm 0.4$, dm2 $= 2.9 \pm 0.5$ PA: di1 $= 1.7 \pm 0.6$, di2 $= 2.0 \pm 0.5$, dc $= 2.7 \pm 0.5$, dm1 $= 2.5 \pm 0.4$, dm2 $= 3.1 \pm 0.6$
H1		*Root length complete; apex width $= 1$ mm* AOA: di1 $= 2.1 \pm 0.3$, di2 $= 2.4 \pm 0.3$, dc $= 3.1 \pm 0.3$, dm1 $= 2.5 \pm 0.4$, dm2 $= 3.2 \pm 0.7$ PA: di1 $= 2.1 \pm 0.3$, di2 $= 2.4 \pm 0.4$, dc $= 3.2 \pm 0.4$, dm1 $= 2.7 \pm 0.5$, dm2 $= 3.5 \pm 0.7$
H2		*Apex just visible/closed* AOA: di1 $= 2.1 \pm 0.2$, di2 $= 2.5 \pm 0.5$, dc $= 3.4 \pm 0.4$, dm1 $= 2.9 \pm 0.5$, dm2 $= 3.7 \pm 0.7$

Mean $\pm$ SD in years. Maxillary and mandibular teeth are pooled. *AOA*, age of attainment; *PA*, predicted age.
Based on Liversidge HM, Molleson T. Variation in crown and root formation and eruption of human deciduous teeth. American Journal of Physical Anthropology 2004;123:172–80.

TABLE 4.2.8 Age of Attainment for Eruption Levels and Corresponding Predicted Age

Tooth	Alveolar Eruption	Midpoint	Occlusal Level
di1	0.3 ± 0.1	0.7 ± 0.1	0.9 ± 0.3
	0.5 ± 0.2	**0.8 ± 0.3**	
di2	0.6 ± 0.4	0.9 ± 0.3	1.2 ± 0.3
	0.8 ± 0.4	**1.1 ± 0.3**	
dc	1.1 ± 0.3	1.4 ± 0.4	2.1 ± 0.4
	1.2 ± 0.4	**1.7 ± 0.5**	
dm1	0.9 ± 0.2	1.2 ± 0.3	1.5 ± 0.3
	1.0 ± 0.3	**1.4 ± 0.3**	
dm2	1.3 ± 0.3	2.0 ± 0.5	2.5 ± 0.5
	1.7 ± 0.5	**2.3 ± 0.5**	

Predicted age is in boldface. Mean ± SD in years. Maxillary and mandibular teeth are pooled.
Adapted from Liversidge HM, Molleson T. Variation in crown and root formation and eruption of human deciduous teeth.
American Journal of Physical Anthropology 2004;123:172—80.

The macro AgeEstimation, provided in the companion website in the homonymous file and in OSTEO, may be used for estimating the age of attainment and the predicted age of individuals based on the data given in Tables 4.2.4 and 4.2.6—4.2.8.

Finally, certain studies have examined tooth length in relation to age instead of making qualitative assessments of the growth stage of a tooth. In this direction, Liversidge et al. (1993) examined the development of mandibular and maxillary deciduous and permanent dentitions in individuals from birth to 5.4 years of age and produced regression equations for age prediction for various teeth. Liversidge and Molleson (1999) later produced regression equations for individuals up to the age of 19 years, in which they combined maxillary and mandibular data. Cardoso (2007a) found the Liversidge et al. method to perform well when multiple mandibular and maxillary permanent teeth are used simultaneously (but see some concerns in Cardoso, 2007b).

An important limitation of all methods estimating age at death from dental development is that, owing to secular changes, the applicability of methods developed based on modern samples in archaeological material is uncertain (Halcrow et al., 2007). In addition, females generally mature earlier than males. However, sex is practically impossible to assess in juvenile skeletal remains; thus, estimating age based on dental development without taking sex into account may cause biases (Molinari et al., 2004). Furthermore, although the impact of extrinsic factors on dental development is smaller than on skeletal development, dental emergence is not as unaffected by external stimuli as dental formation (Holman and Yamaguchi, 2005).

4.3 ADULTS

4.3.1 Fusion of Primary and Secondary Ossification Centers

Most of the secondary ossification centers fuse with the primary ones during adolescence, as described earlier. However, specific centers fuse later in life, making them useful age markers for early adulthood. In particular, the *iliac crest* partially fuses with the rest of the pelvis at the age of 14—22 years, and complete fusion occurs after 17 or 18 years (Webb and Suchey, 1985) (Fig. 4.2.4). The *clavicle* is also extremely useful for aging young adults, as it is the last bone to complete epiphyseal fusion. Scheuer and Black (2000) noted that a flake starts to form on the *medial epiphyseal surface* between 12 and 14 years; this flake starts fusing with the rest of the clavicle between 17 and 21 years and completes fusion by 30 years (Fig. 4.2.6).

4.3.2 Morphology of the Pubic Symphysis

The pubic symphysis is the point at which the two halves of the pelvis articulate anteriorly. From early adulthood the surface of the pubic symphysis starts to change, as can be seen in the male pubic symphyses of Fig. 4.3.1. Todd (1920,

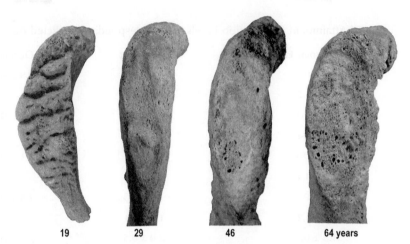

FIGURE 4.3.1 Pubic symphyseal changes in males of known age.

1921) was the first to describe age-related changes in the morphology of the pubic symphysis of white males, which he divided into 10 phases. When Brooks (1955) applied Todd's method to the same skeletal material, she achieved very low accuracy, so she proposed modifications to improve its performance. Subsequently, McKern and Stewart (1957) developed a more complex system, whereby three different components are recorded rather than the symphyseal surface as a whole. Their sample was exclusively male and mostly younger than 35 years. A few years later, Gilbert and McKern (1973) proposed a three-component method for females.

To improve the performance of the pubic symphysis as an age marker, Suchey and Brooks devised new male and female standards that became known as the Suchey–Brooks method (Brooks and Suchey, 1990). This method focuses on the overall morphological change in the symphysis and classifies the observable changes into six phases for each sex, which are visualized, along with the corresponding average age and 95% range, in Figs. 4.3.2 and 4.3.3. The Suchey–Brooks method is currently the preferred one in forensic analyses and osteoarchaeology.

Despite the wide application of this method, it has several limitations. First of all, the limits between successive stages are not clear and there is substantial overlap between them, as seen in Figs. 4.3.2 and 4.3.3. Also, the stages were developed based on modern populations and it is not clear to what degree they can be applied to archaeological material. Finally, it has been noted that this method is accurate for adults up to about 40 years of age. Specifically, the appearance and fusion of the ventral rampart of the pubic symphysis are the main features that make it a valuable aging locus, but this fusion normally occurs before age 35 and all changes after that are degenerative and not strongly correlated with chronological age (Meindl and Russell, 1998; Saunders et al., 1992).

Klepinger et al. (1992) found the Suchey–Brooks method to perform better than earlier aging methods that used the pubic symphysis, but Schmitt (2004) and Fleischman (2013) found it to be inaccurate for old individuals. Finally, Hoppa (2000) stressed the limitations arising from interindividual and interpopulation variation in the timing of the observed morphological changes.

Studies have attempted to refine the Suchey–Brooks method. Berg (2008) reassessed this method for a female sample, adding a seventh stage, as well as redefining stages V and VI. Kimmerle et al. (2008) also provided new age ranges for each phase as well as the age of transition from each phase to the next. More recently, Hartnett (2010a) found significant interobserver error and revised pubic bone phase descriptions and age ranges, as well as proposed a phase VII for individuals in their 70s. In a validation study, Merritt (2014) found that Hartnett's revised method is reliable and improves the accuracy of age estimation, especially among older individuals.

4.3.3 Morphology of the Auricular Surface

Morphological changes on the auricular surface of the ilium have also been found to correlate with biological age. Although age-related changes on the auricular surface were originally noted by Sashin (1930) and later by Kobayashi (1967), Lovejoy et al. (1985) were the first to organize the morphological changes of the auricular surface into eight phases. Each phase covers a 5-year age range, and the final phase includes all individuals older than 60 years. The same phases were used for males and females unless the latter exhibited marked preauricular sulci. The anatomical structures of the auricular surface that are examined in the context of this method are given in Fig. 4.3.4, whereas the age-related changes are given in Box 4.3.1.

FEMALES

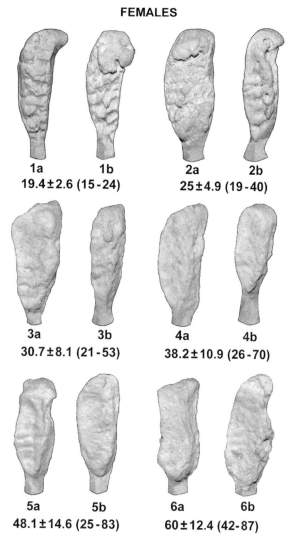

1a	1b	2a	2b
19.4±2.6 (15-24)		25±4.9 (19-40)	

3a	3b	4a	4b
30.7±8.1 (21-53)		38.2±10.9 (26-70)	

5a	5b	6a	6b
48.1±14.6 (25-83)		60±12.4 (42-87)	

FIGURE 4.3.2 Suchey–Brooks stages for females (based on casts by France Casting). Key: The beginning and end of each phase are denoted by "a" and "b," respectively.

In general, in young individuals the auricular surface is finely grained in texture and exhibits regular billowing. In adulthood, surface granularity turns coarser, billowing and striae are reduced, the transverse organization is lost, and the surface shows microporosity. At more advanced ages the surface becomes dense and disorganized and exhibits macroporosity. A brief description of the changes observed in each phase along with the ages that correspond to these phases is given in Table 4.3.1. The original publication should be consulted for more details.

An advantage of auricular surface aging is that this anatomical area is often better preserved than the pubic symphysis, and morphological changes keep occurring even after the age of 50 years. However, a blind test of this method found that the rate at which morphological changes occur is too variable to allow accurate age at death estimation (Murray and Murray, 1991). More recently, Schmitt (2004) noted that this method underestimates age, especially for older individuals, whereas Osborne et al. (2004) found that the 5-year age ranges provided by Lovejoy et al. (1985) are too narrow, correctly classifying only 33% of the sample they examined.

A revised method was developed by Buckberry and Chamberlain (2002) in which surface texture, transverse organization, degree of macro- and microporosity, and morphological changes in the apex and retroauricular areas were scored. Subsequently, the retroauricular area was found not to be an accurate age indicator and was removed from the data set, and the remaining components were scored independently and then summed to generate a composite score. The authors provide a table that assigns the composite scores to stages that correspond to specific age ranges, which are wider than those of Lovejoy et al. (1985). When the Buckberry and Chamberlain method was tested in different samples, the results were contradictory, with Falys et al. (2006) finding it to perform

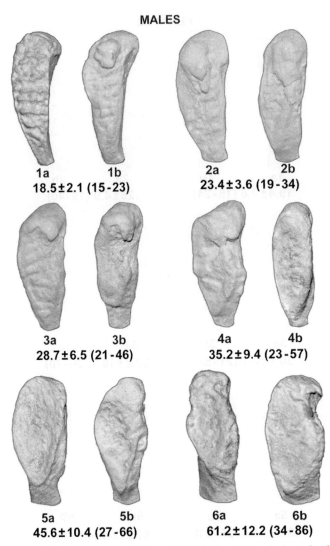

FIGURE 4.3.3 Suchey–Brooks stages for males (based on casts by France Casting). Key: The beginning and end of each phase are denoted by "a" and "b," respectively.

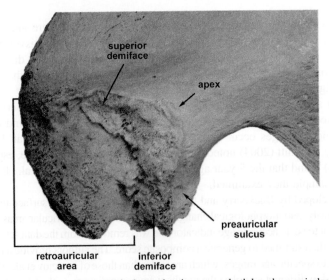

FIGURE 4.3.4 Anatomical structures examined when estimating age at death based on auricular surface morphology.

BOX 4.3.1 Aspects of Auricular Surface Morphology (Lovejoy et al., 1985)

- Porosity
  - Microporosity: tiny perforations
  - Macroporosity: perforations with 1- to 10-mm diameter
- Grain (sandpaper appearance)
- Billowing (transverse ridges)
- Density (compact and smooth subchondral bone)

TABLE 4.3.1 Auricular Surface Phase Descriptions

Phase	Description
Phase 1 (20–24 years)	Billowing and fine granularity; no porosity
Phase 2 (25–29 years)	Decreased billowing and replacement by striae; slightly coarser granularity; no porosity
Phase 3 (30–34 years)	Billowing minimally preserved and replaced by striae; patches of coarse granularity; possibly limited microporosity
Phase 4 (35–39 years)	Uniform coarse granularity; billowing and striae almost eliminated; slight microporosity
Phase 5 (40–44 years)	Decreased granularity and patches of dense surface; no billowing; occasional macroporosity
Phase 6 (45–49 years)	Complete densification and loss of granularity; little or no microporosity and macroporosity; increasingly irregular margins
Phase 7 (50–55 years)	Dense irregular surface; rugged topography; changes in periauricular areas; irregular margins
Phase 8 (60 years and greater)	Irregular surface with subchondral destruction and macroporosity; marginal lipping; marked changes in periauricular areas

Adapted from Lovejoy CO, Meindl RS, Pryzbeck TR, Mensforth RP. Chronological metamorphosis of the auricular surface of the ilium: a new method for the determination of adult skeletal age at death. American Journal of Physical Anthropology 1985;68:15–28.

poorly overall, Moraitis et al. (2014) supporting that it gives reliable results, and Mulhern and Jones (2005) suggesting that it performs better than the original method only for older individuals.

Osborne et al. (2004) proposed an alternative six-phase method, in which each phase corresponds to broader age ranges compared to the 5-year intervals of Lovejoy et al. Igarashi et al. (2005) also developed a new method using a binary recording scheme of presence/absence for 13 variables. The binary scores were used in a multiple regression analysis to obtain an estimated age. According to the authors, their method performs better than previous ones, especially for older individuals.

4.3.4 Suture Closure

At birth the cranium consists of several bones, between which lie sutures (see Chapter 1). These cranial bones fuse together as the sutures gradually close with increasing age. Todd and Lyon were the first to systematically explore cranial suture closure as an age marker, examining endocranial (1924) and ectocranial sutures (1925), whereas a more detailed study was published by Nemeskéri et al. (1960).

Meindl and Lovejoy (1985) published the most widely used aging method based on ectocranial suture closure, described in Box 4.3.2. However, because of the large standard deviations and observed ranges (see Fig. 4.3.6), the authors reached the conclusion that "suture closure can provide valuable estimates of age at death in both archaeological and forensic contexts when used in conjunction with other skeletal age indicators" (Meindl and Lovejoy, 1985, p. 57).

In addition to the aforementioned, Mann et al. (1991) proposed a method for estimating age from the maxillary sutures. The authors observed that the sequence of obliteration of the incisive suture, the anterior and posterior median palatine sutures, and the transverse palatine suture (Fig. 4.3.7) follows the general pattern shown in Table 4.3.2. Ginter (2005) tested this method and found an accuracy rate of 83%, though he stressed that it tends to underestimate age in all age groups and it performs best for older individuals.

BOX 4.3.2 Meindl–Lovejoy (1985) method

Step 1. A series of 1-cm segments is inspected ectocranially on specific sutures or suture sites. These segments are shown in the following figure. Note that these segments belong to two different systems. The *vault system* encompasses suture sites 1–7, and the *lateral–anterior system* includes sites 6–10. Specifically, the segments examined are the following:

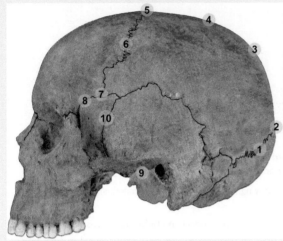

Vault system:

Suture sites: (1) midlambdoid, (2) lambda, (3) obelion, (4) anterior sagittal, (5) bregma, (6) midcoronal, and (7) pterion.

Lateral–anterior system:

Suture sites: (6) midcoronal, (7) pterion, (8) sphenofrontal, (9) inferior sphenotemporal (on the sphenotemporal suture at the level of a line connecting the articular tubercles of the temporomandibular joint; see Fig. 1.7.3 for the location of the sphenotemporal suture), and (10) superior sphenotemporal (2 cm below the intersection of the sphenotemporal suture with the parietal bone).

Step 2. The degree of suture closure is recorded for each segment as follows (Fig. 4.3.5):

0 = open
1 = minimal closure (<50%)
2 = significant closure (>50% but not fully fused)
3 = complete closure

Step 3. A composite score of suture closure is calculated by summing the individual scores for each site within each system. Thus, a separate composite score is obtained for the vault system (range 0–21) and for the lateral–anterior system (range 0–15).

Step 4. The composite score is translated into an approximate age at death based on the tables presented in the original paper (Meindl and Lovejoy, 1985) or using Fig. 4.3.6, which has been drawn from these data. Alternatively, the macro AgeEstimation, provided in the companion website, may be used.

Note: The lateral–anterior system was found to give better results than the vault system (Meindl and Lovejoy, 1985).

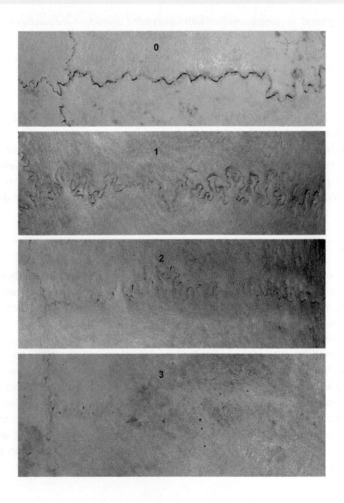

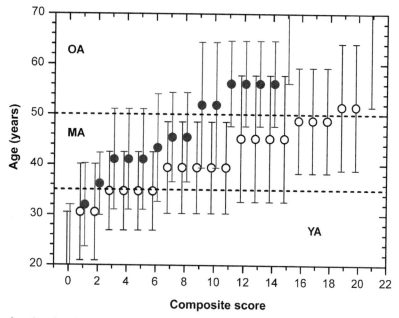

FIGURE 4.3.6 Estimation of age based on the composite score, 0–21 for the vault system (○) and 0–15 for the lateral–anterior system (●), based on the Meindl–Lovejoy method. *YA, young adult; MA, middle adult, OA, old adult.*

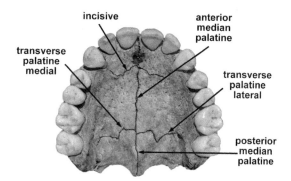

FIGURE 4.3.7 Maxillary sutures used as age markers.

TABLE 4.3.2 Age of Fusion for Maxillary Sutures

Suture	Age (years)
Incisive	20–25
Posterior median palatine	25–35
Transverse palatine lateral	35+
Transverse palatine medial	40+
Anterior median palatine	50+

Adapted from Mann RW, Jantz RL, Bass WM, Willey PS. Maxillary suture obliteration: a visual method for estimating skeletal age. Journal of Forensic Sciences 1991;36:781–91.

Regarding endocranial sutures, Buikstra and Ubelaker (1994) recommend scoring the entire sagittal suture, the left lambdoid, and the left coronal, as shown in Fig. 4.3.8. Overall, endocranial sutures start closing in young adulthood, middle adults exhibit advanced but incomplete closure, and older adults manifest complete fusion.

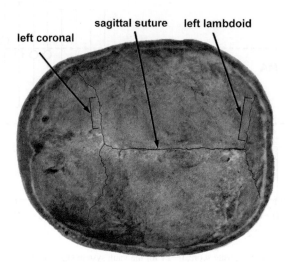

FIGURE 4.3.8 Endocranial sutures examined for age estimation.

An aging method that combines ectocranial, endocranial, and maxillary sutures was developed by Nawrocki (1998). The author recorded suture closure on 27 locations per skull using an ordinal scheme from 0 to 3. Subsequently, he proposed regression equations for the estimation of age based on various combinations of sutural landmarks.

A number of studies evaluated aging methods based on suture closure, and their results are not encouraging (e.g., Hershkovitz et al., 1997; Key et al., 1994). The general conclusion is that although cranial sutures progressively become obliterated, the substantial variability in the rate of suture closure limits the value of this method for age estimation. As a result, suture closure is a useful age indicator only when other criteria are not available or when used in association with other methods, as noted by Meindl and Lovejoy (1985) (see above).

4.3.5 Morphology of the Sternal Rib End

Age-related changes at the sternal rib end have also been explored as age markers (Fig. 4.3.9). Such changes were first noted by Kerley (1970), Semine and Damon (1975), and McCormick (1980), but İşcan et al. (1984, 1985) expanded upon previous work and developed age phases based on morphological changes at the sternal end of the right fourth rib. Specifically, the authors noted that initially the sternal rib end is flat or billowy with rounded edges. Gradually the rim becomes thinner and irregular, and surface porosity and an overall ragged appearance develop. Brief descriptions of the sternal rib-end morphological changes observed with age in males and females are given in Tables 4.3.3 and 4.3.4. The original publication should be consulted for more details, but the method is also described in many standard textbooks such as Ubelaker (1989). In addition, France Casting has produced a series of casts that facilitate the identification of the various phases.

Although the original phases were designed for the right fourth rib, Loth and İşcan (1989) reported that there is no bilateral asymmetry and that ribs 3 and 5 usually exhibit the same phase as rib 4. Dudar (1993) found that the method proposed by İşcan and his colleagues can actually be applied on any rib from the third to the ninth. Loth (1995) tested this method and found it to be overall useful for archaeological samples. Similarly, Saunders et al. (1992) found this method to perform best for individuals under 30 and between 40 and 59 years of age, but to be a poor age marker for individuals older than 60 years. Finally, Cerezo-Román and Hernández Espinoza (2014) found it to generally underestimate age at death.

Attempts to refine this method have been made by Oettlé and Steyn (2000), who adjusted it for South African black males and females by developing new phases and age ranges. In addition, Yoder et al. (2001) suggested the use of a

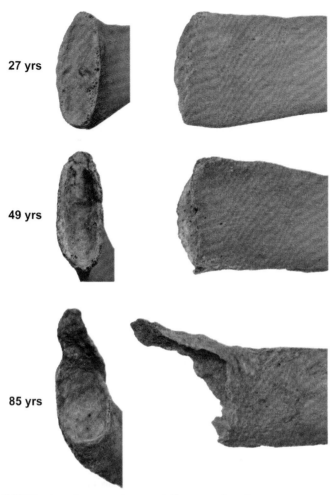

27 yrs

49 yrs

85 yrs

FIGURE 4.3.9   Representative sternal rib-end morphological changes with age.

TABLE 4.3.3 Descriptions of Sternal Rib-End Changes in Males

Phase	Description
Phases 0 and 1 (<19 years)	Pit: Originally flat or billowy, deepening in later stages
	Rim: Regular with occasional scalloping in later stages
	Bone: Smooth and solid
Phases 2 to 4 (20–32 years)	Pit: Increased depth, V shaped but gradually turning moderately wide U shaped
	Walls: Originally thick but growing thinner in later stages
	Rim: Initially scalloped or wavy but more irregular in later stages
	Bone: Overall solid
Phases 5 and 6 (33–55 years)	Pit: Markedly deep and wide U shaped
	Walls: Thin with sharp edges
	Rim: Irregular with projections but no scalloping
	Bone: Increased porosity
Phases 7 and 8 (55 years and greater)	Pit: Very deep and wide U shaped; floor absent or filled with projections
	Walls: Extremely thin with sharp irregular edges and bony projections; occasional "window" formation
	Bone: Very brittle and porous.

Adapted from İşcan MY, Loth SR, Wright RK. Age estimation from the rib by phase analysis: white males. Journal of Forensic Sciences 1984;29: 1094–104.

TABLE 4.3.4 Descriptions of Sternal Rib-End Changes in Females

Phase	Description
Phases 0 and 1 (<15 years)	Pit: Initially flat surface with ridges or billows, but slight deepening and partial loss of the ridges and billows in later stages
	Rim: Regular with rounded edges and slight waviness in later stages
	Bone: Smooth and solid
Phases 2 to 4 (16–32 years)	Pit: Increased depth, initially V shaped but gradually turning narrow U shaped, ridges or billowing possibly still present
	Walls: Thick but growing thinner in later stages
	Rim: Wavy with some scalloping
	Bone: Firm and solid with slight loss of density in later stages
Phases 5 and 6 (33–58 years)	Pit: Increased depth, wider V or U shaped; lined by a plaque-like deposit
	Walls: Thin
	Rim: Irregular, with sharp edges, projections, and no scalloping
	Bone: Lighter and brittle
Phases 7 and 8 (59 years and greater)	Pit: Slight decrease in depth; flared U shaped, with eroded floor, occasionally filled with bony growths
	Walls: Very thin, "window" formation in later stages
	Rim: Irregular with sharp edges and projections
	Bone: Very thin and brittle

Adapted from İşcan MY, Loth SR, Wright RK. Age estimation from the rib by phase analysis: white females. Journal of Forensic Sciences 1985;30:853–63.

composite score obtained by recording sternal rib-end changes on multiple ribs. In addition, Hartnett (2010b) made small changes to the description of the stages, proposed narrower age ranges, suggested new means per phase, and included bone quality and density as variables. However, the author found that variation among individuals of the same age phase was much larger than expected. When testing the Hartnett method, Merritt (2014) noted that it is reliable and gives results comparable to the original method, but it performs better for older adults.

Finally, Kunos et al. (1999) and DiGangi et al. (2009) proposed aging methods based on the first rib. The former method produced low accuracies when tested in independent samples (Kurki, 2005; Schmitt and Murail, 2004). The method by DiGangi et al. evaluated 11 traits focused on the costal face, rib head, and tubercle facet, and found that two of them were the most useful in age estimation: geometric shape of the costal face and surface texture of the tubercle facet. According to the authors, this method can be equally applied to individuals of all ages from adolescence onward; however, the analysis was limited to males, and testing in different assemblages is required before its use can be generalized.

4.3.6 Dentition

4.3.6.1 Dental Wear

As examined in the previous section, the dentition is an important age marker in subadults because the formation and eruption of teeth are largely genetically controlled and well documented. In adults, the dentition may also be used to estimate age, primarily by means of dental wear rates. The calibration of the rate of molar wear in archaeological populations is based on juvenile dentitions. Specifically, the first molar erupts at the age of approximately 6 years, the second at the age of 12 years, and the third at the age of 18 years. Therefore, the amount of wear accumulated on the first molar when the second molar has just erupted indicates how much wear should be expected on a tooth that has been in occlusion for about 6 years. Similarly, when the third molar erupts, the first will have accumulated 12 years of wear, and the second 6 years. Therefore, the different eruption times of the three molars can be used to calibrate dental wear and subsequently estimate an individual's age at death by assessing the number of years during which the observed wear accumulated (Miles, 1963).

Using dental wear as an age indicator has a number of limitations. First of all, molars do not wear at the same rate, because it has been found that the second molar takes around 6½ years to accumulate the same amount of wear levels that the first molar accumulated in 6, whereas the third molar requires 7 years for the same purpose (Miles, 1963). Another important precondition is that a large number of juveniles are required to calibrate the rate of dental wear (Mays, 2010). Moreover, dental wear in juveniles is not necessarily a good indicator of the rate of wear in adults because adults have larger jaw muscles, and increased mechanical loading and subsequent wear compared to subadults (Whittaker, 2000).

Prince et al. (2008) employed a Bayesian approach and concluded that interindividual dental wear variation is too large to allow for accurate age estimation, and dental wear methods should rather be used for grouping individuals into large age classes. More recently, Gilmore and Grote (2012) proposed a modification of the Miles method, which overcomes the issue of using juveniles to calibrate wear rate and may be applied even in heterogeneous samples according to the authors; however, the accuracy of this method has not yet been tested in other samples.

4.3.6.2 The Lamendin Method

Lamendin et al. (1992) proposed a macroscopic method for estimating adult age from single-rooted teeth based on periodontosis and root transparency, both recorded on the labial root surface. The steps followed in this method are described in Box 4.3.3.

Tests of this method have given contradictory results. For example, Ackermann and Steyn (2014) found it to perform poorly, whereas Prince and Ubelaker (2002) concluded that it works well overall. The latter suggested that the performance of the method can be improved further by using separate equations for different sexes and ancestry groups, as follows:

- Black males: Age (years) $= 1.04 \times RH + 0.31 \times P + 0.47 \times T + 1.70$
- White males: Age (years) $= 0.15 \times RH + 0.29 \times P + 0.39 \times T + 23.17$
- Black females: Age (years) $= 1.63 \times RH + 0.48 \times P + 0.48 \times T - 8.41$
- White females: Age (years) $= 1.10 \times RH + 0.31 \times P + 0.39 \times T + 11.82$

In these equations RH is the root height, and the other terms are the same as in the original Lamendin formula (Box 4.3.3). All measurements are in millimeters.

BOX 4.3.3 Steps for Age Estimation From Intact Teeth

1. Extract the tooth carefully.
2. Measure the periodontosis height (distance from the cementoenamel junction to the periodontal attachment line; in skeletal remains this line is yellowish, and stain and dental calculus deposits may be found across its length).

3. Measure the transparency height (distance from the root apex to the maximum height of transparency; viewed under transmitted light).
4. Measure the root height.
5. Apply the following formula:
   Age (years) $= 0.18 \times P + 0.42 \times T + 25.53$,
   where $P = $ (periodontosis height $\times$ 100)/root height and $T = $ (root transparency height $\times$ 100)/root height.
   Note: All measurements are in millimeters.

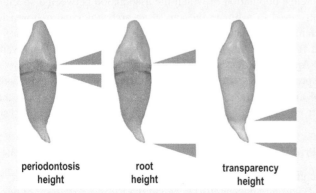

periodontosis height   root height   transparency height

From Lamendin H, Baccino E, Humbert JF, Tavernier JC, Nossintchouk RM, Zerilli A. A simple technique for age estimation in adult corpses: the two criteria dental method. Journal of Forensic Sciences 1992;37:1373–9.

The Lamendin method and its extension by Prince and Ubelaker are implemented in the macro AgeEstimation in the homonymous Excel file or in the OSTEO package.

Among the limitations of these approaches is that root transparency develops later in life; thus such methods are most appropriate for individuals aged 40−65 years. In addition, in skeletal remains, especially of archaeological nature, it may be difficult or even impossible to identify periodontosis height. Furthermore, the aforementioned methods have been found not to give accurate results in cases of skeletal remains that have been buried even for a few years because of the influence of the soil (De Angelis et al., 2015). Finally, when interpreting the obtained results, it must be remembered that poor oral hygiene could accelerate the rate of periodontosis.

4.3.7 Other Age Markers

An area of the pelvis that has received attention as an age marker is the acetabulum. Rissech et al. (2006), based on the work by Rougé-Maillart et al. (2004), identified seven traits that exhibit a high correlation with age in males: acetabular groove, rim shape, rim porosity, apex activity, activity on the outer edge of the acetabular fossa, fossa activity, and fossa porosity. The authors provide detailed descriptions of these traits and photographs, and report an accuracy of 89% when using 10-year intervals and 67% when adopting 5-year intervals. Subsequent testing of this method achieved accuracy rates between 83% and 100% (Rissech et al., 2007); however, the method does not appear to be as accurate for groups geographically distant from the reference sample, although it performs well in individuals older than 40 years (Calce and Rogers, 2011). Calce (2012) revised the Rissech et al. (2006) method using a subset of the original variables, pooling the age classes into three broad groups (young, middle, and old adults) and expanding its application to females. Although the author reported a correct classification rate of 81% when using this method in a North American sample, Mays (2014) found it to perform poorly (45% correct classifications) in British material.

Ríos et al. (2008) proposed a method for age estimation based on the fusion of sacral vertebrae. A more complex technique focused on the sacrum was developed by Passalacqua (2009) and considers both developmental and degenerative changes. A test of the Passalacqua method by Colarusso (2016) concluded that although this method exhibits particularly high accuracy and small interobserver error rates, its large age ranges limit its utility, especially in forensic contexts.

4.3.8 Multifactorial Age Estimation: Transition Analysis

It is generally supported that combining multiple age indicators offers a more accurate age at death estimate than using only one. However, there is no consensus as to the optimal way to combine multiple indicators. Some common practices are to use: (1) the overlap of age ranges provided by different methods, (2) the entire age range provided by different methods, or (3) the lowest range of the method giving the oldest age and the highest range of the method giving the youngest age. However, none of these approaches is statistically valid (Garvin et al., 2012). An approach that appears to overcome this limitation and to effectively combine multiple age indicators is *transition analysis*.

4.3.8.1 The Basis of Transition Analysis

All aging methods have been developed using a modern reference population in which the association between a specific age marker and biological age was assessed and subsequently used to estimate the age of an archaeological or forensic target population. However, the age distribution of the reference population affects the age distribution of the target population. In particular, aging methods tend to replicate the age distribution of the sample on which these methods were developed, a phenomenon known as *age mimicry* (Bocquet-Appel and Masset, 1982).

A way to overcome this issue is by means of Bayesian approaches coupled with transition analysis. Transition analysis estimates the age of transition between successive stages of an age marker, whereas Bayesian approaches compute the conditional probability $\Pr(a|c)$ that the skeletal remains are from an individual who died at age a given that the observed age marker is c, via Bayes's theorem:

$$\Pr(a|c) \propto \Pr(c|a) \mathrm{f}(a) \tag{4.3.1}$$

where $\Pr(c|a)$ is the probability of observing an age marker c given that the individual died at age a, and $\mathrm{f}(a)$ is the age at death distribution of the population we analyze. Note that in Bayesian analysis, $\mathrm{f}(a)$ is called the *prior distribution of ages at death*, because it must be known prior to the estimation of $\Pr(a|c)$.

Eq. (4.3.1) allows the calculation of the maximum-likelihood age at death curve of an individual. The value of a that maximizes this function is the maximum-likelihood estimate of the age at death of the individual. As seen from Eq. (4.3.1), for the computation of $\Pr(a|c)$, we should first estimate $\Pr(c|a)$, usually with a proper regression of c on a using data from a reference population. In addition, the reference population is used for the estimation of $f(a)$, also employed in the computation of $\Pr(c|a)$. Thus, the choice of the reference population is crucial for the correct estimation of $\Pr(c|a)$.

4.3.8.2 The ADBOU Software

Transition analysis is a promising approach for age estimation; however, its implementation requires specialized software. As of this writing, two programs have been created for this purpose: NPHASES2 and ADBOU.

NPHASES2 was created by Lyle Konigsberg and computes the mean age of transition between adjacent stages of a single age indicator and its standard deviation. It is freely available at http://konig.la.utk.edu/nphases2.htm.

ADBOU is the most complete and user-friendly option for transition analysis, as of this writing. It was designed by Boldsen et al. (2002), is freely available to download at http://math.mercyhurst.edu/~sousley/Software/, and may soon be integrated into FORDISC. ADBOU uses three age indicators that are based on five traits of the pubic symphysis, nine traits of the iliac auricular surface, and five cranial sutures. The scoring of these indicators is briefly outlined in Box 4.3.4, whereas Boldsen et al. (2002) offer a detailed account of all the age markers recorded and their character states. The software allows missing values as well as the separate scoring of the right and left sides of the pubic symphysis and auricular surface, and it accepts intermediate scores between phases if necessary. ADBOU calculates a maximum-likelihood estimate of age using either an archaeological or a forensic prior probability function $f(a)$. The archaeological prior originates from 17th-century rural Danish parish records, whereas the forensic prior was drawn from US homicide data (Boldsen et al., 2002). A case study demonstrating the application of ADBOU, coupled with other methods presented in this chapter, is given in Appendix 4.IV.

BOX 4.3.4 Scoring Categories for Input Into ADBOU

Cranial Sutures (Coronal, Sagittal, Lambdoid, Interpalatine, Zygomaticomaxillary)

All Sutures Are Recorded Ectocranially as:

1. Open
2. Juxtaposed (except for interpalatine)
3. Partially obliterated
4. Punctuated
5. Obliterated

Pubic Symphysis

Topography	Texture	Superior Protuberance	Ventral Margin	Dorsal Margin
1. Sharp billows	1. Smooth	1. No protuberance	1. Serrated	1. Serrated
2. Soft, deep billows	2. Coarse	2. Early protuberance	2. Beveled	2. Flattening incomplete
3. Soft, shallow billows	3. Microporosity	3. Late protuberance	3. Rampart formation	3. Flattening complete
4. Residual billows	4. Macroporosity	4. Integrated	4. Rampart completion I	4. Rim
5. Flat			5. Rampart completion II	5. Breakdown
6. Irregular			6. Rim	
			7. Breakdown	

Auricular Surface

Superior/Inferior Topography	Superior/Apical/Inferior Characteristics	Inferior Texture	Superior/Inferior Exostoses	Posterior Exostoses
1. Undulating	1. Billows cover more than 2/3 of the surface	1. Smooth	1. Smooth	1. Smooth
2. Median elevation	2. Billows cover 1/3 to 2/3 of the surface	2. Microporosity	2. Rounded exostoses	2. Rounded exostoses
3. Flat to irregular	3. Billows cover less than 1/3 of the surface	3. Macroporosity	3. Pointed exostoses	3. Pointed spicules
	4. Flat		4. Jagged exostoses	
	5. Bumps		5. Touching exostoses	
			6. Fused	

From Boldsen JL, Milner GR, Konigsberg LW, Wood JW. Transition analysis: a new method for estimating age from skeletons. In: Hoppa RD, Vaupel J, editors. Paleodemography: age distributions from skeletal samples. Cambridge: Cambridge University Press; 2002. p. 73–106.

Although transition analysis is a promising method for age at death estimation, tests of the method revealed that the three age indicators used do not perform equally well; the pubic symphysis performs satisfactorily, whereas the cranial sutures produce the least accurate results. Discussions of the possible reasons for the reduced reliability of ADBOU are presented in Bethard (2005) and Milner and Boldsen (2012).

REFERENCES

Ackermann A, Steyn M. A test of the Lamendin method of age estimation in South African canines. Forensic Science International 2014;236. 192.e1–192.e6.

AlQahtani SJ, Hector MP, Liversidge HM. Brief communication: the London atlas of human tooth development and eruption. American Journal of Physical Anthropology 2010;142:481–90.

AlQahtani SJ, Hector MP, Liversidge HM. Accuracy of dental age estimation charts: Schour and Massler, Ubelaker, and the London atlas. American Journal of Physical Anthropology 2014;154:70–8.

De Angelis D, Mele E, Gibelli D, Merelli V, Spagnoli L, Cattaneo C. The applicability of the Lamendin method to skeletal remains buried for a 16-year period: a cautionary note. Journal of Forensic Sciences 2015;60:S177–81.

Baker BJ, Dupras TL, Tocheri MW. Osteology of infants and children. College Station: Texas A&M University Press; 2005.

Berg GE. Pubic bone age estimation in adult women. Journal of Forensic Sciences 2008;53:569–77.

Bethard JD. A test of the transition analysis method for estimation of age-at-death in adult human skeletal remains [MA thesis]. Knoxville: The University of Tennessee; 2005.

Bocquet-Appel J-P, Masset C. Farewell to paleodemography. Journal of Human Evolution 1982;11:321–33.

Boldsen JL, Milner GR, Konigsberg LW, Wood JW. Transition analysis: a new method for estimating age from skeletons. In: Hoppa RD, Vaupel J, editors. Paleodemography: age distributions from skeletal samples. Cambridge: Cambridge University Press; 2002. p. 73–106.

Brooks ST. Skeletal age at death: the reliability of cranial and pubic age indicators. American Journal of Physical Anthropology 1955;13:567–89.

Brooks S, Suchey JM. Skeletal age determination based on the os pubis: a comparison of the Acsadi-Nemeskeri and Suchey-Brooks methods. Human Evolution 1990;5:227–38.

Buckberry JL, Chamberlain AT. Age estimation from the auricular surface of the ilium: a revised method. American Journal of Physical Anthropology 2002;119:213–39.

Fayetteville, Arkansas: Arkansas Archaeological Survey Report Number 44. In: Buikstra JE, Ubelaker DH, editors. Standards for data collection from human skeletal remains; 1994.

Calce SE. A new method to estimate adult age-at-death using the acetabulum. American Journal of Physical Anthropology 2012;148:11–23.

Calce SE, Rogers TL. Evaluation of age estimation technique: testing traits of the acetabulum to estimate age at death in adult males. Journal of Forensic Sciences 2011;56:302–11.

Cardoso HF. Accuracy of developing tooth length as an estimate of age in human skeletal remains: the deciduous dentition. Forensic Science International 2007a;172:17–22.

Cardoso HF. A test of the differential accuracy of the maxillary versus the mandibular dentition in age estimations of immature skeletal remains based on developing tooth length. Journal of Forensic Sciences 2007b;52:434–7.

Cerezo-Román JI, Hernández Espinoza PO. Estimating age at death using the sternal end of the fourth ribs from Mexican males. Forensic Science International 2014;236. 196.e1–196.e6.

Colarusso T. A test of the Passalacqua age at death estimation method using the sacrum. Journal of Forensic Sciences 2016;61:S22–9.

Demirjian A, Goldstein H. New systems for dental maturity based on seven and four teeth. Annals of Human Biology 1976;3:411–21.

Demirjian A, Goldstein H, Tanner JM. A new system of dental age assessment. Human Biology 1973;42:211–27.

DiGangi EA, Bethard JD, Kimmerle EH, Konigsberg LW. A new method for estimating age-at-death from the first rib. American Journal of Physical Anthropology 2009;138:164–76.

Dudar CJ. Identification of rib number and assessment of intercostal variation at the sternal rib end. Journal of Forensic Sciences 1993;38:788–97.

Falys CG, Schutkowski H, Weston DA. Auricular surface aging: worse than expected? A test of the revised method on a documented historic skeletal assemblage. American Journal of Physical Anthropology 2006;130:508–13.

Fazekas G, Kósa F. Forensic fetal osteology. Budapest: Akadémiai Kiadó; 1978.

Fleischman JM. A comparative assessment of the Chen et al. and Suchey-Brooks pubic aging methods on a North American sample. Journal of Forensic Sciences 2013;58:311–23.

Garvin HM, Passalacqua NV, Uhl NM, Gipson DR, Overbury RS, Cabo LL. Developments in forensic anthropology: age-at-death estimation. In: Dirkmaat DC, editor. A companion to forensic anthropology and archaeology. Chichester: Blackwell Publishing; 2012. p. 202–23.

Gaur R, Kumar P. Effect of undernutrition on deciduous tooth emergence among Rajput children of Shimla District of Himachal Pradesh, India. American Journal of Physical Anthropology 2012;148:54–61.

Gilbert BM, McKern TW. A method for aging the female os pubis. American Journal of Physical Anthropology 1973;38:31–8.

Gilmore CC, Grote MN. Estimating age from adult occlusal wear: a modification of the Miles method. American Journal of Physical Anthropology 2012;149:181–92.

Ginter JK. A test of the effectiveness of the revised maxillary suture obliteration method in estimating adult age at death. Journal of Forensic Sciences 2005;50:1303–9.

Halcrow SE, Tayles N, Buckley HR. Age estimation of children in prehistoric Southeast Asia: are the standards used appropriate? Journal of Archae-

Hartnett KM. Analysis of age-at-death estimation using data from a new, modern autopsy sample — part I: pubic bone. Journal of Forensic Sciences 2010a;55:1145—51.

Hartnett KM. Analysis of age-at-death estimation using data from a new, modern autopsy sample — part II: sternal end of first rib. Journal of Forensic Sciences 2010b;55:1152—6.

Hauspie R, Chrzastek-Spruch H, Verleyen G, Kozlowska M, Suzsanne C. Determinates of growth in body length from birth to 6 years of age: a longitudinal study of Dublin children. International Journal of Anthropology 1994;9:202.

Hershkovitz I, Latimer B, Dutour O, Jellema LM, Wish-Baratz S, Rothschild C, Rothschild BM. Why do we fail in ageing the skull from the sagittal suture? American Journal of Physical Anthropology 1997;103:393—9.

Holman DJ, Yamaguchi K. Longitudinal analysis of deciduous tooth emergence: IV. Covariate effects in Japanese children. American Journal of Physical Anthropology 2005;126:352—8.

Hoppa RD. Population variation in osteological aging criteria: an example from the pubic symphysis. American Journal of Physical Anthropology 2000;111:185—91.

Hoppa RD, FitzGerald CM. From head to toe: integrating studies from bones to teeth in biological anthropology. In: Hoppa RD, FitzGerald CM, editors. Human growth in the past: studies from bones and teeth. Cambridge: Cambridge University Press; 2005. p. 1—32.

Humphrey L. Growth studies of past populations: an overview and an example. In: Cox M, Mays S, editors. Human osteology in archaeology and forensic science. London: Greenwich Medical Media; 2000. p. 23—38.

Igarashi Y, Uesu K, Wakebe T, Kanazawa E. New method for estimation of adult skeletal age at death from the morphology of the auricular surface of the ilium. American Journal of Physical Anthropology 2005;128:324—39.

İşcan MY, Loth SR, Wright RK. Age estimation from the rib by phase analysis: white males. Journal of Forensic Sciences 1984;29:1094—104.

İşcan MY, Loth SR, Wright RK. Age estimation from the rib by phase analysis: white females. Journal of Forensic Sciences 1985;30:853—63.

Kerley ER. Estimation of skeletal age: after about 30 years. In: Stewart TD, editor. Personal identification in mass disasters. Washington: National Museum of Natural History; 1970. p. 57—70.

Key CA, Aiello LC, Molleson T. Cranial suture closure and its implications for age estimation. International Journal of Osteoarchaeology 1994;4:193—207.

Kimmerle EH, Konigsberg LW, Jantz RL, Barabyar JP. Analysis of age-at-death estimation through the use of pubic symphyseal data. Journal of Forensic Sciences 2008;53:558—68.

Klepinger LL, Katz D, Micozzi MS, Carroll L. Evaluation of cast methods for estimating age from the os pubis. Journal of Forensic Sciences 1992;37:763—70.

Kobayashi K. Trends in human life based upon human skeletons from prehistoric to modern times in Japan. Journal of Faculty of Science University of Tokyo 1967;3:107—62.

Kósa F, Castellana C. New forensic anthropological approachment for the age determination of human fetal skeletons on the base of morphometry of vertebral column. Forensic Science International 2005;147(Suppl.):S69—74.

Kunos CA, Simpson SW, Russell KF, Hershkovitz I. First rib metamorphosis: its possible utility for human age-at-death estimation. American Journal of Physical Anthropology 1999;110:303—23.

Kurki H. Use of the first rib for adult age estimation: a test of one method. International Journal of Osteoarchaeology 2005;15:342—50.

Lamendin H, Baccino E, Humbert JF, Tavernier JC, Nossintchouk RM, Zerilli A. A simple technique for age estimation in adult corpses: the two criteria dental method. Journal of Forensic Sciences 1992;37:1373—9.

Lee SE, Lee S-H, Lee J-Y, Park H-K, Kim Y-K. Age estimation of Korean children based on dental maturity. Forensic Science International 2008;178:125—31.

Lewis ME. The bioarchaeology of children. Perspectives from biological and forensic anthropology. Cambridge: Cambridge University Press; 2009.

Liversidge HM. Accuracy of age estimation from developing teeth of a population of known age (0—5.4 years). International Journal of Osteoarchaeology 1994;4:37—45.

Liversidge HM, Molleson T. Developing permanent tooth length as an estimate of age. Journal of Forensic Sciences 1999;44:917—20.

Liversidge HM, Molleson T. Variation in crown and root formation and eruption of human deciduous teeth. American Journal of Physical Anthropology 2004;123:172—80.

Liversidge HM, Dean MC, Molleson TI. Increasing human tooth length between birth and 5.4 years. American Journal of Physical Anthropology 1993;90:307—13.

Loth SR. Age assessment of the Spitalfields cemetery population by rib phase analysis. American Journal of Human Biology 1995;7:465—71.

Loth SR, İşcan MY. Morphological assessment of age in the adult: the thoracic region. In: İşcan MY, editor. Age markers in the human skeleton. Springfield: Charles C. Thomas; 1989. p. 105—35.

Lovejoy CO, Meindl RS, Pryzbeck TR, Mensforth RP. Chronological metamorphosis of the auricular surface of the ilium: a new method for the determination of adult skeletal age at death. American Journal of Physical Anthropology 1985;68:15—28.

Madden G. Age and sex. In: Wilczak CA, Dudar JC, editors. Osteoware™ Software Manual, vol. I. Washington: Smithsonian Institution; 2011. p. 19—44.

Mann RW, Jantz RL, Bass WM, Willey PS. Maxillary suture obliteration: a visual method for estimating skeletal age. Journal of Forensic Sciences 1991;36:781—91.

Maresh MM. Measurements from roentgenograms. In: McCammon RW, editor. Human growth and development. Springfield, IL: Charles C. Thomas; 1970. p. 157—200.

Mays S. The archaeology of human bones. 2nd ed. New York: Routledge; 2010.

Mays S. A test of a recently devised method of estimating skeletal age at death using features of the adult acetabulum. Journal of Forensic Sciences 2014;59:184

McKern TW, Stewart TD. Skeletal age changes in young American males. Natick, Massachusetts: Headquarters Quartermaster Research and Development Command Technical Report EP-45; 1957.

Meindl RS, Lovejoy CO. Ectocranial suture closure: a revised method for the determination of skeletal age at death based on the lateral-anterior sutures. American Journal of Physical Anthropology 1985;68:57−66.

Meindl RS, Russell KF. Recent advances in method and theory in paleodemography. Annual Review of Anthropology 1998;27:375−99.

Merritt CE. A test of Hartnett's revisions to the pubic symphysis and fourth rib methods on a modern sample. Journal of Forensic Sciences 2014;59:703−11.

Miles AEW. Dentition and the estimation of age. Journal of Dental Research 1963;42:255−63.

Milner GR, Boldsen JL. Transition analysis: a validation study with known-age modern American skeletons. American Journal of Physical Anthropology 2012;148:98−110.

Molinari L, Gasser T, Largo RH. TW3 bone age: RUS/CB and gender differences of percentiles for score and score increments. Annals of Human Biology 2004;31:421−35.

Moorrees CFA, Fanning EA, Hunt Jr EE. Formation and resorption of three deciduous teeth in children. American Journal of Physical Anthropology 1963;21:205−13.

Moraitis K, Zorba E, Eliopoulos C, Fox SC. A test of the revised auricular surface aging method on a modern European population. Journal of Forensic Sciences 2014;59:188−94.

Mulhern DM, Jones EB. Test of revised method of age estimation from the auricular surface of the ilium. American Journal of Physical Anthropology 2005;126:61−5.

Murray KA, Murray T. A test of the auricular surface aging technique. Journal of Forensic Sciences 1991;36:1162−9.

Nawrocki SP. Regression formulae for the estimation of age from cranial suture closure. In: Reichs KJ, editor. Forensic osteology: advances in the identification of human remains. Springfield: Charles C. Thomas; 1998. p. 276−92.

Nawrocki SP. The nature and sources of error in the estimation of age at death from the human skeleton. In: Latham KE, Finnegan M, editors. Age estimation of the human skeleton. Springfield: Charles C. Thomas; 2010. p. 79−101.

Nemeskéri J, Harsányi L, Acsádi G. Methoden zur diagnose des lebensalters von skelettfunden. Anthropologischer Anzeiger 1960;24:70−95.

Oettlé AC, Steyn M. Age estimation from sternal ends of ribs by phase analysis in South African blacks. Journal of Forensic Sciences 2000;45:1071−9.

Osborne DL, Simmons TL, Nawrocki SP. Reconsidering the auricular surface as an indicator of age at death. Journal of Forensic Sciences 2004;49:768−73.

Passalacqua NV. Forensic age-at-death estimation from the human sacrum. Journal of Forensic Sciences 2009;54:255−62.

Pechníková M, De Angelis D, Gibelli D, Vecchio V, Cameriere R, Zeqiri B, Cattaneo C. Twins and the paradox of dental-age estimations: a caution for researchers and clinicians. HOMO - Journal of Comparative Human Biology 2014;65:330−7.

Prince DA, Ubelaker DH. Application of Lamendin's adult dental aging technique to a diverse skeletal sample. Journal of Forensic Sciences 2002;47:107−16.

Prince DA, Kimmerle EH, Kongisberg LW. A Bayesian approach to estimate skeletal age-at-death utilizing dental wear. Journal of Forensic Sciences 2008;53:588−93.

Ríos L, Weisensee K, Rissech C. Sacral fusion as an aid in age estimation. Forensic Science International 2008;180:111.e1−111.e7.

Rissech C, Estabrook GF, Cunha E, Malgosa A. Using the acetabulum to estimate age at death of adult males. Journal of Forensic Sciences 2006;51:213−29.

Rissech C, Estabrook GF, Cunha E, Malgosa A. Estimation of age at death for adult males using the acetabulum, applied to four Western European populations. Journal Forensic Sciences 2007;52:774−9.

Rougé-Maillart C, Telmon N, Rissech C, Malgosa A, Rougé D. The determination of male adult age at death by central and posterior coxal analysis: a preliminary study. Journal of Forensic Sciences 2004;49:1−7.

Różyło-Kalinowska I, Kiworkowa-Rączkowska E, Kalinowski P. Dental age in Central Poland. Forensic Science International 2008;174:207−16.

Sashin D. A critical analysis of the anatomy and pathological changes of the sacro-iliac joints. Journal of Bone and Joint Surgery 1930;12:891−910.

Saunders SR, Fitzgerald C, Rogers T, Dudar C, McKillop H. A test of several methods of skeletal age estimation using a documented archaeological sample. Canadian Society of Forensic Science Journal 1992;25:97−118.

Saunders S, DeVito C, Herring A, Southern R, Hoppa R. Accuracy tests of tooth formation age estimations for human skeletal remains. American Journal of Physical Anthropology 1993;92:173−88.

Schaefer M, Black S, Scheuer L. Juvenile osteology: a laboratory and field manual. San Diego: Academic Press; 2008.

Scheuer JL, MacLaughlin-Black SM. Age estimation from the pars basilaris of the fetal and juvenile occipital bone. International Journal of Osteoarchaeology 1994;4:377−80.

Scheuer L, Black S. Developmental juvenile osteology. San Diego: Academic Press; 2000.

Schmitt A. Age-at-death assessment using the os pubis and auricular surface of the ilium: a test on an identified Asian sample. International Journal of Osteoarchaeology 2004;14:1−6.

Schmitt A, Murail P. Is the first rib a reliable indicator of age at death assessment? Test of the method developed by Kunos et al (1999). HOMO-Journal of Comparative Human Biology 2004;54:207−14.

Schour I, Massler M. The development of the human dentition. Journal of American Dental Association 1941;28:1153−60.

Semine AA, Damon A. Costochondral ossification and aging in five populations. Human Biology 1975;47:101−16.

Smith BH. Standards of human tooth formation and dental age assessment. In: Kelley M, Larsen CS, editors. Advances in dental anthropology. New York: Alan R. Liss; 1991. p. 143−68.

Tocheri MW, Molto JE. Aging fetal and juvenile skeletons from Roman period Egypt using basiocciput osteometrics. International Journal of Osteoarchaeology 2002;12:356−63.

Todd TW. Age changes in the pubic bone I: the male white os pubis. American Journal of Physical Anthropology 1920;3:285−334.

Todd TW. Age changes in the pubic bone II-IV: the pubis of the male Negro- White hybrid, the pubis of the White female, the pubis of the female Negro-White hybrid. American Journal of Physical Anthropology 1921;4:1−70.

Todd TW, Lyon DW. Endocranial suture closure, its progress and age relationship: part I.-Adult males of the white stock. American Journal of Physical Anthropology 1924;7:325−84.

Todd TW, Lyon DW. Cranial suture closure, its progress and age relationship: part II.-Ectocranial suture closure in adult males of the white stock. American Journal of Physical Anthropology 1925;8:23−45.

Ubelaker DH. Human skeletal remains: excavation, analysis, interpretation. 2nd ed. Washington: Taraxacum; 1989.

Urzel V, Bruzek J. Dental age assessment in children: a comparison of four methods in a recent French population. Journal of Forensic Sciences 2013;58:1341−7.

Webb PA, Suchey JM. Epiphyseal union of the anterior iliac crest and medial clavicle in a modern multiracial sample of American males and females. American Journal of Physical Anthropology 1985;68:457−66.

Whittaker D. Ageing from the dentition. In: Cox M, Mays S, editors. Human osteology in archaeological and forensic science. London: Greenwich Medical Media; 2000. p. 83−100.

Yoder C, Ubelaker DH, Powell JF. Examination of variation in sternal rib end morphology relevant to age assessment. Journal of Forensic Sciences 2001;46:223−7.

APPENDICES

Appendix 4.I: Age Estimation Recording Protocol: Juveniles

TABLE 4.I.1 Union of Ossification Centers

Skeletal Element	Ossification Centers/Epiphyses	Stage of Union	Age
Frontal bone	Metopic suture		
Occipital bone	Squamous—lateral parts		
	Lateral—basilar parts		
Occipital—sphenoid	Sphenooccipital synchondrosis		
Mandible	Mandibular symphysis		
Sternum	Sternebrae		
Vertebrae	Two halves of the neural arches		
	Neural arches—vertebral centra		
Sacrum	Sacral vertebrae		
Scapula	Coracoid epiphysis		
	Glenoid epiphyses		
	Acromial epiphysis		
	Medial border epiphysis		
	Inferior angle epiphysis		
Clavicle	Medial epiphysis		
	Lateral epiphysis		
Humerus	Proximal epiphysis		
	Distal epiphyses		
Radius	Proximal epiphysis		
	Distal epiphysis		

TABLE 4.I.1 Union of Ossification Centers—cont'd

Skeletal Element	Ossification Centers/Epiphyses	Stage of Union	Age
Ulna	Proximal epiphysis		
	Distal epiphysis		
Os coxa	Ischium—ilium		
	Ischium/ilium—pubis		
	Iliac crest epiphyses		
	Ischial epiphysis for tuberosity		
	Anterior inferior iliac spine epiphysis		
Femur	Head		
	Greater trochanteric epiphysis		
	Lesser trochanteric epiphysis		
	Distal epiphysis		
Tibia	Proximal epiphysis		
	Distal epiphysis		
Fibula	Proximal epiphysis		
	Distal epiphysis		

TABLE 4.I.2 Long-Bone Length

Skeletal Element	Dimension	Equation	Age

TABLE 4.I.3 Dental Development and Eruption

Method	Tooth	Phase/Score	Age
Ubelaker (1989) atlas			
London atlas			
Moorrees et al. (1963)			
Liversidge and Molleson (2004)			
Other (specify)			

Appendix 4.II: Age Estimation Recording Protocol: Adults

TABLE 4.II.1 Adult Age Estimation Based on Pelvic Characters and Sternal Rib-End Morphology

Character	Method	Phase	Age
Morphology of the pubic symphysis	Brooks and Suchey (1990)		
	Other (specify)		
Auricular surface morphology	Lovejoy et al. (1985)		
	Other (specify)		
Sternal rib-end morphology	İşcan et al. (1984, 1985)		
	Other (specify)		

TABLE 4.II.2 Adult Age Estimation Based on Suture Closure

Method	Sutures	Degree of Closure	Age
Meindl and Lovejoy (1985)—vault system	Midlambdoid	—	
	Lambda	—	
	Obelion	—	
	Anterior sagittal	—	
	Bregma	—	
	Midcoronal	—	
	Pterion	—	
	Composite score		
Meindl and Lovejoy (1985)—lateral–anterior system	Midcoronal	—	
	Pterion	—	
	Sphenofrontal	—	
	Inferior sphenotemporal	—	
	Superior sphenotemporal	—	
	Composite score		

Continued

TABLE 4.II.2 Adult Age Estimation Based on Suture Closure—cont'd

Method	Sutures	Degree of Closure	Age
Mann et al. (1991)	Incisive		
	Posterior median palatine		
	Transverse palatine lateral		
	Transverse palatine medial		
	Anterior median palatine		
	Total	—	
Endocranial sutures	Sagittal		—
	Left lambdoid		—
	Left coronal		—
	Total	—	

TABLE 4.II.3 Adult Age Estimation Based on Dentition

Method	Tooth	Periodontosis Height	Transparency Height	Root Height	Age
Dental wear		—	—	—	
Lamendin et al. (1992)					
Prince and Ubelaker (2002)					

TABLE 4.II.4 Adult Age Estimation Using Transition Analysis in ADBOU

Age Marker	Anatomical Structure/Character	Score R Side	Score L Side	Age
Suture closure	Coronal			
	Sagittal			
	Lambdoid			
	Interpalatine			
	Zygomaticomaxillary			
Pubic symphysis	Topography			
	Texture			
	Superior protuberance			
	Ventral margin			
	Dorsal margin			
Auricular surface	Superior topography			
	Inferior topography			
	Superior characteristics			
	Apical characteristics			
	Inferior characteristics			
	Inferior texture			
	Superior exostoses			
	Inferior exostoses			
	Posterior exostoses			

Appendix 4.III: Recording Age Markers in Osteoware

Osteoware allows the recording of age indicators in the Age and Sex module using four data entry tabs: Postcranial Epiphyses, Cranial Sutures, Morphology, and Summary. The information input in each tab is briefly presented in the following paragraphs but the reader may check Madden (2011) for more details and associated photographs. Note that, as mentioned in Appendix 1.III, age-related changes in the deciduous and permanent dentition are recorded in the Dental Inventory/Development/Pathology module, following the scheme proposed by Moorrees et al. (1963).

The first data entry screen that opens by default once the Age and Sex button is clicked is the Postcranial Epiphyses screen (Fig. 4.III.1). This window allows the determination of the degree of epiphyseal union in various secondary centers of ossification in the scapula, clavicle, humerus, radius, ulna, pelvis, sacrum, femur, tibia, fibula, and vertebrae based on a three-scale system: 0, open; 1, partial union; and 2, complete union. In case an epiphysis is missing, the corresponding box is left blank.

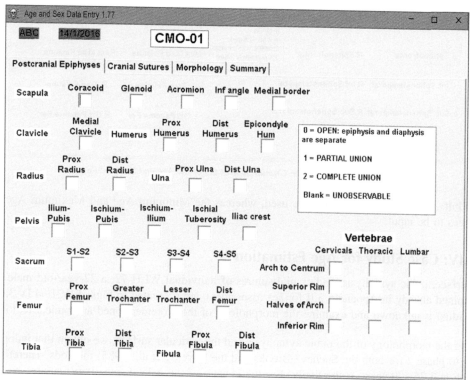

FIGURE 4.III.1   The *Postcranial Epiphyses* tab of the *Age and Sex* module.

The next tab focuses on cranial sutures as an aging method and provides options for recording the degree of closure for ectocranial, endocranial, and palatal (palatine) sutures (Fig. 4.III.2). In addition, for younger individuals, the extent of fusion of primary cranial ossification centers (metopic suture, mental symphysis, parts of the occipital bone—basilar part, lateral parts, squama) may also be recorded. Endocranial, ectocranial, and palatal suture closures are recorded using a four-grade scheme in which 0 is open, 1 is less than 50% closed, 2 is more than 50% and less than 95% closed, and 3 is completely fused. However, for the cranial primary ossification centers, the same recording scheme as for postcranial epiphyses (see previous paragraph) must be used.

The Morphology tab focuses on pelvic and cranial morphology for sex assessment as well as on pelvic and rib morphology for age estimation (see Fig. 3.IV.1). The sex markers recorded in this tab have already been described in Appendix 3.IV. Regarding age, pelvic features examined include the morphology of the pubic symphysis, according to Todd (1920, 1921) and Suchey-Brooks (Brooks and Suchey, 1990), as well as the morphology of the auricular surface. For rib-end morphology, a single rib is to be selected.

The final tab on the Age and Sex Data Entry screen is the Summary. In the Summary Age box, there is a number of predetermined selections for age. When the available skeletal information is too limited for more precise aging, the general

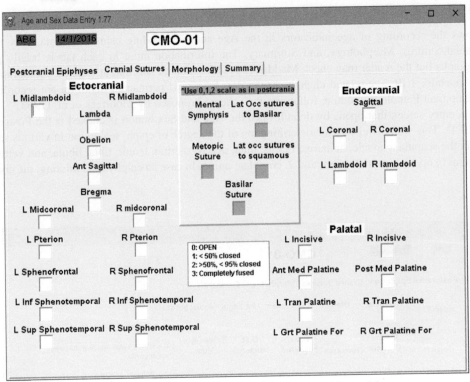

FIGURE 4.III.2 The *Cranial Sutures* tab of the *Age and Sex* module.

categories Subadult, Adult, or Unknown may be used, whereas the Minimum Age and Maximum Age boxes allow for specific age ranges to be input.

Appendix 4.IV: Case Study for Age Estimation

The auricular surface, pubic symphysis, and cranial sutures of individual WLH 72, a 27-year-old male from the Athens Collection, examined already in Appendix 3.II for sex assessment, are presented in Figs. 4.IV.1–4.IV.3. Assume that the age of the individual is unknown and examine the morphology of the aforementioned anatomical regions to estimate it.

By examining the morphology of the pubic symphysis and the auricular surface, we obtain that individual WLH 72 is likely to belong to phase 2 for both the Suchey–Brooks and the Lovejoy et al. (1985) methods. Therefore, his estimated age is 23.4 ± 3.6 and 25–29 years, respectively. For the closure of the palatal (maxillary) sutures we observe that the incisive and the posterior median palatine sutures are fused; therefore the individual is probably 25–35 years of age.

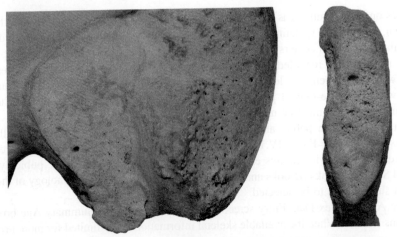

FIGURE 4.IV.1 Morphology of the auricular surface (left) and pubic symphysis (right).

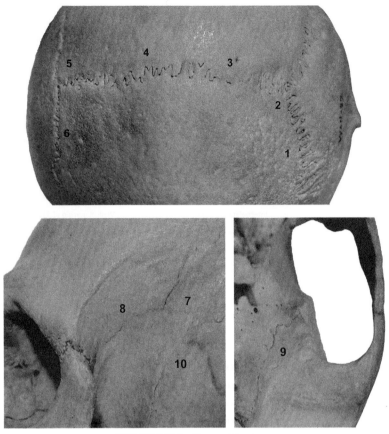

FIGURE 4.IV.2 Ectocranial sutures.

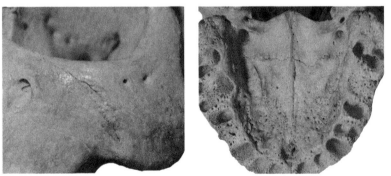

FIGURE 4.IV.3 Zygomaticomaxillary (left) and maxillary (right) sutures.

The recording of the stage of ectocranial suture closure based on the Meindl–Lovejoy method yields the following values:

Suture	1	2	3	4	5	6	7	8	9	10
Score	0	0	2	1	0	0	1	1	1	1

According to these values, we obtain the composite score 4 for both the vault and the lateral–anterior systems. Therefore, the individual's age ranges from 27 to 43 years and from 31 to 51 years, based on each system.

For the application of the ADBOU program, we score the various age indicators given in Box 4.3.4 and input these scores into the ADBOU Age Estimation Program in the Data Table tab as shown in Fig. 4.IV.4. In addition, we enter Sex, Ancestry, and Mortality Model information, in our case, "Male," "White," and "Forensic," and click on "Analyze."

The program computes the point estimates and the corresponding 95% confidence intervals of the age at death of the individual and presents these results along with the maximum-likelihood age at death curves in the Analysis tab (Fig. 4.IV.5). Note that the program computes these results separately for each age indicator as well as for all three indicators simultaneously.

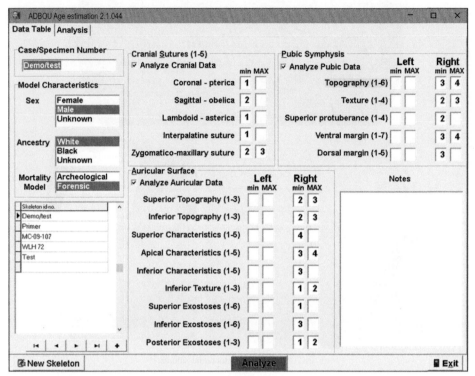

FIGURE 4.IV.4 *Data Table* tab of the ADBOU program and scores used in the study.

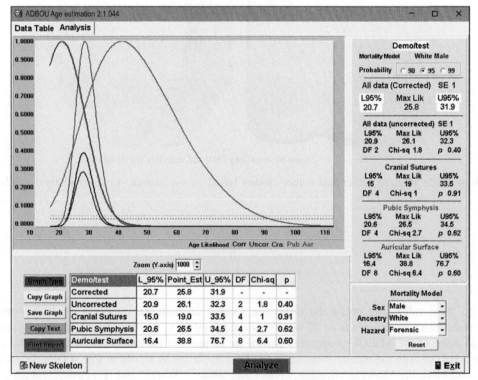

FIGURE 4.IV.5 Graphical output of ADBOU depicting maximum-likelihood age at death curves, the point estimates, and the corresponding 95%

It is seen that ADBOU gives a very good estimation of the age of the individual under study when all age markers are taken into account (Fig. 4.IV.5). The corrected overall point estimation is 25.8 years. However, when each indicator is examined separately, only the pubic symphysis provides an accurate age estimate (26.5 years), whereas cranial sutures underestimate the age of the individual and the auricular surface overestimates it and provides a very broad maximum-likelihood age at death curve.

Table 4.IV.1 summarizes the age estimation according to the adopted methods. Taking into account that the real age of WLH 72 is 27, it is seen that all methods provide a satisfactory age estimation, except for cranial sutures, which over-estimate age when the Meindl—Lovejoy method is adopted and underestimate it in the context of ADBOU. Finally, it is interesting to note that the auricular surface performs rather well when the Lovejoy et al. (1985) method is used, but not as part of ADBOU.

TABLE 4.IV.1 Age Estimation of Individual WLH 72

Method	Age	95% CI
Suchey—Brooks	20—27	
Lovejoy et al. (1985)	25—29	
Palatal sutures	25—35	
Meindl—Lovejoy (lateral—anterior system)	31—51	
Meindl—Lovejoy (vault system)	27—43	
ADBOU (all data)	25.8	20.7—31.9
ADBOU (cranial sutures)	19.0	15.0—33.5
ADBOU (pubic symphysis)	26.5	20.6—34.5
ADBOU (auricular surface)	38.8	16.4—76.7

Chapter 5

Biological Distance

Chapter Outline

Chapter Objectives

By the end of this chapter, the reader will be able to:

- understand the concepts of biological distance (biodistance) and the importance of its estimation in osteoarchaeological studies;
- estimate the biodistances between past groups using metric and nonmetric traits; and
- understand the advantages and limitations of the approaches adopted for the computation of biodistances.

The estimation of the biological distance (biodistance) among skeletal assemblages from past populations or between subgroups within a population is a primary task of osteoarchaeology. The methods used for this purpose are based on the fact that genotypic variation may be phenotypically expressed by means of skeletal morphological and metric traits (Buikstra and Ubelaker, 1994; Ubelaker, 1989). As such, biodistance studies are similar to ancestry studies, discussed in Chapter 3, in the sense that they both focus on assessing the biological affinity of the material under study. However, their specific aims and approaches differ. Specifically, biodistance studies explore the genetic differentiation between populations to study archaeologically relevant questions pertaining to social structure, human mobility, postmarital residence, etc. When certain groups are found to exhibit a small biodistance, this is interpreted as indicative either of a common ancestry of these groups or as a sign of gene flow between them. In contrast, as mentioned in Chapter 3, ancestry assessment in forensic anthropology attempts to identify the ancestral background of the specific individual under study with the aim of assisting his or her identification. As such, in osteoarchaeology the emphasis is on broader patterns at the level of the population, whereas in forensic anthropology the focus is on the individual.

5.1 METRIC METHODS

5.1.1 Cranial Shape and Size as a Proxy for Genotypic Variation

The skeletal element most commonly employed in biodistance studies is the cranium. Studies in animals and humans have found that the dimensions of the craniofacial complex are moderately to highly heritable and determined by multiple genes (Arya et al., 2002; Carson, 2006a; Johannsdottir et al., 2005; Konigsberg and Ousley, 1995; Martínez-Abadías et al., 2009; Sherwood et al., 2008; Sparks and Jantz, 2002). Assessing the control of genetic factors upon cranial morphology is rendered difficult by the fact that the climatic conditions under which an individual lives also influence cranial *form*, that is, the size and shape of the cranium. Some authors have indeed reported a significant climatic effect on the cranium (e.g., Harvati and Weaver, 2006 for the facial bones; Roseman, 2004 for a Siberian population); however, other studies have not identified any such particular connection (e.g., Betti et al., 2009; Manica et al., 2007; Roseman and Weaver, 2007; von Cramon-Taubadel, 2009). To some degree, this discrepancy can been attributed to the type of data analyzed. In particular, a climatic impact has been found mostly in variables that express cranial size. In contrast, studies focusing on cranial shape, whether this stands for the overall shape of the cranium or the shape of specific cranial bones, have found a small or negligible climatic effect (see Betti et al., 2010).

An important complication in assessing climatic impact on cranial form arises from the fact that populations that occupy similar natural environments are often geographically close to one another, which increases the possibility of gene flow between them. Thus, any observed cranial similarities may not necessarily be the outcome of a shared climatic impact but rather the result of gene flow. Betti et al. (2010) analyzed craniometric data using a global sample and focused on measures that are mostly associated with the size and form of the cranium, that is, variables that are believed to be least controlled genetically. Their results suggested that genetic factors actually exert much more influence on the cranium than climate, with the exception of populations occupying particularly cold environments. Thus, cranial measurements can be considered good neutral genetic markers.

With respect to research results examining which specific areas of the cranium reflect genetic factors to a greater degree, Harvati and Weaver (2006) found that the shape of the neurocranium and the temporal bone are good neutral genetic indicators. These conclusions were corroborated by Smith et al. (2007), who also found that the shape of the temporal bone is mostly controlled by genes in Eurasians and Africans, but not when Native Americans were examined. von Cramon-Taubadel (2009) also obtained results that supported the temporal bone as an excellent source of genetic information. Smith (2009) confirmed that the temporal bone is correlated with neutral genetic markers, but found that the same applies to the basicranium, upper facial bones, or even the entire cranium. Other studies have also supported that environmental impact on the shape of the basicranium must be minimal because this anatomical area reflects the shape of the growing brain; thus it cannot be particularly affected by nongenetic parameters (Lieberman et al., 2000a,b). Regarding facial bones, Evteev et al. (2014) found that the morphology of the nasal and maxillary areas is primarily determined climatically, rather than by population history patterns. However, it must be stressed that cranial morphology in this study was captured by means of linear measurements rather than geometric morphometrics (see following sections). Thus, it expressed simultaneously the size and shape of the skeletal elements, and it is unclear if the climatic effect would have been as pronounced had size been controlled for. Finally, it must be noted that another study that employed linear measurements (Herrera et al., 2014) found a high correlation between craniometric variables that captured the entire cranium and mitochondrial DNA data among populations across the Bering strait.

In addition to climatic conditions, a factor that has an impact on cranial shape and size and may complicate the identification of genetic information is mechanical loading, which results from demanding dietary regimes (Spencer and Demes, 1993; Spencer and Ungar, 2000). Mechanical loading may increase the robusticity of certain cranial structures, such as the supraorbital ridges, maxillae, and mandible (Hernández et al., 1997; Holmes and Ruff, 2011). For example, several studies have proposed that the transition from hunting—gathering to agriculture was accompanied by reduced cranial robusticity, smaller facial and occipital bones, a more gracile masticatory complex, and shorter and rounder cranial vaults as a result of reduced muscular activity related to a softer diet (e.g., Larsen, 1995; Paschetta et al., 2010; Pinhasi et al., 2008). Although the overall cranial morphological variation among populations appears to be greater than any activity-induced differentiation (González-José et al., 2005), this is a factor that needs to be taken into consideration when comparisons involve populations with diverse dietary practices.

The above brief discussion illustrates that each researcher should decide which specific areas of the cranium are most pertinent to his or her study, bearing in mind the climatic, biomechanical, and other nongenetic factors that may affect cranial form.

5.1.2 Cranial Digitization

Modern craniometric studies analyze the coordinates of specific *landmarks*, that is, biologically meaningful points, the location of which can be described with Cartesian coordinates. As such, landmark-based morphometrics (or *geometric morphometrics*) allow the effective study of cranial shape and provide information on the spatial relationship of various cranial structures (Rohlf and Marcus, 1993).

The landmarks used in biodistance analysis correspond to developmentally, functionally, structurally, or evolutionarily significant anatomical structures (Ritchmeier et al., 2002). Landmarks that cover the entire cranium are given in Appendix 5.I. The distances between pairs of landmarks constitute *linear measurements*, which may also be used in biodistance studies (see Section 5.1.3). Appendix 5.II gives definitions of the most commonly employed cranial linear measurements.

Landmark coordinates are obtained using 3D scanners or digitizers. During the digitization of a cranium or any other object, it is essential to keep the sample completely still. To digitize the entire cranium, this may be positioned in a way that allows capturing all landmarks (e.g., see the informative video produced by Stephen Ousley: http://math.mercyhurst.edu/ ~sousley/Videos/3Skull-Ousley.mp4). Ousley has also created a software, ThreeSkull, which facilitates recording cranial coordinates. This software is freely available upon request at http://math.mercyhurst.edu/~sousley/Software/, and clear instructions on how to use it are given in the aforementioned video.

Alternatively, the coordinates from one side of the cranium, say the left side, are obtained first, then the cranium is turned over and the other side is digitized. Appendix 5.III shows an example layout of the Excel spreadsheet for data input when each cranial side is digitized separately. This layout is suitable for data pretreatment using the software package Morpheus et al. (Slice, 1998, 2013). When digitizing each cranial side separately, one should always make sure to digitize at least three shared landmarks that lie on the midsagittal plane on both sides of the cranium (e.g., nasion, bregma, lambda). This step allows one to later combine the two halves of the cranium into one single configuration, as the coordinates of the three landmarks create a common plane on which the locations of the remaining landmarks are traced (Lele and Richtsmeier, 2001). The process of putting the two halves of the cranium together using the program Morpheus et al. is described in Appendix 5.IV.

A limitation of the digitization method is that all landmarks must be present in all crania under study. However, in cases in which a landmark is present on one side of the cranium but absent on the other, mirror-imaging methods can be used to construct the missing coordinates (Mardia and Bookstein, 2000). Mirror-imaging can be performed in Morpheus but it is time-consuming and, as it is based on successive superimpositions, to some extent it distorts the obtained and original coordinates. Appendix 5.V presents a simple Excel macro that can estimate the coordinates of missing landmarks using a mirror-imaging technique. Alternative methods by which the coordinates of missing landmarks can be filled in are based on the landmark coordinates of one or more other crania from the same population and include *thin-plate spline* or *multivariate regression*. These methods may be implemented in R, in which there are several functions for this purpose, such as the function estimate.missing of the geomorph library and the function fixLMtps of the Morpho library.

Prior to the use of cranial digitized data in the calculation of biodistances, cranial landmark coordinates need to be submitted to *Generalized Procrustes Analysis* (GPA), that is, preliminary processing that involves scaling, transposition, and rotation, so that all crania become of the same size, are at the same location, and have the same orientation. The criterion used in this process is that the overall sum of squared distances between corresponding landmarks is minimum (Bookstein, 1991). It should be noted that, after scaling, all observed differences among crania relate only to shape and not to size, which is very important given that shape is predominantly an expression of neutral genes instead of environmental factors, as discussed earlier. At this point we should clarify that although size as a factor is removed from the data through GPA, size-related shape variation may still be present (Nicholson and Harvati, 2006). GPA can be performed using various software packages but the simplest one is PAST (Palaeontological Statistics) (Hammer et al., 2001). Appendix 5.VI provides instructions on how to perform GPA in PAST.

For comparisons involving cranial size, the so-called *centroid size* is used. This is the square root of the summed squared distances of all landmarks from their centroid (Bookstein, 1991). Centroid size can be easily calculated using the macro CentroidSize provided in the companion website (see Appendix 5.VII).

5.1.3 Cranial Linear Measurements

Linear measurements are a simpler way of capturing cranial form when 3D scanners or digitizers are not available. As mentioned earlier, linear measurements are distances between pairs of landmarks, and some of the most common ones are defined in Appendix 5.II. It is important to have in mind that such measurements express *both* cranial shape *and* size. Therefore, if a researcher is interested only in the shape component, which, as already discussed, appears to give a more accurate neutral genetic signal, the original measurements should be properly transformed. Several transformations have been proposed and discussed (Jungers et al., 1995). In the simplest approach, to reduce the effect of size, linear measurements are transformed to *Mosimann shape variables* prior to statistical analyses (Darroch and Mosimann, 1985; Mosimann and James, 1979). A Mosimann shape variable is the ratio of any particular measurement of a case to the geometric mean of this case, where the geometric mean (GM) is the nth root of the product of the n measurements of the case. For example, in a data set that contains five variables, the GM per case will be given by:

$$GM = \sqrt[5]{x_1 \cdot x_2 \cdot x_3 \cdot x_4 \cdot x_5} \tag{5.1.1}$$

where x_1, x_2, ..., x_5 are the values of each of the five variables.

For the easy transformation of an initial table of continuous data to Mosimann shape variables the macro DataTransformation, provided in the companion website, may be used. Note that this transformation does not allow for missing values in the data set.

5.1.4 Dental Measurements

In addition to cranial data, dental crown dimensions have been found to be highly heritable based on population and family studies (Dempsey and Townsend, 2001; Townsend, 1980; Townsend et al., 2003, 2009). However, the natural and sociocultural environment also influences dental size and should be taken into consideration in the interpretation of biodistance results (Dempsey and Townsend, 2001; Garn et al., 1979; Potter et al., 1983; Townsend et al., 2012). The dental dimensions most often measured are given in Box 5.1.1.

5.1.5 Euclidean and Mahalanobis Distances

A suitable measure to assess biodistances based on continuous data is the Mahalanobis distance, which is an extension of the Euclidean distance. The Euclidean distance between two single points, A and B, is the length of the line segment connecting them. Thus, if (x_A, y_A) and (x_B, y_B) are the Cartesian coordinates of these two points on the $x-y$ plane, the Euclidean distance between these points is given by:

BOX 5.1.1 Definition of Dental Measurements

- Maximum mesiodistal crown diameter (a)
- Maximum buccolingual crown diameter (b)
- Crown height (c)
- Root length (d)

From Hillson S, FitzGerald C, Flinn H. Alternative dental measurements: proposals and relationships with other measurements. American Journal of Physical Anthropology 2005;126:413–26; White TD, Black MT, Folkens PA. Human osteology. 3rd ed. New York: Elsevier Academic Press; 2011; see also Aubry BS. Technical note: cervical dimensions for in situ and loose teeth: a critique of the Hillson et al. (2005) method. American Journal of Physical Anthropology 2014;154:159–64 for adaptation of the Hillson et al. measurements

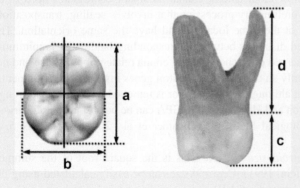

$$d_E = \sqrt{(x_A - x_B)^2 + (y_A - y_B)^2} \tag{5.1.2}$$

If points A and B are defined by r coordinates, A($x_{A1}, x_{A2}, ..., x_{Ar}$) and B($x_{B1}, x_{B2}, ..., x_{Br}$), then their Euclidean distance may be expressed as:

$$d_E = \sqrt{(x_{A1} - x_{B1})^2 + (x_{A2} - x_{B2})^2 + \cdots + (x_{Ar} - x_{Br})^2} \tag{5.1.3}$$

In matrix notation, Eq. (5.1.3) may be written as:

$$d_E = \sqrt{(x_A - x_B)^T (x_A - x_B)} \tag{5.1.4}$$

where $x_A = (x_{A1}, x_{A2}, ..., x_{Ar})^T$, $x_B = (x_{B1}, x_{B2}, ..., x_{Br})^T$, and T denotes the transpose matrix. Thus, $x_A - x_B$ is the column matrix $(x_{A1} - x_{B1}, x_{A2} - x_{B2}, \cdots, x_{Ar} - x_{Br})^T$ and $(x_A - x_B)^T$ is the row matrix $(x_{A1} - x_{B1}, x_{A2} - x_{B2}, \cdots, x_{Ar} - x_{Br})$.

This definition can be extended to include the distance between a point and a group of points, as well as the distance between two groups of points. In these cases the *centroid* of the group is calculated and this point is then used in the aforementioned equations for the calculation of the Euclidean distance (Fig. 5.1.1). Note that the centroid (x_A, y_A) of a group of N points (x_i, y_i), $i = 1, 2, ..., N$, on the $x-y$ plane, is calculated from the average of the x_i and y_i values, that is, x_A is the average value of x_i and, similarly, y_A is the average value of y_i. This definition is straightforwardly extended to groups of points in the r-dimensional space.

When the Euclidean distance is calculated between a point and a group of points or between two groups of points, it may not be an effective distance measure, as visualized in Fig. 5.1.2. In this figure, points A and B have equal Euclidean distances from the groups of points C and D, respectively. However, point B is clearly closer to the points of group D, because the points of this group exhibit greater variances across the x and y axes. Thus, in this case the Euclidean distance is a misleading measure.

When the distribution of the group points is symmetric around the centroid, as in Fig. 5.1.2, the Euclidean distance can be easily corrected to take into account differences in the dispersion of the group points. Because a measure of the dispersion is the standard deviation, s, of the values x_i or y_i, the Euclidean distance may be corrected by division of its value by s:

$$d_{EN} = d_E/s \tag{5.1.5}$$

This corrected distance is called *normalized Euclidean distance*. Thus, in Fig. 5.1.2 the normalized Euclidean distance of point A from group C is greater than that of point B from group D because d_E is the same, but the standard deviation of group D is greater than that of group C. The obtained normalized value, d_{EN}, is, in fact, a limiting case of the Mahalanobis distance, d_M. From the definition of d_{EN}, Eq. (5.1.5), it becomes clear that this distance is effective only when the distribution of the group points is symmetric and, thus, s is the same for all coordinates.

When the distribution is not symmetric, s does not take a single value. A limiting case is depicted in Fig. 5.1.3, which shows the Euclidean distances of two points, A and B, from a group of points, C. The distribution of these points covers the

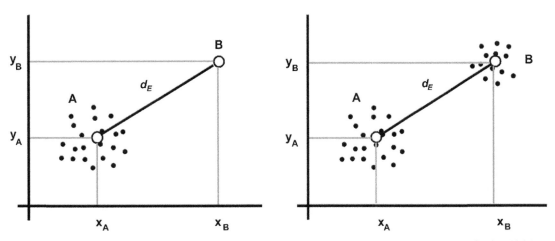

FIGURE 5.1.1 Euclidean distances between a point and a group of points (left), and between two groups of points (right).

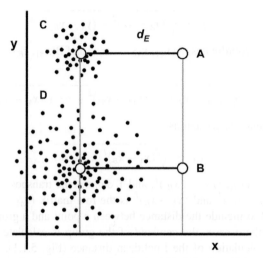

FIGURE 5.1.2 Euclidean distances between points A and B and groups of points C and D, respectively, which exhibit symmetric dispersion of points but with different variance.

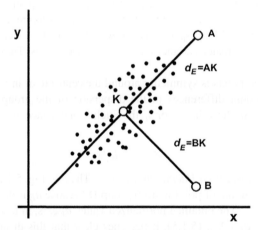

FIGURE 5.1.3 Euclidean distances of two points, A and B, from a group of points, C, exhibiting ellipsoid dispersion of points.

area of an ellipse; point A lies on the major axis of the ellipse and B lies on the corresponding minor axis. K denotes the centroid. By construction, the Euclidean distances of points A and B from C are equal. However, we again observe that point A is much closer to group C than point B. In this case we may correct the Euclidean distance $d_E = $ AK by dividing it by the standard deviation s_{KA} of the projections of all points of group C on the axis that passes through points A and K. Similarly, the Euclidean distance $d_E = $ BK may be corrected by dividing it by the standard deviation s_{KB} of the projections of all points on the axis that passes through points B and K. It is evident that $s_{KA} > s_{KB}$ and therefore the corrected Euclidean distance AK, $d_{EN} = d_E/s_{KA}$, is smaller than that of point B from C, $d_{EN} = d_E/s_{KB}$. These normalized Euclidean distances are again limiting cases of the Mahalanobis distance.

The Mahalanobis distance between a point and a group of points is in general a corrected Euclidean distance that takes into account the variance of the points along the axis that passes from the point and the group centroid. In strict mathematical language, the Mahalanobis distance in r dimensions between a point $x = (x_1, x_2, ..., x_r)^T$ and the centroid $\mu = (\mu_1, \mu_2, ..., \mu_r)^T$ of a group of N points is defined from (Mahalanobis, 1936):

$$d_M = \sqrt{(x - \mu)^T C^{-1}(x - \mu)} \tag{5.1.6}$$

where C^{-1} is the inverse of the variance–covariance matrix of the group of points. Thus, if the kth point in the group is defined from coordinates $(y_{1k}, y_{2k}, ..., y_{rk})$, C is a matrix with elements c_{ij} equal to the covariances between the y_{ik} and the y_{jk} values when k ranges from 1 to N.

In two dimensions, Eq. (5.1.6) may take the analytical expression (De Maesschalck et al., 2000):

$$d_M = \sqrt{\frac{1}{1-\rho^2}\left\{\left(\frac{x_B - \bar{x}}{s_x}\right)^2 + \left(\frac{y_B - \bar{y}}{s_y}\right)^2 - 2\rho\left(\frac{x_B - \bar{x}}{s_x}\right)\left(\frac{y_B - \bar{y}}{s_y}\right)\right\}} \qquad (5.1.7)$$

which calculates the Mahalanobis distance of a point $B(x_B, y_B)$ from a group of points $A(x_i, y_i)$. The centroid of the group of points is located at $(\bar{x}, \bar{y})$, where $\bar{x}$, $\bar{y}$ are the mean values of the x_i, y_i coordinates of the group points. In Eq. 5.1.7, s_x, s_y are the standard deviations of the x_i, y_i values, respectively, and ρ is the covariance of x_i, y_i. In a circular symmetrical distribution of the group points $\rho = 0$, $s_x = s_y = s$, and Eq. (5.1.7) is readily reduced to Eq. (5.1.5), $d_M = d_E/s$.

The Mahalanobis distance between two groups of points is defined similarly from (Mahalanobis, 1936):

$$d_M = \sqrt{(\mu_1 - \mu_2)^T C_{\text{pooled}}^{-1}(\mu_1 - \mu_2)} \qquad (5.1.8)$$

where $\mu_1 = (\mu_{11}, \mu_{12}, ..., \mu_{1r})^T$; $\mu_2 = (\mu_{21}, \mu_{22}, ..., \mu_{2r})^T$; $\mu_{11}, \mu_{12}, ..., \mu_{1r}$ are the mean values of the r variables (measurements) of the first group of points; $\mu_{21}, \mu_{22}, ..., \mu_{2r}$ are the corresponding mean values of the second group; and C_{pooled}^{-1} is the inverse of the pooled variance–covariance matrix of the two groups (Johnson and Wichern, 2007). When more than two groups are involved in the comparisons, the pooled variance–covariance matrix includes all groups.

Note that in osteoarchaeological studies the square of the Mahalanobis distance:

$$d_M^2 = (\mu_1 - \mu_2)^T C_{\text{pooled}}^{-1}(\mu_1 - \mu_2) \qquad (5.1.9)$$

is preferred over the original Mahalanobis distance, Eq. (5.1.8). However, neither the original nor the squared Mahalanobis distance is an unbiased estimator of population divergence (see Section 9.3.7). For this reason, the distance measure most often used is the corrected (for small sample sizes) Mahalanobis d^2 defined from (Sjøvold, 1975):

$$d_{CM}^2 = (\mu_1 - \mu_2)^T C_{\text{pooled}}^{-1}(\mu_1 - \mu_2)\frac{N - g - r - 1}{N - g} - \frac{n_1 + n_2}{n_1 n_2}r \qquad (5.1.10)$$

which is an unbiased estimator of population biodistances. In this expression, N is the total number of cases of all groups, n_1 and n_2 are the number of cases in the two compared groups, g is the total number of groups, and r is the number of variables. Note that owing to the last term in Eq. (5.1.10), negative distances may be calculated when the compared samples come from the same population or from populations that are biologically very similar. Because negative squared distances are physically meaningless, in such cases the negative values are converted to 0.

The statistical significance of the Mahalanobis distances can be estimated by the p-values that test the null hypothesis H_0, $d_M^2 = 0$, with alternative hypothesis H_1, $d_M^2 > 0$ (Section 9.3). The test statistic that may be used is (Sjøvold, 1975):

$$F = \frac{(N - g - r + 1)n_1 n_2 d_M^2}{(N - g)r(n_1 + n_2)} \qquad (5.1.11)$$

which follows the Fisher distribution with r and $N - g - r + 1$ degrees of freedom. In what concerns the corrected Mahalanobis distance calculated from Eq. (5.1.10), its significance can be estimated from the significance of the squared Mahalanobis distance, that is, from Eq. (5.1.11).

The calculation of the Mahalanobis distances from the above equations is quite tedious. This calculation is facilitated via proper software. Appendix 5.VIII offers step-by-step instructions on how to calculate Mahalanobis distances and their significance by means of the macro Biodistances, which is provided in the companion website. Alternatively, Mahalanobis distances (uncorrected for small sample sizes) and their significance may be computed using PAST from the menu Multivariate → Tests → MANOVA → Pairwise → Squared Mahalanobis distances.

5.1.6 Statistical Analysis

The statistical tests that may be employed in the analysis of cranial morphology, based on either linear measurements or digitized coordinates, include:

1. principal component analysis (PCA) to (1) identify clusters of groups from the PC1 versus PC2 plot and (2) reduce the number of variables (when these are more than the number of cases) in order to subsequently use linear discriminant analysis and multivariate analysis of variance and compute Mahalanobis distances;
2. linear discriminant analysis (LDA) to discriminate two or more groups and assign unknown cases to the proper cluster;
3. multivariate analysis of variance (MANOVA) to test if the aforementioned clusters are statistically significantly

4. Mahalanobis distances to calculate the pairwise biodistances among the various populations; and
5. dendrograms and/or multidimensional scaling (MDS) based on the Mahalanobis distances to visualize the biological relationship among populations.

Two case studies are presented in detail in Section 9.9.8, Case Studies 24 and 25. The first concerns linear measurements and the second cranial digitized coordinates. For the correlation between biodistances and temporal and spatial distances, see Section 9.8.4, Case Study 23.

5.2 NONMETRIC TRAITS

5.2.1 Genetic Information and Confounding Factors

Nonmetric traits represent variants of the normal skeletal anatomy that cannot be measured; they are recorded either as present/absent or using ordinal scales for their degree of expression (Berry and Berry, 1967; Tyrrell, 2000). Nonmetric traits do not express pathological conditions and their presence causes no symptoms (Tyrrell, 2000). Alternative terms for nonmetric traits include *discontinuous traits*, *epigenetic traits*, *discrete traits*, *minor variants*, *quasicontinuous traits*, and others (Buikstra and Ubelaker, 1994). Over 400 such traits have been identified in the human skeleton and they exhibit substantial heterogeneity (Mays, 2010).

The genetic control over the expression of nonmetric traits has been explored through studies on laboratory mice (e.g., Grüneberg, 1952; Self and Leamy, 1978), macaques (Cheverud and Buikstra, 1981; McGrath et al., 1984), and humans (e.g., Berry, 1968, 1978; Carson, 2006b; Grüneberg, 1963; Saunders and Popovich, 1978; Sjøvold, 1984; Torgersen, 1951; Velemínský and Dobisíková, 2005). As a result, the heritability of nonmetric traits has been found to range mostly from 0.40 to 0.80, though lower values have also been retrieved (Carson, 2006b; Cheverud and Buikstra, 1981; Mizoguchi, 1977; Scott and Potter, 1984; Sjøvold, 1984; Sofaer et al., 1972; Townsend et al., 1992). Among the traits that appear to exhibit comparatively high heritability are hyperostotic and hypostotic traits as well as dental traits, whereas foramina generally appear to be under weak genetic control (Ansorge, 2001). A study that must be highlighted at this point is that of Ricaut et al. (2010), which tested the correlation between the biodistances obtained based on cranial, postcranial, and dental nonmetric traits and those from genetic data in material from the Egyin Gol necropolis, Mongolia. The authors identified a correlation between the different distance matrices, supporting the utility of nonmetric traits as markers of biological affinity even at an intrapopulation level; however, they stressed that such traits should be employed only when the resolution of the familial relationships is high. On a greater geographic scale, Herrera et al. (2014) identified a high correlation between biodistances obtained from cranial nonmetric traits and genetic distances calculated from Y-chromosomal data for populations across the Bering strait. Similar results were retrieved by Hubbard et al. (2015) in a comparison between biodistances obtained from dental nonmetric traits and DNA data from modern Kenya.

In addition to genes, environmental factors also influence the expression of nonmetric traits. According to Grüneberg's (1952) model of quasicontinuous variation, the expression of the underlying variation in trait expression (genetically and environmentally mediated) is controlled by a threshold; above this threshold the trait is present and variable in expression, whereas below it the character is absent. Under this model the inheritance of nonmetric traits is controlled by multiple genes that interact to produce the final phenotype.

The critical element to note is that although environmental factors to some degree affect trait expression, there does not appear to be a significant impact on population trait frequencies (Scott and Turner, 1997). Therefore, the genetic control over nonmetric trait expression is sufficient to make them useful in osteoarchaeological studies (Berry and Berry, 1967; Brothwell, 2000; Cheverud and Buikstra, 1981; Hauser and De Stefano, 1989; Tyrrell, 2000). Indeed, nonmetric traits have been used extensively in (1) human evolutionary studies (Hanihara, 2008; Manzi et al., 2000), (2) biodistance analysis among archaeological samples (e.g., Donlon, 2000; Hanihara et al., 2003; Leblanc et al., 2008; Nikita et al., 2012; Sutter and Mertz, 2004), and (3) kinship analysis (e.g., Stojanowski and Schillaci, 2006).

Nonmetric traits may be classified into cranial, dental, and postcranial. The first two categories are most commonly employed in osteoarchaeological studies and they are described in the following two sections, whereas postcranial traits are briefly presented in the file "Definition of postcranial nonmetric traits," provided in the companion website.

5.2.2 Recording Cranial Nonmetric Traits

A detailed study of cranial nonmetric traits records the degree of expression of each one in an ordinal scale, as suggestively shown in Appendix 5.IX. In most studies the ordinal scores are subsequently transformed into binary (presence/absence) ones. Unfortunately, it is not clear what degree of expression qualifies each trait as present and this lack of standardization can have a substantial impact on the obtained results. Nikita et al. (2012) successfully employed thresholds suggested by previous scholars and set new ones for certain traits. These thresholds are presented in Table 5.2.1.

After recording, the frequency of each trait is estimated per population. Each trait is recorded only once per individual irrespective of whether it is present unilaterally or bilaterally because there is a high correlation in the expression of nonmetric traits between the two sides of the cranium (McGrath et al., 1984; Sutter and Mertz, 2004). The side with the greatest degree of trait expression is usually preferred during recording. Note that in artificially deformed crania the expression of nonmetric traits, and particularly sutural ossicles, appears to be altered; thus attention should be paid when such crania are examined (van Arsdale and Clark, 2012 and references therein).

In children some nonmetric traits cannot be recorded. For example, the metopic suture can be recorded only after the first few years of life, when it becomes clear whether it will fuse normally or be retained. The scoring of hyperostotic traits in subadults is also potentially problematic as their frequency and degree of expression may increase with age because they involve progressive ossification (Buikstra, 1972).

5.2.3 Recording Dental Nonmetric Traits

The majority of dental nonmetric traits is described in detail in Turner et al. (1991) and Scott and Turner (1997). Appendix 5.X presents representative dental nonmetric traits and a recording scheme for each one. Also, the Anthropology Department at Arizona State University (Tempe, AZ) has produced the Arizona State University Dental Anthropology System (ASUDAS), consisting of casts of teeth that exhibit dental nonmetric traits at different degrees of expression, to facilitate their identification (Fig. 5.2.1). As was the case for cranial nonmetric traits, after the original ordinal scoring of the degree of expression per trait, a present/absent recording may be established, and the frequency of each trait per sample is calculated. In contrast to cranial traits, for dental traits several researchers have proposed thresholds for the presence of each character (e.g., see Table 5.2.2).

Three methods are available for counting dental trait frequencies (Scott, 2008):

- Side count: Trait expression recorded only on the left or right antimere
- Tooth count: Trait expression recorded on all teeth, whether right or left (mostly useful in large assemblages of loose teeth)
- Individual count: Trait expression recorded only on the antimere that exhibits the highest grade of trait expression per individual

Among these three methods, the tooth count is potentially problematic, as it may artificially increase the sample size without providing any substantial new information. Note that the ASUDAS favors the individual count method.

The vast majority of the papers published on human dental morphology focuses on the permanent dentition. Among the researchers who have explored deciduous morphology are Hanihara (1961), Kitagawa (2000), Kitagawa et al. (1995), Lease and Sciulli (2005), Lukacs and Walimbe (1984), Sciulli (1998) and Paul and Stojanowski (2015).

5.2.4 The Mean Measure of Divergence

A common measure to express interpopulation biodistances using nonmetric traits recorded in a binary (presence/absence) format is the mean measure of divergence (MMD). The MMD is a measure of dissimilarity among samples, so the more similar two populations are, the smaller the MMD is. This measure was introduced by statistician C.A.B. Smith for use by Grewal (1962) and it may be expressed as (Sjøvold, 1973):

$$\text{MMD} = \frac{1}{r} \sum_{i=1}^{r} \left\{ (\theta_{1i} - \theta_{2i})^2 - \frac{1}{n_{1i} + 0.5} - \frac{1}{n_{2i} + 0.5} \right\} \tag{5.2.1}$$

Here, r denotes the number of nonmetric traits under study, n_{1i} is the number of individuals from sample 1 in which the presence of trait i is examined, n_{2i} is the number of individuals from sample 2 in which the presence of trait i is examined, and θ_{1i} and θ_{2i} denote the transformed frequencies of each trait per sample. As such, the MMD is the mean value of the measure of divergence calculated using all traits. There are various methods for the estimation of the transformed frequencies: Smith (Grewal, 1962), Freeman–Tukey (1950), and Anscombe (1948) transformations, as well as Bartlett's correction (Green and Suchey, 1976). The Freeman–Tukey transformation is the most widely used and is appropriate even for small sample sizes and low or high trait frequencies (Green and Suchey, 1976). In this transformation θ is estimated from:

TABLE 5.2.1 Expression of Cranial Nonmetric Traits Denoting Their Presence

Trait	Expression Denoting Presence
Metopic suture	If present along more than half of the frontal arc (Dodo, 1974)
Metopic fissure	If present in any of its variants (see Hauser and De Stefano, 1989)
Supranasal suture	If observable irrespective of degree of persistence or shape
Supraorbital osseous structures	No distinction between notches and foramina, present if open to the orbital cavity (Dodo, 1974)
Divided infraorbital foramina	Only complete bridging
Parietal foramina	If observable irrespective of position, size, or number
Divided mental foramina	Only complete division
Ethmoidal foramina	If the posterior foramen is absent
Lesser palatine foramina	If observable irrespective of position, size, shape, or number
Squamous ossicles	If observable irrespective of size or number (Hauser and De Stefano, 1989)
Parietal notch bone	If observable irrespective of predominant position, size, or number (Dodo, 1974)
Epipteric bone	If observable irrespective of size, type of articulation with neighboring bones, or number
Ossicle at asterion	If observable irrespective of predominant position, size, shape, or number (Ossenberg, 1969)
Occipitomastoid wormians	If observable irrespective of exact position, size, or number (Dodo, 1974)
Coronal ossicles	If observable irrespective of position, size, or number
Sagittal ossicles	If observable irrespective of position, size, or number
Lambdoid ossicles	If observable irrespective of position, size, or number
Inca bone	If more than 10 mm of the suture is observable (Dodo, 1974)
Divided occipital condyles	If a deep furrow cutting into the facet from both sides can be seen, even if it does not completely separate the condyle (Hauser and De Stefano, 1989)
Hypoglossal canal bridging	Only complete division (Dodo, 1974)
Mandibular torus	Any expression from weak to strong (Dodo, 1974)
Maxillary torus	Any expression from weak to strong
Auditory torus	Any expression from weak to strong
Palatine torus	Any expression from weak to strong
Aperture at floor of acoustic meatus	At least a pinhole-sized aperture (Hauser and De Stefano, 1989)
Divided parietal bone	If observable for more than 1 cm
Divided temporal squama	If observable for more than 5 mm
Os japonicum	If observable for more than 5 mm (Dodo, 1974)
Marginal tubercle	If projecting for more than 4 mm
Mylohyoid bridging	If an osseous bridge is observable irrespective of location and degree of expression (Dodo, 1974)
Foramen of Vesalius	Only complete division
Foramen oval incomplete	Any kind of communication between the two foramina except for a suture-like gap (Dodo, 1974)
Zygomaxillary tubercle	If projecting for more than 2 mm
Symmetrical thinness of parietal bones	When ranging from slight flattening to a saucer-shaped appearance (Hauser and De Stefano, 1989)

From Nikita E, Mattingly D, Lahr MM. Sahara: barrier or corridor? Nonmetric cranial traits and biological affinities of North African Late Holocene populations. American Journal of Physical Anthropology 2012;147:280–92.

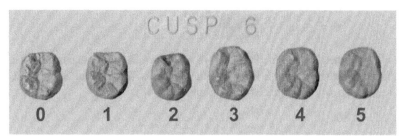

FIGURE 5.2.1   Adapted Arizona State University Dental Anthropology System cast for recording the entoconulid (cusp 6) in mandibular molars.

TABLE 5.2.2 Thresholds for Representative Dental Nonmetric Traits

Trait	Present	Absent
Winging UI1	ASU 1	ASU 2–4
Shoveling UI1	ASU 3–7	ASU 0–2
Double shoveling UI1	ASU 2–6	ASU 0–1
Interruption groove UI2	ASU +	ASU −
Tuberculum dentale UI2	ASU 1–9	ASU 0
Bushman canine UC	ASU 1–3	ASU 0
Distal accessory ridge UC	ASU 2–5	ASU 0–1
Hypocone UM2	ASU 2–5	ASU 0–1
Cusp 5 UM1	ASU 1–5	ASU 0
Carabelli's trait UM1	ASU 2–7	ASU 0–1
Parastyle UM3	ASU 1–5	ASU 0
Enamel extension UM1	ASU 2–3	ASU 0–1
Root number UP1	ASU 1	ASU 2–3
Root number UM2	ASU 3	ASU 1, 2, 4
Peg/reduced/congenital absence UM3	ASU PRC	ASU normal
Lingual cusp LP2	ASU 2–3	ASU 0–1
Groove pattern LM2	ASU Y	ASU +, X
Cusp number LM1	ASU 6	ASU 4–5
Cusp number LM2	ASU 4	ASU 5–6
Deflecting wrinkle LM1	ASU 3	ASU 0–2
Distal trigonid crest LM1	ASU +	ASU −
Protostylid LM1	ASU 1–8	ASU 0
Cusp 7 LM1	ASU 1–5	ASU 0
Tome's root LP1	ASU 4–7	ASU 0–3
Root number LC	ASU 2	ASU 1
Root number LM1	ASU 3	ASU 2
Root number LM2	ASU 1	ASU 2–3
Odontome UP1–P2, LP1–P2	ASU +	ASU −

ASU, Arizona State University Dental Anthropology System; *C*, canine; *I*, incisor; *L*, lower; *M*, molar; *P*, pre-molar; *PRC*, peg-shaped or reduced-sized or congenitally absent; *U*, upper; *1*, first; *2*, second; *3*, third.
From Turner II CG. Late Pleistocene and Holocene population history of East Asia based on dental variation. American Journal of Physical Anthropology 1987;73:305–21.

$$\theta = \frac{1}{2} \sin^{-1}\left(1 - \frac{2k}{n+1}\right) + \frac{1}{2} \sin^{-1}\left(1 - \frac{2(k+1)}{n+1}\right) \tag{5.2.2}$$

where $\sin^{-1}$ is the inverse trigonometric sine function and k shows how many times each trait appears in a sample of n size. Thus $k/n = p$ is the frequency of each trait in a sample. Other scholars (Harris and Sjøvold, 2004; Jackes et al., 2001; Sjøvold, 1977) prefer the transformation suggested by Anscombe (1948):

$$\theta = \sin^{-1}\left(1 - 2\frac{k+3/8}{n+3/4}\right) \tag{5.2.3}$$

The Freeman–Tukey and Anscombe transformations perform equally well and give almost identical results (see Harris and Sjøvold, 2004). In contrast, the old Smith's transformation:

$$\theta = \sin^{-1}\left(1 - \frac{2k}{n}\right) \tag{5.2.4}$$

fails to give correct results at particularly low or high trait frequencies and for this reason it is no longer used.

The MMD is an unbiased estimator of population divergence. When two populations are biologically very close, then $\theta_{1i} \approx \theta_{2i}$ and, therefore, a negative contribution to the MMD may arise from the terms $-1/(n_{1i} + 0.5)$, $-1/(n_{2i} + 0.5)$. In such cases negative MMD values are converted to 0 (Harris and Sjøvold, 2004; Irish, 2006, 2010; Sutter and Verano, 2007).

For the significance of the MMD, the most common test employs the variance of the MMD, when MMD $= 0$, estimated from (Sjøvold, 1973):

$$\sigma^2 = \frac{2}{r^2} \sum_{i=1}^{r} \left(\frac{1}{n_{1i} + 0.5} + \frac{1}{n_{2i} + 0.5}\right)^2 \tag{5.2.5}$$

In this case the test statistic is the ratio:

$$z = \text{MMD}/\sigma \tag{5.2.6}$$

which follows the standard normal distribution. Therefore, if the MMD is at least twice as large as the square root of its variance, then it is statistically significant (Sjøvold, 1977).

The calculation of the MMD from these equations may be performed using the macro Biodistances provided in the companion website. A case study based on this macro is discussed in detail in Appendix 5.XI. Alternatively, the MMD can be computed in R using the StartMMD function of the AnthropMMD library or Konigsberg's R script, tdistR.zip, downloadable from Lyle W. Konigsberg's website: https://50fc25581bb4561d048337efb1525036fe6ae84e.googledrive. com/host/0B-YNQGBRIWzxfmtwSUZreXpWTk1kVDA1TDVpVEZkd2ZhZnUzbEt6WjJDTTRlNEsyWU1ST0E/.

However, we should stress that before the calculation of the MMD, data should be properly edited to meet the requirements of this measure. The data editing procedure is described in Section 5.2.6.

5.2.5 Nonmetric Mahalanobis Distances

Nikita (2015) showed that if nonmetric traits are recorded using ordinal scores, a good biodistance measure is the Mahalanobis distance, Eq. (5.1.9), and, in the case of groups with small sizes, the corrected Mahalanobis distance, Eq. (5.1.10), computed directly from the ordinal data. This suggests that the ordinal scores adopted for nonmetric traits may code an underlying continuous variable. These distances may be denoted as ordinal Mahalanobis distance (OMD) and corrected ordinal Mahalanobis distance (COMD). The significance of these biodistance measures may be assessed by means of Eq. (5.1.11), although permutations or similar techniques should be adopted for more confidence in cases of data sets with many missing values.

If the ordinal data are transformed to binary ones, then Mahalanobis-type distances may be defined as follows. The Freeman–Tukey and Anscombe transformations convert the binary scores of each trait to normally distributed variables. Therefore, the MMD is strictly valid for data sets of uncorrelated traits, that is, data sets in which the covariances between the variables (traits) are equal to zero. To take into account intercorrelated traits, an extension of the Mahalanobis distance to binary data is required. This was attempted by Konigsberg (1990), who proposed an elegant version of the Mahalanobis distance for binary data, based on the assumption that the binary nonmetric traits code an underlying continuous variable that follows the normal distribution with unit standard deviation. This assumption constitutes the *Threshold Model*.

Subsequently, under the validity of this model, the threshold value z_{qj} of trait j in sample q may be estimated using the probit function from:

$$z_{qj} = \text{probit}(p_{qj}) \tag{5.2.7}$$

where p_{qj} is the percentage of presences for trait j in sample q. In this case, if we have data from two samples, 1 and 2, that is, values p_{1j} and p_{2j}, the difference $z_{1j} - z_{2j}$ is equal to the difference in the mean values of the normal distributions with unit standard deviation from which samples 1 and 2 derive. Therefore, we may define a Euclidean distance between samples 1 and 2 from:

$$d_E = \sqrt{(z_1 - z_2)^T (z_1 - z_2)} \tag{5.2.8}$$

where $z_1 = (\mu_{11}, \mu_{12}, ..., \mu_{1r})^T$; $z_2 = (\mu_{21}, \mu_{22}, ..., \mu_{2r})^T$; $\mu_{11}, \mu_{12}, ..., \mu_{1r}$ are the mean values of z_{1j} of the first sample; and $\mu_{21}, \mu_{22}, ..., \mu_{2r}$ are the corresponding mean values of z_{2j} of the second sample.

To extend this distance measure to a proper Mahalanobis-type distance, we need to define a variance—covariance matrix. Note that in this matrix all diagonal elements will be equal to 1, because, according to the threshold model, the variances of the underlying continuous variables are equal to 1. The nondiagonal elements are the covariances between traits i and j, that is, the nondiagonal elements are equal to $cov(z_i, z_j)$. To estimate $cov(z_i, z_j)$, we note that the Pearson correlation coefficient, r_{ij}, is given by:

$$r_{ij} = \frac{cov(z_i, z_j)}{s_i s_j} = cov(z_i, z_j) \tag{5.2.9}$$

where s_i and s_j are the standard deviations of traits i and j, which under the threshold model are equal to 1. Eq. (5.2.9) is valid for the underlying continuous variable, which is coded by the binary variable. Because the continuous data set is unknown, we should approximate r_{ij} from the binary nonmetric traits. Konigsberg, in his pioneer work in 1990, approximates r_{ij} through tetrachoric coefficients. Thus, the following Mahalanobis-type distance (TMD) is defined:

$$d_{TM}^2 = (z_1 - z_2)^T T_{\text{pooled}}^{-1} (z_1 - z_2) \tag{5.2.10}$$

where T_{pooled}^{-1} is the inverse of the pooled within-group tetrachoric correlation matrix between all traits. Specifically, for traits i and j the number of pairs 0—0, 0—1, 1—0, and 1—1 among all cases is calculated, and in the resulting 2×2 table the tetrachoric correlation coefficient is estimated using a proper algorithm, usually Brown's algorithm (1977). The tetrachoric correlation coefficients between all traits form an $r \times r$ matrix for each sample. The tetrachoric T_{pooled} matrix is then formed by pooling the individual matrices. The pooling procedure may accept different sample sizes as well as missing values by using weighted average correlation coefficients.

An alternative Mahalanobis-type distance arises if we approximate r_{ij} by the Pearson correlation coefficient calculated directly from the binary traits i and j. In this case the modified Mahalanobis distance (RMD) is expressed as:

$$d_{RM}^2 = (z_1 - z_2)^T R_{\text{pooled}}^{-1} (z_1 - z_2) \tag{5.2.11}$$

where R_{pooled}^{-1} is the inverse of the pooled within-group correlation matrix, that is, the matrix with the Pearson correlation coefficients estimated between all traits.

In a 2015 study by Nikita (2015) the aforementioned distance measures, including the MMD, were critically reviewed based on artificial data sets and it was shown that they offer overall a satisfactory estimation of the bio-distance between samples provided that the number of statistically nonsignificant distances is very small. Special attention should be paid to the TMD, Eq. (5.2.10), because its values might exhibit ill-conditioned problems especially when the number of traits is large. In this case a simple solution to detect abnormal TMDs is to disturb the diagonal elements of the pooled tetrachoric matrix used in the TMD by a very small random noise with a maximum value of 0.025. When the system is ill-conditioned, the difference in the TMD values recorded with and without noise is usually high, much higher than 10%. The test statistics used for Mahalanobis-type distances, that is, Eq. (5.1.11), do not give reliable p-values for the TMD and RMD. Thus, permutations or similar techniques should also be adopted provided that there are no ill-conditioned problems for the TMD.

All the Mahalanobis-type distances presented in this section and the corresponding p-values can be easily computed using the macro Biodistances, provided in the companion website. The OMD/COMD are computed as the corresponding MD/CMD discussed in Appendix 5.VIII. For the RMD and TMD a case study is presented in detail in

Appendix 5.XI. The TMD may be alternatively computed in R using Konigsberg's R script, tdistR.zip. Data requirements for the computation of Mahalanobis-type distances are fewer than for the MMD and are presented in the next section.

5.2.6 Data Analysis

5.2.6.1 Preliminary Editing of Nonmetric Traits

Once the frequency of each trait in a sample has been calculated, for the computation of the MMD, it is common practice to perform data editing, which involves the following steps:

1. Traits that exhibit only missing values in one or more samples under study are eliminated.
2. Traits that exhibit a particularly high (>0.95) or low (<0.05) frequency within one or more samples under study may be eliminated. Alternatively, Harris and Sjøvold (2004) recommend the use of Bartlett's correction, which entails the replacement of $p = 0$ with $p = 1/4n$, and $p = 1$ with $p = 1 - 1/4n$, where p denotes the trait frequency.
3. All nondiagnostic traits, that is, all traits that are not significantly different between at least one pair of samples because they are either too rare or too common in all groups are removed from the data set (Harris and Sjøvold, 2004). The reason is that, whereas such traits should have a small or negligible contribution to the MMD, because of the correction factor, $-1/(n_{1i} + 0.5) - 1/(n_{2i} + 0.5)$, their contribution becomes negative, which is biologically meaningless. These traits may be detected using χ^2 or Fisher's exact tests.
4. All traits that exhibit a statistically significant intercorrelation with one another may be dropped from the data set because, as already mentioned, the MMD is valid under the assumption that there are no intercorrelated traits (Irish, 2010 and references therein). There are several strategies to determine trait intercorrelations. The best of them is by means of Kendall's tau-b correlation coefficients calculated from the original nondichotomized ordinal data (Irish, 2010). Alternatively, tetrachoric correlations of dichotomized data or even Pearson's correlations may be used as an approximation of the tetrachoric correlations. Traits that exhibit correlation coefficients greater than 0.5 or traits that demonstrate a statistically significant intercorrelation (*p*-value < .05) should be removed from the data set. It should be stressed that although removing intercorrelated traits is standard practice, a 2015 study found that the inclusion of such traits does not appear to affect the validity of the MMD results (Nikita, 2015).
5. Sexual dimorphism should also be tested if males and females are going to be pooled in the biodistance analyses, because some nonmetric traits exhibit different frequencies in each sex.

These steps can be easily implemented by means of the DataEditing macro in the homonymous Excel file or from the menu Add-ins → OSTEO → Data pre-treatment → Data editing for the MMD from the OSTEO file (see companion website). A description and application of this macro are given in Appendix 5.XI.

For the calculation of the Mahalanobis distances for nonmetric traits (d^2_{RM} and d^2_{TM}), traits that exhibit only missing values within one or more samples must also be removed from the data set. Note that for traits that are always present or absent within a certain sample, the value of p_{qj} in Eq. (5.2.7) is either 1 or 0, and therefore z_{qj} values cannot be calculated. In this case we may adopt Bartlett's correction, discussed earlier, or Konigsberg's suggestion to substitute 0 with $1/2n$ and 1 with $1 - (1/2n)$ (see script tdistR.zip on Konigsberg's website).

OMD and COMD require no preliminary data editing except for the elimination of traits that exhibit only missing values within one or more samples. However, we should take into account that these distances, as well as all Mahalanobis-type distances (but not the MMD), cannot be calculated if the number of variables exceeds the number of cases.

5.2.6.2 Statistical Treatment

After data editing, the MMD and nonmetric Mahalanobis distances are calculated. Subsequently, dendrograms are plotted based on the Mahalanobis distances and the MMD to visualize the biodistance among populations, whereas metric or nonmetric MDS can be used on the Mahalanobis data and the MMD to visualize the biodistances among populations (see Sections 9.9.6 and 9.9.7, Case Study 27).

5.3 R-MATRIX ANALYSIS

An approach that complements biodistance analyses and allows one to explore genetic similarities within and between populations is R-matrix analysis. For g populations, the R-matrix is a square matrix consisting of g rows and g columns, the elements of which are calculated from (Relethford and Harpending, 1994; Relethford et al., 1997):

$$R_{ij} = \frac{(p_i - \bar{p})(p_j - \bar{p})}{\bar{p}(1 - \bar{p})} \tag{5.3.1}$$

where p_i and p_j are the allele frequencies in populations i and j and $\bar{p}$ is the mean allele frequency over all populations. According to Konigsberg (2006), the off-diagonal elements of this matrix can be defined as average kinship coefficients between populations, and the diagonal elements as kinship coefficients within populations. Thus, positive R_{ij} values characterize pairs of populations that are similar to each other, whereas the inverse applies for negative values (Relethford and Harpending, 1994; Relethford et al., 1997).

A quantity closely related to the R-matrix is the fixation index, F_{st}. F_{st} was introduced by Sewall Wright (1951) and expresses the total variation among populations (Relethford and Harpending, 1994). The values of this index range from 0 to 1. For two populations a zero F_{st} value suggests that none of the observed variation can be attributed to differences in allele frequencies between the populations. Thus, a relatively small F_{st} value for a group of populations indicates that these populations were experiencing significant gene flow. Based on the R-matrix, the F_{st} value may be estimated from:

$$F_{st} = \sum_{i=1}^{g} w_i R_{ii} \tag{5.3.2}$$

where the weighting factors, w_i, are estimated based on the size of the populations from which the samples originate. If this information is not available, w_i are approximated by $1/g$.

Once the R-matrix of a group of samples/populations has been computed, it may be further analyzed using principal coordinates analysis (Section 9.9.7). This analysis may be performed using the macro PCoA, provided in the companion website in the homonymous Excel file. The two-dimensional plot between the first two "Coordinates" shows the relative biological positions of the samples. Note that the same information is obtained when we apply MDS on a matrix of biodistances, that is, on the MD, CMD, MMD, etc. Finally, from the R-matrix we may compute a generalized squared distance using:

$$d_{ij}^2 = R_{ii} + R_{jj} - 2R_{ij} \tag{5.3.3}$$

and analyze it as the biodistances presented in the previous sections.

To estimate the F_{st} and the R-matrix from continuous craniometric data as well as from nonmetric binary data, we may adopt the following approaches.

5.3.1 Continuous Data

According to Relethford and Blangero (1990) and Relethford et al. (1997), the F_{st} value may be estimated from:

$$F_{st} = \sum_{i=1}^{g} w_i C_{ii} \bigg/ \left(1 + \sum_{i=1}^{g} w_i C_{ii}\right) \tag{5.3.4}$$

where again $w_i = 1/g$ and C_{ii} are the diagonal elements of the C-matrix computed from:

$$C_{ij} = (x_i - \mu)^T P^{-1} (x_j - \mu)(1/2r) \tag{5.3.5}$$

Here, r is the number of metric traits; x_i, x_j are the mean vectors of groups i and j; μ is the vector of total means over all groups; and P^{-1} is the inverse of the pooled within-group covariance matrix. Note that $w_i = 1/g$ may be used for the calculation of both μ and P. Note also that to include the average heritability, h^2, in the calculations, matrix P is multiplied by h^2. Once the F_{st} and C-matrix have been obtained, the R-matrix is calculated from:

$$R = C(1 - F_{st}) \tag{5.3.6}$$

An unbiased R-matrix is obtained if the term $1/2n_i$, n_i being the number of cases in the ith group, is subtracted from the diagonal element R_{ii}, computed from Eq. (5.3.6), for each i (Relethford et al., 1997). Note that Relethford et al. (1997) provide equations for the computation of the standard deviations of the F_{st} and R_{ij}.

5.3.2 Binary Data

According to Irish (2010) and Konigsberg (2006), to estimate the F_{st} and the R-matrix from nonmetric binary data, the following approach may be adopted. First, a C-matrix is calculated directly from the MMD or the Mahalanobis distances by means of the following equation:

$$C = -(I - 1w^T)d^2(I - 1w^T)^T/4r \qquad (5.3.7)$$

where I is a $g \times g$ identity matrix and g is the number of populations, 1 is a $g \times 1$ column vector of 1's, d^2 is a $g \times g$ matrix of squared distances based on traits (MMD, TMD, or RMD), and w is a $g \times 1$ column vector of relative population sizes in which all elements are approximated by $1/g$. Subsequently, the F_{st} and the R-matrix may be estimated from Eqs. (5.3.4) and (5.3.6), respectively. Note that the C-matrix in Eq. (5.3.7) has been divided by $2r$ in comparison to the corresponding matrix presented by Irish (2010), to make the expressions of F_{st} and R given in Irish's paper identical to those of Eqs. (5.3.4) and (5.3.6).

The aforementioned methods for computing the F_{st} and R-matrix are implemented in the macro Fst, which is provided in the companion website in the Excel files Fst and OSTEO. Its application is straightforward (see Appendices 5.VIII and 5.XI). Note also that a freely available software for F_{st} and R-matrix calculations for metric traits is RMET 5.0, authored by John Relethford. This software can be downloaded from http://employees.oneonta.edu/relethjh/programs/ and an application of this program is presented in Appendix 5.VIII.

REFERENCES

Alt KW, Türp JC. Hereditary anomalies. In: Alt KW, Rösing FW, Teschler-Nicola M, editors. Dental anthropology. Fundamentals, limits and prospects. New York: Springer; 1998. p. 95−128.

Anscombe FJ. The transformation of Poisson, binomial, and negative-binomial data. Biometrika 1948;35:246−54.

Ansorge H. Assessing non-metric skeleton characters as a morphological tool. Zoology 2001;104:268−77.

Arya R, Duggirala R, Comuzzie AG, Puppala S, Modem S, Busi BR, Crawford MH. Heritability of anthropometric phenotypes in caste populations of Visakhapatnam, India. Human Biology 2002;74:325−44.

Aubry BS. Technical note: cervical dimensions for in situ and loose teeth: a critique of the Hillson et al. (2005) method. American Journal of Physical Anthropology 2014;154:159−64.

Berry RJ. Biology and nonmetrical variation in mice and men. In: Brothwell DR, editor. The skeletal biology of earlier human populations. Oxford: Pergamon; 1968. p. 103−33.

Berry AC. Anthropological and family studies on minor variants of the dental crown. In: Butler PM, Joysey KA, editors. Development, function and evolution of teeth. London: Academic Press; 1978. p. 81−98.

Berry AC, Berry RJ. Epigenetic variation in the human cranium. Journal of Anatomy 1967;101:361−79.

Betti L, Balloux F, Hanihara T, Manica A. Distance from Africa, not climate, explains within-population phenotypic diversity in humans. Proceedings of the Royal Society Series B: Biological Sciences 2009;276:809−14.

Betti L, Balloux F, Hanihara T, Manica A. The relative role of drift and selection in shaping the human skull. American Journal of Physical Anthropology 2010;141:76−82.

Bookstein FL. Morphometric tools for landmark data. Cambridge: Cambridge University Press; 1991.

Brothwell D. Studies on skeletal and dental variation: a view across two centuries. In: Cox M, Mays S, editors. Human osteology in archaeology and forensic science. London: Greenwich Medical Media, Ltd.; 2000. p. 1−6.

Brown MB. Algorithm AS 116: the tetrachoric correlation and its asymptotic standard error. Applied Statistics 1977;26:343−51.

Buikstra JE. Techniques for coping with the age-regressive nature of nonmetric traits. American Journal of Physical Anthropology 1972;37:431−2.

Buikstra JE, Ubelaker DH, editors. Standards for data collection from human skeletal remains. Fayetteville, Arkansas: Arkansas Archaeological Survey Report Number 44; 1994.

Carson EA. Maximum likelihood estimation of human craniometric heritabilities. American Journal of Physical Anthropology 2006a;131:169−80.

Carson EA. Maximum-likelihood variance components analysis of heritabilities of cranial nonmetric traits. Human Biology 2006b;78:383−402.

Cheverud JM, Buikstra JE. Quantitative genetics of skeletal nonmetric traits in the rhesus macaques on Cayo Santiago. I. Single trait heritabilities. American Journal of Physical Anthropology 1981;54:43−9.

Darroch JN, Mosimann JE. Canonical and principal components of shape. Biometrika 1985;72:241−52.

De Maesschalck R, Jouan-Rimbaud D, Massart DL. The Mahalanobis distance. Chemometrics and Intelligent Laboratory Systems 2000;50:1−18.

Dempsey PJ, Townsend GC. Genetic and environmental contributions to variation in human tooth size. Heredity 2001;86:685−93.

Dodo Y. Non-metrical cranial traits in the Hokkaido Ainu and the northern Japanese of recent times. Journal of the Anthropology Society of Nippon 1974;82:31−51.

Donlon DA. The value of infracranial nonmetric variation in studies of modern *Homo sapiens*: an Australian focus. American Journal of Physical Anthropology 2000;113:349−68.

Evteev A, Cardini AL, Morozova I, O'Higgins P. Extreme climate, rather than population history, explains mid-facial morphology of Northern Asians. American Journal of Physical Anthropology 2014;153:449−62.

Freeman MF, Tukey JW. Transformations related to the angular and square root. The Annals of Mathematical Statistics 1950;21:607−11.

Garn S, Osborne R, McCabe K. The effect of prenatal factors on crown dimensions. American Journal of Physical Anthropology 1979;51:665−78.

Godde K. An examination of proposed causes of auditory exostoses. International Journal of Osteoarchaeology 2010;20:486−90.

González-José R, Ramírez-Rozzi F, Sardi M, Martínez-Abadías N, Hernández M, Pucciarelli HM. Functional−cranial approach to the influence of economic strategy on skull morphology. American Journal of Physical Anthropology 2005;128:757−71.

Green RF, Suchey JM. The use of inverse sine transformations in the analysis of non-metric cranial data. American Journal of Physical Anthropology 1976;45:61−8.

Grewal MS. The rate of genetic divergence in the C57BL strain of mice. Genetical Research 1962;3:226−37.

Grüneberg H. Genetical studies on the skeleton of the Mouse IV. Quasi-continuous variations. Journal of Genetics 1952;51:95−114.

Grüneberg H. The Pathology of development: a study of inherited skeletal disorders in animals. New York: Wiley-Liss; 1963.

Hammer Ø, Harper DAT, Ryan PD. PAST: paleontological statistics software package for education and data analysis. Paleontologia Electronica 2001;4:1−9.

Hanihara K. Criteria for classification of crown characters of the human deciduous dentition. Journal of the Anthropological Society of Nippon 1961;69:27−45.

Hanihara T. Morphological variation of major human populations based on nonmetric dental traits. American Journal of Physical Anthropology 2008;136:169−82.

Hanihara T, Ishida H, Dodo Y. Characterization of biological diversity through analysis of discrete cranial traits. American Journal of Physical Anthropology 2003;121:241−51.

Harris EF. Carabelli's trait and tooth size of human maxillary first molars. American Journal of Physical Anthropology 2007;132:238−46.

Harris EF, Sjøvold T. Calculation of Smith's mean measure of divergence for intergroup comparisons using nonmetric data. Dental Anthropology 2004;17:83−93.

Harvati K, Weaver TD. Human cranial anatomy and the differential preservation of population history and climate signatures. The Anatomical Record Part A 2006;288:1225−33.

Hauser G, De Stefano GF. Epigenetic variants of the human skull. Stuttgart: E. Schweizarbart'sche Verlagsbuchhandlung; 1989.

Hernández M, Lalueza C, García-Moro C. Fueguian cranial morphology: the adaptation to a cold, harsh environment. American Journal of Physical Anthropology 1997;103:103−17.

Herrera B, Hanihara T, Godde K. Comparability of multiple data types from the Bering strait region: cranial and dental metrics and nonmetrics, mtDNA, and Y-chromosome DNA. American Journal of Physical Anthropology 2014;154:334−48.

Hillson S. Dental anthropology. Cambridge: Cambridge University Press; 1996.

Hillson S. Teeth. Cambridge: Cambridge University Press; 2005.

Hillson S, FitzGerald C, Flinn H. Alternative dental measurements: proposals and relationships with other measurements. American Journal of Physical Anthropology 2005;126:413−26.

Holmes MA, Ruff CB. Dietary effects on development of the human mandibular corpus. American Journal of Physical Anthropology 2011;145:615−28.

Howells WW. Cranial variation in man. A study by multivariate analysis of patterns of difference among recent human populations. Cambridge MA: Harvard University Press; 1973.

Howells WW. Skull shapes and the map. Cambridge, MA: Harvard University Press; 1989.

Hubbard AR, Guatelli-Steinberg D, Irish JD. Do nuclear DNA and dental nonmetric data produce similar reconstructions of regional population history? An example from modern Coastal Kenya. American Journal of Physical Anthropology 2015;157:295−304.

Irish JD. Who were the ancient Egyptians? Dental affinities among Neolithic through post-dynastic peoples. American Journal of Physical Anthropology 2006;129:529−43.

Irish JD. The mean measure of divergence: its utility in model-free and model-bound analyses relative to the Mahalanobis D^2 distance for nonmetric traits. American Journal of Human Biology 2010;22:378−95.

Jackes M, Silva AM, Irish J. Dental morphology: a valuable contribution to our understanding of prehistory. Journal of Iberian Archaeology 2001;3:97−119.

Johannsdottir B, Thorarinsson F, Thordarson A, Magnusson TE. Heritability of craniofacial characteristics between parents and offspring estimated from lateral cephalograms. American Journal of Osthodontics and Dentofacial Orthopedics 2005;127:200−7.

Johnson RA, Wichern DW. Applied multivariate statistical analysis. 6th ed. New Jersey: Prentice Hall; 2007.

Jungers WL, Falsetti AB, Wall CE. Shape, relative size, and size-adjustments in morphometrics. Yearbook of Physical Anthropology 1995;38:137−61.

Kitagawa Y. Nonmetric morphological characters of deciduous teeth in Japan: diachronic evidence of the past 4000 years. International Journal of Osteoarchaeology 2000;10:242−53.

Kitagawa Y, Manabe Y, Oyamada J, Rokutanda A. Deciduous dental morphology of the prehistoric Jomon people of Japan: comparison of nonmetric characters. American Journal of Physical Anthropology 1995;97:101−11.

Konigsberg LW. Analysis of prehistoric biological variation under a model of isolation by geographic and temporal distance. Human Biology 1990;62:49−70.

Konigsberg LW. A post-Neumann history of biological and genetic distance studies in bioarchaeology. In: Buikstra JE, Beck LA, editors. Bioarchaeology: the contextual analysis of human remains. New York: Academic Press; 2006. p. 263−79.

Konigsberg LW, Ousley SD. Multivariate quantitative genetics of anthropometric traits from the Boas data. Human Biology 1995;67:481−98.

Larsen CS. Biological changes in human populations with agriculture. Annual Review of Anthropology 1995;24:185−213.

Lease LR, Sciulli PW. Discrimination between European-American and African-American children based on deciduous dental metrics and morphology. American Journal of Physical Anthropology 2005;126:56−60.

Leblanc SA, Turner B, Morgan ME. Genetic relationships based on discrete dental traits: basketmaker II and Mimbres. International Journal of Osteoarchaeology 2008;18:109−30.

Lele SR, Richtsmeier JT. An invariant approach to statistical analysis of shapes. London: Chapman and Hall/CRC; 2001.

Lieberman DE, Ross CR, Ravosa M. The primate cranial base: ontogeny, function, and integration. Yearbook of Physical Anthropology 2000a;43:117−69.

Lieberman DE, Mowbray KM, Pearson OM. Basicranial influences on overall cranial shape. Journal of Human Evolution 2000b;38:291−315.

Lukacs JR, Walimbe SR. Deciduous dental morphology and the biological affinities of a late Chalcolithic skeletal series from western India. American Journal of Physical Anthropology 1984;65:23−30.

Mahalanobis PC. On the generalised distance in statistics. Proceedings of the National Institute of Science of India 1936;12:49−55.

Manica A, Amos W, Balloux F, Hanihara T. The effect of ancient population bottlenecks on human phenotypic variation. Nature 2007;448:346−8.

Manzi G, Gracia A, Arsuaga JL. Cranial discrete traits in the middle Pleistocene humans from Sima de los Huesos (Sierra de Atapuerca. Spain). Does hypostosis represent any increase in 'ontogenetic stress' along the Neanderthal lineage? Journal of Human Evolution 2000;38:425−46.

Mardia KV, Bookstein FL. Statistical assessment of bilateral symmetry of shapes. Biometrika 2000;87:285−300.

Martin R. Lehrbuch der Anthropologie. Jena: Verlag von Gustav Fischer; 1928.

Martínez-Abadías N, Esparza M, Sjøvold T, González-José R, Santos M, Hernández M. Heritability of human cranial dimensions: comparing the evolvability of different cranial regions. Journal of Anatomy 2009;214:19−35.

Mayhall JT. Dental morphology: techniques and strategies. In: Katzenberg MA, Saunders SR, editors. Biological anthropology of the human skeleton. New York: Wiley Liss; 2000. p. 103−34.

Mays S. The archaeology of human bones. 2nd ed. London: Routledge; 2010.

McGrath JW, Cheverud JM, Buikstra JE. Genetic correlations between sides and heritability of asymmetry for nonmetric traits in rhesus macaques. American Journal of Physical Anthropology 1984;64:401−11.

Mizoguchi Y. Genetic variability in tooth crown characters: analysis by the tetrachoric correlation method Bulletin of the National Science Museum. Series D 1977;3:37−62.

Moore-Jansen PH, Jantz RL. Data collection procedures for forensic skeletal material. Report of Investigations No.48. Knoxville: University of Tennessee; 1989.

Mosimann JE, James FC. New statistical methods for allometry with application to Florida red-winged blackbirds. Evolution 1979;33:444−59.

Nicholson E, Harvati K. Quantitative analysis of human mandibular shape using three-dimensional geometric morphometrics. American Journal of Physical Anthropology 2006;131:368−83.

Nikita E. A critical review of the Mean Measure of Divergence and Mahalanobis Distances using artificial data and new approaches to estimate bio-distances from non-metric traits. American Journal of Physical Anthropology 2015;157:284−94.

Nikita E, Mattingly D, Lahr MM. Sahara: barrier or corridor? Nonmetric cranial traits and biological affinities of North African Late Holocene populations. American Journal of Physical Anthropology 2012;147:280−92.

Okumura MM, Boyadjian CH, Eggers S. Auditory exostoses as an aquatic activity marker: a comparison of coastal and inland skeletal remains from tropical and subtropical regions of Brazil. American Journal of Physical Anthropology 2007;132:558−67.

Ossenberg NS. Discontinuous morphological variation in the human cranium [Ph.D. thesis]. University of Toronto; 1969.

Paschetta C, de Azevedo S, Castillo L, Martínez-Abadías N, Hernández M, Lieberman DE, González-José R. The influence of masticatory loading on craniofacial morphology: a test case across technological transitions in the Ohio Valley. American Journal of Physical Anthropology 2010;141:297−314.

Paul KS, Stojanowski CM. Performance analysis of deciduous morphology for detecting biological siblings. American Journal of Physical Anthropology 2015;157:615−29.

Pinhasi R, Eshed V, Shaw P. Evolutionary changes in the masticatory complex following the transition to farming in the Southern Levant. American Journal of Physical Anthropology 2008;135:136−48.

Potter RHY, Rice JP, Dahlberg AA, Dahlberg T. Dental size traits within families: path analysis for first molar and lateral incisor. American Journal of Physical Anthropology 1983;61:283−9.

Relethford JH. Genetic drift and anthropometric variation in Ireland. Human Biology 1991;63:155−65.

Relethford JH, Blangero J. Detection of differential gene flow from patterns of quantitative variation. Human Biology 1990;62:5−25.

Relethford JH, Harpending HC. Craniometric variation, genetic theory, and modern human origins. American Journal of Physical Anthropology 1994;95:249−70.

Relethford JH, Crawford MH, Blangero J. Genetic drift and gene flow in post-famine Ireland. Human Biology 1997;69:443−65.

Ricaut F, Auriol V, von Cramon-Taubadel N, Keyser C, Murail P, Ludes B, Crubézy E. Comparison between morphological and genetic data to estimate biological relationship: the case of the Egyin Gol necropolis (Mongolia). American Journal of Physical Anthropology 2010;143:355−64.

Ritchmeier JT, DeLeon VB, Lele SR. The promise of geometric morphometrics. Yearbook of Physical Anthropology 2002;45:63−91.

Rohlf FJ, Marcus LF. A revolution in morphometrics. Trends in Ecology and Evolution 1993;8:129−32.

Roseman CC. Detecting interregionally diversifying natural selection on modern human cranial form by using matched molecular and morphometric data. Proceedings of the National Academy of Sciences United States of America 2004;101:12824−9.

Roseman CC, Weaver TD. Molecules versus morphology? Not for the human cranium. BioEssays 2007;29:1185

Saunders SR, Popovich F. A family study of two skeletal variants: atlas bridging and clinoid bridging. American Journal of Physical Anthropology 1978;49:193—204.

Sciulli PW. Evolution of the dentition in prehistoric Ohio Valley Native Americans: II. morphology of the deciduous dentition. American Journal of Physical Anthropology 1998;106:189—205.

Scott GR. Dental morphology. In: Katzenberg MA, Saunders SR, editors. Biological anthropology of the human skeleton. 2nd ed. New York: Wiley-Liss; 2008. p. 265—98.

Scott GR, Potter RHY. An analysis of tooth crown morphology in American white twins. Anthropologie 1984;22:223—31.

Scott GR, Turner CG. The anthropology of modern teeth: dental morphology and its variation in recent human populations. Cambridge: Cambridge University Press; 1997.

Self GS, Leamy LJ. Heritability of quasicontinuous skeletal traits in a randombred population of House mice. Genetics 1978;88:109—20.

Sherwood RJ, Duren DL, Demerath EW, Czerwinski SA, Siervogel RM, Towne B. Quantitative genetics of modern human cranial variation. Journal of Human Evolution 2008;54:909—14.

Sjøvold T. The occurrence of minor non-metrical variants in the skeleton and their quantitative treatment for population comparisons. HOMO-Journal of Comparative Human Biology 1973;24:204—33.

Sjøvold T. Some notes on the distribution and certain modifications of Mahalanobis generalized distance. Journal of Human Evolution 1975;4:549—58.

Sjøvold T. Non—metrical divergence between skeletal populations. The theoretical foundation and biological importance of C. A. B. Smith's mean measure of divergence. OSSA 1977;4(Suppl.):1—133.

Sjøvold T. A report on the heritability of some cranial measurements and nonmetric traits. In: van Vark GN, Howells WW, editors. Multivariate statistical methods in physical anthropology. Dordrecht: D. Reidel; 1984. p. 223—46.

Slice DE. Morpheus et al.: software for morphometric research. Stony Brook: State University of New York, Department of Ecology and Evolution; 1998.

Slice DE. Morpheus et al.: java edition. Department of Scientific Computing. Tallahassee, Florida, U.S.A: The Florida State University; 2013.

Smith HF. Which cranial regions reflect molecular distances reliably inhumans? Evidence from three-dimensional morphology. American Journal of Human Biology 2009;21:36—47.

Smith HF, Terhune CE, Lockwood CA. Genetic, geographic, and environmental correlates of human temporal bone variation. American Journal of Physical Anthropology 2007;134:312—22.

Sofaer JA, MacLean CJ, Bailit HL. Heredity and morphological variation in early and late developing human teeth of the same morphological class. Archives of Oral Biology 1972;17:811—6.

Sparks CS, Jantz RL. A reassessment of human cranial plasticity: boas revisited. Proceedings of the National Academy of Sciences of the United States of America 2002;99:14636—9.

Spencer MA, Demes B. Biomechanical analysis of masticatory system configuration in Neandertals and Inuits. American Journal of Physical Anthropology 1993;91:1—20.

Spencer MA, Ungar PS. Craniofacial morphology, diet and incisor use in three Native American populations. International Journal of Osteoarchaeology 2000;10:229—41.

Stojanowski CM, Schillaci MA. Phenotypic approaches for understanding patterns of intracemetery biological variation. Yearbook of Physical Anthropology 2006;49:49—88.

Sutter RC, Mertz L. Nonmetric cranial trait variation and prehistoric biocultural change in the Azapa Valley, Chile. American Journal of Physical Anthropology 2004;123:130—45.

Sutter RC, Verano JW. Biodistance analysis of the Moche sacrificial victims from Huaca de la Luna plaza 3C: matrix method test of their origins. American Journal of Physical Anthropology 2007;132:193—206.

Torgersen J. The developmental genetics and evolutionary meaning of the metopic suture. American Journal of Physical Anthropology 1951;9:193—210.

Townsend GC. Heritability of deciduous tooth size in Australian Aboriginals. American Journal of Physical Anthropology 1980;53:297—300.

Townsend GC, Richards LC, Brown T, Burgess VB, Travan GR, Rogers JR. Genetic studies of dental morphology in South Australian twins. In: Smith P, Tchernov E, editors. Structure, function and evolution of teeth. London: Freund Publishing House Ltd; 1992. p. 501—18.

Townsend G, Richards L, Hughes T. Molar intercuspal dimensions: genetic input to phenotypic variation. Journal of Dental Research 2003;82:350—5.

Townsend G, Hughes T, Luciano M, Bockmann M, Brook A. Genetic and environmental influences on human dental variation: a critical evaluation of studies involving twins. Archives of Oral Biology 2009;54:S45—51.

Townsend G, Bockmann M, Hughes T, Brook A. Genetic, environmental and epigenetic influences on variation in human tooth number, size and shape. Odontology 2012;100:1—9.

Turner II CG. The dentition of arctic peoples [Ph.D. thesis]. Madison University of Wisconsin; 1967.

Turner II CG. Late Pleistocene and Holocene population history of East Asia based on dental variation. American Journal of Physical Anthropology 1987;73:305—21.

Turner II CG, Nichol CR, Scott GR. Scoring procedures for key morphological traits of the permanent dentition: the Arizona State University Dental Anthropology System. In: Kelley MA, Larsen CS, editors. Advances in dental anthropology. New York: Wiley-Liss; 1991. p. 13—32.

Tyrrell A. Skeletal non-metric traits and the assessment of inter- and intra-population diversity: past problems and future potential. In: Cox M, Mays S, editors. Human osteology in archaeology and forensic science. London: Greenwich Medical Media, Ltd; 2000. p. 289—306.

Ubelaker DH. Human skeletal remains: excavation, analysis, interpretation. 2nd ed. Washington: Taraxacum; 1989.

van Arsdale AP, Clark JL. Re-examining the relationship between cranial deformation and extra-sutural bone formation. International Journal of Osteoarchaeology 2012;22:119—26.

Velemínský P, Dobisíková M. Morphological likeness of the skeletal remains in a Central European family from 17th to 19th century. HOMO-Journal of Comparative Human Biology 2005;56:173—96.

von Cramon-Taubadel N. Congruence of individual cranial bone morphology and neutral molecular affinity patterns in modern humans. American Journal of Physical Anthropology 2009;140:205—15.

Weidenreich F. The dentition of sinanthropus pekinensis: a comparative odontography of the hominids. Peiping: Palaeolontologica Sinica; 1937. p. 1—180. New Series D No 1.

White TD, Black MT, Folkens PA. Human osteology. 3rd ed. New York: Elsevier Academic Press; 2011.

Williams-Blangero S, Blangero J. Anthropometric variation and the genetic structure of the Jirels. Human Biology 1989;61:1—12.

Wright S. The genetical structure of populations. Annals of Eugenics 1951;15:323—54.

APPENDICES

Appendix 5.I: Definitions of Cranial Landmarks

The following landmarks have been selected primarily from Howells (1973), Martin (1928), and Moore-Jansen and Jantz (1989). The reader may check these sources for more detailed instructions on the exact location of each landmark as well as for descriptions of additional ones. Figs. 5.I.1—5.I.4 present the landmarks given in this appendix in the cranial views that show them more clearly.

1. Glabella: The most anteriorly projecting point lying on the midsagittal plane, between the superciliary arches
2. Nasion: The point of intersection of the frontonasal and the internasal suture
3. Rhinion: The inferiormost point of the internasal suture
4. Alare: The lateralmost point on the margin of the nasal aperture
5. Nariale: The inferiormost point on the margin of the nasal aperture
6. Nasospinale: The point of intersection between the midsagittal plane and a line tangent to the most inferior points on the margin of the nasal aperture
7. Subspinale: The point at the deepest curvature of the maxillae below the anterior nasal spine
8. Prosthion: The anteriormost point of the maxillary alveolar border in the midsagittal plane
9. Alveolare: The inferiormost point of the alveolar border in the midsagittal plane
10. Maxillofrontale: The point of intersection between the inner orbital margin and the frontomaxillary suture

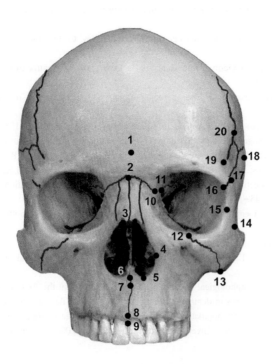

1 = Glabella
2 = Nasion
3 = Rhinion
4 = Alare
5 = Nariale
6 = Nasospinale
7 = Subspinale
8 = Prosthion
9 = Alveolare
10 = Maxillofrontale
11 = Dacryon
12 = Zygoorbitale
13 = Zygomaxillare anterior
14 = Jugalia
15 = Ectoconchion
16 = Frontomalare orbitale
17 = Frontomalare temporale
18 = Euryon
19 = Frontotemporale
20 = Stephanion

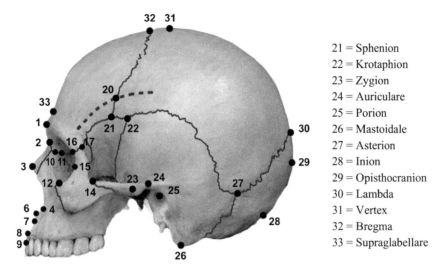

21 = Sphenion
22 = Krotaphion
23 = Zygion
24 = Auriculare
25 = Porion
26 = Mastoidale
27 = Asterion
28 = Inion
29 = Opisthocranion
30 = Lambda
31 = Vertex
32 = Bregma
33 = Supraglabellare

FIGURE 5.1.2   Cranial landmarks; lateral view.

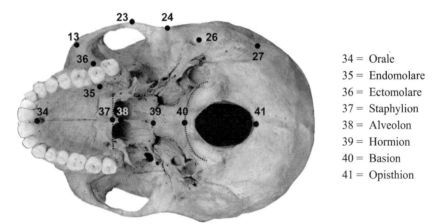

34 = Orale
35 = Endomolare
36 = Ectomolare
37 = Staphylion
38 = Alveolon
39 = Hormion
40 = Basion
41 = Opisthion

FIGURE 5.1.3   Cranial landmarks; basal view.

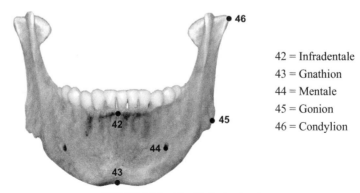

42 = Infradentale
43 = Gnathion
44 = Mentale
45 = Gonion
46 = Condylion

FIGURE 5.1.4   Mandibular landmarks.

11. Dacryon: The apex of the lacrimal fossa, impinging on the frontal bone
12. Zygoorbitale: The point of intersection between the orbital margin and the zygomaxillary suture
13. Zygomaxillare anterior: The point of intersection between the zygomaxillary suture and the point of attachment of the masseter muscle
14. Jugalia: The points at the deepest curvature between the frontal and the temporal processes of the zygomatic bones
15. Ectoconchion: The point on the lateral orbital margin where an axis parallel to the superior orbital margin divides the orbit into two equal halves
16. Frontomalare orbitale: The point of intersection between the frontozygomatic suture and the inner orbital rim
17. Frontomalare temporale: The lateralmost point of the frontozygomatic suture
18. Euryon: The lateralmost point on the cranial vault, located either on the parietals or on the superior part of the temporals; determined osteometrically
19. Frontotemporale: The point on the superior temporal line, lying at the base of the zygomatic process of the frontal bone
20. Stephanion: The point of intersection between the coronal suture and the temporal line
21. Sphenion: The anteriormost point on the sphenoparietal suture
22. Krotaphion: The posteriormost point on the sphenoparietal suture
23. Zygion: The lateralmost point on each zygomatic arch
24. Auriculare: The point at the deepest curvature of the root of the zygomatic process
25. Porion: The superiormost point on the margin of the external auditory meatus
26. Mastoidale: The inferiormost point on the mastoid process when orienting the cranium in the Frankfort horizontal
27. Asterion: The point of intersection between the temporal, parietal, and occipital bones
28. Inion: The point at the base of the external occipital protuberance at the midsagittal plane
29. Opisthocranion: The posteriormost point of the cranium in the midsagittal plane; determined osteometrically as the most distant point from the glabella
30. Lambda: The point of intersection between the lambdoidal suture and the sagittal suture
31. Vertex: The superiormost point of the skull when this is oriented in the Frankfort horizontal
32. Bregma: The point of intersection between the sagittal and the coronal sutures
33. Supraglabellare: The point of maximum convexity on the frontal bone above the glabella
34. Orale: The midline point of the line connecting the lingualmost surfaces of the maxillary central incisors
35. Endomolare: The medialmost point of the alveolar process at the level of the second maxillary molars
36. Ectomolare: The lateralmost point of the alveolar process at the level of the second maxillary molars
37. Staphylion: The midline point of a line connecting the anteriormost invaginations of the posterior margins of the palatine bones
38. Alveolon: The point of intersection between the midsagittal plane and a line connecting the posterior borders of the alveolar crests
39. Hormion: The posteriormost point of the vomer
40. Basion: The landmark pointed to by the apex of the occipital condyles, anterior to the foramen magnum, in the midline (Howells, 1973, p. 166)
    Note: Other scholars define basion as the anteriormost point of the foramen magnum in the midsagittal plane (e.g., Moore-Jansen and Jantz, 1989, p. 50).
41. Opisthion: The posteriormost point of the foramen magnum in the midsagittal plane
42. Infradentale: The anteriormost point of the mandibular alveolar border in the midsagittal plane
43. Gnathion: The inferiormost point of the mandibular body in the midsagittal plane
44. Mentale: The anteriormost point of the mental foramen
45. Gonion: The point of intersection between the inferior margin of the mandibular corpus and the posterior margin of the ramus
46. Condylion: The lateralmost point on the mandibular condyle

Appendix 5.II: Definitions of Cranial Linear Measurements

The following cranial measurements have been selected from Howells (1989) and Moore-Jansen and Jantz (1989). The reader may consult the original books to obtain more detailed information on the definition of each measurement as well as definitions of additional cranial dimensions. Note that most definitions are based on cranial landmarks, which are defined in Appendix 5.I. Figs. 5.II.1–5.II.4 depict the linear cranial measurements described in this appendix in the cranial views that show them more clearly. Instruments commonly used in osteometry are given in Appendix 6.I. *Note:* The measurements

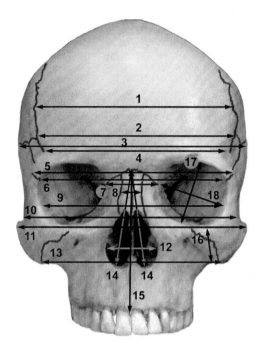

1 = Maximum frontal breadth (XFB)
2 = Bistephanic breadth (STB)
3 = Maximum cranial breadth (XCB)
4 = Minimum frontal breadth (WFB)
5 = Upper facial breadth (UFBR)
6 = Bifrontal breadth (FMB)
7 = Interorbital breadth (DKB)
8 = Least nasal breadth (WNB)
9 = Biorbital breadth (EKB)
10 = Bijugal breadth (JUB)
11 = Bizygomatic breadth (ZYB)
12 = Nasal breadth (NLB)
13 = Bimaxillary breadth (ZMB)
14 = Nasal height (NLH)
15 = Nasion-prosthion height or upper facial height (NPH)
16 = Cheek height (WMH)
17 = Orbital height (OBH)
18 = Orbital breadth (OBB)

FIGURE 5.II.1 Cranial measurements; anterior view.

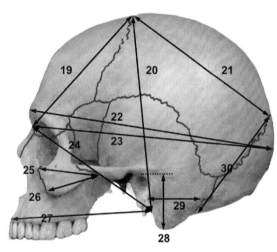

19 = Frontal chord (FRC)
20 = Basion-bregma height (BBH)
21 = Parietal chord (PAC)
22 = Glabello-occipital length (GOL)
23 = Nasio-occipital length (NOL)
24 = Basion-nasion length or Cranial base length (BNL)
25 = Malar length, maximum (XML)
26 = Malar length, inferior (IML)
27 = Basion-prosthion length (BPL)
28 = Mastoid height (MDH)
29 = Mastoid width (MDB)
30 = Occipital chord (OCC)

FIGURE 5.II.2 Cranial measurements; lateral view. Important note: The arrows that end at the anterior of the mastoid process for measurements 20, 24, and 27 actually point to the basion, while the arrow that ends at the posterior of the mastoid process for measurement 30 actually points to the opisthion.

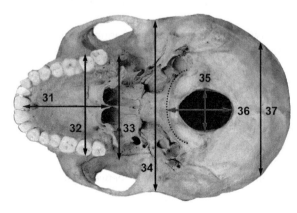

31 = Maxillo-alveolar length (MAL)
32 = Palate breadth, external, or Maxillo-alveolar breadth (MAB)
33 = Minimum cranial breadth (WCB)
34 = Biauricular breadth (AUB)
35 = Foramen magnum breadth (FOB)
36 = Foramen magnum length (FOL)
37 = Biasterionic breadth (ASB)

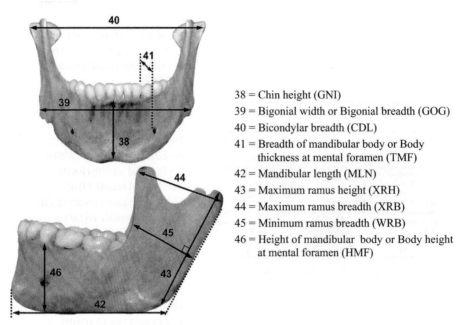

38 = Chin height (GNI)
39 = Bigonial width or Bigonial breadth (GOG)
40 = Bicondylar breadth (CDL)
41 = Breadth of mandibular body or Body thickness at mental foramen (TMF)
42 = Mandibular length (MLN)
43 = Maximum ramus height (XRH)
44 = Maximum ramus breadth (XRB)
45 = Minimum ramus breadth (WRB)
46 = Height of mandibular body or Body height at mental foramen (HMF)

FIGURE 5.II.4 Mandibular measurements.

1. Maximum frontal breadth (XFB): The maximum breadth of the frontal bone, obtained along the coronal suture, perpendicular to the sagittal plane
2. Bistephanic breadth (STB): The distance between the right and the left stephanion
3. Maximum cranial breadth (XCB)*: The distance between the right and the left euryon
4. Minimum frontal breadth (WFB)*: The distance between the right and the left frontotemporale
5. Upper facial breadth (UFBR)*: The distance between the right and the left frontomalare temporale
6. Bifrontal breadth (FMB): The distance between the right and the left frontomalare orbitale
7. Interorbital breadth (DKB)*: The distance between the right and the left dacryon (Howells, 1989, p. 6)
   Note: Other authors define this measurement as the distance between the two maxillofrontalia (e.g., Moore-Jansen and Jantz, 1989, p. 64).
8. Least nasal breadth (WNB): The minimum transverse breadth across the nasal bones
9. Biorbital breadth (EKB)*: The distance between the right and the left ectoconchion
10. Bijugal breadth (JUB): The distance between the two jugalia
11. Bizygomatic breadth (ZYB)*: The maximum breadth along the zygomatic arches, perpendicular to the sagittal plane
12. Nasal breadth (NLB)*: The maximum breadth of the nasal aperture
13. Bimaxillary breadth (ZMB): The distance between the right and the left zygomaxillare anterior
14. Nasal height (NLH)*: The distance between nasion and nariale (Howells, 1989, p. 5)
    Note: Other authors measure this distance between the nasion and the nasospinale (e.g., Moore-Jansen and Jantz, 1989, p. 62).
15. Nasion–prosthion height or upper facial height (NPH or UFHT according to the FORDISC abbreviation)*: The distance between nasion and prosthion
16. Cheek height (WMH): The minimum distance between the inferior orbital margin and the inferior maxillary margin
17. Orbital height (OBH)*: The distance between the superior and the inferior orbital margins, perpendicular to the long axis of the orbit
18. Orbital breadth (OBB)*: The distance between ectoconchion and dacryon (Howells, 1989, p. 5).
    Note: Other authors define this measurement as the distance between ectoconchion and maxillofrontale (e.g., Moore-Jansen and Jantz, 1989, p. 63).
19. Frontal chord (FRC)*: The distance between nasion and bregma
20. Basion–bregma height (BBH)*: The distance between bregma and basion
21. Parietal chord (PAC)*: The distance between bregma and lambda
22. Glabello–occipital length (maximum cranial length) (GOL)*: The distance between glabella and opisthocranion
23. Nasio–occipital length (NOL): The distance between nasion and opisthocranion

24. Basion—nasion length or cranial base length (BNL)*: The distance between nasion and basion
25. Malar length, maximum (XML): The length of the zygomatic bone measured as the distance between the inferiormost point of the zygotemporal suture and the zygoorbitale
26. Malar length, inferior (IML): The distance between the zygomaxillare anterior and the inferiormost point on the zygo-temporal suture
27. Basion—prosthion length (BPL)*: The distance between prosthion and basion
28. Mastoid height (MDH)*: The length of the mastoid process below, and perpendicular to the Frankfort horizontal
29. Mastoid width (MDB): The width of the mastoid process at its base
30. Occipital chord (OCC)*: The distance between lambda and opisthion
31. Maxillo—alveolar length (MAL)*: The distance between prosthion and alveolon
32. Palate breadth, external, or maxillo—alveolar breadth (MAB)*: The maximum breadth across the alveolar borders, wherever found, perpendicular to the sagittal plane
33. Minimum cranial breadth (WCB): Cranial breadth at the base of the temporal fossa
34. Biauricular breadth (AUB)*: The least exterior breadth across the roots of the zygomatic processes, wherever found
35. Foramen magnum breadth (FOB)*: The breadth of the foramen magnum at the point of greatest curvature of its lateral margins
36. Foramen magnum length (FOL)*: The distance between basion and opisthion
    Note: Many scholars place the basion at the midline of the anterior border of the foramen magnum, whereas others place it at the area pointed to by the apex of the occipital condyles. The dimension depicted in Fig. 5.II.3 follows the latter definition.
37. Biasterionic breadth (ASB)*: The distance between the right and the left asterion
38. Chin height (GNI)*: The distance between infradentale and gnathion
39. Bigonial width or bigonial breadth (GOG)*: The distance between the right and the left gonion
40. Bicondylar breadth (CDL)*: The distance between the right and the left condylion
41. Breadth of mandibular body or body thickness at mental foramen (TMF)*: The maximum breadth of the mandibular body in the region of the mental foramen
42. Mandibular length (MLN)*: The distance between the anteriormost point of the chin and the central point on the pro-jected straight line along the posterior border of the two mandibular angles
43. Maximum ramus height (XRH)*: The distance between the superiormost point of the mandibular condyle and gonion
44. Maximum ramus breadth (XRB): The distance between the anteriormost point on the mandibular ramus and the pos-teriormost point of the condyle
45. Minimum ramus breadth (WRB)*: The minimum breadth of the mandibular ramus, measured perpendicular to the ramus height
46. Height of mandibular body or body height at mental foramen (HMF)*: The distance between the alveolar process and the inferior border of the mandible, measured at the level of the mental foramen

Appendix 5.III: Recording Protocol for Cranial Landmarks

A freely available software for the recording of cranial landmark coordinates is ThreeSkull, designed by Stephen Ousley and accessible at http://math.mercyhurst.edu/~sousley/Software/. For cranial landmarks recorded separately on each side of the cranium, the Excel spreadsheet depicted in Fig. 5.III.1 may be used. This layout is suitable for data pretreatment using the software package Morpheus et al. (see Appendix 5.IV).

In Fig. 5.III.1 we observe that the label of each landmark should be given as: p "landmark label." Each side should have the same landmarks. All bilateral landmarks should end in either R or L depending on whether they belong to the right or left side. The number 999 indicates missing values. Vacant cells will be filled in during the digitization process. If there are missing landmarks, they are also indicated by 999. At least three landmarks that lie on the midsagittal plane must be digitized on both sides of the cranium. In the layout of Fig. 5.III.1 these landmarks are the nasion, bregma, and lambda. As already pointed out, this step allows one to combine the two halves of the cranium into one single configuration. Finally, in the layout of Fig. 5.III.1 there are 37 landmarks; however, depending on the study, more or fewer landmarks may be employed. Note that the template shown in Fig. 5.III.1 is also provided in the companion website.

	A	B	C	D	E	F
1	LEFT SIDE			x	y	z
2	1	nasion	p "nasion"			
3	2	bregma	p "bregma"			
4	3	lambda	p "lambda"			
5	4	glabella	p "glabella"			
6	5	nasofrontaleL	p "nasofrL"			
7	6	dacryonL	p "dacryonL"			
8	7	alareL	p "alareL"			
9	8	subspinale	p "subspin"			
10	9	prosthion	p "prosthion"			
11	10	zygoorbitaleL	p "zygoorbL"			
12	11	zygomaxillareL	p "zygomaxL"			
13	12	zygotemporaleL	p "zygotempL"			
14	13	zygionL	p "zygionL"			
15	14	frontomalareL	p "frontomL"			
16	15	sphenionL	p "sphenionL"			
17	16	krotaphionL	p "krotaphL"			
18	17	euryonL	p "euryonL"			
19	18	auriculareL	p "auric-L"			
20	19	porionL	p "porionL"			
21	20	asterionL	p "astL"			
22	21	opistocranion	p "opistocran"			
23	22	inion	p "inion"			
24	23	vertex	p "vertex"			
25	24	nasofrontaleR	p "nasofrR"	999	999	999
26	25	dacryonR	p "dacryonR"	999	999	999
27	26	alareR	p "alareR"	999	999	999
28	27	zygoorbitaleR	p "zygoorbR"	999	999	999
29	28	zygomaxillareR	p "zygomaxR"	999	999	999
30	29	zygotemporaleR	p "zygotempR"	999	999	999
31	30	zygionR	p "zygionR"	999	999	999
32	31	frontomalareR	p "frontomR"	999	999	999
33	32	sphenionR	p "sphenionR"	999	999	999
34	33	krotaphionR	p "krotaphR"	999	999	999
35	34	euryonR	p "euryonR"	999	999	999
36	35	auriculareR	p "auric-R"	999	999	999
37	36	porionR	p "porionR"	999	999	999
38	37	asterionR	p "astR"	999	999	999

	A	B	C	D	E	F
41	RIGHT SIDE			x	y	z
42	1	nasion	p "nasion"			
43	2	bregma	p "bregma"			
44	3	lambda	p "lambda"			
45	4	glabella	p "glabella"	999	999	999
46	5	nasofrontaleL	p "nasofrL"	999	999	999
47	6	dacryonL	p "dacryonL"	999	999	999
48	7	alareL	p "alareL"	999	999	999
49	8	subspinale	p "subspin"	999	999	999
50	9	prosthion	p "prosthion"	999	999	999
51	10	zygoorbitaleL	p "zygoorbL"	999	999	999
52	11	zygomaxillareL	p "zygomaxL"	999	999	999
53	12	zygotemporaleL	p "zygotempL"	999	999	999
54	13	zygionL	p "zygionL"	999	999	999
55	14	frontomalareL	p "frontomL"	999	999	999
56	15	sphenionL	p "sphenionL"	999	999	999
57	16	krotaphionL	p "krotaphL"	999	999	999
58	17	euryonL	p "euryonL"	999	999	999
59	18	auriculareL	p "auric-L"	999	999	999
60	19	porionL	p "porionL"	999	999	999
61	20	asterionL	p "astL"	999	999	999
62	21	opisthocranion	p "opistocran"	999	999	999
63	22	inion	p "inion"	999	999	999
64	23	vertex	p "vertex"	999	999	999
65	24	nasofrontaleR	p "nasofrR"			
66	25	dacryonR	p "dacryonR"			
67	26	alareR	p "alareR"			
68	27	zygoorbitaleR	p "zygoorbR"			
69	28	zygomaxillareR	p "zygomaxR"			
70	29	zygotemporaleR	p "zygotempR"			
71	30	zygionR	p "zygionR"			
72	31	frontomalareR	p "frontomR"			
73	32	sphenionR	p "sphenionR"			
74	33	krotaphionR	p "krotaphR"			
75	34	euryonR	p "euryonR"			
76	35	auriculareR	p "auric-R"			
77	36	porionR	p "porionR"			
78	37	asterionR	p "astR"			

FIGURE 5.III.1 Excel spreadsheet for recording three-dimensional cranial coordinates.

Appendix 5.IV: Combining the Two Digitized Halves of a Cranium Into One Single Configuration Using Morpheus et al.

When an object is digitized as two separate halves, these can be combined into one single configuration using GPA. GPA is the process by which the objects to be compared are scaled, rotated, and translated so that they all have the same scale and are in the same location, with the same orientation. By treating the right and the left sides of the cranium as two separate objects with three shared landmarks (nasion, bregma, lambda) and performing GPA on them, each side is moved around in space so that these three landmarks taken from one side of the cranium coincide in space with the corresponding landmarks on the other side. In this way the two halves are combined into a single cranium.

GPA can be performed in various software packages, but Morpheus et al. is a good option as it allows the visualization of the landmark coordinates as points in the three-dimensional space and subsequently the confirmation that the data have been correctly collected. Morpheus et al. can be downloaded from its homepage, which is http://morphlab.sc.fsu.edu/software/morpheus/.

When digitizing cranium, it is convenient to save the recorded x, y, z coordinates in an Excel file (Fig. 5.III.1). Once this is done, the data are copied and pasted into a text file. Morpheus accepts only a specific format of data input and the appropriate template with no data is shown in Fig. 5.IV.1. In this figure "DIM 3" indicates that three-dimensional data are being input for each object, and "Missing 999" suggests that the value "999" has been employed to denote missing values.

Fig. 5.IV.2 presents the same template once the coordinates of one individual have been copied and pasted from Excel. When transferring data from Excel to the Morpheus text template, do not use any special paste options and make sure to copy the label of each landmark from Excel along with the coordinates. The text file may look "messy" once the data have been pasted but do not use spaces or tabs to align them.

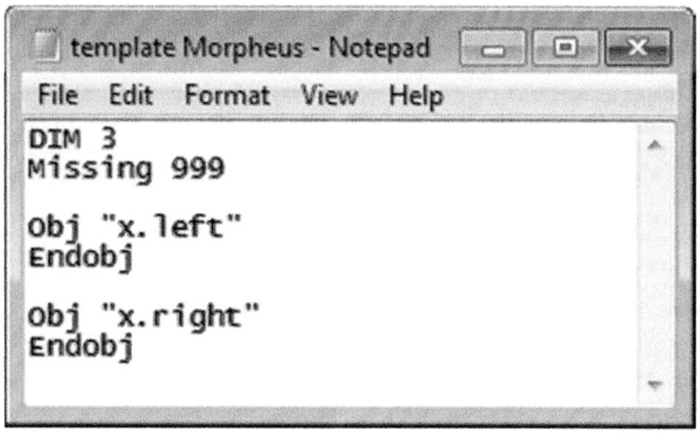

```
DIM 3
Missing 999

Obj "x.left"
Endobj

Obj "x.right"
Endobj
```

FIGURE 5.IV.1 Morpheus template with no data.

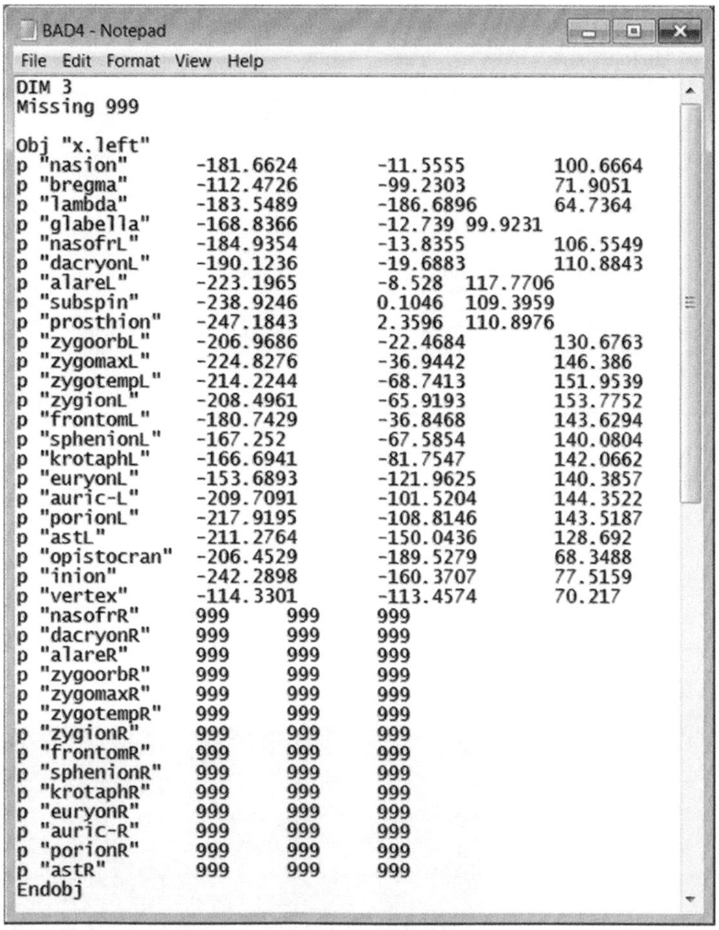

```
DIM 3
Missing 999

Obj "x.left"
p "nasion"      -181.6624      -11.5555        100.6664
p "bregma"      -112.4726      -99.2303        71.9051
p "lambda"      -183.5489      -186.6896       64.7364
p "glabella"    -168.8366      -12.739 99.9231
p "nasofrL"     -184.9354      -13.8355        106.5549
p "dacryonL"    -190.1236      -19.6883        110.8843
p "alareL"      -223.1965      -8.528  117.7706
p "subspin"     -238.9246      0.1046  109.3959
p "prosthion"   -247.1843      2.3596  110.8976
p "zygoorbL"    -206.9686      -22.4684        130.6763
p "zygomaxL"    -224.8276      -36.9442        146.386
p "zygotempL"   -214.2244      -68.7413        151.9539
p "zygionL"     -208.4961      -65.9193        153.7752
p "frontomL"    -180.7429      -36.8468        143.6294
p "sphenionL"   -167.252       -67.5854        140.0804
p "krotaphL"    -166.6941      -81.7547        142.0662
p "euryonL"     -153.6893      -121.9625       140.3857
p "auric-L"     -209.7091      -101.5204       144.3522
p "porionL"     -217.9195      -108.8146       143.5187
p "astL"        -211.2764      -150.0436       128.692
p "opistocran"  -206.4529      -189.5279       68.3488
p "inion"       -242.2898      -160.3707       77.5159
p "vertex"      -114.3301      -113.4574       70.217
p "nasofrR"     999     999     999
p "dacryonR"    999     999     999
p "alareR"      999     999     999
p "zygoorbR"    999     999     999
p "zygomaxR"    999     999     999
p "zygotempR"   999     999     999
p "zygionR"     999     999     999
p "frontomR"    999     999     999
p "sphenionR"   999     999     999
p "krotaphR"    999     999     999
p "euryonR"     999     999     999
p "auric-R"     999     999     999
p "porionR"     999     999     999
p "astR"        999     999     999
Endobj
```

FIGURE 5.IV.2 Part of the Morpheus template filled in with the coordinates of one individual.

Once the data have been put into the Morpheus template, run Morpheus and from the File menu select "Open" and choose the template for the individual you want to analyze. Note that in the Files of Type drop-down menu the option "All Files" should be selected because the template is in a .txt format. You will obtain the image shown in Fig. 5.IV.3, in which you can inspect the points of each side in three-dimensional space.

Subsequently, use the menu Process → Points → Superimposition → GPA (GLS)—Generalized Procrustes Analysis. Then select Process → Points → Superimposition → Restore → Scale. Finally, use the menu Save → Objects → Grand mean and select to save the results as a text file.

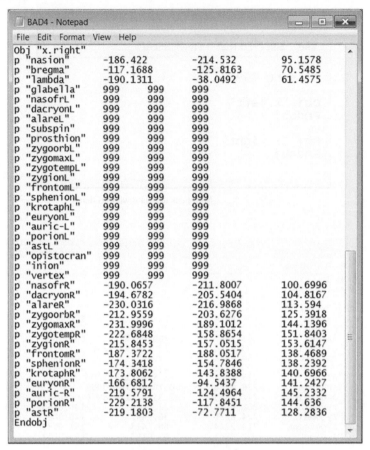

FIGURE 5.IV.2   Cont'd

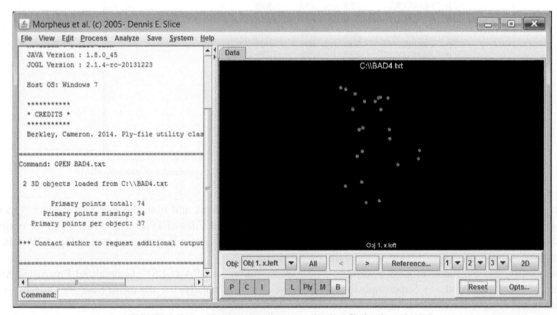

FIGURE 5.IV.3   Morpheus interface once the data file has been loaded.

```
GM-BAD4 - Notepad                                    ─  □  ✕

File  Edit  Format  View  Help
VERSION 3
DIM 3
MISSING 999.0

OBJ "GrandMean"
P "nasion"     12.186116   61.308958   -15.700855
P "bregma"     81.549592  -26.150467   -44.444294
P "lambda"     10.058258 -114.279236   -51.687689
P "glabella"   24.891996   60.120096   -16.352204
P "nasofrL"     8.793196   59.023596    -9.720404
P "dacryonL"    3.604996   53.170796    -5.391004
P "alareL"    -29.467904   64.331096     1.495296
P "subspin"   -45.196004   72.963696    -6.879404
P "prosthion" -53.455704   75.218696    -5.377704
P "zygoorbL"  -13.240004   50.390696    14.400996
P "zygomaxL"  -31.099004   35.914896    30.110696
P "zygotempL" -20.495804    4.117796    35.678596
P "zygionL"   -14.767504    6.939796    37.499896
P "frontomL"   12.985696   36.012296    27.354096
P "sphenionL"  26.476596    5.273696    23.805096
P "krotaphL"   27.034496   -8.895604    25.790896
P "euryonL"    40.039296  -49.103404    24.110396
P "auric-L"   -15.980504  -28.661304    28.076896
P "porionL"   -24.190904  -35.955504    27.243396
P "astL"      -17.547804  -77.184504    12.416696
P "opistocran" -12.724304 -116.668804   -47.926504
P "inion"     -48.561204  -87.511604   -38.759404
P "vertex"     79.398496  -40.598304   -46.058304
P "nasofrR"     7.290017   60.669218   -20.879208
P "dacryonR"    1.547748   56.168422   -25.797155
P "alareR"    -34.382803   67.999719   -20.606792
P "zygoorbR"  -21.337387   61.100705   -40.392053
P "zygomaxR"  -45.021244   53.641083   -57.958720
P "zygotempR" -39.151672   29.145978   -78.593831
P "zygionR"   -33.048415   28.537803   -82.543245
P "frontomR"   -0.467274   53.131621   -64.247388
P "sphenionR"  10.848316   23.058469   -79.871312
P "krotaphR"   10.310564   13.900903   -86.350974
P "euryonR"    15.067634  -31.036843  -107.304256
P "auric-R"   -35.897741   -4.930823   -86.512852
P "porionR"   -45.342596  -11.864881   -86.142125
P "astR"      -33.394199  -59.109613   -91.132982
ENDOBJ
```

FIGURE 5.IV.4 Output of Morpheus showing the grand mean coordinates.

The obtained output is given in Fig. 5.IV.4. Note that the coordinates obtained after GPA are different from the original ones. These new coordinates (GrandMean) may be transferred to a new Excel spreadsheet or any other software for subsequent statistical analysis.

If we now open the grand mean text file using Morpheus, we can inspect the single configuration of the cranium. Two different aspects (anterior and superior) of this configuration are given in Fig. 5.IV.5.

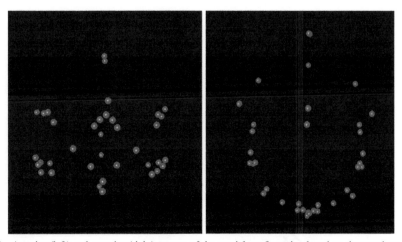

FIGURE 5.IV.5 Anterior (left) and superior (right) aspects of the cranial configuration based on the grand mean (Fig. 5.IV.4).

Appendix 5.V: Computing the Coordinates of Missing Landmarks Using Mirror-Imaging

The equation of a plane in the three-dimensional Euclidean space may be expressed as:

$$z = Ax + By + C \tag{5.V.1}$$

where A, B, and C are constants and x, y, and z are the coordinates of every point on this plane. Consider a point P outside this plane with coordinates (x_1, y_1, z_1) (Fig. 5.V.1). The coordinates (x_1', y_1', z_1') of the reflection point P′ of P may be calculated from:

$$x_1' = x_1 - 2\lambda A \tag{5.V.2}$$

$$y_1' = y_1 - 2\lambda B \tag{5.V.3}$$

$$z_1' = z_1 + 2\lambda \tag{5.V.4}$$

where:

$$\lambda = \frac{Ax_1 + By_1 - z_1 + C}{A^2 + B^2 + 1} \tag{5.V.5}$$

The plane constants A, B, and C are easily determined if the coordinates of three or more points that lie on this plane are known. Thus A, B, and C may be determined by a least-squares fitting to the plane equation $z = Ax + By + C$, that is, using the z value as a dependent variable and the x and y values as independent ones. In the case of a cranium, the points that can be used for the determination of the plane constants A, B, and C may be (1) the three points that represent the coordinates of nasion, bregma, and lambda, that is, the points that are usually employed for determining a common plane so that the two sides of the digitized cranium are combined into a single configuration; (2) the coordinates of all landmarks that are located on the symmetry (midsagittal) plane of the cranium; and (3) the coordinates of the midpoint of the pairs of landmarks located symmetrically on the midsagittal plane. Note that the midpoint coordinates of a left−right pair of landmarks with coordinates (x_L, y_L, z_L) and (x_R, y_R, z_R), respectively, are $x = (x_L + x_R)/2$, $y = (y_L + y_R)/2$, and $z = (z_L + z_R)/2$.

It is seen that if the reflection plane is known, that is, if constants A, B, and C have been estimated, the calculation of the coordinates of a reflection point is straightforward, based on Eqs. (5.V.2)−(5.V.5). For example, consider the following coordinates of nasion, bregma, and lambda:

	x	y	z
Nasion	19.514	49.903	12.431
Bregma	111.651	−24.157	−2.965
Lambda	37.07	−128.231	−21.085

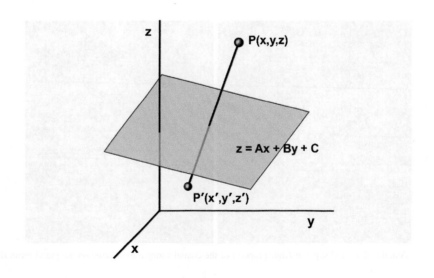

If these values are fitted to $z = Ax + By + C$, the plane equation is given by:

$$z = -0.01723x + 0.18645y + 3.4626$$

Suppose now that the coordinates of dacryonL are missing, whereas those of dacryonR are $x_1 = 12.016$, $y_1 = 40.531$, and $z_1 = 2.354$. Based on these values, we obtain $\lambda = 8.1722$. Therefore, the missing coordinates are:

$$x_1' = x_1 - 2\lambda A = 12.016 - 2 \times 8.1722 \times (-0.01723) = 12.298$$

$$y_1' = y_1 - 2\lambda B = 40.531 - 2 \times 8.1722 \times 0.18645 = 37.484$$

$$z_1' = z_1 + 2\lambda = 2.3541 + 2 \times 8.1722 = 18.698$$

If the number of the reflections required is large, the aforementioned procedure is time-consuming. For this reason, the macro Reflection has been written in Excel VBA to speed up the calculations and it is provided in the companion website. The macro can be run either directly from the homonymous Excel file or from the OSTEO package using the menu Add-ins → OSTEO → Data pre-treatment → Data mirroring. It offers two options: a manual and an automatic calculation of the reflection points.

When the macro is run in the manual mode, in the first dialog box the user should select the region of the landmarks that are used for the determination of the mirroring plane. These landmarks may be the x, y, and z coordinates of nasion, bregma, and lambda and/or the coordinates of landmarks that are located on the midsagittal plane of the cranium, while coordinates of the midpoint of pairs of bilateral landmarks may also be included. All these landmarks should be located in a rectangular region without vacant cells. In the next dialog box the range of the landmarks that are going to be reflected is selected. Again, these landmarks should be located in a rectangular region without vacant rows between them. In the last dialog box we click on the cell that will be the top left corner of the table of results, which are the coordinates of the missing landmarks.

When the auto mode is selected, the layout of the spreadsheet should have the form shown in Fig. 5.V.2, left. In particular, the landmarks should be in one column, in the format they acquire when a Morpheus .txt file is opened in Excel (see Fig. 5.V.2, column B or H), whereas the landmark coordinates should be in three successive columns on the right. The nasion, bregma, and lambda (or whichever landmarks are used to define a common plane for the two digitized halves of the cranium) should be located in the first three lines. The pairs of left−right landmarks should have precisely the same name and format, but end in L or R, respectively. For example, dacryonL and dacryonR or dacryon-L and dacryon-R, but not dacryonL and dacryon-R.

When the auto mode runs, a dialog box appears that allows the selection of one of three options. The landmarks used for the determination of the reflection plane will be (1) the landmarks located in the first three lines, (2) the previous landmarks plus all the landmarks that are located on the midsagittal plane of the cranium, or (3) all previous landmarks plus the coordinates of the midpoints of all pairs of bilateral landmarks. In the next input dialog box click on the label of the first landmark (cell B6 in Fig. 5.V.2) in the column of landmarks. The macro fills all missing values automatically and provides a final option to present the equation of the symmetry plane. Fig. 5.V.2, right, shows the results obtained when the macro is run using option "2".

Appendix 5.VI: Performing Generalized Procrustes Analysis in PAST

PAST is a free statistical software package that can be used, among others, to perform GPA. For this purpose, the x, y, and z coordinates of all landmarks of each individual should occupy one single row and be arranged in successive columns. Therefore, we first need to rearrange the data obtained from Morpheus.

This rearrangement may be performed in PAST as follows. We input the grand mean values (only the values, not the labels) for each individual in a PAST spreadsheet by copying them from the Excel spreadsheet and pasting them into PAST. Make sure the "Select" option is activated in the Click mode panel before pasting. Then select columns A, B, and C and use the menu Edit → Rearrange → Grouped columns to multivar. In the dialog box that appears type in the number "3" so that you indicate that every landmark occupies three columns. Then click on "OK" and the data will be automatically rearranged in one row. This process is repeated to separate PAST spreadsheets for each individual and in the end the data are copied and pasted into a single PAST spreadsheet that will include all individuals, with each occupying one row.

An alternative approach is the following. Copy all grand mean Morpheus files into Excel spreadsheets. Then open all these spreadsheets and run the TransposeLandmarks macro, provided in the companion website, from the

	A	B	C	D	E	F	G	H	I	J	K
1	VERSION	3					VERSION	3			
2	DIM	3					DIM	3			
3	MISSING	999					MISSING	999			
4											
5	OBJ	GrandMean					OBJ	GrandMean			
6	P	nasion	12.1861	61.309	-15.701		P	nasion	12.1861	61.309	-15.701
7	P	bregma	81.5496	-26.15	-44.444		P	bregma	81.5496	-26.15	-44.444
8	P	lambda	10.0583	-114.28	-51.688		P	lambda	10.0583	-114.28	-51.688
9	P	glabella	24.892	60.12	-16.352		P	glabella	24.892	60.12	-16.352
10	P	nasofrL	8.7932	59.024	-9.7204		P	nasofrL	8.7932	59.024	-9.7204
11	P	dacryonL	3.605	53.171	-5.391		P	dacryonL	3.605	53.171	-5.391
12	P	alareL	-29.468	64.331	1.4953		P	alareL	-29.468	64.331	1.4953
13	P	subspin	-45.196	72.964	-6.8794		P	subspin	-45.196	72.964	-6.8794
14	P	prosthion	-53.456	75.219	-5.3777		P	prosthion	-53.456	75.219	-5.3777
15	P	zygoorbL					P	zygoorbL	-14.167	50.137	13.6154
16	P	zygomaxL					P	zygomaxL	-33.036	35.316	32.3091
17	P	zygotempL	-20.496	4.1178	35.6786		P	zygotempL	-20.496	4.1178	35.6786
18	P	zygionL	-14.768	6.9398	37.4999		P	zygionL	-14.768	6.9398	37.4999
19	P	frontomL	12.9857	36.012	27.3541		P	frontomL	12.9857	36.012	27.3541
20	P	sphenionL	26.4766	5.2737	23.8051		P	sphenionL	26.4766	5.2737	23.8051
21	P	krotaphL	27.0345	-8.8956	25.7909		P	krotaphL	27.0345	-8.8956	25.7909
22	P	euryonL	40.0393	-49.103	24.1104		P	euryonL	40.0393	-49.103	24.1104
23	P	auric-L	-15.981	-28.661	28.0769		P	auric-L	-15.981	-28.661	28.0769
24	P	porionL	-24.191	-35.956	27.2434		P	porionL	-24.191	-35.956	27.2434
25	P	astL	-17.548	-77.185	12.4167		P	astL	-17.548	-77.185	12.4167
26	P	opistocran	-12.724	-116.67	-47.927		P	opistocran	-12.724	-116.67	-47.927
27	P	inion	-48.561	-87.512	-38.759		P	inion	-48.561	-87.512	-38.759
28	P	vertex	79.3985	-40.598	-46.058		P	vertex	79.3985	-40.598	-46.058
29	P	nasofrR	7.29002	60.669	-20.879		P	nasofrR	7.29002	60.669	-20.879
30	P	dacryonR	1.54775	56.168	-25.797		P	dacryonR	1.54775	56.168	-25.797
31	P	alareR	-34.383	68	-20.607		P	alareR	-34.383	68	-20.607
32	P	zygoorbR	-21.337	61.101	-40.392		P	zygoorbR	-21.337	61.101	-40.392
33	P	zygomaxR	-45.021	53.641	-57.959		P	zygomaxR	-45.021	53.641	-57.959
34	P	zygotempR	-39.152	29.146	-78.594		P	zygotempR	-39.152	29.146	-78.594
35	P	zygionR	-33.048	28.538	-82.543		P	zygionR	-33.048	28.538	-82.543
36	P	frontomR	-0.4673	53.132	-64.247		P	frontomR	-0.4673	53.132	-64.247
37	P	sphenionR	10.8483	23.058	-79.871		P	sphenionR	10.8483	23.058	-79.871
38	P	krotaphR	10.3106	13.901	-86.351		P	krotaphR	10.3106	13.901	-86.351
39	P	euryonR	15.0676	-31.037	-107.3		P	euryonR	15.0676	-31.037	-107.3
40	P	auric-R	-35.898	-4.9308	-86.513		P	auric-R	-35.898	-4.9308	-86.513
41	P	porionR	999	999	999		P	porionR	-38.829	-13.575	-83.003
42	P	astR	-33.394	-59.11	-91.133		P	astR	-33.394	-59.11	-91.133
43	ENDOBJ						ENDOBJ				

FIGURE 5.V.2   Data set arrangement for the auto mode of the Reflection macro (left) and obtained results (right).

homonymous Excel file or from the menu Add-ins → OSTEO → Data pre-treatment → Transpose of Landmarks from the OSTEO file. In the input data dialog box click on the cell at the upper left corner of the landmarks data table, that is, on the cell with the value x1 (cell C6 in Fig. 5.VI.1). Next click on the output cell and the macro will arrange the landmarks in one row as $x_1, y_1, z_1, x_2, y_2, z_2, \ldots$ (Fig. 5.VI.1). This process is repeated for every file with grand

	A	B	C	D	E	F	G	H	I	J	K	L	M
1	VERSION	3											
2	DIM	3											
3	MISSING	999											
4													
5	OBJ	GrandMean											
6	P	nasion	12.1861	61.309	-15.701		12.1861	61.309	-15.701	81.5496	-26.15	-44.444	10.0583
7	P	bregma	81.5496	-26.1505	-44.444								
8	P	lambda	10.0583	-114.279	-51.688								
9	P	glabella	24.892	60.1201	-16.352								
10	P	nasofrL	8.7932	59.0236	-9.7204								
11	P	dacryonL	3.605	53.1708	-5.391								

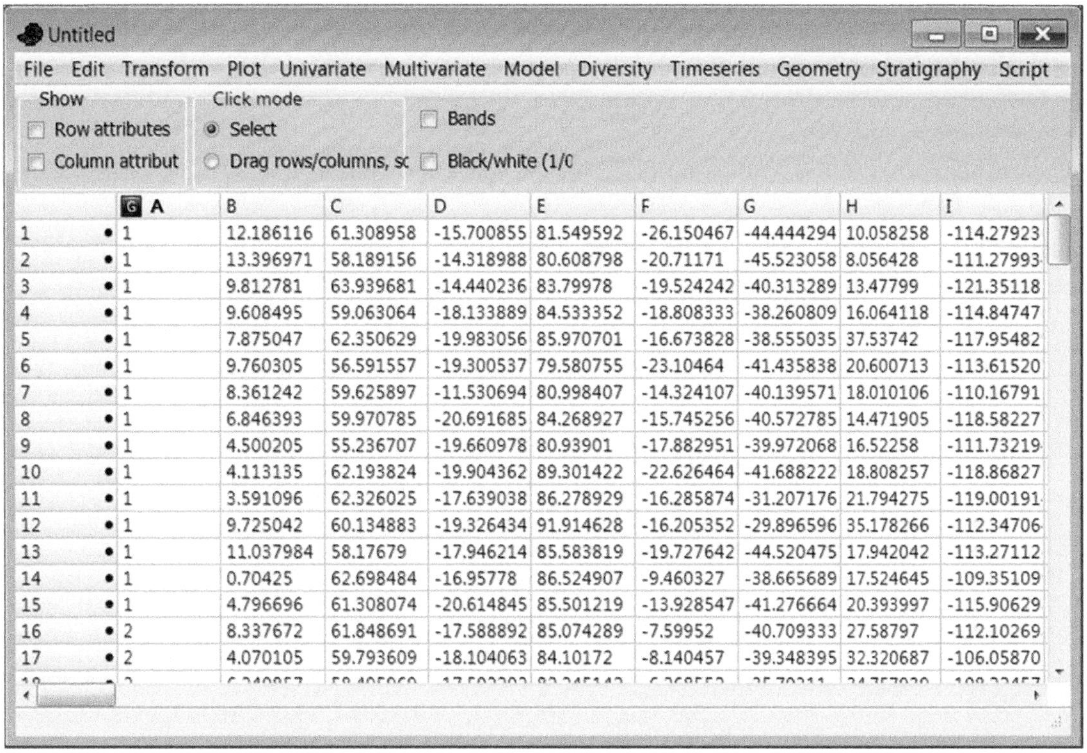

	A	B	C	D	E	F	G	H	I
1	1	12.186116	61.308958	-15.700855	81.549592	-26.150467	-44.444294	10.058258	-114.27923
2	1	13.396971	58.189156	-14.318988	80.608798	-20.71171	-45.523058	8.056428	-111.27993
3	1	9.812781	63.939681	-14.440236	83.79978	-19.524242	-40.313289	13.47799	-121.35118
4	1	9.608495	59.063064	-18.133889	84.533352	-18.808333	-38.260809	16.064118	-114.84747
5	1	7.875047	62.350629	-19.983056	85.970701	-16.673828	-38.555035	37.53742	-117.95482
6	1	9.760305	56.591557	-19.300537	79.580755	-23.10464	-41.435838	20.600713	-113.61520
7	1	8.361242	59.625897	-11.530694	80.998407	-14.324107	-40.139571	18.010106	-110.16791
8	1	6.846393	59.970785	-20.691685	84.268927	-15.745256	-40.572785	14.471905	-118.58227
9	1	4.500205	55.236707	-19.660978	80.93901	-17.882951	-39.972068	16.52258	-111.73219
10	1	4.113135	62.193824	-19.904362	89.301422	-22.626464	-41.688222	18.808257	-118.86827
11	1	3.591096	62.326025	-17.639038	86.278929	-16.285874	-31.207176	21.794275	-119.00191
12	1	9.725042	60.134883	-19.326434	91.914628	-16.205352	-29.896596	35.178266	-112.34706
13	1	11.037984	58.17679	-17.946214	85.583819	-19.727642	-44.520475	17.942042	-113.27112
14	1	0.70425	62.698484	-16.95778	86.524907	-9.460327	-38.665689	17.524645	-109.35109
15	1	4.796696	61.308074	-20.614845	85.501219	-13.928547	-41.276664	20.393997	-115.90629
16	2	8.337672	61.848691	-17.588892	85.074289	-7.59952	-40.709333	27.58797	-112.10269
17	2	4.070105	59.793609	-18.104063	84.10172	-8.140457	-39.348395	32.320687	-106.05870

FIGURE 5.VI.2 Part of a PAST spreadsheet with the cranial coordinates of multiple individuals.

mean data and the results are copied and pasted to a PAST spreadsheet (Fig. 5.VI.2). Note that in the arrangement shown in Fig. 5.VI.2, column A contains the grouping variable, which denotes the sample to which each individual belongs. This variable is redundant for performing GPA, but necessary if multivariate statistical analyses are conducted on the data using PAST. Note that in the latter case the data type of the first variable must be defined as Group from the Column Attributes check box.

Once the data are arranged as shown in Fig. 5.VI.2, proceed to perform GPA. Note that before GPA, it is advisable to make a copy of the original data set because the original coordinates will be automatically replaced by the Procrustes coordinates. To perform GPA, select all columns except for the first one, which is the grouping variable, and use the menu Transform → Landmarks → Procrustes (2D + 3D). In Dimensionality activate the 3D option and click on "OK."

You will observe that the values of the original data set have been altered. This is because the impact of position, size, and orientation has been removed from the original coordinates. The new coordinates are known as *Procrustes coordinates*. Before proceeding to the statistical analysis, further transform these coordinates to the so-called *Procrustes residuals*, which represent approximate tangent space coordinates. In other words, after GPA, a mean cranial shape, the *consensus shape configuration*, is obtained. The Procrustes residuals are the deviations of each landmark from this consensus configuration. The Procrustes residuals can be calculated if you select all columns except for the first one, the column of the grouping variable, and use Transform → Subtract mean. The coordinates are once again modified and this is the data set that can be used in all statistical analyses (Fig. 5.VI.3). Be very careful *first to convert the original coordinates to Procrustes coordinates and then to Procrustes residuals*, not the other way around.

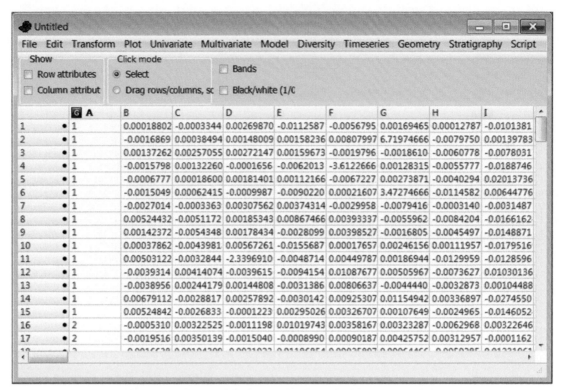

FIGURE 5.VI.3   Part of the data set after Generalized Procrustes Analysis.

Appendix 5.VII: Calculating the Centroid Size

For the calculation of the centroid size using the CentroidSize macro, provided in the companion website, the data should be arranged in an Excel spreadsheet so that each individual occupies a single row and the *x*, *y*, and *z* coordinates of each landmark occupy successive columns (Fig. 5.VII.1). Missing values are allowed provided that they are indicated by the value 999. To compute the centroid size, open the file CentroidSize and return to the Excel spreadsheet that contains your data. Then run the CentroidSize macro from the menu Developer → Macros. Alternatively, you may use the OSTEO macro via Add-ins → OSTEO → Data analysis → Centroid size calculation. The first dialog box informs you that the data should be arranged as shown in Fig. 5.VII.1. In the next dialog box select the range of cells that include only coordinate data, whereas in the final dialog box click on the cell that will be the upper left corner of the range in which the results will appear.

	A	B	C	D	E	F	G	H	I	J	K	L	M
1	individual	x1	y1	z1	x2	y2	z2	x3	y3	z3	x4	y4	z4
2	1	28.998	45.061	6.131	97.884	-43.607	-12.503	999	999	999	999	999	999
3	2	29.368	50.115	2.212	101.992	-40.714	-13.158	25.683	-138.38	-18.564	78.774	28.534	-7.352
4	3	22.421	43.224	-1.723	103.304	-28.287	-14.691	39.77	-127	-11.019	71.492	33.07	-7.029
5	4	26.709	48.245	5.129	95.738	-35.429	-17.886	28.854	-125.66	-24.763	70.514	37.096	-4.94
6	5	19.89	53.21	6.903	103.824	-22.072	-12.697	53.15	-129.03	-24.001	74.358	34.726	2.435
7	6	27.383	44.907	6.72	96.746	-42.552	-22.024	25.255	-130.68	-29.267	72.076	28.811	2.253
8	7	28.334	40.853	6.158	95.546	-38.047	-25.046	22.994	-128.62	-33.32	64.758	33.996	-5.894
9	8	21.514	43.872	0.671	96.579	-32.404	-22.039	36.167	-121.57	-18.123	62.98	36.519	-6.203
10	9	28.035	47.884	5.972	102.022	-35.58	-19.901	31.7	-137.41	-25.887	71.965	34.164	-1.796
11	10	23.982	44.88	4.264	98.907	-32.992	-15.863	30.438	-129.03	-23.234	62.083	38.448	-2.321
12	11	999	999	999	102.083	-29.487	-13.606	53.649	-130.77	-22.715	73.367	34.133	-1.932

FIGURE 5.VII.1   Data arrangement for the calculation of centroid size.

	No	Size	Normalized Size
14			
15	1	80.48	56.91
16	2	161.47	80.74
17	3	149.17	74.58
18	4	152.42	76.21
19	5	156.62	78.31
20	6	154.55	77.27
21	7	152.09	76.04
22	8	146.05	73.03
23	9	161.04	80.52
24	10	153.91	76.96
25	11	123.43	71.26

FIGURE 5.VII.2 Centroid size results.

The obtained results are shown in Fig. 5.VII.2. The values in the column *Size* give the total Euclidean distance of all coordinates from their centroid per individual, that is, the centroid size, whereas *Normalized Size* is the centroid size divided by the square root of the number of landmarks.

Important note: To calculate the centroid size, it is essential to use the raw coordinates, prior to GPA.

Appendix 5.VIII: A Case Study on Calculating Mahalanobis Distances Using Continuous Data

This appendix presents the calculation of Mahalanobis distances using cranial linear measurements. The same issue is explored more thoroughly in Chapter 9, Case Study 24, whereas an example employing digitized coordinates is given in Chapter 9, Case Study 25. The data set analyzed here is given in Table 5.VIII.1; it is artificial and presents the cranial

TABLE 5.VIII.1 Cranial Dimensions of Four Samples

Sample	XCB	BBH	BPL	NLH	Sample	XCB	BBH	BPL	NLH
1	127	139	91	51	3	140	130	93	45
1	128	132	92	52	3	132	132	91	55
1	131	132	99	50	3	145	129	86	54
1	119	130	98	50	3	134	123	93	52
1	128	145	96	58	3	132	126	98	51
1	137	138	87	55	3	134	126	87	59
1	141	133	107	48	3	128	129	85	58
1	124	143	96	48	3	142	135	96	57
1	131	136	105	57	3	153	127	92	43
1	138	132	99	50	3	138	130	88	48
2	139	143	98	54	4	140	144	97	58
2	128	134	92	50	4	146	135	105	57
2	137	138	93	46	4	137	145	109	58
2	134	131	109	48	4	152	131	112	57
2	130	134	100	48	4	151	132	95	59
2	147	135	99	50	4	152	138	90	52
2	139	139	98	45	4	133	138	90	59
2	138	149	98	55					
2	137	134	91	48					
2	124	135	95	61					

BBH, Basion—bregma height; *BPL*, basion—prosthion length; *NLH*, nasal height; *XCB*, maximum cranial breadth.

dimensions of four samples. Given that cranial shape is largely determined genetically, we can compare the four samples with respect to their cranial dimensions and draw conclusions concerning the biological affinities of the parental populations. Note that for simplicity, we are analyzing the raw data instead of Mosimann shape variables.

To calculate the Mahalanobis distance between each pair of samples, we may use the macro Biodistances, provided in the companion website. This macro can be run either directly from the homonymous Excel file or from the OSTEO package using the menu Add-ins → OSTEO → Data Analysis → Calculation of Biodistances.

The data should be arranged in an Excel spreadsheet in five successive columns. The first column is for the grouping variable. This variable takes integer values starting from 1. The integers should be arranged in ascending order, that is, all individuals belonging to sample 1 must be placed first, the individuals belonging to sample 2 must lie below those of sample 1, and so on. The variables of the cranial dimensions should be in successive columns on the right of the grouping variable. Missing values are allowed and indicated by a specified integer.

We open the Excel file Biodistances or OSTEO, return to the spreadsheet that contains our data, and run the Biodistances macro as described earlier. In the dialog box that appears, we type in "0" because we are interested in calculating biodistances for continuous data (Fig. 5.VIII.1). We click on "OK" and in the new dialog box we click on "Yes" so long as we have arranged the data as indicated earlier. Note that this window informs us that missing values can be supported by the macro and these should be indicated using any integer that will be defined in the next window. Make sure this integer is not equal to any value in the data set.

In the Data Input box that appears, we click on the first cell of the grouping variable and then click on "OK." In the Results Output box we click on any cell to indicate the upper left corner of the output range.

Part of the obtained results are shown in Fig. 5.VIII.2. These results include the squared Euclidean distance (ED), the normalized ED (EDN), the p-value of the EDN (p-EDN), the squared Mahalanobis distance (MD), the corrected MD

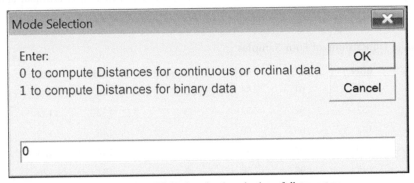

FIGURE 5.VIII.1 Dialog box for the selection of distance type.

Squared Euclidean and Mahalanobis distances for continuous or ordinal data						
MD pooled matrix determinant = 651659.310955053						
Missing values indicator = -1						
Pairs	ED	EDN	p-EDN	MD/OMD	CMD/CO	p-MD/CMD
1-2	27.5	0.66598	0.50421	0.58984	0	0.61771
1-3	145.35	3.57883	0.00129	5.65909	4.00166	0.00073
1-4	234.125	3.89185	0.00299	8.36877	6.12935	0.00019
2-3	122.35	3.41208	0.00188	5.85871	4.17103	0.00058
2-4	133.425	2.99087	0.01515	6.50953	4.55181	0.00103
3-4	224.764	4.99521	0.00039	8.57004	6.30012	0.00016
Squared Mahalanobis distance (MD/OMD)						
		1	2	3	4	
	1	0	0.58984	5.65909	8.36877	
	2	0.58984	0	5.85871	6.50953	
	3	5.65909	5.85871	0	8.57004	
	4	8.36877	6.50953	8.57004	0	

(CMD), and the corresponding *p*-value (p-MD/CMD). The MD, its corrected expression, and the EDN are also given in a matrix format.

Note that the ED between two groups of points is defined by:

$$d_E^2 = (\mu_1 - \mu_2)^T(\mu_1 - \mu_2) = (\mu_{11} - \mu_{21})^2 + (\mu_{12} - \mu_{22})^2 + \cdots + (\mu_{1r} - \mu_{2r})^2 \qquad (5.VIII.1)$$

where $\mu_{11}, \mu_{12}, \ldots, \mu_{1r}$ are the mean values of the r variables (measurements) of the first group of points and $\mu_{21}, \mu_{22}, \ldots, \mu_{2r}$ are the corresponding mean values of the second group, whereas the corresponding EDN is calculated from:

$$d_{EN}^2 = \left(\frac{\mu_{11} - \mu_{21}}{s_1}\right)^2 + \left(\frac{\mu_{12} - \mu_{22}}{s_2}\right)^2 + \cdots + \left(\frac{\mu_{1r} - \mu_{2r}}{s_r}\right)^2 \qquad (5.VIII.2)$$

where s_j is the standard deviation of the jth variable in the two samples. The *p*-values of the Mahalanobis distance are calculated from Eq. (5.1.11), whereas the *p*-values of the normalized Euclidean distance are estimated from the χ^2 test statistic:

$$\chi^2 = \frac{n_1 n_2 d_{EN}^2}{(n_1 + n_2)} \qquad (5.VIII.3)$$

which follows the χ^2 distribution with r degrees of freedom.

We notice that the distance between samples 1 and 2 is rather small, whereas all others are much larger and statistically significant (p-value $< .05$). In contrast to them, the distance between samples 1 and 2 does not appear to be statistically significant (p-value $> .05$). However, we should stress that the *p*-values shown in Fig. 5.VIII.2 come from multiple comparisons and, therefore, they should be corrected by setting a higher significance threshold for the individual comparisons (see Section 9.5.1). This correction may be performed by means of the *Holm–Bonferroni* method, which is implemented in the macro Holm–Bonferroni. We may run this macro either directly from the homonymous Excel file or from the OSTEO package using the menu Add-ins → OSTEO → Data analysis → Holm–Bonferroni correction. In the dialog box that appears we select the range of *p*-values that should be corrected. The range of p-EDN values may be selected first and then the macro is rerun and the range of p-MD/CMD values is selected. The corrected *p*-values are depicted in Fig. 5.VIII.3. We again observe that all distances are statistically significant except that between samples 1 and 2.

To verify the *p*-values given in Fig. 5.VIII.2, we may use the permutation method. This may be done using the program MD_CMD_ED_EDN&p-values.exe in the folder DistancesForContinuousOrdinalDataC. This program is provided in the companion website and estimates *p*-values using permutations in C++. Detailed instructions on how to use this program are given in the relevant file. The data input file is shown in Fig. 5.VIII.4 and the results are given in Fig. 5.VIII.5. Note that in the Results file, OMD and COMD indicate that the same macro can also be applied to ordinal data. We observe that the obtained *p*-values agree with those calculated from the test statistics (Fig. 5.VIII.2). Again the *p*-values obtained from the permutation method should be corrected for multiple comparisons and this may be done by means of the Holm–Bonferroni correction.

To compute the F_{st} and R-matrix, we may use the RMET 5.0 program by Relethford, which is downloadable from http://employees.oneonta.edu/relethjh/programs/. The program is based on the work carried out by Williams-Blangero and Blangero (1989), Relethford and Blangero (1990), Relethford (1991), and Relethford et al. (1997) and it is accompanied by a detailed Read Me file.

The input data file should have a specific format, as shown in Fig. 5.VIII.6. It may be created using Microsoft Notepad and saved as a .met file. The first line is a title to describe the data, and the second line includes two

Pairs	rawp-values		p-values after Holm-Bonferroni correction	
	p-EDN	p-MD/CMD	p-EDN	p-MD/CMD
1-2	0.50421	0.61771	0.50421	0.61771
1-3	0.00129	0.00073	0.00647	0.00234
1-4	0.00299	0.00019	0.00896	0.00096
2-3	0.00188	0.00058	0.00753	0.00234
2-4	0.01515	0.00103	0.03031	0.00234
3-4	0.00039	0.00016	0.00231	0.00096

FIGURE 5.VIII.3 *p*-values corrected using the Holm–Bonferroni method.

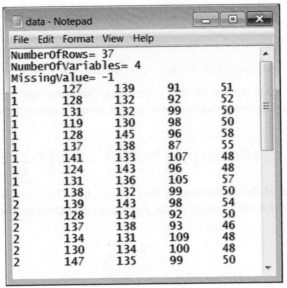

FIGURE 5.VIII.4 Part of the data input file for the calculation of *p*-values using permutations.

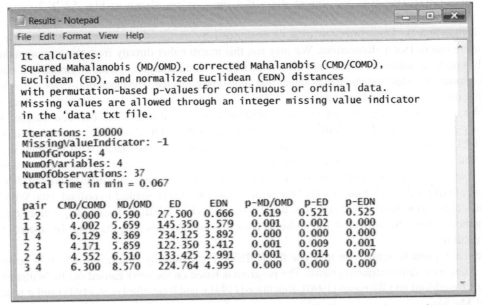

FIGURE 5.VIII.5 Biodistances and corresponding *p*-values obtained by means of permutations.

numbers, the number of samples and the number of variables, separated by a space. The lines that follow are the *population* lines, *variable* lines, and then the data. The population lines are equal to the number of samples and each one must contain three values separated by commas. The first is the sample label, the second is the sample code, and the third is an estimate of the size of the population from which the sample comes. If such an estimation is not possible, use "1". The variable lines are equal to the number of variables in the data set and each one is the label of each variable. Finally, for the data layout, the grouping variable must be the first variable followed by the variables that express cranial measurements. Note that the initial raw cranial measurements must be converted into *z* scores (see Section 9.9.1).

To use the program, we first open the data input file from File → Open, then from the menu Analysis → Options we enter an average Heritability, whereas from the menu Analysis → Run we select the samples and the variables used and run the program. Some of the obtained results, rearranged and formatted, are shown in Fig. 5.VIII.7.

CranialLinearData - Notepad

File   Edit   Format   View   Help

```
Cranial linear data
4 4
sample1,1,1
sample2,2,1
sample3,3,1
sample4,4,1
XCB
BBH
BPL
NLH
1        -1.124797571      0.732486485      -0.739150135      -0.332713233
1        -1.004862383      -0.445861339     -0.589704479      -0.124062561
1        -0.64505682       -0.445861339     0.456415111       -0.541363904
1        -2.084279072      -0.782532146     0.306969455       -0.541363904
1        -1.004862383      1.742498906      0.008078144       1.127841466
1        0.074554306       0.564151082      -1.336932758      0.501889453
1        0.554295057       -0.277525935     1.651980357       -0.958665246
1        -1.484603134      1.405828099      0.008078144       -0.958665246
1        -0.64505682       0.227480275      1.353089045       0.919190795
1        0.194489494       -0.445861339     0.456415111       -0.541363904
2        0.314424681       1.405828099      0.306969455       0.293238781
2        -1.004862383      -0.109190532     -0.589704479      -0.541363904
```

FIGURE 5.VIII.6   Part of the data input file to the RMET software.

Fig. 5.VIII.7, left, shows the unbiased R-matrix when the heritability is equal to 1 and the matrix of the generalized distances (GD) based on the R-matrix. As discussed in Section 5.3.1, positive values in the R-matrix indicate samples that come from populations that are more similar to each other than on average (samples 1 and 2), whereas negative values correspond to pairs of samples that are less similar to each other than on average. The program computes two F_{st} values associated with the R-matrix, a raw and an unbiased value: $F_{st} = 0.2145$ and unbiased $F_{st} = 0.1591$. An interesting feature of the GDs is that they are highly correlated to the MD and CMD computed earlier (Figs. 5.VIII.2 and 5.VIII.5). Specifically, the correlation coefficient between GD and MD is 0.995 and that between GD and CMD is 0.994. Thus, all these distances provide essentially the same information, at least in the example under study.

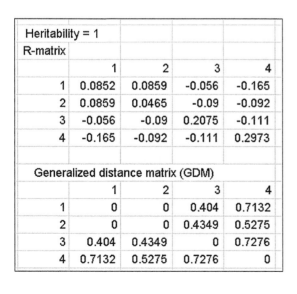

Heritability = 1			
R-matrix			
	1	2	3	4
1	0.0852	0.0859	-0.056	-0.165
2	0.0859	0.0465	-0.09	-0.092
3	-0.056	-0.09	0.2075	-0.111
4	-0.165	-0.092	-0.111	0.2973
Generalized distance matrix (GDM)			
	1	2	3	4
1	0	0	0.404	0.7132
2	0	0	0.4349	0.5275
3	0.404	0.4349	0	0.7276
4	0.7132	0.5275	0.7276	0

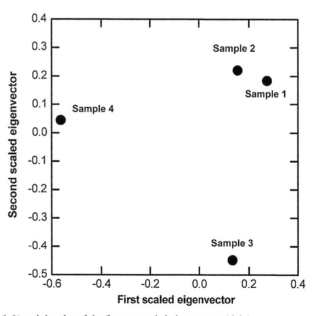

FIGURE 5.VIII.7   R-matrix and generalized distances (left) and the plot of the first two scaled eigenvectors (right).

Apart from the aforementioned computations, the RMET program performs principal coordinates analysis on the R-matrix and presents the first two scaled coordinates. The plot based on these two coordinates shows the relative positions of the samples and closely resembles the corresponding MDS plots (compare Figs. 5.VIII.7, right, and 9.9.11). Note that distant pairs of populations correspond to negative R_{ij} values, whereas neighboring pairs correspond to positive R_{ij} values.

The RMET program does not allow for missing values. Missing values are allowed in the Fst macro provided that the pooled within-group covariance matrix P can be computed. The macro can run either from the Fst Excel file or from OSTEO via the menu Add-ins $\rightarrow$ OSTEO $\rightarrow$ Data analysis $\rightarrow$ Fst and R-matrix computation. In both cases we select the option for continuous data. In data arrangement one column should be the grouping variable starting from 1. The continuous variables should be in successive columns on the right of the grouping variable. Note that raw data do not need to be transformed to z scores. All cases belonging to the same group must occupy successive rows and the groups must be arranged in ascending order. When running this option, in the dialog boxes that appear we enter the heritability and an integer missing value indicator, and click on the cell with the first grouping variable. We obtain F_{st}, R-matrix, and GD-matrix identical to those of RMET. To perform principal coordinates analysis, we may use the macro PCoA, provided in the companion website in the homonymous Excel file. We run this macro from Developer $\rightarrow$ Macros $\rightarrow$ PCoA, select the entire range of the R-matrix values, and draw the two-dimensional plot between the first two Coordinates. We obtain a plot practically identical to that of Fig. 5.VIII.7, right, but there is a different scaling of the axes.

For further practice and research purposes, the macro DataCreationForBiodistances, provided in the companion website, can be used to generate artificial continuous, ordinal, and binary data. The continuous data follow the multivariate normal distribution with known variance–covariance matrix, whereas the ordinal and binary data code the continuous ones. The data sets may include missing values.

Appendix 5.IX: Definitions of Cranial Nonmetric Traits

Definitions and suggested recording schemes for some of the most frequently used cranial nonmetric traits are given in this appendix. The reader may consult Hauser and De Stefano (1989) for a thorough presentation of cranial nonmetric traits and their anatomy, function, development, genetics, and inter- and intrapopulation variation, as well as medical implications.

In this appendix, the location of various cranial nonmetric traits is indicated in Figs. 5.IX.1–5.IX.5 and, subsequently, these are briefly described. In addition, a scoring system is provided for each trait, which is a simplified version of the recording scheme proposed by Hauser and De Stefano (1989).

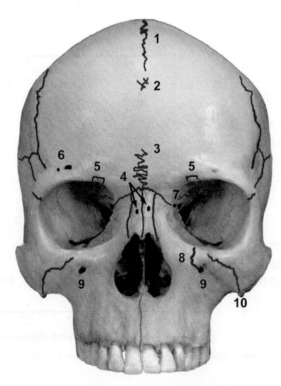

1 = metopic suture
2 = metopic fissure
3 = supranasal suture
4 = nasal foramina
5 = supraorbital notches
6 = supraorbital foramina
7 = ethmoidal foramina
8 = infraorbital suture
9 = infraorbital foramina
10 = zygomaxillary tubercle

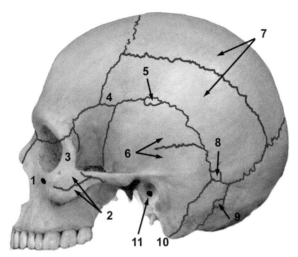

1 = zygomatico-facial foramen
2 = divided zygomatic bone
3 = marginal tubercle
4 = frontotemporal articulation
5 = squamous ossicle
6 = divided temporal squama
7 = divided parietal bone
8 = parietal notch bone
9 = occipitomastoid ossicle
10 = squamomastoid suture
11 = external auditory
torus/exostosis

FIGURE 5.IX.2   Cranial nonmetric traits; lateral view.

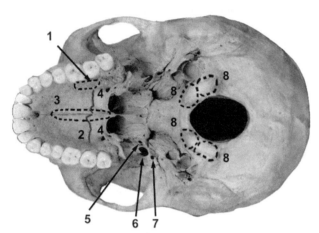

1 = maxillary torus
2 = transverse palatine suture
3 = palatine torus
4 = lesser palatine foramina
5 = foramen of Vesalius
6 = oval foramen
7 = spinous foramen
8 = divided occipital condyles

FIGURE 5.IX.3   Cranial nonmetric traits; basal view.

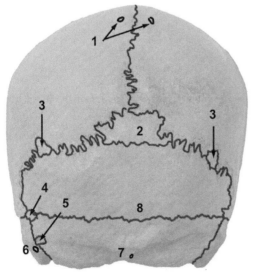

1 = parietal foramina
2 = ossicle at lambda
3 = lambdoid ossicles
4 = ossicle at asterion
5 = occipitomastoid ossicle
6 = mastoid foramen
7 = occipital foramen
8 = inca bone

FIGURE 5.IX.4   Cranial nonmetric traits; posterior view.

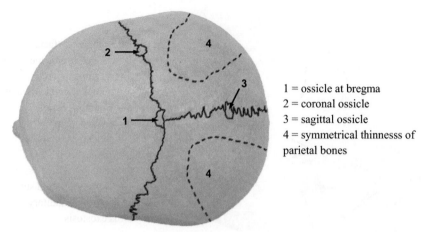

1 = ossicle at bregma
2 = coronal ossicle
3 = sagittal ossicle
4 = symmetrical thinnesss of
parietal bones

FIGURE 5.IX.5 Cranial nonmetric traits; superior view.

Metopic suture (*sutura metopica*): This suture is located on the midline of the frontal bone, connecting the bregma to the nasion (Fig. 5.IX.1). It is present in all individuals at birth because the frontal bone originally consists of two halves. These usually fuse by the end of the fourth year but in some cases the suture may persist during adulthood.

Scoring:
1. Degree of expression
   a. Partial persistence
   b. Complete persistence

Metopic fissure (*fissura metopica*): This is a metopic fontanelle that corresponds to a long extension of the great fontanelle persisting until late fetal life. Remnants of it may occur into adulthood (Fig. 5.IX.1).

Scoring:
1. Expression
   a. Suture
   b. Fissure
   c. Fontanelle bone

Supranasal suture (*sutura supranasalis*): This is a short zigzag suture in the area of the glabella (Fig. 5.IX.1). Note that it is not part of a metopic suture, because these are generally less complex.

Scoring:
1. Degree of expression
   a. Open
   b. Closing
   c. Closed

Nasal foramina (*foramina nasalia*): These foramina are situated near the center of the nasal bones (Fig. 5.IX.1).

Scoring:
1. Number
   a. 1
   b. >1
2. Size of the largest
   a. Small (<0.3 mm)
   b. Medium (0.3−1.2 mm)
   c. Large (>1.2 mm)

Supraorbital osseous structures (*structurae osseae supraorbitales*): These include notches and foramina that allow the passage of nerves and vessels (Fig. 5.IX.1).

Scoring:
1. Expression
   a. Notch
   b. Foramen
2. Number
   a. 1
   b. >1
3. Size of the largest
   a. Small notches (<1 mm); small foramina (<0.3 mm)
   b. Medium notches (1−2.5 mm); medium foramina (0.3−1.2 mm)
   c. Large notches (>2.5 mm); large foramina (>1.2 mm)

Ethmoidal foramina (*foramina ethmoidalia*): The *anterior ethmoid foramen* lies on the medial orbital wall and the *posterior ethmoid foramen* lies behind the anterior one (Fig. 5.IX.1).

Scoring:
1. Expression
   a. No posterior foramen
   b. One posterior foramen
   c. Multiple posterior foramina

Infraorbital suture (*sutura infraorbitalis*): This suture may appear along the infraorbital canal (Fig. 5.IX.1).

Scoring:
1. Degree of expression
   a. Partial persistence (orbital or facial)
   b. Complete persistence

Infraorbital foramen (*foramen infraorbitale*): This foramen is situated below the infraorbital margin on the maxilla, above the canine fossa. It is usually a single structure but it is occasionally divided or additional foramina may be present in this area (Fig. 5.IX.1).

Scoring:
1. Number of foramina
   a. 1
   b. >1
2. Degree of division
   a. Minimal (lingula partially dividing the foramen)
   b. Strong (complete division)
   c. Extreme (two separate canals)

Zygomaxillary tubercle (*tuberculum zygomaxillare*): This tubercle is located on the inferior margin of the zygomaxillary suture (Fig. 5.IX.1).

Scoring:
1. Degree of expression
   a. Minimal (<2 mm)
   b. Moderate (2−4 mm)
   c. Pronounced (>4 mm)

Zygomaticofacial foramen (*foramen zygomaticofaciale*): One or more foramina may occur on the external (facial) surface of the zygomatic bone (Fig. 5.IX.2).

Scoring:
1. Number
   a. 1
   b. >1
2. Size of the largest
   a. Small (<0.3 mm)
   b. Medium (0.3−1.2 mm)

Divided zygomatic bone (*os japonicum*): The zygomatic bone may be divided by one or two sutures (Fig. 5.IX.2).

Scoring:

1. Degree of division
   a. Partial
   b. Complete

Marginal tubercle (*tuberculum marginale*): The temporal border of the frontal process of the zygomatic bone often exhibits a tubercle below the frontozygomatic suture (Fig. 5.IX.2).

Scoring:

1. Degree of expression
   a. Weak (<4 mm)
   b. Medium (4–7 mm)
   c. Strong (>7 mm)

Frontotemporal articulation (*articulato frontotemporalis*): The pattern of contact between the sphenoid and the parietal exhibits considerable variability (Fig. 5.IX.2).

Scoring:

1. Expression
   a. Complete articulation
   b. Incomplete articulation

Divided temporal squama (*squama temporali partita*): On rare occasions the temporal squama may be completely or partially divided by a horizontal or, less often, a vertical suture (Fig. 5.IX.2).

Scoring:

1. Degree of division
   a. Partial
   b. Complete

Divided parietal bone (*os parietale partitum*): The parietal bone is occasionally completely or partially divided by accessory sutures (Fig. 5.IX.2).

Scoring:

1. Degree of division
   a. Trace (<1 cm)
   b. Partial (>1 cm)
   c. Complete
2. Number of parts
   a. 2
   b. 3
   c. Multiple

Squamomastoid suture (*sutura squamomastoidea*): This is a suture that marks the junction between the squamous and the petrous portions of the temporal bone and separates the anterior and the posterior parts of the mastoid process (Fig. 5.IX.2).

Scoring:

1. Degree of expression
   a. Trace (sutural persistence in 1/5 to 1/3 of the length of the mastoid process)
   b. Partial (sutural persistence in 1/3 to 3/4 of the length of the mastoid process)
   c. Complete (sutural persistence in >3/4 of the length of the mastoid process)

External auditory exostosis/torus (*torus auditivus*): This is a bony nodule within the external auditory meatus (Fig. 5.IX.2). Research has supported that this trait is largely controlled environmentally. In particular, auditory exostoses are linked to cold water reaching the inner canal, as well as to cold atmospheric temperatures combined with wind chill (Okumura et al., 2007; but see Godde, 2010).

Scoring:
1. Degree of expression
   a. Weak (small)
   b. Strong (well developed)
   c. Excessive (partial or complete occlusion of the meatus)

Maxillary torus (*torus maxillaris*): This trait may be expressed as bony nodules or even as a moundlike elevation of the lingual aspect of the maxillary alveolar process in the molar area (Fig. 5.IX.3).

Scoring:
1. Size
   a. Small
   b. Large

Transverse palatine suture (*sutura palatine transversa*): This suture connects the maxillae with the palatine bones (Fig. 5.IX.3).

Scoring:
1. Maximum sutural shape extension
   a. Absent
   b. Small (<0.5 mm)
   c. Medium (0.5−1 mm)
   d. Large (>1 mm)

Palatine torus (*torus palatinus*): This is an osseous prominence along the median suture of the hard palate (Fig. 5.IX.3).

Scoring:
1. Size
   a. Trace
   b. Medium
   c. Strong

Lesser palatine foramina (*foramina palatine minora*): These foramina are found on the palatine bones, at the posterior section of the palate (Fig. 5.IX.3).

Scoring:
1. Number
   a. 1
   b. >1
2. Size of the largest
   a. Small (<0.3 mm)
   b. Medium (0.3−1.2 mm)
   c. Large (>1.2 mm)

Retropterygoid apertures in the greater wing (*aperturae retropterygoideae alae majoris*): The oval and the spinous foramina on the basicranium may communicate. Also, sometimes the oval foramen may be divided in two, in which case the anterior part is called the *foramen of Vesalius* (Fig. 5.IX.3).

Scoring:
1. Degree of expression of the spinous and oval foramina
   a. Complete expression of both foramina
   b. Partial incompleteness of the oval foramen
   c. Confluent oval and spinous foramina
2. Degree of expression of the venous part of the oval foramen
   a. Trace of separation
   b. Incomplete separation
   c. Complete separation—foramen of Vesalius

Divided occipital condylar facet (*facies condylaris bipartite*): The surface of the occipital condyles may be divided anteromedially and posterolaterally (Fig. 5.IX.3). The bone separating the two halves has a coarse surface and sharp edges. On rare occasions the occipital condyles may be divided into more than two parts.

Scoring:
1. Degree of division
   a. Partial
   b. Complete

Parietal foramen (*foramen parietale*): Foramina penetrate the parietals and lie in the obelion area, near or in the sagittal suture (Fig. 5.IX.4).

Scoring:
1. Number
   a. 1
   b. >1
2. Size
   a. Small (<0.3 mm)
   b. Medium (0.3−1.2 mm)
   c. Large (>1.2 mm)

Mastoid foramen (*foramen mastoideum*): This foramen represents the external aperture of the mastoid canal (Fig. 5.IX.4). Occasionally there may be multiple foramina in this area.

Scoring:
1. Number of foramina
   a. 1
   b. >1
2. Size of the largest
   a. Small (<1 mm)
   b. Medium (1−2 mm)
   c. Large (>2 mm)

Occipital foramen (*foramen occipitale*): This foramen occurs on the occipital squama, near the external occipital protuberance (Fig. 5.IX.4).

Scoring:
1. Size
   a. Small (<0.3 mm)
   b. Medium (0.3−1.2 mm)
   c. Large (>1.2 mm)

Inca bone (*os incae*): When a transverse suture (*sutura Mendoza*) occurs along the highest nuchal line, dividing the occipital squama, the osseous segment above this suture is called *complete Inca bone* (Fig. 5.IX.4). This suture may occasionally be incomplete, in which case the result is called *partial Inca bone*.

Scoring:
1. Degree of division
   a. Partial Inca bone
   b. Complete Inca bone

Symmetrical thinness of the parietal bones (*depression biparietalis circumscripta*): This trait is generally expressed bilaterally and is usually located above the temporal ridge (Fig. 5.IX.5).

Scoring:
1. Degree of expression
   a. Weak
   b. Medium
   c. Strong

Sutural ossicles (*ossicula suturarum*): These ossicles permit minimal movement of the cranial bones during birth and allow for postnatal bone growth.

A. **Squamous ossicles** (*ossicula suturae squamosae*): These ossicles are found in the suture between the temporal and the parietal bone (Fig. 5.IX.2).

Scoring:
1. Number
   a. 1
   b. >1
2. Size of the largest
   a. Small (largest diameter <1 cm, area <0.5 cm^2)
   b. Large (largest diameter >1 cm, area >0.5 cm^2)

B. **Parietal notch bone** (*ossiculum incisurae parietalis*): This ossicle is located on the angle that is formed at the anterior third of the suture that articulates the parietal bone with the mastoid part of the temporal bone (Fig. 5.IX.2).

Scoring:
1. Number
   a. 1
   b. >1
2. Size of the largest
   a. Small (largest diameter <1 cm, area <0.5 cm^2)
   b. Large (largest diameter >1 cm, area >0.5 cm^2)

C. **Ossicle at asterion** and **occipitomastoid ossicles** (*ossiculum fonticuli posterolateralis et ossicula suturae occipitomastoideae*): These ossicles are located either on the asterion or on the occipitomastoid suture (Fig. 5.IX.2).

Scoring:
1. Number
   a. 1
   b. >1
2. Size of the largest
   a. Small (largest diameter <1 cm, area <0.5 cm^2)
   b. Large (largest diameter >1 cm, area >0.5 cm^2)

D. **Coronal ossicles** (*ossicula suturae coronalis*): These are ossicles located on the coronal suture (Fig. 5.IX.5).

Scoring:
1. Number
   a. 1
   b. >1
2. Size of the largest
   a. Small (largest diameter <1 cm, area <0.5 cm^2)
   b. Large (largest diameter >1 cm, area >0.5 cm^2)

E. **Ossicle at bregma** (*ossiculum fonticuli maioris*): This ossicle is located on bregma (Fig. 5.IX.5). It may provide protection for the brain in the late fetal period and early infancy.

Scoring:
1. Number
   a. 1
   b. >1
2. Size of the largest
   a. Small (largest diameter <1 cm, area <0.5 cm^2)
   b. Large (largest diameter >1 cm, area >0.5 cm^2)

F. **Sagittal ossicles** (*ossicula suturae sagittalis*): These ossicles are located on the sagittal suture (Fig. 5.IX.5).

Scoring:
1. Number
   a. 1
   b. >1

2. Size of the largest
   a. Small (largest diameter <1 cm, area <0.5 cm^2)
   b. Large (largest diameter >1 cm, area >0.5 cm^2)

G. Ossicle at lambda (*ossiculum fonticuli minoris*): This ossicle is located on lambda (Fig. 5.IX.4).

Scoring:
1. Number
   a. 1
   b. >1
2. Size of the largest
   a. Small (largest diameter <1 cm, area <0.5 cm^2)
   b. Large (largest diameter >1 cm, area >0.5 cm^2)

Appendix 5.X: Definitions of Dental Nonmetric Traits

This appendix presents some of the most commonly used dental traits and their recording schemes, which have been reproduced with permission from Turner et al. (1991). The reader may consult Scott and Turner (1997) for a detailed description of a broad range of dental nonmetric traits, as well as Turner et al. (1991) for a thorough presentation of recording standards.

Incisors

Winging: Winging occurs when the distal end of the labial surface of the maxillary central incisors is rotated outward. Counterwinging, in which the distal end of the incisors is rotated inward, should not be recorded, as it is often the result of dental crowding. This trait should preferably be recorded in the maxillary central incisors (Scott and Turner, 1997).

Scoring (Turner et al., 1991, p. 14):
1. Bilateral winging
2. Unilateral winging
3. Straight (no winging)
4. Counterwinging

Shovel-shaped incisors: Shovel-shaped incisors (Fig. 5.X.1) exhibit prominent mesial and distal ridges lingually, as well as a deep lingual fossa (Mayhall, 2000). The determination of the degree of shoveling can be done visually but certain researchers have also measured the depth of the lingual fossa. This trait should preferably be recorded in the maxillary central incisors (Scott and Turner, 1997).

Scoring (Turner et al., 1991, pp. 14–15):
0. None (lingual surface is essentially flat)
1. Faint (very slight elevations of the mesial and distal aspects of lingual surface can be seen and palpated)
2. Trace (elevations are easily seen)
3. Semishovel (stronger ridging is present and there is a tendency for ridge convergence at the cingulum)
4. Semishovel (convergence and ridging are stronger than in grade 3)
5. Shovel (strong development of ridges, which almost come into contact at the cingulum)

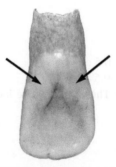

FIGURE 5.X.1   Shovel-shaped incisor.

6. Marked shovel (strongest development; mesial and distal lingual ridges are sometimes in contact at the cingulum)
7. Barrel (only in maxillary second incisors; expression exceeds grade 6)

Double shoveling: This trait is characterized by mesial and distal ridges on the labial surface of the maxillary incisors and canines, irrespective of whether strong lingual ridges are also present. It is preferentially recorded on the maxillary first incisors (Scott and Turner, 1997).

Scoring (Turner et al., 1991, p. 15):
0. None (labial surface is smooth)
1. Faint (mesial and distal ridging can be seen in strong contrasting light)
2. Trace (ridging is more easily seen and palpated)
3. Semi-double shovel (ridging can be readily palpated)
4. Double shovel (ridging is pronounced on at least one-half of the total crown height)
5. Pronounced double shovel (ridging is very prominent and may occur from the occlusal surface to the cementoenamel junction)
6. Extreme double shovel

Labial curvature: The labial surface of the upper incisors may range from flat to markedly convex (Fig. 5.X.2). Ideally, this trait should be assessed at a location approximately 2/3 of the distance up from the cementoenamel junction (Turner et al., 1991). It may be scored in the maxillary central or lateral incisor (Scott and Turner, 1997).

Scoring (Turner et al., 1991, p. 15):
0. Labial surface is flat
1. Labial surface exhibits trace convexity
2. Labial surface exhibits weak convexity
3. Labial surface exhibits moderate convexity
4. Labial surface exhibits pronounced convexity

Interruption groove: Grooves may dissect the mesial or distal marginal ridges (Fig. 5.X.3) or occur on the cingulum of the lingual surface of the maxillary incisors (Turner, 1967). The focal tooth for the scoring of this trait is the maxillary lateral incisor (Scott and Turner, 1997).

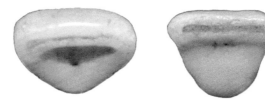

FIGURE 5.X.2   Different degrees of expression for labial curvature.

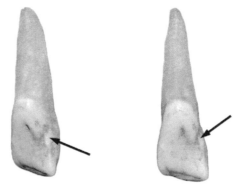

FIGURE 5.X.3   Interruption groove on the mesiolingual border.

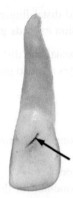

FIGURE 5.X.4 Tuberculum dentale.

Scoring (Turner et al., 1991, p. 16):

0. None
M. An interruption groove occurs on the mesiolingual border
D. An interruption groove occurs on the distolingual border
MD. Grooves occur on both the mesiolingual and the distolingual borders
Med. A groove occurs in the medial area of the cingulum

Tuberculum dentale: This feature appears on the lingual surface of the maxillary incisors and canines (Fig. 5.X.4). It varies considerably in expression and may even appear as a free cusp (Hillson, 1996). The focal tooth for its study is the maxillary second incisor (Scott and Turner, 1997).

Scoring (Turner et al., 1991, p. 16):

0. No expression
1. Faint ridging
2. Trace ridging
3. Strong ridging
4. Pronounced ridging
5-. A weakly developed cuspule is attached to either the mesiolingual or the distolingual marginal ridge; cuspule apex is not free
5. Weakly developed cuspule with a free apex
6. Strong cusp with a free apex

Peg-shaped incisors: The maxillary lateral incisors may exhibit smaller size than normal and the morphology of their crown may occasionally deviate from the standard (Scott and Turner, 1997).

Scoring (Turner et al., 1991, p. 20):

0. Normal-sized incisor
1. Incisor reduced in size but with normal crown form
2. Peg-shaped incisor (very reduced in size and lacking normal crown morphology)

Canines

Distal accessory ridge: A ridge may be present on the lingual surface of the maxillary and mandibular canines between the median ridge and the distal marginal ridge. This trait should be preferentially recorded on the maxillary canines (Scott and Turner, 1997).

Scoring (Turner et al., 1991, p. 17):

0. Distal accessory ridge absent
1. Accessory ridge very faint
2. Accessory ridge weakly developed
3. Accessory ridge moderately developed
4. Accessory ridge strongly developed
5. Very pronounced accessory ridge

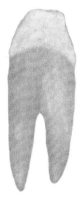

FIGURE 5.X.5   Double-rooted canine.

Bushman canine (mesial canine ridge): The mesiolingual marginal ridge of the maxillary canines may occasionally be larger than the distal one and it may even merge with the tuberculum dentale (Scott and Turner, 1997).

Scoring (Turner et al., 1991, pp. 16–17):
0. Mesial and distal lingual ridges are the same size, neither is attached to the tuberculum dentale if present
1. Mesiolingual ridge is larger than the distolingual, and is weakly attached to the tuberculum dentale
2. Mesiolingual ridge is larger than the distolingual, and is moderately attached to the tuberculum dentale
3. Mesiolingual ridge is much larger than the distolingual, and is fully incorporated into the tuberculum dentale

Lower canine root number: The mandibular canines may exhibit two roots instead of one (Fig. 5.X.5) (Turner, 1967).
Scoring (Turner et al., 1991, p. 24):
1. One root
2. Two roots (free for more than 1/4 to 1/3 of the total lingual root length)

Premolars

Odontomes: The maxillary and mandibular premolars may exhibit a conical projection on the median occlusal ridge of the buccal cusp (Scott and Turner, 1997).

Scoring (Turner et al., 1991, p. 21):
0. Odontome absent
1. Odontome present

Upper premolar root number: The maxillary premolars may exhibit one, two (Fig. 5.X.6), or even three roots (Turner, 1967). The focal tooth for the recording of this trait is the maxillary first premolar (Scott and Turner, 1997).

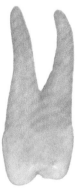

FIGURE 5.X.6   Double-rooted premolar.

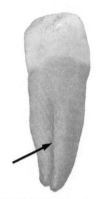

FIGURE 5.X.7 Tome's root.

Scoring (Turner et al., 1991, p. 20):

1. One root (tip may be bifurcated)
2. Two roots (separate roots must be greater than 1/4 to 1/3 of the total root length)
3. Three roots (length defined as in grade 2)

Distosagittal ridge (Uto-Aztecan premolar): The distal margin of the buccal cusp of the maxillary first premolars may exhibit a buccalward rotation along with an associated fossa or pit (Turner et al., 1991).

Scoring (Turner et al., 1991, p. 18):

0. Normal premolar form
1. Distosagittal ridge is present

Tome's root: The roots of the mandibular first premolars may exhibit deep grooves (Fig. 5.X.7) or partial or complete division (Scott and Turner, 1997).

Scoring (Turner et al., 1991, pp. 24−25):

0. Developmental grooving is absent or, if present, shallow with rounded rather than V-shaped indentation
1. Developmental groove is present and has a shallow V-shaped cross section
2. Developmental groove is present and has a moderately deep V-shaped cross section
3. Developmental groove is present, V-shaped, and deep; groove extends at least 1/3 of total root length
4. Developmental grooving is deeply invaginated on both the mesial and the distal borders
5. Two free roots are present and separate for at least 1/4 to 1/3 of the total root length

Lower premolar lingual cusp variation: The lingual cusps of the mandibular premolars exhibit variation in size and shape, because one, two, or three cusps with variable size may be present (Fig. 5.X.8). The mandibular second premolar is the focal tooth for the study of this trait (Scott and Turner, 1997).

Scoring (Turner et al., 1991, pp. 21−22):

A. No lingual cusp
0. One lingual cusp (size and form may vary a great deal but a tip can be seen)

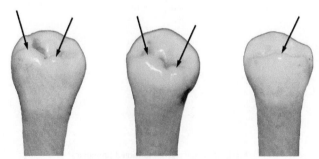

FIGURE 5.X.8 Various degrees of expression for lingual cusp variation (grade 3, left; grade 2, middle; grade 0, right).

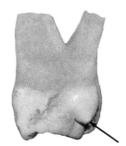

FIGURE 5.X.9   Carabelli's trait.

1. One or two lingual cusps
2. Two lingual cusps; mesial cusp is much larger than distal cusp
3. Two lingual cusps; mesial cusp is larger than distal cusp
4. Two lingual cusps; mesial and distal cusps are equal in size
5. Two lingual cusps; distal cusp is larger than mesial cusp
6. Two lingual cusps; distal cusp is much larger than mesial cusp
7. Two lingual cusps; distal cusp is very much larger than mesial cusp
8. Three lingual cusps; each is about the same size
9. Three lingual cusps; mesial cusp is much larger than medial and/or distal cusp

Molars

Carabelli's trait: This trait occurs on the lingual surface of the mesiolingual cusp (protocone) of the maxillary molars (Fig. 5.X.9) (Buikstra and Ubelaker, 1994; Harris, 2007). Its form ranges from a slight elevation of the enamel to a large cusp. The maxillary first molar is the focal tooth for the study of this trait (Mayhall, 2000; Scott and Turner, 1997).

Scoring (Turner et al., 1991, p. 19):
0. The lingual aspect of the mesiolingual cusp is smooth
1. A groove is present
2. A pit is present
3. A small Y-shaped depression is present
4. A large Y-shaped depression is present
5. A small cusp without a free apex occurs (the distal border of the cusp does not contact the lingual groove separating cusps 1 and 4)
6. A medium-sized cusp with an attached apex making contact with the medial lingual groove is present
7. A large free cusp is present

Upper molar root number: Upper molars normally have three roots. However, some teeth may be one-rooted or two-rooted (Fig. 5.X.10). The focal tooth for the study of this trait is the maxillary second molar (Scott and Turner, 1997).

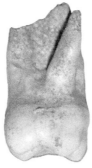 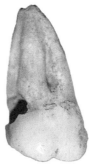

FIGURE 5.X.10   Double-rooted (left) and single-rooted (right) maxillary molars.

Scoring (Turner et al., 1991, p. 20):
1. One root (tip may be bifurcated with deeply inset developmental grooves)
2. Two roots (separate roots must be greater than 1/4 to 1/3 of the total root length)
3. Three roots (length defined as in grade 2)
4. Four roots (length defined as in grade 2)

Enamel extensions: These are apical projections of the enamel and may be traced lingually or buccally (Fig. 5.X.11). Occasionally they are found associated with *enamel pearls* (spherical masses of enamel). The focal tooth is the maxillary or mandibular first molar (Scott and Turner, 1997).

Scoring (Turner et al., 1991, p. 19):
0. Enamel border is straight or rarely curved toward the crown
1. A faint, approximately 1-mm-long extension projects toward and along the root
2. A medium-sized, approximately 2-mm-long extension
3. A lengthy extension, generally >4 mm in length, is present

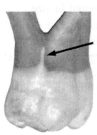

FIGURE 5.X.11   Enamel extension on maxillary molar.

Hypocone: This trait has the form of a distolingual cusp of varying size on the maxillary molars (Fig. 5.X.12). The focal tooth for studying hypocone variation is the maxillary second molar (Scott and Turner, 1997).

Scoring (Turner et al., 1991, p. 18):
0. No hypocone (site is smooth)
1. Faint ridging present at the site
2. Faint cuspule present
3. Small cusp present
3.5. Moderate-sized cusp present
4. Large cusp present
5. Very large cusp present

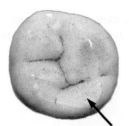 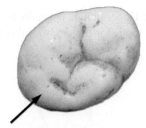

FIGURE 5.X.12   Different degrees of expression for hypocone.

Metaconule: This is an occlusal tubercle between the metacone and the hypocone, and ranges from a tiny cuspule to a prominent cusp (Fig. 5.X.13). The focal tooth for its study is the maxillary first molar (Scott and Turner, 1997).

Scoring (Turner et al., 1991, pp. 18–19):
0. Site of cusp 5 is smooth (only a single distal groove present separating cusps 3 and 4)
1. Faint cuspule present
2. Trace cuspule present

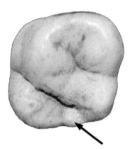

FIGURE 5.X.13   Metaconule

3. Small cuspule present
4. Small cusp present
5. Medium-sized cusp present

Protostylid (tubercle of Bolk): This trait is found on the buccal surface of the mesiobuccal cusps of the mandibular molars. Its expression displays about the same range of variation as Carabelli's trait (Mayhall, 2000; Scott and Turner, 1997). The focal tooth for its study is the mandibular first molar (Scott and Turner, 1997).

Scoring (Turner et al., 1991, pp. 23–24):
0. No expression (smooth buccal surface)
1. A pit occurs in the buccal groove
2. Buccal groove is curved distally
3. A faint secondary groove extends mesially from the buccal groove
4. Secondary groove is slightly more pronounced
5. Secondary groove is stronger and can easily be seen
6. Secondary groove extends across most of the buccal surface of the mesiobuccal cusp
7. A cusp with a free apex occurs

Anterior fovea: A deep triangular depression may occasionally be present distal to the mesial marginal ridge of the mandibular molars, with the mesial marginal ridge and the mesial accessory ridges of the protoconid and metaconid forming the boundaries of this triangle (Fig. 5.X.14). The focal tooth to study is the mandibular first molar (Scott and Turner, 1997).

Scoring (Turner et al., 1991, p. 22):
0. Anterior fovea is absent
1. A weak ridge connects the mesial aspects of cusps 1 and 2 producing a faint groove
2. The connecting ridge is larger and the resulting groove deeper than in grade 1
3. Groove is longer than in grade 2
4. Groove is very long and mesial ridge is robust

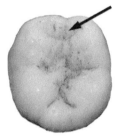

FIGURE 5.X.14   Anterior fovea.

Tuberculum intermedium (metaconulid): A seventh cusp may lie in the lingual groove between the mesiolingual and the distolingual cusps of the mandibular molars (Fig. 5.X.15) (Mayhall, 2000). The focal tooth for study is the mandibular first molar (Scott and Turner, 1997).

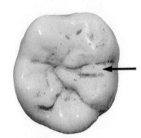

FIGURE 5.X.15   Tuberculum intermedium.

Scoring (Turner et al., 1991, p. 24):

0. No occurrence of cusp 7

1. Faint cusp is present

1A. Faint tipless cusp 7 occurs displaced as a bulge on the lingual surface of cusp 2

2. Cusp 7 is small

3. Cusp 7 is medium sized

4. Cusp 7 is large

Tuberculum sextum (entoconulid): This is an additional cusp between the hypoconulid and the entoconid (Fig. 5.X.16) (Mayhall, 2000). Note that there is some doubt as to whether this trait should be recorded in the absence of the hypoconulid (Scott and Turner, 1997). The focal tooth for study is the mandibular first molar (Scott and Turner, 1997).

Scoring (Turner et al., 1991, p. 24):

0. Absent

1. Cusp 6 much smaller than cusp 5

2. Cusp 6 smaller than cusp 5

3. Cusp 6 equal in size to cusp 5

4. Cusp 6 larger than cusp 5

5. Cusp 6 much larger than cusp 5

Lower molar root number: The lower molars may have one (Fig. 5.X.17) to three roots (Turner, 1967).

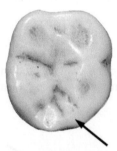

FIGURE 5.X.16   Tuberculum sextum.

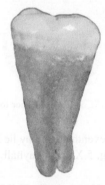

FIGURE 5.X.17   Single-rooted lower molar.

Scoring (Turner et al., 1991, p. 25):

1. One root (root tip may be bifurcated)
2. Two roots (two separate roots exist for at least 1/4 to 1/3 of the total root length)
3. Three roots (a third root is present on the distolingual aspect, it may be very small but is usually about 1/3 the size of the normal distal root)

Hypoconulid: This is a distal or distobuccal cusp on the mandibular molars (Fig. 5.X.18). The focal tooth is the mandibular second molar (Scott and Turner, 1997).

Scoring (Turner et al., 1991, p. 24):

0. No occurrence of cusp 5
1. Cusp 5 is present and very small
2. Cusp 5 is small
3. Cusp 5 is medium sized
4. Cusp 5 is large
5. Cusp 5 is very large

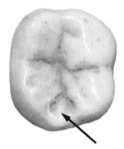

FIGURE 5.X.18 Hypoconulid.

Groove pattern: In the mandibular molars the pattern of the grooves on the occlusal surface varies (Fig. 5.X.19). The mandibular second molar is the focal tooth for this trait (Turner et al., 1991).

Scoring[1] (Turner et al., 1991, pp. 22–23):

Y. Metaconid and hypoconid are in contact
+. All four cusps are in contact
X. Protoconid and entoconid are in contact

Deflecting wrinkle: This is an angulation that occasionally appears on the median occlusal ridge of the mesiolingual cusp of the mandibular molars (Weidenreich, 1937). The focal tooth for study is the mandibular first molar (Scott and Turner, 1997).

Scoring (Turner et al., 1991, p. 23):

0. Absent (medial ridge of mesiolingual cusp is straight)
1. Mesiolingual cusp medial ridge is straight, but shows a midpoint constriction

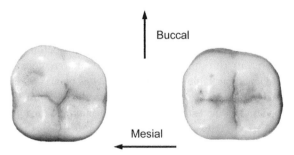

Buccal

Mesial

FIGURE 5.X.19 Groove pattern X (left) and + (right).

---

1. See Fig. 1.8.8 for cusp names.

2. Mesiolingual cusp medial ridge is deflected distally, but does not make contact with the distolingual cusp

3. Mesiolingual cusp medial ridge is deflected distally, forming an L-shaped ridge; the medial ridge contacts the distolingual cusp

Entire Dentition

Supernumerary teeth: Sometimes additional teeth may appear anywhere in the maxilla and mandible as separate structures or fused to other teeth (Alt and Türp, 1998; Scott and Turner, 1997). These often have an anomalous form, although they may look like their neighboring teeth (Hillson, 2005).

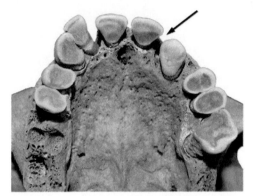

FIGURE 5.X.20 Agenesis of left maxillary lateral incisor.

Agenesis: Sometimes one or more teeth may never erupt (Fig. 5.X.20) (Scott and Turner, 1997). This trait has two expressions: hypodontia and anodontia. Hypodontia refers to the absence of specific teeth, whereas anodontia is the congenital absence of the entire dentition (Alt and Türp, 1998). The most frequently congenitally missing teeth are the third molars and the maxillary lateral incisors.

Scoring (Turner et al., 1991, p. 21):

0. Tooth is present

1. Tooth is congenitally absent

Appendix 5.XI: A Case Study of the Treatment of Nonmetric Traits

The artificial data given in Table 5.XI.1 present the cranial nonmetric traits of four male samples. The aim is to calculate the biodistances between all pairs of samples to draw conclusions about the biological affinity of the parental populations. Note that these data are already in a binary present/absent format, where 1 = present, 2 = absent, and 3 = missing.

For this data set to be analyzed using the macro Biodistances, already used for continuous data in Appendix 5.VIII, the spreadsheet layout must be similar to that of Table 5-XI.1. That is, it is essential to have a grouping variable, i.e., a variable that denotes the sample to which each individual belongs. This variable should be in the far left column and use integers, starting from 1, to define the groups. In addition, as was the case for the continuous data set, all individuals belonging to the same sample must be given in successive rows and in ascending order from sample 1 onward. Finally, for the application of the macro Biodistances, it is necessary to use the following coding for the expression of each trait: 1 = present, 2 = absent, and 3 = missing.

Note that often nonmetric binary data arise from ordinal data using a certain threshold value for each trait. This procedure can be facilitated using the macro Threshold, provided in the homonymous Excel file in the companion website. This macro transforms an initial rectangular table of ordinal data to binary variables coded either as 1 = present, 2 = absent, and 3 = missing (Mode 1) or 1 = present, 0 = absent, and blank = missing (Mode 2). The threshold values used for the transformation should be arranged in a single row. When running the macro, either directly from the Threshold Excel file or using the menu Add-ins → OSTEO → Data pre-treatment → Transformation of ordinal data to binary, in the first input dialog box we select the mode, in the Input Data dialog box we select the entire range of cells that contain the original ordinal data including a first row of labels, in the Input threshold values dialog box we select the entire row of the threshold values, and in the final dialog box we click on the cell that will be the upper left corner of the range in which the binary data together with their labels will appear.

TABLE 5.XI.1 Cranial Nonmetric Traits of Four Male Samples

Sample	Metopic Suture	Supranasal Suture	Supraorbital Structures	Parietal Foramina	Ethmoidal Foramina	Coronal Ossicles	Squamous Ossicles
1	2	1	1	1	1	1	2
1	2	1	1	1	1	1	2
1	2	1	2	1	2	1	2
1	2	1	1	1	1	2	2
1	2	2	1	1	2	1	2
1	2	1	3	1	1	1	2
1	1	1	3	2	1	2	2
1	2	1	1	2	1	1	2
1	1	2	2	1	2	1	2
1	1	1	1	1	1	2	2
1	2	3	1	2	1	1	2
1	2	3	2	1	2	1	2
2	2	1	2	1	3	2	1
2	2	2	2	2	3	2	2
2	2	2	1	2	3	1	2
2	1	2	1	1	3	2	1
2	2	1	1	1	1	2	2
2	3	2	2	2	3	2	1
2	3	2	2	1	3	2	1
2	2	2	1	1	3	2	2
2	1	2	2	3	2	1	2
2	2	1	1	1	2	2	2
3	1	2	1	1	2	2	1
3	1	2	1	2	2	2	1
3	2	2	1	2	2	2	1
3	1	2	1	2	2	1	1
3	2	1	1	1	1	2	1
3	1	2	2	2	1	2	1
3	1	2	1	2	1	2	1
3	1	2	1	2	1	2	1
3	3	1	2	1	2	2	1
3	3	2	1	1	1	1	1
3	1	2	1	2	2	1	1
4	2	2	1	2	1	2	1
4	1	1	1	2	1	2	2
4	2	1	1	3	2	2	2
4	1	2	1	2	2	2	1
4	1	2	2	1	2	2	2

Continued

TABLE 5.XI.1 Cranial Nonmetric Traits of Four Male Samples—cont'd

Sample	Metopic Suture	Supranasal Suture	Supraorbital Structures	Parietal Foramina	Ethmoidal Foramina	Coronal Ossicles	Squamous Ossicles
4	2	2	1	2	2	1	1
4	2	2	2	1	2	1	1
4	3	1	1	2	2	2	2
4	1	2	2	2	2	2	2
4	3	2	3	3	1	2	2
4	1	3	2	2	2	2	1
4	1	3	1	2	2	2	2
4	2	2	1	1	2	2	2
4	3	1	1	2	2	3	1

As described in detail in Section 5.2.6, preliminary data editing of nonmetric traits is usually performed, especially prior to the calculation of the MMD. The data editing process may involve the detection of (1) traits with only missing values even within one single sample, (2) traits that exhibit a particularly high (>0.95) or low (<0.05) frequency, (3) non-diagnostic traits, and (4) traits that exhibit a statistically significant intercorrelation with one another. These tasks may be performed by means of the DataEditing macro in the homonymous Excel file or from Add-ins → OSTEO → Data pretreatment → Data editing for the MMD. In more detail, the data editing process may proceed as follows.

First we arrange the data in an Excel spreadsheet in eight successive columns, adopting the layout of Table 5.XI.1; run the DataEditing macro; and in the Mode Selection dialog box select option "1" (Fig. 5.XI.1) to identify traits with only missing values within at least one sample. Such traits must be eliminated from the calculation of all biodistances. The next dialog box gives instructions on how the data need to be arranged and, so long as they have the proposed arrangement, we click on "Yes". In the new dialog box we click on the cell with the first value of the grouping variable and then click on "OK". If there are traits with only missing values in at least one sample, these traits are colored red and the following warning appears at the bottom of the data table: "DATA EDITING-1: Traits indicated with red exhibit only missing values and they should be eliminated." If there are no such traits, the above warning turns to the message: "DATA EDITING-1: There are no traits with only missing values," as in the present case (Fig. 5.XI.2).

Subsequently, we rerun the DataEditing macro and in the Mode Selection dialog box we select option "2" to detect traits with high (>0.95) or low (<0.05) frequency. In the Input Threshold Value dialog box we type in "5" ($p = 5/100 = 0.05$) to define the threshold value that determines whether a frequency ($p = k/n$) is low ($p < 0.05$) or high ($p > 1 - 0.05$). In the next dialog box for Data Input we click on the cell with the first grouping value, and click "OK."

Certain cells may automatically turn red (Fig. 5.XI.3). The traits that exhibit red cells may be eliminated from the calculation of the MMD. In our example, we may delete the squamous ossicles from the data set. Note that the frequency of squamous ossicles appears to be differentiated between samples. Because this is an important piece of information, as it shows that samples 1 and 3 differ completely with respect to the frequency of squamous ossicles, the elimination of this

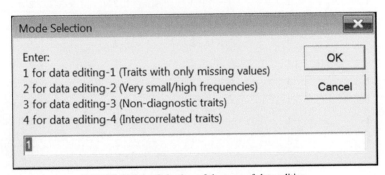

FIGURE 5.XI.1 Selection of the type of data editing.

	A	B	C	D	E	F	G	H
43	4	1	2	2	2	2	2	2
44	4	3	2	3	3	1	2	2
45	4	1	3	2	2	2	2	1
46	4	1	3	1	2	2	2	2
47	4	2	2	1	1	2	2	2
48	4	3	1	1	2	2	3	1
49								
50	**DATA EDITING-1: There are no traits with only missing values**							
51								

FIGURE 5.XI.2 Message that there are no traits with only missing values within at least one sample.

	A	B	C	D	E	F	G	H
1	sample	metopic suture	supra-nasal suture	supra-orbital structures	parietal foramina	ethmoidal foramina	coronal ossicles	squamous ossicles
2	1	2	1	1	1	1	1	2
3	1	2	1	1	1	1	1	2
4	1	2	1	2	1	2	1	2
5	1	2	1	1	1	1	2	2
6	1	2	2	1	1	2	1	2
7	1	2	1	3	1	1	1	2
8	1	1	1	3	2	1	2	2
9	1	2	1	1	2	1	1	2
10	1	1	2	2	1	2	1	2
11	1	1	1	1	1	1	2	2
12	1	2	3	1	2	1	1	2
13	1	2	3	2	1	2	1	2
14	2	2	1	2	1	3	2	1
15	2	2	2	2	2	3	2	2
16	2	2	2	1	2	3	1	2
17	2	1	2	1	1	3	2	1
18	2	2	1	1	1	1	2	2
19	2	3	2	2	2	3	2	1
20	2	3	2	2	1	3	2	1
21	2	2	2	1	1	3	2	2
22	2	1	2	2	3	2	1	2
23	2	2	1	1	1	2	2	2
24	3	1	2	1	1	2	2	1

FIGURE 5.XI.3 Part of the Excel spreadsheet showing traits that may be eliminated because of very high or low frequencies.

trait is not suggested. Instead, we can either ignore this step of data editing or we can apply Bartlett's correction to the computation of the MMD.

We rerun the DataEditing macro and once we reach the window Binary Mode Selection, we type in "3" so that the nondiagnostic traits are identified. Note that to find nondiagnostic traits, we need to leave at least one empty column to the left of the data set; otherwise a warning message appears. We again click on the cell with the first value of the grouping variable and obtain the results shown in Fig. 5.XI.4. Now, we may delete all columns/variables with noncolored cells, because these columns contain nondiagnostic traits. To identify nondiagnostic traits, the macro performs all pairwise comparisons per trait among samples using χ^2 or Fisher's exact tests. A nondiagnostic trait is one for which none of these comparisons is statistically significant. In our case, there is only one nondiagnostic trait, the supraorbital structures, which may be deleted for the computation of the MMD.

The final step is to test if the remaining variables are significantly intercorrelated. We rerun the DataEditing macro and in the Binary Mode Selection dialog box we select option "4". The dialog box that appears provides two options. The intercorrelated traits may be determined by means of Kendall's tau-b correlations or Pearson's correlations. The first option tests for intercorrelations using the original data set of ordinally recorded nonmetric traits. In addition, it presupposes that all missing values in the data set are indicated with an integer, such as -1. The data arrangement should be similar to that already adopted for binary data. The second option, Pearson's correlations, is applied directly to the binary data.

	group	present/absence	metopic suture	supra-nasal suture	supra-orbital structures	parietal foramina	ethmoidal foramina	coronal ossicles	squamous ossicles
51	1	1	3	8	7	9	8	9	0
52	1	2	9	2	3	3	4	3	12
53	2	1	2	3	5	6	1	2	4
54	2	2	6	7	5	3	2	8	6
55	3	1	7	2	9	4	5	3	11
56	3	2	2	9	2	7	6	8	0
57	4	1	6	4	9	3	3	2	6
58	4	2	5	8	4	9	11	11	8

DATA EDITING-3 (NON-DIAGNOSTIC TRAITS)
Columns without marked cells may be deleted
p-values without correction for multiple comparisons

pair	metopic suture	supra-nasal suture	supra-orbital structures	parietal foramina	ethmoidal foramina	coronal ossicles	squamous ossicles
1 - 2	1	0.0376	0.6499	1	0.5253	0.0300	0.0287
1 - 3	0.0300	0.0089	0.6351	0.0995	0.4136	0.0391	7.40E-07
1 - 4	0.2138	0.0427	1	0.0391	0.0447	0.0048	0.0171
2 - 3	0.0567	0.6351	0.1827	0.2198	1	1	0.0039
2 - 4	0.3521	1	0.4173	0.0872	1	1	1
3 - 4	0.3742	0.6404	0.6494	0.6668	0.3892	0.6299	0.0029

FIGURE 5.XI.4 Results for nondiagnostic traits.

When the first option is selected, in the first input box we click on the cell of the first value of the grouping variable, in the second dialog box we define the integer that denotes missing values, and then we click on the output cell. The macro computes the Kendall tau-b values, τ_B, for all pairwise comparisons between the r traits and presents these values in the form of an $r \times r$ matrix. Based on this matrix, we can assess which traits exhibit high τ_B values and we may delete them. It is advisable to delete one trait at a time.

When the second option is selected, in the first input box we click on the cell of the first value of the grouping variable and in the second dialog box we type in the level of significance for the intercorrelated comparisons. Note that the level of significance, a, is entered on a scale of 0–100, and therefore for the usually adopted value $a = 0.05$, we type in "5". Finally, we click on the output cell.

For the data set we examine, the macro gives the results shown in Fig. 5.XI.5. It is seen that the macro computes all pairwise Pearson's r correlation coefficients, their raw p-values, and the corresponding adjusted p-values using the Holm–Bonferroni method. The results are presented in three $r \times r$ matrices and based on these matrices we can identify and remove traits that exhibit a statistically significant intercorrelation. The macro identifies the trait that exhibits the greatest number of statistically nonsignificant p-values. This trait, if present, is highlighted in red and a message appears stating that the trait may be removed from the data set. We delete the trait and repeat the above process until there are no statistically significantly intercorrelated traits. Alternatively, we can delete the traits that exhibit high r or small p-values. During this process we must be careful to avoid overediting, which may result in important information loss. In addition, as already mentioned, the presence of intercorrelated traits does not appear to affect the validity of the MMD values substantially (Nikita, 2015).

In Fig. 5.XI.5 we observe that there are no high r values, although there are several statistically significant raw p-values. However, when the Holm–Bonferroni correction is applied, no traits appear to be significantly intercorrelated, so no further traits need to be eliminated from the data set for the calculation of the MMD.

Now that we have completed the preliminary editing of the data set, we can proceed to the calculation of the MMD using the remaining variables. This may be done by the Biodistances macro using option "1" in the Binary Mode Selection box. We obtain the results shown in Fig. 5.XI.6 where Bartlett's correction has been selected. The corresponding results based on all seven traits are shown in Fig. 5.XI.7 because data editing options "2"–"4" are not required for the calculation of Mahalanobis-type distances. We observe that the macro calculates the MMD, the squared Mahalanobis-type distances RMD and TMD, as well as the p-values for the MMD (p-MMD) calculated by means of Eq. (5.2.6) and the p-values for RMD and TMD using Eq. (5.1.11). Note that the p-values for the RMD and TMD are not reliable,

DATA EDITING-4 (INTERCORRELATED TRAITS)

Pearson's correlation coefficients

	metopic suture	supra-nasal suture	parietal foramina	ethmoidal foramina	coronal ossicles	squamous ossicles
metopic suture	1	-0.3694942	-0.3705	-0.148522	-0.2854	0.287213
supra-nasal suture	-0.369	1	0.26569	0.325	-0.0347	-0.37258
parietal foramina	-0.37	0.26569371	1	0.0235997	0.1294	-0.22751
ethmoidal foramina	-0.149	0.325	0.0236	1	-0.0572	-0.12532
coronal ossicles	-0.285	-0.0346688	0.1294	-0.057231	1	-0.18014
squamous ossicles	0.2872	-0.3725797	-0.2275	-0.12532	-0.1801	1

Uncorrected intercorrelation p-values

	metopic suture	supra-nasal suture	parietal foramina	ethmoidal foramina	coronal ossicles	squamous ossicles
metopic suture	0	0.02656353	0.02204	0.3944945	0.0742	0.07234
supra-nasal suture	0.0266	0	0.09751	0.0531071	0.8275	0.013875
parietal foramina	0.022	0.09751069	0	0.8897317	0.4082	0.137484
ethmoidal foramina	0.3945	0.05310714	0.88973	0	0.7293	0.441001
coronal ossicles	0.0742	0.82745703	0.40823	0.7292949	0	0.230916
squamous ossicles	0.0723	0.01387497	0.13748	0.4410014	0.2309	0

Holm-Bonferroni corrected p-values

	metopic suture	supra-nasal suture	parietal foramina	ethmoidal foramina	coronal ossicles	squamous ossicles
metopic suture	0	0.34532584	0.30858	1	0.7957	0.795743
supra-nasal suture	0.3453	0	0.8776	0.6372856	1	0.208125
parietal foramina	0.3086	0.87759618	0	1	1	1
ethmoidal foramina	1	0.63728564	1	0	1	1
coronal ossicles	0.7957	1	1	1	0	1
squamous ossicles	0.7957	0.20812454	1	1	1	0

There are no traits to be eliminated

FIGURE 5.XI.5 Results for intercorrelated traits.

especially when many traits are being analyzed, and, therefore, these values must be obtained using the permutation method. Note also that negative MMD values are turned to zeros.

It is seen that the obtained biodistances with and without data editing (Figs. 5.XI.6 and 5.XI.7) do not appear to be substantially different. This is because only one trait has been eliminated during data editing. In a data set with many traits, in which the number of nondiagnostic characters may be large, this may not be the case.

To apply permutations for the computation of p-values, we may use the .exe file MMD_RMD_TMD&p-values in the folder DistancesForBinaryDataC, provided in the companion website. The data input file is shown in Fig. 5.XI.8 and the results obtained are given in Fig. 5.XI.9. Note that the command "Bartlett = 1" indicates the application of Bartlett's

MMD with Freeman-Tukey transformation & Mahalanobis-type D^2 distances							
Bartlett's correction used			Disturbance noise= 0.025				
Pair	MMD	p-MMD	RMD	p-RMD (Sjovold)	TMD	TMD-disturbed	p-TMD (Sjovold)
1-2	0.331	0.006	10.511	3.8E-05	8.030	7.996	0.010
1-3	1.312	0	19.287	8.4E-09	16.868	16.934	3.2E-05
1-4	0.705	8.8E-15	13.578	2.0E-07	10.001	9.904	0.000
2-3	0.287	0.016	6.671	0.002	6.471	6.467	0.030
2-4	0	0.614	2.165	0.187	1.828	1.816	0.404
3-4	0.195	0.022	5.663	0.001	5.689	5.666	0.008

MMD with Freeman-Tukey transformation & Mahalanobis-type D^2 distances							
Bartlett's correction used				Disturbance noise= 0.025			
Pair	MMD	p-MMD	RMD	p-RMD (Sjovold)	TMD	TMD-disturbed	p-TMD (Sjovold)
1-2	0.276	0.010	10.522	8.6E-05	8.177	8.191	0.020
1-3	1.108	0	20.784	2.4E-08	18.310	18.171	0.000
1-4	0.580	7E-12	13.936	9.3E-07	10.017	10.040	0.001
2-3	0.276	0.011	8.444	0.001	8.980	8.968	0.014
2-4	0	0.625	2.664	0.137	2.088	2.090	0.409
3-4	0.154	0.042	6.053	0.001	6.842	6.824	0.008
MMD							
group	1	2	3	4			
1	0	0.276	1.108	0.580			
2	0.276	0	0.276	0			
3	1.108	0.276	0	0.154			
4	0.580	0	0.154	0			
RMD							
	1	2	3	4			
1	0	10.522	20.784	13.936			
2	10.522	0	8.444	2.664			
3	20.784	8.444	0	6.053			
4	13.936	2.664	6.053	0			
TMD							
	1	2	3	4			
1	0	8.177	18.310	10.017			
2	8.177	0	8.980	2.088			
3	18.310	8.980	0	6.842			
4	10.017	2.088	6.842	0			

FIGURE 5.XI.7 Calculated biodistances using all seven traits.

correction to the computation of the MMD. The program provides the MMD and the two squared Mahalanobis-type distances, RMD and TMD. In addition, it provides the *p*-values of the distances calculated from the permutation method. We observe that after the Holm–Bonferroni correction the only statistically significant biodistances are those between sample 1 and all other groups (Fig. 5.XI.10).

Another interesting observation is the following: The MMD, RMD, and TMD are highly correlated (Section 9.8.4, Case Study 23). Therefore, at least in the example under study, these three distance measures basically provide the same

```
data - Notepad                                                    [_] [□] [X]

File   Edit   Format   View   Help

NumberOfRows= 47
NumberOfVariables= 7
Bartlett= 1
1        2        1        1        1        1        1        2
1        2        1        1        1        1        1        2
1        2        1        2        1        2        1        2
1        2        1        1        1        1        2        2
1        2        2        1        1        1        1        2
1        2        1        3        1        1        1        2
1        1        1        3        2        1        2        2
1        2        1        1        2        1        1        2
1        1        2        2        1        2        1        2
1        1        1        1        1        1        2        2
1        2        3        1        1        2        1        2
1        2        3        2        1        1        1        2
2        2        1        2        1        3        2        1
```

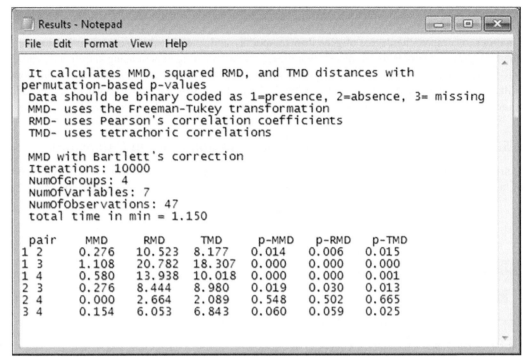

FIGURE 5.XI.9   Calculated biodistances employing all seven traits and their *p*-values using the permutation method.

pair	p-RMD	p-HB
1 2	0.006	0.024
1 3	0	0
1 4	0	0
2 3	0.03	0.09
2 4	0.502	0.502
3 4	0.059	0.118

FIGURE 5.XI.10   Uncorrected and corrected *p*-values for RMD using the Holm–Bonferroni method.

information concerning population biodistances. However, because this is not always the case (Nikita, 2015), the correlation among these distances should always be tested. For the visualization of the biodistances we may apply *Hierarchical Cluster Analysis* and/or MDS. These techniques are described in Sections 9.9.6 and 9.9.7, and their application to the TMD is presented in Section 9.9.8, Case Study 27.

Finally, we may calculate the F_{st} and the R-matrix using the macro Fst, either from the homonymous Excel file or from the OSTEO package using the menu Add-ins → OSTEO → Data analysis → Fst and R-matrix computation, and selecting the option for binary data. The biodistances should be in a squared matrix format, as in Fig. 5.XI.7, bottom. In the first dialog box we select the squared region of the biodistance values and in the next dialog box we type in the number of traits. The results obtained for the RMD are shown in Fig. 5.XI.11. Note that we obtain just one F_{st} value. Individual F_{st}

RMD				
	1	2	3	4
1	0	10.522	20.784	13.936
2	10.522	0	8.444	2.664
3	20.784	8.444	0	6.053
4	13.936	2.664	6.053	0

Fst =	0.2179	Number of traits =		7

Genetic relationship (R-) matrix

	1	2	3	4
1	0.414	-0.045	-0.2361	-0.133
2	-0.045	0.0842	-0.0563	0.01694
3	-0.236	-0.056	0.2749	0.01759
4	-0.133	0.0169	0.0176	0.0985

values are of limited importance. They become meaningful when we examine large data sets of populations from different time periods and/or geographical areas. In such cases it is interesting to compare the F_{st} values obtained from diverse populations in order to compare the degree of gene flow temporally and spatially. As discussed in Section 5.3, a relatively small F_{st} value for a group of populations indicates that these populations were experiencing significant gene flow. In what concerns the R-matrix, as discussed earlier, positive values in this matrix indicate samples that come from populations that are more similar to each other than on average (samples 2—4 and 3—4), whereas negative values correspond to pairs of samples that are less similar to each other than on average (samples 1—2, 1—3, 1—4, and 2—3).

Appendix 5.XII: Recording Nonmetric Traits and Craniometrics in Osteoware

Dental nonmetric traits can be recorded in Osteoware in the Dental Morphology tab, shown in Fig. 5.XII.1. When clicking on each trait, a description of the various character states appears in the box in the lower left corner of the data entry window.

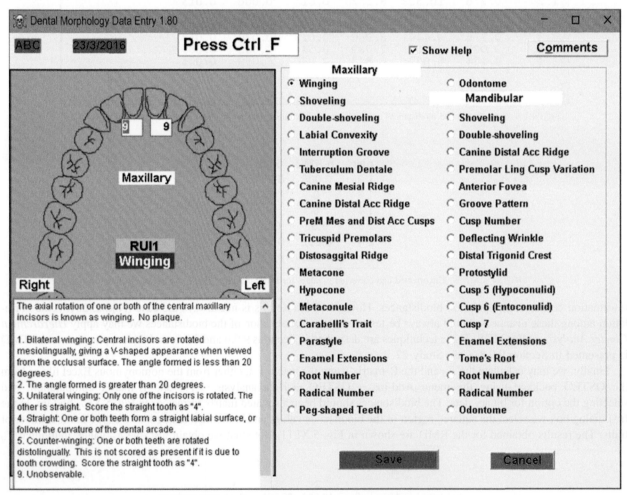

FIGURE 5.XII.1 Osteoware data entry screen for dental nonmetric traits.

Osteoware allows the recording of cranial nonmetric traits in the Cranial Nonmetrics tab. Various facial, lateral, basilar, and mandibular traits may be recorded by clicking on the appropriate tabs. For example, Fig. 5.XII.2 shows the facial nonmetric traits. The character states for each trait are provided from a drop-down menu when clicking on the data entry window for each trait.

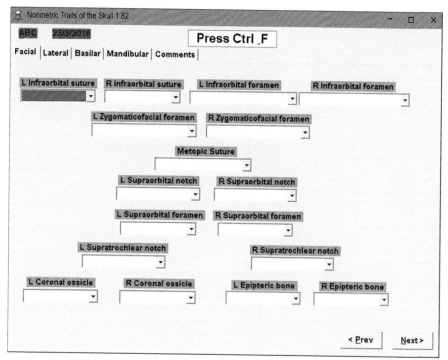

FIGURE 5.XII.2   Osteoware data entry screen for facial nonmetric traits.

Finally, cranial and mandibular measurements are recorded using the Craniometrics tab (Fig. 5.XII.3). Most of these measurements are defined in Appendix 5.II.

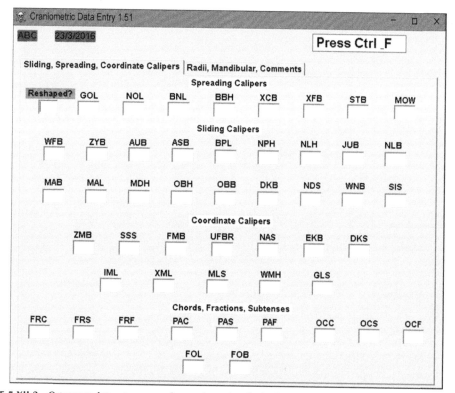

FIGURE 5.XII.3   Osteoware data entry screen for craniometrics obtained using sliding, spreading, and coordinate calipers.

Chapter 6

Growth Patterns

Chapter Outline

Chapter Objectives

By the end of this chapter, the reader will be able to:

- understand the mechanisms that affect human growth;
- use methods for the study of growth patterns in past populations;
- take various postcranial measurements; and
- perform calculations to obtain stature and body mass estimates.

The growth of individuals is genetically controlled; however, environmental conditions associated with elevated stress, such as malnutrition or increased disease load, can result in growth disruption. This disruption may take the form of a decelerated bone growth rate, delayed maturation, prolonged growth, or decreased adult size (Larsen, 2015). As such, growth studies performed on osteoarchaeological material can offer important insights into the stress experienced by past societies and the effectivity of the buffering mechanisms they had developed for coping (Eveleth and Tanner, 1991; Hoppa and FitzGerald, 2005; Ulijaszek et al., 1998). Traditionally, osteoarchaeological studies of growth patterns employ long-bone lengths or stature estimates. However, measurements of different bone dimensions, as well as the study of different growth-related parameters (e.g., cortical bone thickness, body mass, cross-sectional geometry), could offer interesting insights into growth in the past (e.g., Mays et al., 2009; Newman and Gowland, 2015; Ruff et al., 2013). Appendix 6.I presents measurements that may be obtained from postcranial elements, including lengths and other dimensions, whereas Appendix 6.II outlines the recording of postcranial measurements in Osteoware.

This chapter presents the basic principles and methods adopted in osteoarchaeological studies of growth patterns, describes methods for the estimation of stature and body mass, and outlines linear measurements of the axial and appendicular skeleton. In addition to their use in growth studies, stature and body mass are particularly important in forensic contexts, as they can assist in the identification of unknown individuals.

Fazekas and Kósa (1978) and Schaefer et al. (2008) are excellent sources for juvenile measurements and age assessment standards based on morphological and metric characters from the fetal stage onward. The reader may study these textbooks for a more in-depth understanding of the development of the juvenile skeleton.

6.1 GROWTH IN HUMAN POPULATIONS

The term *growth* describes the changes that occur in body size from the fetal stage until early adulthood. Growth is not a uniform process; rather it is characterized by alternating periods of intense and slow activity. The two periods during which growth is particularly rapid are infancy and adolescence (Fig. 6.1.1) (Crews and Bogin, 2010; Hoppa and FitzGerald, 2005). However, even during stages of overall rapid growth, there are intermittent periods of no growth (Lampl, 2005), highlighting the complexity of the growth process.

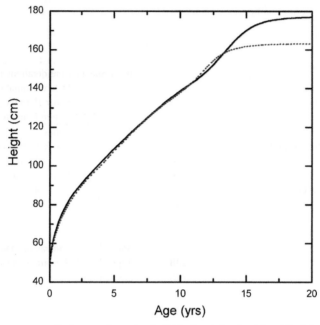

FIGURE 6.1.1 Median height versus age smoothed curves for males (*solid line*) and females (*dotted line*) from birth to 20 years. *Drawn from US Centers for Disease Control data.*

A point that must be stressed is that the aforementioned general pattern expresses primarily the growth of long bones in length. However, different patterns may be observed depending upon the aspect of skeletal growth under examination (see review in Gosman et al., 2011). For example, bone diameter and cortical thickness keep increasing until approximately 30 years of age, rather than ceasing in early adulthood (Baxter-Jones et al., 2011), whereas bone mineral content reaches its highest levels in the third decade of life and decreases dramatically in postmenopausal women (Heaney et al., 2000). Additional changes in bone size and mass occur throughout life as adaptations to mechanical stress and various diseases (see Chapters 7 and 8).

6.2 GROWTH PATTERNS AS A STRESS MARKER

Modern growth studies employing juveniles from various ethnic and social backgrounds have shown that multiple factors can affect growth patterns, such as diet (Foster et al., 2005; Leonard et al., 2000), infectious diseases (Moffat, 2003; Worthen et al., 2001), urbanization and associated overcrowding (Tanner and Eveleth, 1976), physiological stress (Eveleth and Tanner, 1991), and climatic conditions (Panter-Brick, 1997). The impact of these factors on the skeleton is not uniform throughout the growth period; rather it alters with age (Duren et al., 2013; Scheuer and Black, 2000, 2004). In addition, some of these stressors have a synergistic relationship. For instance, individuals suffering from malnutrition are more susceptible to infectious diseases, and gastrointestinal infections reduce the absorption of essential nutrients (Scrimshaw, 2003).

When the aforementioned stressors are not effectively buffered, they affect an individual's growth, rendering growth patterns a useful indicator of the health and life quality of past populations (see review in Lewis, 2006; Saunders, 2008). The reason growth is affected by these stressors is that juveniles under stress must invest their energy in tissue maintenance and immune response, rather than growth, resulting in delayed growth and maturation and reduced stature (Humphrey, 2000a,b; King and Ulijaszek, 2005; McDade et al., 2008). It should be kept in mind that the mere presence of stressful factors does not necessarily result in a disruption of growth patterns because the magnitude and duration of the impact of the stressful factor, as well as the potential of the population to cope with it, also determine the final outcome (Humphrey, 2000a).

A point to be noted is that bones do not grow at the same rate. For example, cranial bones grow faster than postcranial elements, axial skeletal growth is more advanced than appendicular growth, and more distal appendicular elements are more advanced than the proximal ones (Sinclair, 1989). As a result, the growth of different parts of the skeleton is more susceptible to stressors during different periods; thus, the same insult will produce different levels of stunting in different skeletal elements. Therefore, differences in body proportions may also provide interesting insights into past stress episodes (Zakrzewski, 2003).

It must also be emphasized that, in addition to the information drawn regarding stress during the early years of an individual's life, when growth is taking place, growth pattern studies can reveal interesting information about susceptibility to various diseases during adulthood. Indeed, several studies have identified a connection between growth disruption during the juvenile stage and cardiovascular disease, hypertension, type 2 diabetes, obesity, and overall morbidity and mortality later in life (e.g., Bogin et al., 2007; Cameron and Demerath, 2002). Paleopathological research has also identified a connection between childhood indicators of stress, such as growth stunting and enamel hypoplasia (see Chapter 8), and reduced adult longevity (e.g., Armelagos et al., 2009 and references therein; Watts, 2011, 2013, 2015).

6.3 CATCH-UP AND CATCH-DOWN GROWTH

Two phenomena that must be taken into account in growth pattern studies are *catch-up* and *catch-down* growth. As mentioned earlier, during a stressful period, an individual's growth rate slows down. However, once the stressor is eliminated, the individual may catch up with his or her peers by exhibiting a much faster growth rate. For catch-up growth to occur, adequate nutrients should be available. In the opposite case, the growth rate cannot increase; rather it stays the same but extends over a longer period of time (Bogin, 1999; Tanner, 1981). In contrast to earlier suggestions that catch-up growth can occur only in early childhood, it appears that it may also manifest during preadolescence (Adair, 1999) and adolescence (Prentice et al., 2013).

In catch-down growth, growth velocity decreases because of a disruption in the normal growth pattern (Humphrey, 2010). Stini (1975) interpreted this as a *developmental adaptation* because smaller individuals require less nutrition, thus they have better chances of survival, and the work of Frisancho et al. (1973) appears to support this scenario. However, others argue that growth retardation most likely represents a short-term adjustment (*acclimatization*) rather than an evolutionary adaptation (Beaton, 1989).

6.4 OSTEOARCHAEOLOGICAL APPLICATIONS

Johnston (1962) was the first to examine the growth patterns of past populations, focusing on the Indian Knoll Native American population. Initially the focus of osteoarchaeological growth pattern studies was on comparing past populations with one another, or past and modern groups, as well as on exploring the underlying factors that produce the observed growth pattern differences (e.g., Mensforth, 1985; Saunders et al., 1993; Steyn and Henneberg, 1996; Stloukal and Hánaková, 1978; review of additional studies in Saunders, 2008).

More recently, studies have highlighted the multidimensionality of human growth disruption and the need to combine paleopathological, osteological, physiological, and isotopic methods in the effective study of past growth patterns, as well as the need to take into account the natural and cultural environment of past groups while interpreting the obtained results. In this direction, an interesting case study is that of Arcini et al. (2014), who employed stature analysis coupled with isotopic data and concluded that the decrease in stature from medieval to early 19th century Swedish groups cannot be attributed to dietary factors, in contrast to the evidence provided by historical records. Similarly, Clark et al. (2014) combined stature analysis, as an indicator of stress during late childhood, with linear enamel hypoplasia, as an indicator of stress during early childhood (see Chapter 8), to explore the impact of the intensification of rice agriculture in prehistoric Asia. The authors identified a health improvement in the early stages of agricultural intensification in this area, which they attributed to the fact that rice agriculture allowed individuals to maintain a nutritious diet and buffer environmental stressors. However, health deterioration was identified in later periods and it was attributed to environmental changes and subsequent sociocultural transformations. As a final example, Klaus and Tam (2009) combined multiple childhood stress indicators, namely linear enamel hypoplasias, periostitis, porotic hyperostosis (see Chapter 8), femoral growth velocity, and terminal adult stature, to test the impact of Spanish colonization on indigenous populations on the north coast of Peru. The authors identified increased porotic hyperostosis and periostitis and decreased subadult growth in the postcontact sample compared to the precontact one, which they attributed to increased stress due to the Spanish colonization.

6.5 METHODOLOGICAL APPROACHES

Modern growth studies employ longitudinal data to assess how the body size of an individual changes with increasing age. However, in osteoarchaeological assemblages, growth data are cross-sectional, because there is only one measurement (or a set of measurements) representing the body size of each individual at the age of his or her death. As such, osteoarchaeological studies do not provide true growth curves; rather, broad growth patterns are identified by comparing the growth profiles of various groups with one another or with modern standards (Lewis, 2006).

6.5.1 Skeletal Expressions of Stress With Regard to Growth Patterns

6.5.1.1 Small Size for Age

Studies of living children have demonstrated that small size for age indicates stressful environmental conditions (Bogin, 1999; Eveleth and Tanner, 1991). Divergence between an individual's skeletal age and his or her dental age is commonly used for inferring environmental stress in past groups (e.g., Cardoso, 2007; Hummert and Van Gerven, 1983; Mensforth, 1985). This approach is based on the fact that environmental stress affects skeletal development more than dental development (Cardoso, 2007; but see for example Holman and Yamaguchi, 2005). Typically, the comparison between skeletal and dental growth is performed by means of plotting skeletal size against dental age (e.g., Conceição and Cardoso, 2011).

6.5.1.2 Prolonged Skeletal Growth

Studies in developing countries have found that undernourished children exhibit a prolonged growth period, as it takes them longer to reach full growth compared to their nonstressed peers (Bogin, 1999). Variation in the duration of skeletal growth can be explored by comparing the percentage of adult size achieved by individuals at different ages. Using this approach, the end point of growth of each group under study is standardized and emphasis is placed on growth rate rather than on absolute bone size at specific age intervals (Humphrey, 1998, 2010). As it is impossible to know the exact size each juvenile would have reached in adulthood, a mean adult size is calculated per population by averaging the size of all adults in the sample (Humphrey, 2000b, 2010). It must be noted that Shapland and Lewis (2013) proposed an alternative approach for examining pubertal timing as evidence of a prolonged growth period. Instead of focusing on the dimensions of long bones, the authors examined the stage of mineralization of the mandibular canine root, as well as the stage of union of ossification centers of the hand bones, os coxae, and radius (see Chapter 4), and compared these among various groups.

6.5.2 Practical Considerations

Most growth studies are based on plotting long-bone lengths (or percentage of adult size attained) against age (Hoppa, 2000). Depending on the research question, all long bones may be measured and plotted against age, especially given that different bones are affected to different extents by environmental stressors, as discussed earlier. When only one element is examined, this is usually the femur because the growth of the bones of the lower limbs appears to be more sensitive to stress compared to those of the upper limbs (Sciulli, 1994). However, in addition to long-bone length, other skeletal measurements (e.g., cranial or vertebral dimensions) and markers of bone growth (e.g., cross-sectional geometric properties, bone density) may be adopted (Mays et al., 2009; Newman and Gowland, 2015; Ruff et al., 2013).

Dental age is used as a proxy for chronological age as it is less affected by environmental stressors, as mentioned above. It has been suggested that it may be preferable to employ tooth length as an age indicator (e.g., Liversidge et al., 1993), rather than using the methods proposed by Moorrees et al. (1963) and Ubelaker (1989) and other similar approaches. This method has the advantage that the age proxy is now a continuous variable rather than an ordinal one (Cardoso and Garcia, 2009). See Chapter 4 for a review of dental aging methods.

Separate growth profiles can be drawn for each tooth or an overall dental age can be calculated as the mean age obtained from all available teeth per skeleton. Once skeletal dimensions are plotted against dental age/tooth length, regression equations are fitted to the data points of each sample. Differences in the slope of the produced regression equations are indicative of a difference in the growth pattern between groups. To explore the existence of such differences, analysis of covariance (ANCOVA) may by used with skeletal size as the dependent variable, site as the grouping factor, and age as the covariate. See Chapter 9 on how to perform regression analysis and ANCOVA.

6.5.3 Comparative Material

Studies in growth patterns compare the growth of a certain group against that of a different past or modern assemblage. Comparative data from past populations can be found in the literature but should be used cautiously because different studies have employed different aging methods (Lewis, 2006). Comparative data from modern populations are obtained from radiographs of children of known chronological age. The data presented by Maresh (1955, 1970) are often used for this purpose. These data include measurements for all six long bones and were collected during a longitudinal study of children aged between 2 months and 18 years from Denver, Colorado.

Schillaci et al. (2012) examined how efficient the Maresh data are in expressing the growth patterns of healthy populations. For this purpose, they compared the Maresh data against the World Health Organization (WHO) international child growth standard. The authors found that the Maresh reference data generally agree with the WHO standard, and therefore may be used as comparative material in growth patterns; however, they were not effective enough in assessing stunting.

6.6 LIMITATIONS OF GROWTH PATTERN STUDIES

Growth pattern studies in past populations suffer from serious limitations that should be taken into consideration when designing any relevant project and when interpreting the obtained results:

1. Osteoarchaeological assemblages are cross-sectional and, therefore, it is impossible to explore growth rate variations, in contrast to modern longitudinal studies (Humphrey, 2010; Saunders, 2008).
2. Catch-up growth and catch-down growth may hinder the interpretation of observed patterns (see Section 6.3).
3. Wood et al. (1992) argued that growth pattern variation in past groups actually represents differences in mortality levels. Specifically, the authors highlighted the fact that during periods of high mortality, both tall and short people die, but during periods of low mortality, only the most vulnerable group members die, and these are usually shorter, falsely making the overall population appear to be of reduced size. Saunders and Hoppa (1993) addressed this issue by performing a literature review on survivors and nonsurvivors. They found that although there is a significant stature difference between the two groups, the actual femoral length difference is on the order of millimeters. These findings were interpreted as suggestive that the effect of mortality bias on juvenile long-bone lengths is actually minimal.
4. Owing to secular trends, comparisons between archaeological and modern growth profiles to identify retarded growth can be misleading. Secular trends express the changes that occur in the size and shape of the human body over a period of time, and are generally associated with variations in socioeconomic conditions (Henneberg, 1992; Tobias, 1975). The rate of secular trends is not uniform across the world, whereas their impact is not constant throughout the growth period. For instance, Hermanussen et al. (2010) suggest that the factors that produce a secular trend for increased height are influential only during early childhood and late adolescence. In addition, it must be stressed that different parts of the body express different secular trends. Meadows Jantz and Jantz (1999) found that secular change is expressed more pronouncedly in males than in females, in the lower limbs than in the upper limbs, and in distal segments than in proximal ones.
5. Age assessment based on the dentition may be problematic given interpopulation variation in tooth formation and emergence schedules (Humphrey, 2010; Saunders, 2008). Important in this respect is the finding that more recent populations tend to exhibit earlier dental development (Vucic et al., 2014).
6. When examining long-bone lengths, data from different assemblages must be comparable by always including either the entire bone length (diaphysis and fused epiphyses) or only the diaphysis. This naturally depends upon the age groups under examination and it may be preferable to examine children separate from adolescents, even if this limits the identification of growth patterns that span the entire juvenile stage. An additional complication arises when one epiphysis has fused with the diaphysis but the other is still unfused. If such individuals are to be included in the analyses, measurements should be obtained to ensure that either the entire bone or only the diaphyseal segment is measured.

6.7 STATURE ESTIMATION

As mentioned earlier, the majority of osteoarchaeological studies of growth patterns employ linear measurements of the long bones. As different elements are affected to different degrees by environmental stressors, separate plots may be drawn depicting each bone versus age, so that different patterns can be identified. However, in cases of small assemblages, stature estimates based on different skeletal elements may be preferably adopted instead of long-bone lengths. This approach has the advantage of increasing the sample size, although it introduces additional error into the calculations (Lewis, 2006). Given the importance of stature in growth pattern studies, as well as in the identification of individuals in forensic contexts, *anatomical* and *mathematical* methods for calculating stature have been developed and are presented here.

6.7.1 Anatomical Methods

Anatomical methods measure the height of various skeletal elements from the feet to the cranium and calculate stature by summing these measurements and adding a correction factor for the missing soft tissue. Dwight (1894) was the first to propose such a method, and Fully (1956) later proposed a similar but simpler approach. The Fully method has been found to under-estimate stature (Bidmos, 2005; King, 2004), so subsequently Raxter et al. (2006) provided clarifications regarding the obtained measurements and proposed a different soft tissue correction (Box 6.7.1). The method by Raxter et al. is currently the most frequently adopted approach of anatomical stature estimation. Further research highlighted the impact of age on the soft tissue correction factor (Raxter et al., 2007), proposed additional correction factors for supernumerary vertebrae (Raxter and Ruff, 2010), and made adjustments for cases in which certain skeletal elements could not be measured (Auerbach, 2011).

More recently, Bidmos and Manger (2012) suggested that ancestry may affect the soft tissue correction used in such methods, as they found a substantial stature underestimation in their sample of indigenous South African males when using the Raxter et al. (2006) soft tissue correction factors. Their new proposed formula is:

$$\text{Living stature} = 1.037 \times \text{TSH} + 20.56 \tag{6.7.1}$$

where TSH is the total skeletal height (in cm) (but see Ruff et al., 2012a for critique).

Anatomical methods have the advantage of being robust to population and individual variation in body proportions due to climatic, nutritional, genetic, and other factors, as well as to age-related stature loss. In addition, such methods can be adopted even when the sex and ancestry of the individual are unknown, and provide more accurate estimates compared to approaches that use only a limited number of skeletal elements. An important limitation of anatomical methods is that they require an excellent preservation of most of the skeleton.

6.7.2 Mathematical Methods

Mathematical methods comprise regression equations with which stature is estimated using certain bone dimensions. Regression methods are based on the correlation between stature and body segments, mostly long-bone lengths. In particular, such methods usually measure the overall stature, as well as the length of individual bones in cadavers, or adopt anatomical methods to calculate stature. Subsequently, they use regression analysis to determine how long-bone length can predict stature. In general, the femur is most commonly employed in such methods because it contributes most to stature, followed by the tibia and humerus (Wilson et al., 2010). Although regression equations can employ multiple skeletal elements simultaneously (multiple regression), a problem of multicollinearity arises because many bone measurements are intercorrelated to one another. A way to overcome the issue of multicollinearity is to sum the measurements of different bones.

After the bones are measured, the measurements are put into the appropriate regression formula. Linear regression is described in Chapter 9. In general, the linear regression equation for stature estimation from a skeletal measurement has the following form:

$$\text{Stature} = a + bx$$

where a is the y intercept of the line, b is the slope, and x is the bone measurement. Note that a few scholars have utilized curvilinear models (Agnihotri et al., 2007).

Karl Pearson was the first to apply linear regression to estimate stature in a French population (Pearson, 1899). The equations most often found in the literature are those of Trotter and Gleser (1952, 1958, 1977) and Trotter (1970). The original paper (Trotter and Gleser, 1952) was based on American whites and blacks who died in World War II and whose skeletal remains were part of the Terry Collection. In 1958, Trotter and Gleser reevaluated their equations using skeletal

BOX 6.7.1 Method of Raxter et al. (2006) (Revised Version of the Fully, 1956, Method)

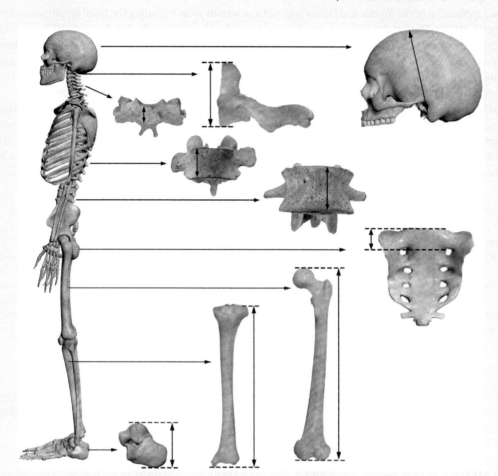

Definitions of obtained measurements, illustrated in the figure above:

- Cranial height: Distance between bregma and basion
- C2 height: Distance between the superiormost point of the odontoid process and the inferiormost point of the anteroinferior rim of the vertebral body
- C3−C7 height: Maximum height of each body, measured in the anterior third, medially to the superiorly curving edges of the centrum
- T1−T12 height: Maximum height of each body, anteriorly to the costal facets and pedicles
- L1−L5 height: Maximum height of each body, anterior to the pedicles, without including any associated swelling
- S1 height: Maximum height between the promontory and the point of articulation between the first and second sacral vertebra at the midsagittal plane

- Femoral bicondylar length (Appendix 6.I)
- Tibial length (maximum morphological length; Appendix 6.I)
- Talus−calcaneus height: Distance between a line tangent to the lateral and medial edges of the talar trochlea and the inferiormost point of the calcaneal tuber when the talus and the calcaneus are articulated

After summing these dimensions to obtain the *skeletal height*, apply one of the following equations to estimate *living stature* (dimensions in centimeters, age in years):

- Living stature $= 1.009 \times$ (skeletal height) $- 0.0426 \times$ age $+ 12.1$
- Living stature $= 0.996 \times$ (skeletal height) $+ 11.7$

material of Americans who died during the Korean War. In this case, a few "Mongoloids," Mexicans, and Puerto Ricans were also available and used in the analyses.

Despite the broad application of the Trotter and Gleser equations, a serious issue regarding the tibial length measurement has been noted by Jantz et al. (1995). The authors observed that the maximum tibial length described by Trotter and Gleser (1952) is not the same as the measurement used by the same authors to produce their 1952 regression equations. Specifically, although the authors claim to have measured the tibia from the lateral part of the lateral condyle to the tip of the medial malleolus, their measurement did not actually include the malleolus, rather it extended only to the talar surface. Jantz et al. (1995) could not determine if the same issue applied to the tibial measurement used in the Trotter and Gleser (1958) publication.

Formulae to estimate stature have been published for a number of populations across the world, and representative studies are given as online supplementary material in Tables S.2.1–S.2.5 by continent. When regression equations are not available for the population of interest, the most appropriate reference sample and corresponding equations should be adopted (but see Albanese et al., 2016 for a critique of population-specific equations). Note that stature estimation based on mathematical methods may also be performed using FORDISC (Box 6.7.2).

BOX 6.7.2 FORDISC

FORDISC was briefly described in Chapter 3 as a software package used for ancestry assessment by means of discriminant function analysis. The same software can be used for stature estimation provided that the epiphyses have fused to the diaphysis (Jantz and Ousley, 2005). As was the case for ancestry assessment, skeletal measurements are entered in the program and the appropriate reference sample is selected (see Chapter 3 for an outline of the available reference samples in FORDISC). FORDISC then calculates the stature of the individual and reports selected prediction intervals. Note that in cases in which ancestry is unknown, the entire reference sample can be used in stature estimation; however, this practice results in larger standard errors compared to population-specific equations.

As an example of mathematical stature estimation, Fig. 6.7.1 presents stature versus maximum femoral length (MFL) for pooled males and females from the Athens Collection (Nikita and Chovalopoulou, 2016). This figure also depicts the reduced major axis regression line (see Chapter 9) obtained from:

$$\text{Stature} = 30.29 + 3 \times \text{MFL} \tag{6.7.2}$$

where stature and MFL are in centimeters. In addition, the regression line obtained from the equation proposed by Ruff et al. (2012b):

$$\text{Stature} = 40.5 + 2.77 \times \text{MFL} \tag{6.7.3}$$

is also included in Fig. 6.7.1. Eq. (6.7.3) was obtained based on a broad sample of Holocene European populations and it can be seen that it actually describes very satisfactorily the Greek data.

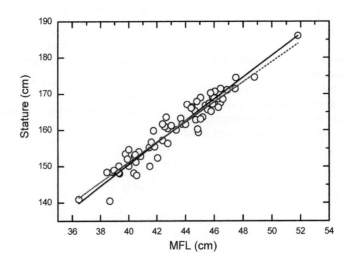

Equations proposed by Ruff et al. (2012b), Sjøvold (1990), and Trotter and Glesser (1952) are used to estimate stature in the macro StatureEstimation, provided in the companion website in the homonymous Excel file or in the OSTEO software through the menu Add-Ins → OSTEO → Estimation → Stature estimation.

Because regression methods employ only one or a few bone lengths, they are generally not as accurate as anatomical methods, which use all skeletal elements that contribute to stature. Moreover, regression methods cannot effectively account for abnormal or pathological changes in anatomy (e.g., kyphosis) and proportions (variations in allometric relationships). Finally, the relationship between stature and individual bones may exhibit substantial variability at an intra- and interpopulation level; thus caution should be exerted in selecting the most appropriate equation each time.

6.7.3 Special Considerations in Stature Estimation

6.7.3.1 Stature Estimation Using Skeletal Elements Other Than the Long Bones

A number of studies have used skeletal elements other than the long bones for stature estimation, namely hand and foot bones, the sternum, spinal segments, and the cranium. Representative examples can be found in the companion website in Tables S.2.1–S.2.5. In most cases, the relationship between these elements and stature is not as strong as that for long bones, and the resulting estimates exhibit greater error. In addition, in the examination of small bones, measurement errors may affect significantly the final estimate, and activity-induced osseous alterations, may also have a large impact in elements such as the hand bones. Overall, it is not advisable to use such methods unless no long bones can be measured.

6.7.3.2 Stature Estimation Using Fragmentary Long Bones

A series of papers has explored the potential of fragmentary long bones in stature estimation. Some of the papers in Tables S.2.2–S.2.5 belong to this category. Such approaches are based on the correlation that exists between a bone's segment length and its total length. Some of these methods estimate stature directly from the dimensions of specific bone segments (Bidmos, 2008a,b, 2009; Chibba and Bidmos, 2007; Holland, 1992), but most use two consecutive regression equations: the first to estimate the maximum bone length based on segment dimensions, and the second to estimate stature from the maximum bone length (de Mendonça, 2000; Koshy et al., 2002; Simmons et al., 1990; Steele, 1970; Steele and McKern, 1969; Wright and Vásquez, 2003). Methods that directly calculate stature from bone segment dimensions are generally preferable as they introduce less error into the estimates by eliminating the need to adopt two consecutive regression equations in stature estimation (e.g., Bidmos, 2009).

The earliest study adopting bone segments in stature estimation was performed by Müller (1935), who identified specific segments on the humerus, radius, and tibia and then determined the proportion of each segment to total bone length. One of the most commonly cited publications is that of Steele (1970), who devised bone length estimation regression equations based on fragmentary femora, tibiae, and humeri. Given the population-specific character of regression analyses, the reader may check the studies given in Tables S.2.2–S.2.5, as well as the literature more broadly, to determine if other studies provide equations that are temporally and geographically closer to his or her sample under study.

6.7.3.3 Age-Related Stature Loss

With increasing age, bone and soft tissue loss occurs, resulting in gradually decreasing stature. This decrease is estimated to be around 6 mm per decade after the age of 30 years (Sjøvold, 2000). Therefore, age-related losses may affect stature estimates, especially for elderly individuals, and should be taken into consideration. Note that because in osteoarchaeological studies we are primarily interested in the peak height of the individual, potential underestimations of age-at-death height due to age losses are not particularly important; however, such losses may confound the correct identification of individuals in forensic contexts.

Various methods have been used for correcting stature estimates for advanced age. Trotter and Gleser (1951) proposed subtracting 0.06 cm for each year over the age of 30. This approach assumes that age-related stature loss progresses linearly, which has been disputed (Hertzog et al., 1969). Galloway (1988) identified a roughly linear stature loss beginning at around 45 years of age, and recommended subtracting 0.16 cm for each year over 45. Two years later, the same author proposed two alternative age-related stature loss corrections (Galloway, 1990):

$$[((\text{age} - 45) \times 0.10) - 0.03] \times (\text{maximum height})/100 \qquad (6.7.4)$$

or

$$[((age - 45) \times 0.10) + (maximum\ height) \times 0.02 - 3.41] \times (maximum\ height)/100 \qquad (6.7.5)$$

where maximum height is in centimeters.

Cline et al. (1989) found that in their sample from Tucson, Arizona, age-related stature decrease begins earlier in males, but the rate of decline is much higher in females, mostly due to osteoporosis. The authors subsequently proposed sex-specific equations to account for age-related stature decline. Giles (1991) stressed that secular trends may also play a role in the sense that older people may appear shorter because they are compared against younger generations, which tend to be taller as a result of improved living conditions. Subsequently, Giles (1991) proposed new values to be subtracted from maximum stature estimates at different ages. Note that, as mentioned in Section 6.7.1 on anatomical stature estimation methods, Raxter et al. (2006) also suggested using the formula that takes age into account (see Box 6.7.1).

More recently, Niskanen et al. (2013) proposed new corrections based on a sample of males and females from the Terry Collection, taking into account that stature loss begins at the age of 40 and follows a quadratic, rather than a linear, pattern. For individuals younger than 40 years, the authors propose the estimation of cadaveric stature (CSTA) from the equation:

$$CSTA = 1.039 \times SKH - 0.075 \times age + 13.127 \qquad (6.7.6)$$

where SKH is the skeletal height, that is, stature calculated using the anatomical method but, in contrast to Raxter et al. (2006), vertebral body heights should be measured at the anterior midline. For individuals older than 40 years, the following equation should be used instead:

$$CSTA = 1.043 \times SKH - 0.103 \times age + 14.586 \qquad (6.7.7)$$

When the age of the individuals is unknown but it can be grossly assessed that they are younger than 40 years, CSTA can be estimated from:

$$CSTA = 1.051 \times SKH - 8.136 \qquad (6.7.8)$$

A problem with the proposed age corrections for stature in all equations except Eq. (6.7.8) is that it is not possible to estimate age in adults with the accuracy required for their application. This is particularly the case for older individuals, for which the issue of bone loss is most crucial. In addition, age-related stature loss varies at an intra- and interpopulation level as it depends upon bone density, activity patterns, and other factors; thus no single correction can be successfully applied in all cases.

6.7.3.4 Stature Estimation in Juveniles

Stature estimation in juveniles is problematic because juvenile bone lengths are derived from the diaphysis, the epiphyses, and the cartilage growth plate between them. However, in skeletal remains it is not possible to estimate the height of the growth plate as its thickness varies at different developmental periods, as well as between individuals (Lewis, 2006). Another serious limitation is the fact that sex and ancestry are almost impossible to assess in juvenile skeletal remains, rendering the use of mathematical methods of limited validity. In addition, given the overall rapid growth of the skeleton during childhood and adolescence, the regression lines for stature estimation cannot be straight; therefore, the obtained regression equations are more complex (Kromeyer-Hauschild and Jaeger, 2000; Smith and Buschang, 2004, 2005). Finally, and in association with these limitations, limb proportions change throughout growth, which, coupled with the inaccuracies of aging methods based on skeletal remains, restricts stature estimates.

Despite the difficulties entailed in stature estimation in juveniles, numerous attempts have been made in this direction. Representative studies are provided in the companion website in Table S.2.6. Estimations of fetal and child stature were first attempted by Balthazard and Dervieux (1921), Olivier (1969), and Olivier and Pineau (1958, 1960). Among the more recent studies, those by Ruff (2007) and Smith (2007) are noteworthy. Both authors used data from the Denver growth study, which mostly included white children. Ruff (2007) examined radiographs of 10 males and 10 females for each age group from age 1 to 17. Lengths of humeri, radii, femora, and tibiae were used to generate regression equations for stature estimation at each age, pooling male and female data. For younger children, regression equations were based solely on diaphyseal lengths, whereas for older children the entire bone, including the diaphysis and epiphyses, was examined. Sciulli and Blatt (2008) tested the performance of this method and obtained overall accurate results. Note that the equations by Ruff (2007) are used for stature estimation in the macro StatureEstimation, provided in the companion website.

The macro may be run either through its homonymous Excel file or through OSTEO using the menu Add-Ins → OSTEO → Estimation → Stature estimation.

The Smith (2007) study included children 3–10 years of age; thus only diaphyseal lengths were measured. Equations were produced for combined sexes as well as separately for males and females, but the resulting standard errors were high. It must be stressed that this study suffered from two limitations. First, no correction for magnification was used for any of the measurements obtained from radiographs, which will lead to an underestimation of stature when the derived equations are applied to osteological material. Second, the proposed equations were not age specific, rather they were based on a pooled sample of children aged 3–10 years, which decreases their accuracy considering the substantial changes that occur in limb proportions during this developmental period (Ruff, 2007).

6.7.3.5 Forensic Stature Issues and Circadian Variation

In forensic contexts, Ousley (1995) noted that there is often a difference between forensic stature (i.e., stature recorded on a person's ID or driving license), measured stature (stature estimated based on skeletal remains), and biological stature (the actual stature of the individual). A serious limitation of forensic stature is that individuals, especially males and short individuals of either sex, tend to report their stature as higher than in reality (Giles and Hutchinson, 1991). In addition, a first driving license may be obtained in adolescence/early adulthood when growth is still taking place; therefore the final biological stature of the individual may be greater than the forensic one (Byers, 2010). The potential impact of forensic stature biases should be taken into consideration when stature estimations are used for individuation in forensic material.

Circadian or diurnal variation in stature, that is, a change in stature throughout the day, is another issue to be considered, because stature appears to be greater in the morning and slightly decreased after a few hours of standing upright, due to the compression of intervertebral discs (Krishan et al., 2009). However, it must be stressed that circadian variation is minimal compared to the overall error in skeletal stature estimates.

6.8 BODY MASS ESTIMATION

Body mass predicted from skeletal remains could provide another indicator of overall population health, as numerous studies of living populations have used body mass as a measure of nutrition and well-being (Bogin, 1999; Eveleth and Tanner, 1991). For the estimation of body mass from skeletal remains two principal approaches may be followed: *mechanical* and *morphometric* (Auerbach and Ruff, 2004; Ruff, 2002). Mechanical approaches are based on the relationship that exists between body mass and the dimensions of skeletal elements that support the body. In particular, such methods are based on the biomechanics of load bearing on the diaphysis and articular surfaces of the long bones of the lower limb, particularly the femoral head (Auerbach and Ruff, 2004; Grine et al., 1995; Kurki et al., 2010; Ruff et al., 2006). Commonly adopted equations for body mass estimation from femoral head diameter are those of McHenry (1992) for small-bodied individuals, Grine et al. (1995) for large-bodied individuals, and Ruff et al. (1991) for modern US samples. Depending on the body size of the individual(s) under study, one of these equations or the average estimate of all three may be employed (e.g., Auerbach and Ruff, 2004; Kurki et al., 2010). Alternatively, population-specific equations have been proposed for various groups. Representative studies for body mass estimation in extinct hominins and modern humans are given in the companion website in Tables S.3.1 and S.3.2 for adults and juveniles, respectively. Note that the equations by Ruff et al. (1991, 2005, 2012b), and Squyres and Ruff (2015) for adults, as well as those by Ruff (2007) for subadults, can be applied using the macro BodyMassEstimation either directly from the homonymous Excel file or through OSTEO via the menu Add-Ins → OSTEO → Estimation → Body mass estimation.

Moore (2008) noted that a potential limitation of mechanical approaches is that it is unclear to what extent the observed differences in the dimensions of the bones of the lower limbs are due to variation in body mass or to activity patterns. However, Ruff et al. (1991) and Lieberman et al. (2001) have shown that joint size is less plastic in relation to loading compared to other anatomical areas of the long bones; thus the femoral head diameter is expected to be minimally affected by activity patterns.

Morphometric methods view the body as a cylinder, whereby the stature of the individual is equal to the height of the cylinder and biiliac breadth gives the diameter of the cylinder (Ruff, 1994, 2000). The advantage of such methods is that they do not assume that there is a consistent biomechanical relationship between body mass and bone size (Auerbach and

Ruff, 2004; Kurki et al., 2010). On the other hand, their main disadvantage is that they require very good skeletal preservation, including an intact pelvis, which is extremely rare, especially in archaeological contexts.

Special note must be made to the study by Robbins et al. (2010) and Robbins Schug et al. (2013), who estimated juvenile body mass using femoral cross-sectional geometric data (see Chapter 7 for a discussion on cross-sectional geometry). Their approach is based on the correlation that exists between body weight and femoral midshaft bone mass during ontogeny (Ruff, 2003a,b, 2005; Ruff et al., 2006).

Finally, Moore (2008) proposed ways of estimating body mass, combining femoral cross-sectional geometric properties and bone mineral density with the macroscopic study of degenerative articular changes in the spine and lower limb. The author focused mainly on calculating body mass extremes of emaciation and obesity, and the optimum methods were found to be those that combined the cross-sectional area of the proximal femur and bone mineral density data, while pathologies complemented the prediction of obesity.

REFERENCES

Adair LS. Filipino children exhibit catch-up growth from age 2 to 12 years. The Journal of Nutrition 1999;129:1140–8.

Agnihotri AK, Purwar B, Googoolye K, Agnihotri S, Jeebun N. Estimation of stature by foot length. Journal of Forensic and Legal Medicine 2007;14:279–83.

Albanese J, Osley SE, Tuck A. Do group-specific equations provide the best estimates of stature? Forensic Science International 2016;261:154–8.

Arcini C, Ahlström T, Tagesson G. Variations in diet and stature: are they linked? Bioarchaeology and paleodietary Bayesian mixing models from Linköping, Sweden. International Journal of Osteoarchaeology 2014;24:543–56.

Armelagos GJ, Goodman RH, Harper KN, Blakey ML. Enamel hypoplasia and early mortality: bioarchaeological support for the Barker hypothesis. Evolutionary Anthropology 2009;18:261–71.

Auerbach BM. Methods for estimating missing human skeletal element osteometric dimensions employed in the revised Fully technique for estimating stature. American Journal of Physical Anthropology 2011;145:67–80.

Auerbach BM, Ruff CB. Human body mass estimation: a comparison of "morphometric" and "mechanical" methods. American Journal of Physical Anthropology 2004;125:331–42.

Balthazard V, Dervieux D. Études anthropologiques sur le foetus humain. Annales de Médecine Légale 1921;1:37–42.

Baxter-Jones AD, Faulkner RA, Forwood MR, Mirwald RL, Bailey DA. Bone mineral accrual from 8 to 30 years of age: an estimation of peak bone mass. Journal of Bone and Mineral Research 2011;26:1729–39.

Beaton GH. Small but healthy? Are we asking the right question? Human Organization 1989;48:30–9.

Bidmos MA. On the non-equivalence of documented cadaver lengths to living stature estimates based on Fully's method on bones in the Raymond A. Dart collection. Journal of Forensic Sciences 2005;50:1–6.

Bidmos MA. Stature reconstruction using fragmentary femora in South Africans of European descent. Journal of Forensic Sciences 2008;53:1044–8.

Bidmos MA. Estimation of stature using fragmentary femora in indigenous South Africans. International Journal of Legal Medicine 2008;122:293–9.

Bidmos MA. Fragmentary femora: evaluation of the accuracy of the direct and indirect methods in stature reconstruction. Forensic Science International 2009;192. 131.e1–131.e5.

Bidmos MA, Manger PR. New soft tissue correction factors for stature estimation: results from magnetic resonance imaging. Forensic Science International 2012;214. 212.e1–212.e7.

Bogin B. Patterns of human growth. 2nd ed. Cambridge: Cambridge University Press; 1999.

Bogin B, Silva MIV, Rios L. Life history trade-offs in human growth: adaptation or pathology? American Journal of Human Biology 2007;19:631–42.

Buikstra JE, Ubelaker DH, editors. Standards for data collection from human skeletal remains; 1994. Arkansas Archeological Survey Research Series no. 44.

Byers SN. Introduction to forensic anthropology. 4th ed. Boston: Prentice Hall; 2010.

Cameron N, Demerath E. Critical periods in human growth and their relationship to diseases of aging. Yearbook of Physical Anthropology 2002;45:159–84.

Cardoso HFV. Environmental effects on skeletal versus dental development: using a documented subadult skeletal sample to test a basic assumption in human osteological research. American Journal of Physical Anthropology 2007;132:223–33.

Cardoso HFV, Garcia S. The not-so-dark ages: ecology for human growth in medieval and early twentieth century Portugal as inferred from skeletal growth profiles. American Journal of Physical Anthropology 2009;138:136–47.

Chibba K, Bidmos MA. Using tibia fragments from South Africans of European descent to estimate maximum tibia length and stature. Forensic Science International 2007;169:145–51.

Clark AL, Tayles N, Halcrow SE. Aspects of health in prehistoric mainland Southeast Asia: indicators of stress in response to the intensification of rice agriculture. American Journal of Physical Anthropology 2014;153:484–95.

Cline MG, Meredith KE, Boyer JT, Burrows B. Decline of height with age in adults in a general population sample: estimating maximum height and distinguishing birth cohort effects from actual loss of stature with aging. Human Biology 1989;61:415–25.

Conceição ELN, Cardoso HFV. Environmental effects on skeletal versus dental development II: further testing of a basic assumption in human osteological research. American Journal of Physical Anthropology 2011;144:463–70.

Crews DE, Bogin B. Growth, development, senescence, and aging: a life history perspective. In: Larsen CS, editor. A companion to biological anthropology. Malden: Wiley-Blackwell; 2010. p. 124–52.

de Mendonça MC. Estimation of height from the length of long bones in a Portuguese adult population. American Journal of Physical Anthropology 2000;112:39–48.

Duren DL, Seselj M, Froehle AW, Ramzi W, Nahhas RW, Richard J, Sherwood RJ. Skeletal growth and the changing genetic landscape during childhood and adulthood. American Journal of Physical Anthropology 2013;150:48–57.

Dwight T. Methods of estimating the height from parts of the skeleton. Medical Record 1894;46:293–6.

Eveleth PB, Tanner JM. Worldwide variation in human growth. 2nd ed. Cambridge: Cambridge University Press; 1991.

Fazekas G, Kósa F. Forensic fetal osteology. Budapest: Akadémiai Kiadó; 1978.

Foster Z, Byron E, Reyes-Garcia V, Huanca T, Vadez V, Apaza L, Pérez E, Tanner S, Gutierrez Y, Sandstrom B, Yakhedts A, Osborn C, Godoy RA, Leonard WR. Physical growth and nutritional status of Tsimane' Amerindian children of lowland Bolivia. American Journal of Physical Anthropology 2005;126:343–51.

Frisancho AR, Sanchez J, Pallardel D, Yanez L. Adaptive significance of small body size under poor socio-economic conditions in southern Peru. American Journal of Physical Anthropology 1973;39:255–62.

Fully G. Un nouvelle méthode de détermination de la taille. Annales de Médecine Légale 1956;35:266–73.

Galloway A. Estimating actual height in the older individual. Journal of Forensic Sciences 1988;33:126–36.

Galloway A. Stature loss among an older United States population and its relation to bone mineral status. American Journal of Physical Anthropology 1990;83:467–76.

Giles E. Corrections for age in estimating older adults' stature from long bones. Journal of Forensic Sciences 1991;36:898–901.

Giles E, Hutchinson DL. Stature- and age-related bias in self-reported stature. Journal of Forensic Sciences 1991;36:765–80.

Gosman JH, Stout SD, Larsen CS. Skeletal biology over the life span: a view from the surfaces. Yearbook of Physical Anthropology 2011;54:86–98.

Grine FE, Jungers WL, Tobias PV, Pearson OM. Fossil *Homo* femur from, Berg Aukas, northern Namibia. American Journal of Physical Anthropology 1995;97:151–85.

Heaney RP, Abrams S, Dawson-Hughes B, Looker A, Marcus R, Matkovic V, Weaver C. Peak bone mass. Osteoporosis International 2000;11:985–1009.

Henneberg M. Continuing human evolution: bodies, brains and the role of variability. Transactions of the Royal Society of South Africa 1992;48:159–82.

Hermanussen M, Godina E, Ruhli FJ, Blaha P, Boldsen JL, Van Buuren S, MacIntyre M, Aßmann C, Ghosh A, De Stefano GF, Sonkin VD, Tresguerres JAF, Meigen C, Scheffler C, Geiger C, Liebermann LS. Growth variation, final height and secular trend. HOMO-Journal of Comparative Human Biology 2010;61:277–84.

Hertzog KP, Garn SM, Hempy III HO. Partitioning the effects of secular trend and aging on adult stature. American Journal of Physical Anthropology 1969;31:111–5.

Holland TD. Estimation of adult stature from fragmentary tibias. Journal of Forensic Sciences 1992;37:1223–9.

Holman DJ, Yamaguchi K. Longitudinal analysis of deciduous tooth emergence: IV. covariate effects in Japanese children. American Journal of Physical Anthropology 2005;126:352–8.

Hoppa RD. Population variation in osteological aging criteria: an example from the pubic symphysis. American Journal of Physical Anthropology 2000;111:185–91.

Hoppa RD, FitzGerald CM, editors. Human growth in the past: studies from bones and teeth. Cambridge: Cambridge University Press; 2005.

Hummert JR, Van Gerven DP. Skeletal growth in a medieval population from Sudanese Nubia. American Journal of Physical Anthropology 1983;60:471–8.

Humphrey LT. Patterns of growth in the modern human skeleton. American Journal of Physical Anthropology 1998;105:57–72.

Humphrey LT. Interpretations of the growth of past populations. In: Derevenski JS, editor. Children and material culture. London: Routledge; 2000. p. 193–205.

Humphrey LT. Growth studies of past populations: an overview and an example. In: Cox M, Mays S, editors. Human osteology in archaeology and forensic science. London: Greenwich Medical Media; 2000. p. 25–38.

Humphrey LT. Linear growth variation in the archaeological record. In: Thompson JL, Krovitz GE, Nelson AJ, editors. Patterns of growth and development in the genus *Homo*. Cambridge: Cambridge University Press; 2010. p. 144–69.

Jantz RL, Ousley SD. Fordisc 3.0 personal computer forensic discriminant functions. Knoxville: The University of Tennessee; 2005.

Jantz RL, Hunt DR, Meadows L. The measure and mismeasure of the tibia: implications for stature estimation. Journal of Forensic Sciences 1995;40:758–61.

Johnston FE. Growth of long bones of infants and young children at Indian Knoll. American Journal of Physical Anthropology 1962;20:249–54.

King KA. A test of the Fully anatomical method of stature estimation. American Journal of Physical Anthropology 2004;(Suppl. 38):125.

King SE, Ulijaszek SJ. Invisible insults during growth and development: contemporary theories and past populations. In: Hoppa RD, Fitzgerald CM, editors. Human growth in the past: studies from bones and teeth. Cambridge: Cambridge University Press; 2005. p. 161–82.

Klaus HD, Tam ME. Contact in the Andes: bioarchaeology of systemic stress in colonial Mórrope, Peru. American Journal of Physical Anthropology 2009;138:356–68.

Koshy S, Vettivel S, Selvaraj KG. Estimation of length of calcaneum and talus from their bony markers. Forensic Science International 2002;129:200–4.

Krishan K, Sidhu MC, Kanchan T, Menezes RG, Sen J. Diurnal variation in stature — is it more in children or adults? Bioscience Hypotheses 2009;2:174—5.

Kromeyer-Hauschild K, Jaeger U. Growth studies in Jena, Germany: changes in sitting height, biacromial and bicristal breadth in the past decenniums. American Journal of Human Biology 2000;12:646—54.

Kurki HK, Ginter JK, Stock JT, Pfeiffer S. Body size estimation of small-bodied humans: applicability of current methods. American Journal of Physical Anthropology 2010;141:169—80.

Lampl M. Grandma's right: a sleeping baby may be a growing baby American Journal of Physical Anthropology 2005;(Suppl. 40):134.

Larsen CS. Bioarchaeology: interpreting behavior from the human skeleton. 2nd ed. Cambridge: Cambridge University Press; 2015.

Leonard WR, Dewalt KM, Stansbury JP, McCaston MK. Influence of dietary quality on the growth of highland and coastal Ecuadorian children. American Journal of Human Biology 2000;12:825—37.

Lewis ME. The bioarchaeology of children: perspectives from biological and forensic anthropology. Cambridge: Cambridge University Press; 2006.

Lieberman DE, Devlin ME, Pearson OM. Articular area responses to mechanical loading: effects of exercise, age, and skeletal location. American Journal of Physical Anthropology 2001;116:266—77.

Liversidge HM, Dean MC, Molleson TI. Increasing human tooth length between birth and 5.4 years. American Journal of Physical Anthropology 1993;90:307—13.

Maresh MM. Linear growth of long bones of extremities from infancy through adolescence. American Journal of Diseases in Childhood 1955;89:725—42.

Maresh MM. Measurements from roentgenograms. In: McCammon RW, editor. Human growth and development. Springfield: Charles C. Thomas; 1970. p. 157—200.

Martin R. Lehrbuch der Anthropologie. Jena: Verlag von Gustav Fischer; 1928.

Mays S, Ives R, Brickley M. The effects of socioeconomic status on endochondral and appositional bone growth, and acquisition of cortical bone in children from 19th century Birmingham, England. American Journal of Physical Anthropology 2009;140:410—6.

McDade TW, Reyes-García V, Tanner S, Huanca T, Leonard WR. Maintenance versus growth: investigating the costs of immune activation among children in lowland Bolivia. American Journal of Physical Anthropology 2008;136:478—84.

McHenry HM. Body size and proportions in early hominids. American Journal of Physical Anthropology 1992;87:407—31.

Meadows Jantz LM, Jantz RL. Secular change in long bone length and proportion in the United States, 1800—1970. American Journal of Physical Anthropology 1999;110:57—67.

Mensforth RP. Relative tibia long bone growth in the Libben and Bt-5 prehistoric skeletal populations. American Journal of Physical Anthropology 1985;68:247—62.

Moffat T. Diarrhea, respiratory infections, protozoan gastrointestinal parasites, and child growth in Kathmandu, Nepal. American Journal of Physical Anthropology 2003;122:85—97.

Moore MK. Body mass estimation from the human skeleton [Ph.D. dissertation]. Knoxville: The University of Tennessee; 2008.

Moore-Jansen PH, Jantz RL. Data collection procedures for forensic skeletal material. Report of Investigations No. 48. Knoxville: University of Tennessee; 1989.

Moorrees CFA, Fanning EA, Hunt EE. Formation and resorption of three deciduous teeth in children. American Journal of Physical Anthropology 1963;21:205—13.

Mulhern D. Postcranial metrics. In: Wilczak CA, Dudar CJ, editors. Osteoware software manual, vol. I. Washington: Smithsonian Institution; 2011. p. 46—62.

Müller G. Zur Bestimmung der Lange beschadigter Extremitatenknochen. Anthropologischer Anzeiger 1935;12:70—2.

Newman SL, Gowland RL. Brief communication: the use of non-adult vertebral dimensions as indicators of growth disruption and non-specific health stress in skeletal populations. American Journal of Physical Anthropology 2015;158:155—64.

Nikita E, Chovalopoulou M-E. Regression equations for the estimation of stature and body mass using a Greek documented skeletal collection. In: Hellenic society for biological sciences 38th annual meeting, Kavala, 26th—28th May; 2016.

Niskanen M, Maijanen H, McCarthy D, Junno J-A. Application of the anatomical method to estimate the maximum adult stature and the age-at-death stature. American Journal of Physical Anthropology 2013;152:96—106.

Olivier G. Practical anthropology. Springfield: Charles C. Thomas; 1969.

Olivier G, Pineau H. Détermination de l'âge du foetus et de l'embryon. Achaeologie et Anatomie (La Semaine des Hôpitaux) 1958;6:21—8.

Olivier G, Pineau H. Nouvelle détermination de la taille foetale d'apres les longueurs diaphysaires des os longs. Annales de Médecine Légale 1960;40:141—4.

Ousley S. Should we estimate biological or forensic stature? Journal of Forensic Sciences 1995;40:768—73.

Panter-Brick C. Seasonal growth patterns in rural Nepali children. Annals of Human Biology 1997;24:1—18.

Pearson K. Mathematical contribution to the theory of evolution: on the reconstruction of the stature of prehistoric races. Philosophical Transactions of the Royal Society of London. Series A 1899;192:169—244.

Prentice AM, Ward KA, Goldberg GR, Jarjou LM, Moore SE, Fulford AJ, Prentice A. Critical windows for nutritional interventions against stunting. The American Journal of Clinical Nutrition 2013;97:911—8.

Raxter MH, Ruff CB. The effect of vertebral numerical variation on anatomical stature estimates. Journal of Forensic Sciences 2010;55:464—6.

Raxter MH, Auerbach BM, Ruff CB. Revision of the Fully technique for estimating statures. American Journal of Physical Anthropology 2006;130:374—84.

Raxter MH, Ruff CB, Auerbach BM. Technical note: revised Fully stature estimation technique. American Journal of Physical Anthropology 2007;133:817−8.

Robbins G, Sciulli PW, Blatt SH. Estimating body mass in subadult human skeletons. American Journal of Physical Anthropology 2010;143:146−50.

Robbins Schug G, Gupta S, Cowgill LW, Sciulli PW, Blatt S. Panel regression formulas for stature and body mass estimation in immature skeletons, without reference to specific age estimates. Journal of Archaeological Science 2013;40:3076−86.

Ruff CB. Morphological adaptation to climate in modern and fossil hominids. Yearbook of Physical Anthropology 1994;37:65−107.

Ruff CB. Body mass prediction from skeletal frame size in elite athletes. American Journal of Physical Anthropology 2000;113:507−17.

Ruff CB. Variation in human body size and shape. Annual Review of Anthropology 2002;31:211−32.

Ruff CB. Growth in bone strength, body size, and muscle size in a juvenile longitudinal sample. Bone 2003;33:317−29.

Ruff CB. Ontogenetic adaptation to bipedalism: age changes in femoral to humeral length and strength proportions in humans, with a comparison to baboons. Journal of Human Evolution 2003;45:317−49.

Ruff CB. Growth tracking of femoral and humeral strength from infancy through late adolescence. Acta Paediatrica 2005;94:1030−7.

Ruff C. Body size prediction from juvenile skeletal remains. American Journal of Physical Anthropology 2007;133:698−716.

Ruff CB, Scott WW, Liu AYC. Articular and diaphyseal remodeling of the proximal femur with changes in body mass in adults. American Journal of Physical Anthropology 1991;86:397−413.

Ruff C, Niskanen M, Junno J-A, Jamison P. Body mass prediction from stature and bi-iliac breadth in two high latitude populations, with application to earlier higher latitude humans. Journal of Human Evolution 2005;48:381−92.

Ruff CB, Holt B, Trinkaus E. Who's afraid of the big bad Wolff? "Wolff's law" and bone functional adaptation. American Journal of Physical Anthropology 2006;129:484−98.

Ruff CB, Raxter M, Auerbach B. Comment on Bidmos and Manger, "new soft tissue correction factors for stature estimation: results from magnetic resonance imaging". Forensic Science International 2012;222:e42−3.

Ruff CB, Holt BM, Niskanen M, Sladék V, Berner M, Garofalo E, Garvin HM, Hora M, Maijanen H, Niinimäki S, Salo K, Schuplerová E, Tompkins D. Stature and body mass estimation from skeletal remains in the European Holocene. American Journal of Physical Anthropology 2012;148:601−17.

Ruff CB, Garofalo E, Holmes MA. Interpreting skeletal growth in the past from a functional and physiological perspective. American Journal of Physical Anthropology 2013;150:28−37.

Saunders SR. Juvenile skeletons and growth-related studies. In: Katzenberg MA, Saunders SR, editors. Biological anthropology of the human skeleton. 2nd ed. Hoboken: Wiley-Liss; 2008. p. 117−47.

Saunders SR, Hoppa RD. Growth deficit in survivors and non-survivors: biological correlates of mortality bias in subadult skeletal samples. Yearbook of Physical Anthropology 1993;36:127−51.

Saunders S, Hoppa R, Southern R. Diaphyseal growth in a nineteenth century skeletal sample of subadults from St Thomas' Church Belleville, Ontario. International Journal of Osteoarchaeology 1993;3:265−81.

Schaefer M, Black S, Scheuer L. Juvenile osteology. A laboratory and field manual. New York: Elsevier Academic Press; 2008.

Scheuer L, Black S. Development and ageing of the juvenile skeleton. In: Cox M, Mays S, editors. Human osteology in archaeology and forensic science. London: Greenwich Medical Media, Ltd.; 2000. p. 9−22.

Scheuer L, Black S. The juvenile skeleton. New York: Academic Press; 2004.

Schillaci MA, Sachdev HPS, Bhargava SK. Technical note: comparison of the Maresh reference data with the WHO international standard for normal growth in healthy children. American Journal of Physical Anthropology 2012;147:493−8.

Sciulli P. Standardization of long bone growth in children. International Journal of Osteoarchaeology 1994;4:257−9.

Sciulli PW, Blatt SH. Evaluation of juvenile stature and body mass prediction. American Journal of Physical Anthropology 2008;136:387−93.

Scrimshaw NS. Historical concepts of interactions, synergism and antagonism between nutrition and infection. Journal of Nutrition 2003;133:316S−21S.

Shapland F, Lewis ME. Brief communication: a proposed osteological method for the estimation of pubertal stage in human skeletal remains. American Journal of Physical Anthropology 2013;151:302−10.

Simmons T, Jantz RL, Bass WM. Stature estimation from fragmentary femora: a revision of the Steele method. Journal of Forensic Sciences 1990;35:628−36.

Sinclair DC. Human growth after birth. 5th ed. Oxford: Oxford University Press; 1989.

Sjøvold T. Estimation of stature from long bones utilizing the line of organic correlation. Human Evolution 1990;5:431−47.

Sjøvold T. Stature estimation from the skeleton. In: Siegel JA, Saukko PJ, Knupfer GC, editors. Encyclopedia of forensic sciences, vol. I. San Diego: Academic Press; 2000. p. 276−84.

Smith SL. Stature estimation of 3−10 year-old children from long bone lengths. Journal of Forensic Sciences 2007;52:538−46.

Smith SL, Buschang PH. Variation in longitudinal diaphyseal long bone growth in children three to ten years of age. American Journal of Human Biology 2004;16:648−57.

Smith SL, Buschang PH. Longitudinal models of long bone growth during adolescence. American Journal of Human Biology 2005;17:731−45.

Squyres N, Ruff CB. Body mass estimation from knee breadth, with application to early hominins. American Journal of Physical Anthropology 2015;158:198−208.

Steele DG. Estimation of stature from fragments of long limb bones. In: Stewart TD, editor. Personal identification in mass disasters. Washington: Smithsonian Institution; 1970. p. 85−97.

Steele DG, McKern TW. A method for assessment of maximum long bone length and living stature from fragmentary long bones. American Journal of Physical Anthropology 1969;31:215—28.

Steyn M, Henneberg M. Skeletal growth of children from the iron age site at K2 (South Africa). American Journal of Physical Anthropology 1996;100:389—96.

Stini WA. Adaptive strategies of human populations under nutritional stress. In: Watts ES, Johnston FE, Lasker GW, editors. Biosocial interrelations in population adaptation. Paris: Mouton; 1975. p. 19—41.

Stloukal M, Hánaková H. The length of long bones in ancient Slavonic populations with particular consideration to the questions of growth. HOMO-Journal of Comparative Human Biology 1978;29:53—69.

Tanner JM. Catch-up growth in man. British Medical Bulletin 1981;37:233—8.

Tanner JM, Eveleth PB. Urbanisation and growth. In: Harrison GA, Gibson JB, editors. Man in urban environments. Oxford: Oxford University Press; 1976. p. 144—66.

Tobias PV. Stature and secular trend among southern African Negroes and San (Bushmen). The South African Journal of Medical Sciences 1975;40:145—64.

Trotter M. Estimation of stature from intact long limb bones. In: Stewart TD, editor. Personal identification in mass disasters. Washington: Smithsonian Institution; 1970. p. 71—84.

Trotter M, Gleser GC. The effect of aging on stature. American Journal of Physical Anthropology 1951;9:311—24.

Trotter M, Gleser GC. Estimation of stature from long bones of American whites and Negroes. American Journal of Physical Anthropology 1952;10:463—514.

Trotter M, Gleser G. A re-evaluation of estimation of stature based on measurements of stature taken during life and of long bones after death. American Journal of Physical Anthropology 1958;16:79—123.

Trotter M, Gleser G. Corrigenda to "Estimation of stature from long limb bones of American whites and Negroes." American Journal of Physical Anthropology 1977;47:355—6.

Ubelaker DH. Human skeletal remains. Excavation, analysis, interpretation. 2nd ed. Washington: Taraxacum; 1989.

Ulijaszek SJ, Johnston FE, Preece MA, editors. The Cambridge Encyclopedia of human growth and development. Cambridge: Cambridge University Press; 1998.

Vucic S, de Vries E, Eilers PHC, Willemsen SP, Kuijpers MAR, Prahl-Andersen B, Jaddoe VWV, Hofman A, Wolvius EB, Ongkosuwito EM. Secular trend of dental development in Dutch children. American Journal of Physical Anthropology 2014;155:91—8.

Watts R. Non-specific indicators of stress and their relationship to age-at-death in medieval York: using stature and vertebral canal neural size to examine the effects of stress occurring during different stages of development. International Journal of Osteoarchaeology 2011;21:568—76.

Watts R. Childhood development and adult longevity in an archaeological population from Barton-upon-Humber, Lincolnshire, England. International Journal of Paleopathology 2013;3:95—104.

Watts R. The long-term impact of developmental stress. Evidence from later medieval and post-medieval London (AD1117—1853). American Journal of Physical Anthropology 2015;158:569—80.

Wilson RJ, Herrmann NP, Jantz LM. Evaluation of stature estimation from the database for forensic anthropology. Journal of Forensic Sciences 2010;55:684—9.

Wood JW, Milner GR, Harpending HC, Weiss KM. The osteological paradox. Problems of inferring prehistoric health from skeletal samples. Current Anthropology 1992;33:343—70.

Worthen C, Flinn M, Leone D, Quinlan R, England B. Parasite load, growth, fluctuating asymmetry, and stress hormone profiles among children in a rural Caribbean village. American Journal of Physical Anthropology 2001;(Suppl. 32):167.

Wright LE, Vásquez MA. Estimating the length of incomplete long bones: forensic standards from Guatemala. American Journal of Physical Anthropology 2003;120:233—51.

Zakrzewski SR. Variation in ancient Egyptian stature and body proportions. American Journal of Physical Anthropology 2003;121:219—29.

APPENDICES

Appendix 6.I: Postcranial Measurements

This appendix presents representative postcranial bone dimensions that can be measured in the axial and appendicular skeleton. More detailed measurements can be obtained depending on the type of questions one wishes to answer. Most descriptions here follow the guidelines of Martin (1928), as well as Moore-Jansen and Jantz (1989), reproduced in Buikstra and Ubelaker (1994).

The measurements described here refer to adult remains. For adolescents, the same measurements may be used provided that the secondary ossification centers have fused with the primary ones. For younger individuals, most of the following measurements may be obtained, excluding the secondary ossification centers, as long as the necessary landmarks can be identified. Note that, Fazekas and Kosá (1978) present a series of measurements for juvenile bones, reproduced

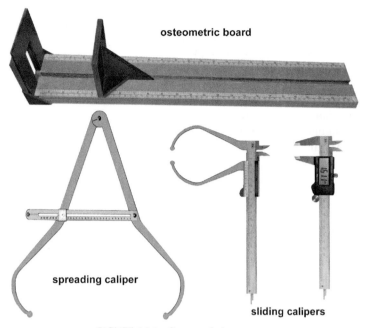

FIGURE 6.I.1 Osteometric instruments.

in Buikstra and Ubelaker (1994). Representative osteometric instruments used for obtaining these measurements are shown in Fig. 6.I.1.

Sternum (Fig. 6.I.2)

1. Manubrial length (#2, Martin, 1928, p. 1004)
2. Length of the corpus sterni (#3, Martin, 1928, p. 1004)
3. Maximum manubrial breadth (#4, Martin, 1928, p. 1004)
4. Minimum manubrial breadth (#6, Martin, 1928, p. 1004)
5. Maximum breadth of corpus sterni (#5, Martin, 1928, p. 1004)
6. Total manubrium−sternal length (#1, Martin, 1928, p. 1004)

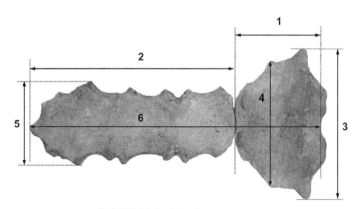

FIGURE 6.I.2 Sternal measurements.

Vertebrae (Fig. 6.I.3)

1. Superior dorsoventral body diameter (#4, Martin, 1928, p. 999)
2. Superior transverse body diameter (#7, Martin, 1928, p. 999)
3. Vertebral canal length (#10, Martin, 1928, p. 1000)
4. Vertebral canal breadth (#11, Martin, 1928, p. 1000)
5. Inferior transverse body diameter (#8, Martin, 1928, pp. 999–1000)
6. Inferior dorsoventral body diameter (#5, Martin, 1928, p. 999)
7. Ventral body height (#1, Martin, 1928, p. 998)
8. Total height of axis (#1a, Martin, 1928, p. 998)

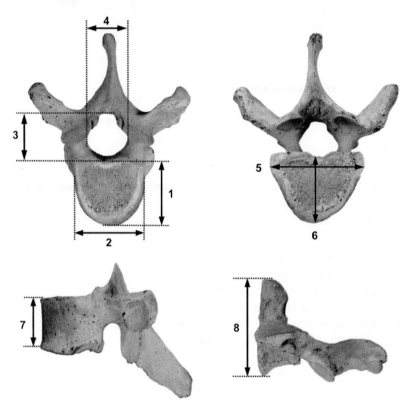

FIGURE 6.I.3 Vertebral measurements.

Sacrum (Fig. 6.I.4)

1. Maximum anterior breadth (#5, Martin, 1928, p. 1001)
2. Breadth at inferior sacral foramina (#10, Martin, 1928, p. 1001)
3. Middle breadth (#9, Martin, 1928, p. 1001)
4. Maximum anterior height (#2, Martin, 1928, p. 1001; #53, Moore-Jansen and Jantz, 1989, p. 76)
5. Auricular surface height (#14, Martin, 1928, p. 1002)
6. Auricular surface breadth (#15, Martin, 1928, p. 1002)
7. Anterosuperior breadth (#4, Martin, 1928, p. 1001; #54, Moore-Jansen and Jantz, 1989, p. 76)
8. Maximum transverse base diameter (#19, Martin, 1928, p. 1002; #55, Moore-Jansen and Jantz, 1989, p. 76)
9. Sagittal base diameter (#18, Martin, 1928, p. 1002)

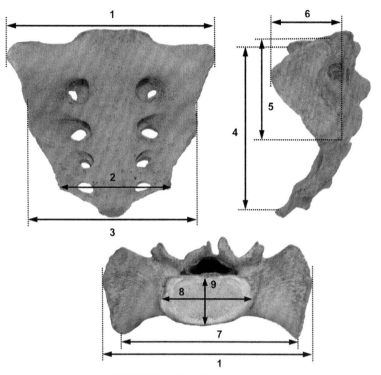

FIGURE 6.I.4   Sacral measurements.

Clavicle (Fig. 6.I.5)

1. Maximum length (#1, Martin, 1928, p. 1005; #35, Moore-Jansen and Jantz, 1989, p. 70)
2. Midshaft circumference (#6, Martin, 1928, p. 1006)
3. Superoinferior (vertical) midshaft diameter (#4, Martin, 1928, p. 1006; #37, Moore-Jansen and Jantz, 1989, p. 70)
4. Anteroposterior (sagittal) midshaft diameter (#5, Martin, 1928, p. 1006; #36, Moore-Jansen and Jantz, 1989, p. 70)

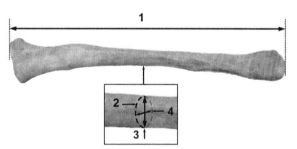

FIGURE 6.I.5   Clavicular measurements.

Scapula (Fig. 6.I.6)

1. Height (maximum length) (#1, Martin, 1928, p. 1006; #38, Moore-Jansen and Jantz, 1989, p. 71)
2. Breadth (#2, Martin, 1928, p. 1006; #39, Moore-Jansen and Jantz, 1989, p. 71)
3. Spine length (#7, Martin, 1928, p. 1008)
4. Axillary border length (#3, Martin, 1928, p. 1008)
5. Cranial border length (or infraspinous line length) (#5a, Martin, 1928, p. 1008)
6. Supraspinous line length (#6a, Martin, 1928, p. 1008)
7. Maximum glenoid fossa length (#12, Martin, 1928, p. 1008)
8. Maximum glenoid fossa breadth (#13, Martin, 1928, p. 1008)

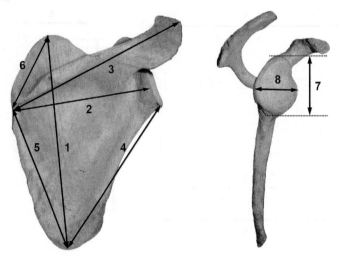

FIGURE 6.1.6 Scapular measurements.

Humerus (Figs. 6.1.7–6.1.9)

1. Maximum length (#1, Martin, 1928, p. 1010; #40, Moore-Jansen and Jantz, 1989, p. 72)
2. Total length or biomechanical length (#2, Martin, 1928, p. 1010)
3. Midshaft circumference (#7a, Martin, 1928, p. 1011)
4. Maximum midshaft diameter (#5, Martin, 1928, p. 1011; #43, Moore-Jansen and Jantz, 1989, p. 73)
5. Minimum midshaft diameter (#6, Martin, 1928, p. 1011; #44, Moore-Jansen and Jantz, 1989, p. 73)
6. Vertical head diameter (#10, Martin, 1928, p. 1011; #42, Moore-Jansen and Jantz, 1989, p. 72)
7. Proximal transverse diameter (#3, Martin, 1928, p. 1010)
8. Anteroposterior head diameter (#9, Martin, 1928, p. 1011)
9. Epicondylar breadth (#4, Martin, 1928, pp. 1010–1011; #41, Moore-Jansen and Jantz, 1989, p. 72)
10. Distal articular breadth (#12a, Martin, 1928, p. 1012)
11. Olecranon fossa breadth (#14, Martin, 1928, p. 1012)
12. Minimum trochlear breadth (#13, Martin, 1928, p. 1012)

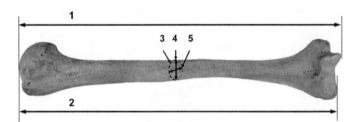

FIGURE 6.1.7 Humeral measurements.

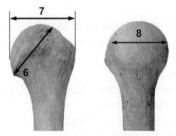

FIGURE 6.1.8 Humeral measurements.

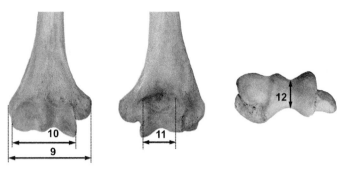

FIGURE 6.I.9 Humeral measurements.

Ulna (Figs. 6.I.10 and 6.I.11)

1. Maximum length (#1, Martin, 1928, p. 1017; #48, Moore-Jansen and Jantz, 1989, p. 74)
2. Physiological length (#2, Martin, 1928, p. 1018; #51, Moore-Jansen and Jantz, 1989, p. 75)
3. Minimum circumference (#3, Martin, 1928, p. 1018; #52, Moore-Jansen and Jantz, 1989, p. 75)
4. Maximum anteroposterior (dorsovolar) diameter (#11, Martin, 1928, p. 1020; #49, Moore-Jansen and Jantz, 1989, p. 75)
5. Mediolateral (transverse) diameter, perpendicular to #4 (#12, Martin, 1928, p. 1020; #50, Moore-Jansen and Jantz, 1989, p. 75)
6. Olecranon anteroposterior diameter (#7, Martin, 1928, p. 1019)
7. Olecranon—coronoid process distance (#7(1), Martin 1928, p. 1019)

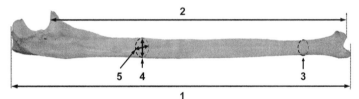

FIGURE 6.I.10 Ulnar measurements.

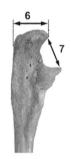

FIGURE 6.I.11 Ulnar measurements.

Radius (Fig. 6.I.12)

1. Maximum length (#1, Martin, 1928, p. 1014; #45, Moore-Jansen and Jantz, 1989, p. 73)
2. Midshaft circumference (#5(5), Martin 1928, p. 1015)
3. Mediolateral (transverse) midshaft diameter (#4a, Martin, 1928, p. 1015; #47, Moore-Jansen and Jantz, 1989, p. 74)
4. Anteroposterior (sagittal) midshaft diameter (#5a, Martin, 1928, p. 1015; #46, Moore-Jansen and Jantz, 1989, p. 74)
5. Minimum circumference (#3, Martin, 1928, p. 1015)

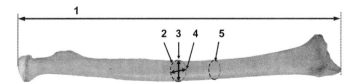

Os Coxa (Fig. 6.I.13)

1. Height (maximum length) (#1, Martin, 1928, p. 1031; #56, Moore-Jansen and Jantz, 1989, p. 77)
2. Iliac breadth (maximum breadth) (#12, Martin, 1928, p. 1033; #57, Moore-Jansen and Jantz, 1989, p. 77)
3. Iliac length (#9, Martin, 1928, p. 1032)
4. Acetabular height (#22, Martin, 1928, p. 1033)
5. Ischial length (#16, Martin, 1928, p. 1033; #59, Moore-Jansen and Jantz, 1989, p. 78)
6. Pubic length (#17, Martin, 1928, p. 1033; #58, Moore-Jansen and Jantz, 1989, p. 77)
7. Obturator foramen length (#20, Martin, 1928, p. 1033)
8. Obturator foramen breadth (#21, Martin, 1928, p. 1033)

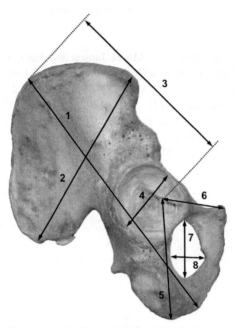

FIGURE 6.I.13 Os coxal measurements. *Note*: The point within the acetabum used for obtaining measurements #3, 5 and 6 marks the intersection of ilium, pubis, and ischium.

Femur (Figs. 6.I.14—6.I.16)

1. Maximum length (#1, Martin, 1928, p. 1037; #60, Moore-Jansen and Jantz, 1989, p. 78)
2. Subtrochanteric mediolateral (transverse) diameter (#9, Martin, 1928, p. 1040; #65, Moore-Jansen and Jantz, 1989, p. 80)
3. Subtrochanteric anteroposterior (sagittal) diameter (#10, Martin, 1928, p. 1040; #64, Moore-Jansen and Jantz, 1989, p. 79)
4. Midshaft circumference (#8, Martin, 1928, p. 1040; #68, Moore-Jansen and Jantz, 1989, p. 80)
5. Mediolateral (transverse) midshaft diameter (#7, Martin, 1928, p. 1039; #67, Moore-Jansen and Jantz, 1989, p. 80)

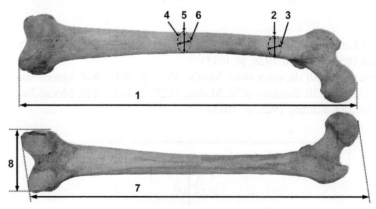

FIGURE 6.I.14 Femoral measurements.

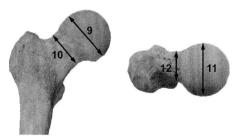

FIGURE 6.I.15 Femoral measurements.

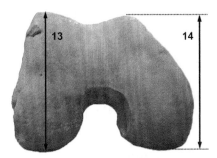

FIGURE 6.I.16 Femoral measurements.

6. Anteroposterior (sagittal) midshaft diameter (#6, Martin, 1928, p. 1039; #66, Moore-Jansen and Jantz, 1989, p. 80)
7. Physiological (bicondylar or oblique) length (#2, Martin, 1928, pp. 1037−1038; #61, Moore-Jansen and Jantz, 1989, p. 79)
8. Epicondylar breadth (#21, Martin, 1928, p. 1041; #62, Moore-Jansen and Jantz, 1989, p. 79)
9. Vertical head diameter (#18, Martin, 1928, p. 1041)
10. Superoinferior neck diameter (#15, Martin, 1928, p. 1041)
11. Transverse head diameter (#19, Martin, 1928, p. 1041)
12. Anteroposterior neck diameter (#16, Martin, 1928, p. 1041)
13. Anteroposterior lateral condyle diameter (#23, Martin, 1928, p. 1042)
14. Anteroposterior medial condyle diameter (#24, Martin, 1928, p. 1042)

Tibia (Figs. 6.I.17 and 6.I.18)

1. Maximum length (#1a, Martin, 1928, p. 1049)
2. Maximum morphological length (or total length) (#1, Martin, 1928, pp. 1048−1049; #69, Moore-Jansen and Jantz, 1989, p. 81)
3. Biomechanical length (#2, Martin, 1928, p. 1049)
4. Midshaft circumference (#10, Martin, 1928, p. 1050)
5. Mediolateral midshaft diameter (#9, Martin, 1928, p. 1050)
6. Anteroposterior midshaft diameter (#8, Martin, 1928, p. 1050)
7. Circumference at nutrient foramen (#10a, Martin, 1928, p. 1050; #74, Moore-Jansen and Jantz, 1989, p. 82)

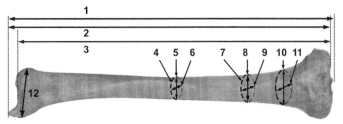

FIGURE 6.I.17 Tibial measurements.

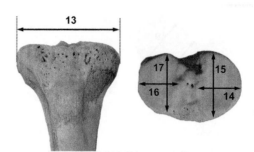

FIGURE 6.I.18 Tibial measurements.

8. Mediolateral (transverse) diameter at nutrient foramen (#9a, Martin, 1928, p. 1050; #73, Moore-Jansen and Jantz, 1989, p. 82)
9. Anteroposterior diameter at nutrient foramen (#8a, Martin, 1928, p. 1050)
10. Mediolateral diameter at tuberosity (#5, Martin, 1928, p. 1049)
11. Anteroposterior diameter at tuberosity (#4, Martin, 1928, p. 1049)
12. Maximum distal epiphyseal breadth (#6, Martin, 1928, p. 1049; #71, Moore-Jansen and Jantz, 1989, p. 81)
13. Maximum proximal epiphyseal breadth (#3, Martin, 1928, p. 1049; #70, Moore-Jansen and Jantz, 1989, p. 81)
14. Medial condyle breadth (#3a, Martin, 1928, p. 1049)
15. Medial condyle depth (#4a, Martin, 1928, p. 1049)
16. Lateral condyle breadth (#3b, Martin, 1928, p. 1049)
17. Lateral condyle depth (#4b, Martin, 1928, p. 1049)

Fibula (Fig. 6.I.19)

1. Maximum length (#1, Martin, 1928, p. 1052; #75, Moore-Jansen and Jantz, 1989, p. 82)
2. Midshaft circumference (#4, Martin, 1928, p. 1053)
3. Maximum midshaft diameter (#2, Martin, 1928, p. 1052; #76, Moore-Jansen and Jantz, 1989, p. 83)
4. Minimum midshaft diameter (#3, Martin, 1928, p. 1053)

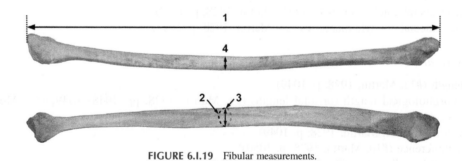

FIGURE 6.I.19 Fibular measurements.

Appendix 6.II: Recording Postcranial Metrics in Osteoware

The Postcranial Metrics module in Osteoware allows the input of postcranial metrics for adults, as well as cranial and postcranial metrics for subadults (Mulhern, 2011). When one clicks on the "Postcranial Metrics" button, a window pops up, wherein the user should select whether the input measurements will be for immature or adult remains, depending upon whether the epiphyses have fused with the diaphysis or not.

When one selects the "Adult" option and clicks on "Go," the Data Entry window shown in Fig. 6.II.1 appears. It can be seen that adult metrics are input in three different tabs, one for the clavicle, scapula, humerus, and radius; another one for the ulna, sacrum, innominate, and femur; and a last one for the tibia, fibula, and calcaneus. By default, left-side measurements are input first; however, by clicking on the "Other side" button, right-side measurements can be input. Most

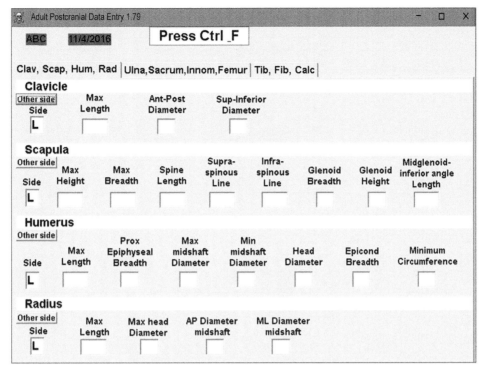

FIGURE 6.II.1   Part of the data entry screen for clavicular, scapular, humeral, and radial adult measurements.

measurements that may be recorded using Osteoware have already been described in Appendix 6.I and the reader can find figures depicting all of them in Mulhern (2011).

When the immature data entry selection is made, both cranial and postcranial measurements can be input in three tabs: one for cranial data, another one for the upper body and the pelvis, and a final one for the lower body (Fig. 6.II.2). Note that the cranial measurements are appropriate only for fetuses and infants and have been obtained from Buikstra and Ubelaker (1994). Postcranial measurements can generally be used for subadults of any age provided that the epiphyses have not yet fused to the diaphysis; however, iliac and ischial width should be measured only in individuals younger than 1 year of age.

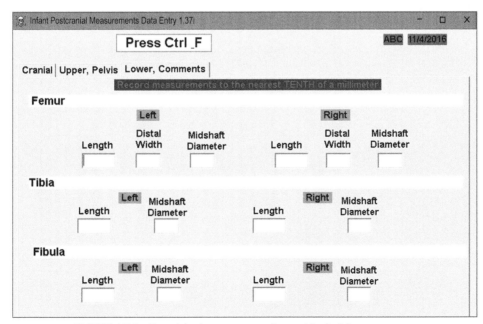

FIGURE 6.II.2   Part of the data entry screen for cranial subadult measurements.

measurements that may be recorded using Osteoware have already been described in Appendix 6.2 and the reader can find approx depictions all of them in Multhern (2011).

When the immature data entry selection is made, both cranial and postcranial measurements can be input in three tabs: one for cranial only, another one for the upper body and the pelvis, and a final one for the lower body (Fig. 6.11.2). Note that the cranial measurements are appropriate only for femora and tibiae and have been obtained from Buitstra and Ubelaker (1994). Postcranial measurements can generally be used for subadults of any age provided that the epiphyses have not yet fused to the diaphysis; however, tibial and ischial width should be measured only in individuals younger than 1 year of age.

Chapter 7

Activity Patterns

Chapter Outline

Chapter Objectives

By the end of this chapter, the reader will be able to:

- understand the properties of living bone that allow the skeleton to reflect past activity patterns;
- record entheseal changes on the long bones of the upper and lower limbs;
- calculate cross-sectional geometric properties of long-bone diaphyses;
- record dental wear in an ordinal and continuous manner;
- determine which statistical tests should be adopted to explore activity patterns at intra- and interpopulation levels; and
- understand the limitations of currently available methods.

Assessment of the activity patterns of an individual based on his or her skeletal remains is based on the fact that bone, as a living tissue, can adapt its form depending on the mechanical loads imposed on it, whereas teeth provide a permanent record of the dietary habits of individuals as well as of extramasticatory activities that involved the mouth. As such, the study of human skeletal remains may provide insights into the social status of individuals and, more importantly, allow intra- and interpopulation comparisons regarding subsistence patterns and overall life quality. Note that activity markers are primarily of use in osteoarchaeological studies; however, in a forensic context, they could assist to some extent in the identification of an unknown individual (Klepinger, 2006). This chapter presents the main methods used for the study of activity patterns from skeletal remains, namely, entheseal changes, cross-sectional geometric properties, and dental wear. Note that osteoarthritis is also a potentially useful activity marker, but this is briefly discussed in Chapter 8.

7.1 ENTHESEAL CHANGES

7.1.1 Anatomical Information

Each muscle attaches on the bones at two sites, the *insertion* and the *origin*. The origin typically lies proximally and is rather stable during muscle contraction, whereas the insertion lies distally and is more movable during contraction. The site where the muscles connect with the bone via ligaments or tendons is called *enthesis*. Figs. 7.1.1−7.1.7[1] outline the

---

1. In Figs. 7.1.1−7.1.7 muscle origins are given in green and muscle insertions in blue. For additional entheses, see White et al. (2011).

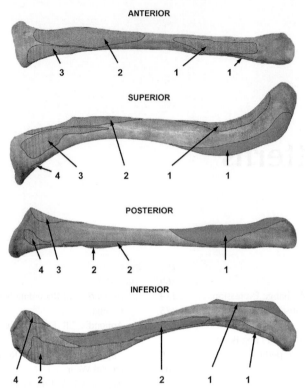

ANTERIOR

SUPERIOR

POSTERIOR

INFERIOR

FIGURE 7.1.1 Clavicular entheses. Origins: *1* = deltoideus, *2* = pectoralis major, *3* = sternocleidomastoideus, *4* = sternohyoid. Insertions: *1* = trapezius, *2* = subclavius. *Based on White TD, Black MT, Folkens PA. Human osteology. 3rd ed. San Diego: Academic Press; 2011.*

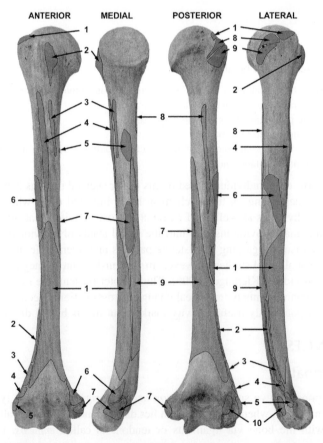

ANTERIOR   MEDIAL   POSTERIOR   LATERAL

FIGURE 7.1.2 Humeral entheses. Origins: *1* = brachialis, *2* = brachioradialis, *3* = extensor carpi radialis longus, *4* = extensor carpi radialis brevis, *5* = common origin of extensors, *6* = pronator teres, *7* = common origin of flexors, *8* = triceps brachii (lateral head), *9* = triceps brachii (medial head), *10* = anconeus. Insertions: *1* = supraspinatus, *2* = subscapularis, *3* = latissimus dorsi, *4* = pectoralis major, *5* = teres major, *6* = deltoideus,

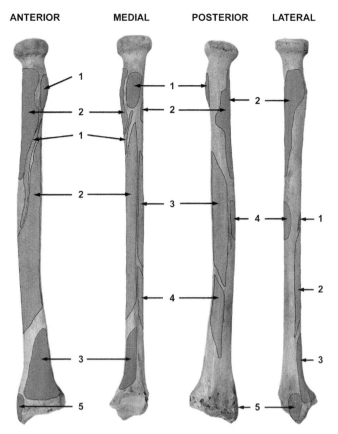

FIGURE 7.1.3 Radial entheses. Origins: *1* = flexor digitorum superficialis, *2* = flexor pollicis longus, *3* = abductor pollicis longus, *4* = extensor pollicis brevis. Insertions: *1* = biceps brachii, *2* = supinator, *3* = pronator quadratus, *4* = pronator teres, *5* = brachioradialis. *Based on White TD, Black MT, Folkens PA. Human osteology. 3rd ed. San Diego: Academic Press; 2011.*

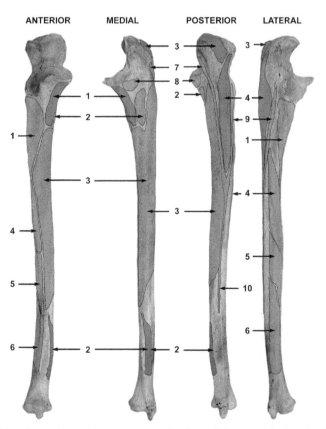

FIGURE 7.1.4 Ulnar entheses. Origins: *1* = supinator, *2* = pronator teres, *3* = flexor digitorum profundus, *4* = abductor pollicis longus, *5* = extensor

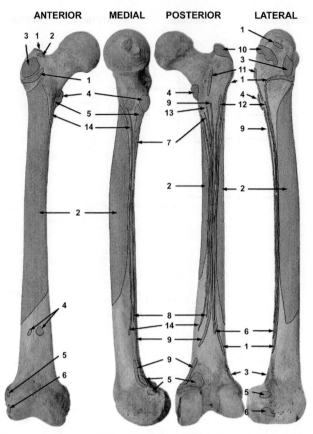

FIGURE 7.1.5 Femoral entheses. Origins: *1* = vastus medialis, *2* = vastus lateralis, *3* = vastus intermedius, *4* = articularis genu, *5* = plantaris, *6* = gastrocnemius. Insertions: *1* = piriformis, *2* = oburator internus and gemelli, *3* = gluteus minimus, *4* = psoas major, *5* = iliacus, *6* = popliteus, *7* = pectineus, *8* = adductor magnus, *9* = biceps femoris, *10* = gluteus medius, *11* = quadratus femoris, *12* = gluteus maximus, *13* = adductor longus, *14* = adductor brevis. *Based on White TD, Black MT, Folkens PA. Human osteology. 3rd ed. San Diego: Academic Press; 2011.*

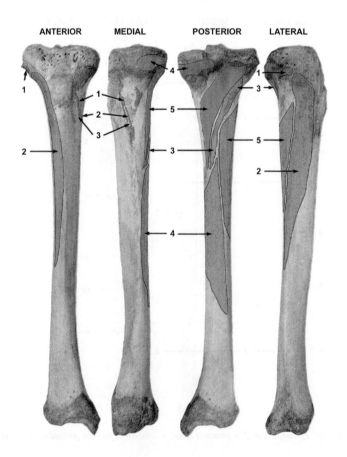

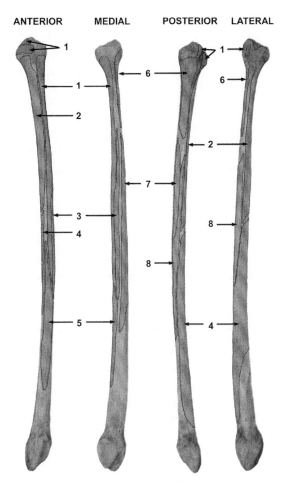

ANTERIOR   MEDIAL   POSTERIOR   LATERAL

FIGURE 7.1.7   Fibular entheses. Origins: *1* = extensor digitorum longus, *2* = fibularis longus, *3* = extensor hallucis longus, *4* = fibularis brevis, *5* = fibularis tertius, *6* = soleus, *7* = tibialis posterior, *8* = flexor hallucis longus. Insertions: *1* = biceps femoris. *Based on White TD, Black MT, Folkens PA. Human osteology. 3rd ed. San Diego: Academic Press; 2011.*

locations of indicative entheses on the long bones. When there is increased mechanical loading applied on the entheses during muscle activity, the skeleton responds by new bone formation, bone resorption, or a combination of the two. Fig. 7.1.8 presents the formation of new osseous tissue on entheses in the proximal tibia and radius.

Several terms have been proposed to describe the osseous changes observed in entheses, such as enthesopathies (e.g., Crubézy et al., 2002; Mariotti et al., 2004), musculoskeletal stress markers (Hawkey and Merbs, 1995), occupational stress markers (Kennedy, 1989), and others. The term *enthesopathy* implies a modification of pathological nature, whereas the terms *musculoskeletal stress markers* and *occupational stress markers* imply that the causative factor of the morphological changes seen in entheses is activity. As discussed in the following sections, alterations occurring on the entheses are multifactorial in etiology, thus in this chapter the more generic term *entheseal changes* (ECs) will be employed, as recommended by Jurmain and Villotte (2010).

Entheses belong to two different categories depending on the type of tissue at the attachment site, *fibrous* or *fibro-cartilaginous* (Benjamin et al., 2006) (Table 7.1.1). Fibrous entheses are mostly located on long-bone diaphyses, where there is a large attachment surface and the soft tissue does not move substantially during muscle usage. Fibrocartilaginous entheses are found near the epiphyseal articular surfaces of the long bones as well as on flat, short, and irregular bones; they have a small attachment area and exhibit substantial mobility of the soft tissue during joint usage.

In fibrous entheses the soft tissues (tendons or ligaments) attach to the bone through collagen fibers directly or via a layer of periosteum. In contrast, fibrocartilaginous entheses are composed of four histological zones: (1) tendon or ligament, (2) uncalcified fibrocartilage, (3) calcified fibrocartilage, and (4) subchondral bone. Between zones (2) and (3) lies the so-called *tidemark*, a regular calcification front (Benjamin et al., 1986, 2002). Note that the aforementioned structure

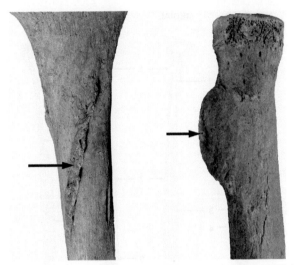

FIGURE 7.1.8 Entheseal changes on the soleus (proximal posterior tibia, left) and biceps brachii (proximal anterior radius, right).

TABLE 7.1.1 Selected Fibrocartilaginous and Fibrous Entheses on the Long Bones

Location		Enthesis
		Fibrocartilaginous
Upper limbs	Humerus	**Origins:** Common origin of extensors, common origin of flexors **Insertions:** Supraspinatus, subscapularis, infraspinatus, teres minor
	Radius	**Insertions:** Biceps brachii, brachioradialis
	Ulna	**Insertions:** Brachialis, triceps brachii
Lower limbs	Femur	**Origins:** Gastrocnemius **Insertions:** Gluteus minimus, psoas major, iliacus, popliteus, gluteus medius
		Fibrous
Upper limbs	Humerus	**Origins:** Triceps brachii (lateral head) **Insertions:** Latissimus dorsi, pectoralis major, teres major, deltoideus
	Radius	**Insertions:** Pronator quadratus, pronator teres, supinator
Lower limbs	Femur	**Origins:** Vastus medialis, vastus lateralis **Insertions:** Gluteus maximus, adductor magnus
	Tibia	**Origins:** Soleus

From Benjamin M, Toumi H, Suzuki D, Redman S, Emery P, McGonagle D. Microdamage and altered vascularity at the enthesis-bone interface provides an anatomic explanation for bone involvement in the HLA-B27-associated spondylarthritides and allied disorders. Arthritis and Rheumatism 2007;56:224–33; Davis CB, Shuler KA, Danforth ME, Herndon KE. Patterns of interobserver error in the scoring of entheseal changes. International Journal of Osteoarchaeology 2013;23:147–51; Lieverse AR, Bazaliiskii VI, Goriunova OI, Weber AW. Lower limb activity in the Cis-Baikal: entheseal changes among Middle Holocene Siberian foragers. American Journal of Physical Anthropology 2013;150:421–32; and Villotte S, Castex D, Couallier V, Dutour O, Knüsel CJ, Henry-Gambier D. Enthesopathies as occupational stress markers: evidence from the upper limb. American Journal of Physical Anthropology 2010a;142:224–34.

characterizes the innermost part of fibrocartilaginous entheses, whereas the periphery shows less fibrocartilage and the collagen fibers of the tendons and ligaments attach directly to the periosteum (Benjamin et al., 1986; Villotte, 2012).

7.1.2 Factors Affecting Entheseal Change Expression

ECs are multifactorial in etiology, as their expression is affected by mechanical loading, age, body size, sex, diet, and metabolic, genetic, and pathological factors (especially diffuse idiopathic skeletal hyperostosis, seronegative spondyloarthropathies, and other bone-forming diseases) (Benjamin and McGonagle, 2001; Jurmain et al., 2011; Milella et al., 2012; Niinimäki, 2011; Niinimäki and Sotos, 2013; Weiss, 2003, 2004; Weiss et al., 2012; Wilczak, 1998). Regarding the factors other than mechanical loading, several studies have supported that the primary factor affecting ECs is age (see

Alves Cardoso and Henderson, 2010; Milella et al., 2012; Nagy, 1998; Niinimäki, 2011; Weiss, 2003, 2004, 2007). Entheseal morphology changes gradually with time until the age of 40–50 years (Robb, 1998) or 60 years (Shaibani et al., 1993). The observed age changes may be the result of cumulative activity patterns or the outcome of tissue degeneration occurring with increasing age. Moreover, entheseal morphology differs between males and females. Although this differentiation may be attributed to sexual division of labor, and thus be indicative of daily activity patterns, it has also been linked to the different weights and sizes (Weiss, 2003, 2004, 2007), as well as hormonal differences, between the two sexes (Niinimäki, 2011; Wilczak, 1998). Finally, body size affects ECs because bigger individuals exhibit more pronounced changes (Niinimäki, 2011; Weiss, 2003, 2004, 2007). This may be explained by the fact that individuals with greater body size require more effort for movement.

With respect to the use of ECs as activity indicators, when the entheses are subjected to mechanical loading, for instance, because of increased muscular activity, blood circulation increases and osteoblastic activity is activated so there is bone hypertrophy at the attachment site (e.g., Parfitt, 2004). As such, the morphology of the entheseal sites has the potential to offer information about the intensity of past activities, despite the nonoccupational factors that affect EC morphology outlined above. Although reservations have been expressed regarding the validity of ECs as activity markers (e.g., Alves Cardoso and Henderson, 2010; Djukic et al., 2015; Jurmain et al., 2011; Milella et al., 2012), the correlation between ECs and daily activities has been confirmed by kinematic, ergonomic, and electromyographic studies (Kuorinka and Forcier, 1995); sports medicine studies (Shaw and Benjamin, 2007); and studies in documented osteological collections (Niinimäki, 2012; Villotte et al., 2010a; Yonemoto, 2016). For this reason, several researchers study ECs as a means of examining the levels of activity of past groups at inter- and intrapopulation levels (e.g., Eshed et al., 2004; Havelková et al., 2011; Lieverse et al., 2009; Niinimäki, 2011; Villotte et al., 2010a,b).

An important development, which generated renewed interest in the study of ECs as activity indicators, has been the acknowledgment that entheses can be anatomically distinguished as fibrous or fibrocartilaginous, as mentioned earlier (Benjamin and McGonagle, 2001; Benjamin et al., 2002). Studies on samples of known sex, age, and occupational status, as well as on archaeological material, found that fibrocartilaginous entheses correlate more strongly with activity patterns than fibrous ones, particularly in individuals younger than 50 years of age (Havelková et al., 2011; Villotte et al., 2010a,b; Weiss, 2015). This result has been corroborated by scholars who found that excessive mechanical stress can affect the fibrocartilaginous tissue structure, especially the tidemark (Benjamin et al., 2006). This may be attributed to the fact that in fibrocartilaginous entheses mechanical loading produces localized changes at the tidemark, whereas in fibrous entheses mechanical loading is dispersed across the bone surface (Benjamin et al., 2002). Differences between trabecular and cortical bone modeling and remodeling rates may also be important, as muscles in fibrocartilaginous entheses are most often attached to trabecular bone via tendons, while muscles in fibrous entheses attach directly to cortical bone (Benjamin et al., 2002). These findings indicate that variability in the changes observed in some fibrocartilaginous entheses can offer useful information on activity-induced changes when appropriately studied (e.g., controlling for age, sex, and body size).

7.1.3 Recording Schemes and Statistical Analysis

Many researchers have examined the most efficient way to record ECs. Some propose ordinal schemes and others opt for simple presence/absence (see Appendix 7.I for a presentation of various recording protocols). More recently, it has become clear that it is not that straightforward to define what *normal* and *altered* entheses look like; thus it is very difficult to establish appropriate recording methods (see discussion in Villotte and Knüsel, 2013). Specifically, in a healthy fibrocartilaginous enthesis the tidemark is "a smooth, well-defined imprint on the bone, without vascular foramina, and with a regular margin" (Villotte et al., 2010a, p. 226). However, this definition is not valid for all fibrocartilaginous entheses (Villotte and Knüsel, 2013). Moreover, the definition of a healthy fibrous enthesis is very difficult because of a lack of clinical and anatomical data (Alves Cardoso and Henderson, 2010; Villotte, 2006). Also, fibrous entheses are characterized by rather coarse surfaces even when the individual is very young (Villotte, 2009). Therefore, it appears that the changes observed in each type of enthesis are not suggestive of the same underlying mechanisms.

A 2015 study by Michopoulou et al. (2015) tested the correlation between ECs recorded using binary and ordinal schemes and activity patterns deduced by means of archival data and long-bone cross-sectional geometric properties (see Section 7.2). The authors did not find a systematic correlation between ECs and activity when controlling for the effects of age and body mass. However, they identified that age and body mass appeared to affect right- and left-sided elements differently, which was interpreted as suggestive of an underlying activity effect. The authors concluded that activity patterns must affect ECs and highlighted the need for more refined recording protocols.

When entheses are recorded as binary dichotomies (present/absent), they can be statistically analyzed by means of χ^2 test/Fisher's exact test (see Section 9.6). When using ordinal scales, the Wilcoxon test can be used to ascertain whether side dominance exists, whereas the Mann–Whitney test can be adopted to evaluate differences between males and females, and Kruskal–Wallis test for interpopulation comparisons. These tests are described in Sections 9.4 and 9.5. In addition to these traditional statistical tests, Villotte et al. (2010a) and Nikita (2014) proposed the use of generalized linear models (GLM) and generalized estimating equations (GEE), which are types of regression analyses, but without presupposing that all variables are continuous. These analyses have the advantage that they can take into account multiple variables simultaneously and test the impact of each variable while controlling for the effects of the remaining ones. Section 9.7.7, Case Study 16, demonstrates in practice the use of GLM and GEE for the analysis of EC data, whereas the macro Data-Creation_EC, provided in the companion website, can be used to generate artificial data sets that simulate EC data.

7.2 LONG-BONE CROSS-SECTIONAL GEOMETRIC PROPERTIES

7.2.1 Impact of Mechanical Loading on Long-Bone Cross-Sectional Geometric Properties

Physical activity affects the cross-sectional geometry (CSG) of long-bone diaphyses given that the skeleton, as a living tissue, deposits new bone along the axes that are subjected to increased mechanical stress (Ruff et al., 2006). On the other hand, prolonged immobilization, and subsequent reduction in the mechanical loading applied on the skeleton, decreases the rate of bone remodeling and makes the skeleton more fragile (Giangregorio and Blimkie, 2002; Schlecht et al., 2012). The concept that bone structure adapts to mechanical loading is often referred to as *Wolff's law* (Wolff, 1892). However, Wolff's law has limitations reviewed in Bertram and Swartz (1991), and a more appropriate term to describe the aforementioned process is *bone functional adaptation* (Ruff et al., 2006).

Biomechanics, the application of mechanical principles to biological systems, can contribute to the assessment of mechanical loading on the bones (Ruff, 2008). The effect of physical activity on bone CSG properties may be explained by means of mechanostat theory and beam theory. According to the mechanostat theory (Frost, 1987), if mechanical loading reaches certain threshold values, bone mass is increased via bone remodeling. Note that the maintenance of healthy bone mass levels in adults depends upon the continued effects of normal mechanical loadings established earlier in development (Ferretti et al., 1998; Ruff et al., 2006). Based on beam theory, under mechanical stress, long-bone diaphyses behave similar to engineering beams (Huiskes, 1982); thus the overall shape of the cross section of a skeletal element plays an important role in determining bending and torsional rigidity (Lieberman et al., 2004; Ruff et al., 2006). The adaptation of bone structure is accomplished through the deposition and resorption of bone tissue so that mechanical integrity is maintained (Frost, 1964, 1988a,b; Skerry, 2006).

To examine these general principles in mathematical terms, we first need to have a clear understanding of the types of stress that may be applied on a human long bone. Bone is anisotropic, that is, it exhibits different material properties under different directions of loading (Currey, 2006). Fig. 7.2.1 visualizes the various forces that may be applied on bone, namely tension, compression, shear, torsion, bending, or a combination of these. Note that a tensile force produces narrowing and elongation, whereas a compressive one has the opposite effect, causing shortening and extension; a shear force results in bone sliding failure along a plane parallel to the direction of the force; a torsional force causes angulation and, if excessive, spiral fractures, whereas a bending force generates all alterations produced in compression, tension, and shear.

In engineering, *stress*, σ, is the average force per unit area, i.e., the average force F acting normal to a cross-sectional area A of a specimen divided by A:

$$\sigma = F/A \tag{7.2.1}$$

Strain, ε, is the response of a system when stress is applied to it. It is defined as the extent of deformation, ΔL, in the direction of the applied force divided by the initial length, L, of the material (Fig. 7.2.2):

$$\varepsilon = \Delta L/L \tag{7.2.2}$$

For small deformations, *Hooke's law* applies:

$$\sigma = E\varepsilon \tag{7.2.3}$$

where E is the *elastic modulus* of the material. The range of deformations in which Hooke's law is valid is called the *elastic range*. The end of this range is the *elastic limit*, i.e., the limit beyond which the material will no longer return to its original shape when the load is removed. Beyond the elastic range lies the *plastic range*, where there is no linear relationship between σ and ε. If stress keeps being applied on the material, then the material breaks, a phenomenon known as *failure*

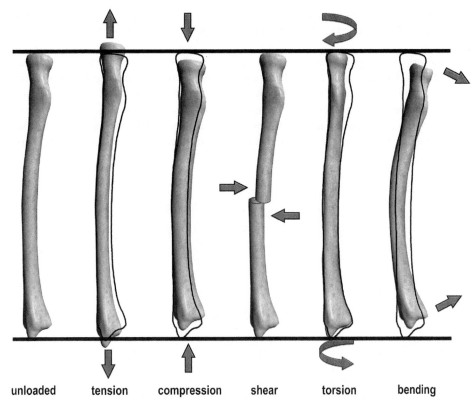

unloaded   tension   compression   shear   torsion   bending

FIGURE 7.2.1   Modes of loading on the radius. The solid outline of the bone indicates its original state.

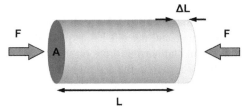

FIGURE 7.2.2   Definition of stress and strain.

(Fig. 7.2.3). Two important terms to note are *rigidity*, which expresses the resistance of an element to deformation prior to failure, and *strength*, which expresses the load required in order for the bone to fail (Ruff, 2008).

From Eqs. (7.2.1)−(7.2.3) it becomes clear that the cross-sectional area A of a skeletal element is a measure of the rigidity of this element. For the same material (in our case bone tissue), the bigger the surface area A, the smaller the stress,

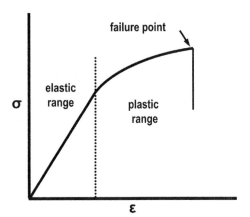

σ (Eq. (7.2.1)), and subsequently, the smaller the strain, ε (Eq. (7.2.3)), and, finally, the smaller the deformation, ΔL (Eq. (7.2.2)). As such, among the CSG properties that are studied in skeletal analyses is the total subperiosteal area (*TA*) (Ruff, 2008).

The aforementioned principles apply mainly to forces that result in tension, compression, or shear. The situation is different for bending forces. Consider that a long bone can be represented as a homogeneous cylinder and a tangential force (bending force) is applied to it, as in Fig. 7.2.4. We observe the following: The surface area that lies in the same direction as the bending force (inner surface) is in compression and decreases in size, whereas the surface area on the opposite side (outer surface) is in tension and increases in size. In Fig. 7.2.4 these areas are marked with − and +, respectively. In the interior of the beam, there is an area where neither compression nor tension is applied. This area is called the *neutral plane*.

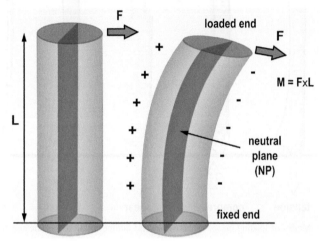

FIGURE 7.2.4 Simple bending of a cylinder due to tangential force *F*. *L*, length; *M*, bending moment.

Fig. 7.2.5 presents part of the longitudinal cross section of the bent beam of Fig. 7.2.4. Owing to the bending force, as mentioned, the right part of the beam has shrunk and the left has expanded. As a result, the bending force is creating compressive forces on the right part of the beam and tensile forces on the left. These forces are perpendicular to the cross section of the beam. The intensity of these forces is zero in the neutral plane and increases linearly with increasing distance from this plane. In Fig. 7.2.5 these forces are expressed as stress, σ, that is, their magnitude has been divided by the area of the cross section.

The bending stresses, σ, are subject to the *bending stress equation* or *flexure formula*:

$$\sigma = Mc/I \tag{7.2.4}$$

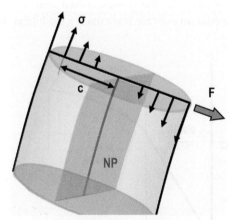

FIGURE 7.2.5 Longitudinal cross section of the bended beam of Fig. 7.2.4. *c*, distance from the neutral plane; *F*, tangential force; *NP*, trace of the neutral plane; σ, stress.

where M is the bending moment, i.e., the product $F \times L$; c is the distance from the neutral plane; and I is the *second moment of area*, also known as *moment of inertia of plane area, area moment of inertia,* or *second area moment.* This quantity is very important in anthropological studies because it is a measure of the bending rigidity of a long bone. Indeed, from Eq. (7.2.4) it is seen that the greater the value of I is, the smaller the bending stresses, and thus the more resistant the bone against bending deformations.

For the calculation of the second moment of area, we subdivide the cross-sectional area into a great number of subregions of area ΔA_i (Fig. 7.2.6) and then sum all ΔA_i values, each one multiplied by the square of its distance from the neutral axis, i.e., from the trace of the neutral plane on the cross section:

$$I = \sum_i y_i^2 \Delta A_i \qquad (7.2.5)$$

Thus, the strict mathematical definition of I is:

$$I = \iint_A y^2 dx dy \qquad (7.2.6)$$

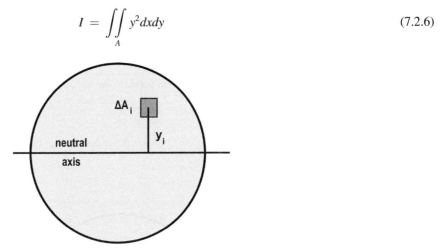

FIGURE 7.2.6 Calculation of the second moment of area. ΔA_i, area of subregions; y_i, distance from the neutral axis.

Note that a long bone is not a solid beam because its interior is occupied by a hollow cavity, the medullary cavity. Therefore, during the calculation of the second moment of area, the empty area in the cross section of the diaphysis should be taken into account; thus subregions of area ΔA_i should not lie in the hollow space of the medullary cavity (Fig. 7.2.7). However, it must be stressed that the effect of the medullary cavity on the calculation of I is rather small in bones. For example, if we assume a circular cross section with r_p and r_e periosteal and endosteal radii, respectively, then the second moment of area is given by:

$$I = \frac{1}{4}\pi\left(r_p^4 - r_e^4\right) \qquad (7.2.7)$$

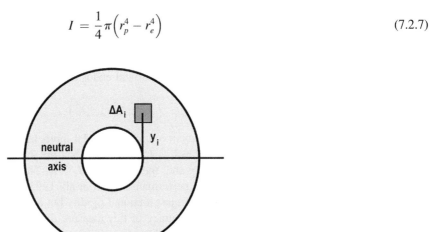

FIGURE 7.2.7 Calculation of the second moment of area in the presence of a hollow interior area. ΔA_i, area of subregions; y_i, distance from the neutral axis.

and because $r_p^4 \gg r_e^4$, the effect of the endosteal radius is small. For example, if $r_p = 1.5$ cm and $r_e = 0.7$ cm, then:

$$I = \frac{1}{4}\pi\left(1.5^4 - 0.7^4\right) = \frac{1}{4}\pi(5.06 - 0.24) = 3.79 \ \text{cm}^4 \tag{7.2.8}$$

If we ignore the existence of the medullary cavity, we obtain $I = 3.98$ cm^4, that is, an error of the order of 5%.

Because the cross section of human bones is not circular, we calculate various second moments of area. In particular, I_x expresses rigidity to anteroposteriorly imposed bending loads, whereas I_y expresses rigidity to loads applied on the mediolateral plane. In addition, the maximum (I_{max}) and minimum (I_{min}) second moments of area express maximum and minimum bending rigidity, respectively.

Often the second moments of area are not calculated to be used per se but to estimate the ratios I_x/I_y and I_{max}/I_{min}. These ratios reflect cross-sectional shape as they show the distribution of cortical bone with regard to different axes (Ruff, 2008 and references therein). The interpretation of these ratios is not always easy (Ruff and Larsen, 2001). I_{max}/I_{min} provides no information on the orientation of maximum/minimum bending rigidity, whereas I_x/I_y depends on the orientation of the diaphysis during data collection (Shaw and Stock, 2009a; Stock and Pfeiffer, 2001). If the preservation of the skeletal material is fair, the anteroposterior and mediolateral axes can be identified with certainty during the orientation of the diaphysis, so the aforementioned restrictions do not apply. However, it is generally preferable to calculate both indexes as they provide different information (Ruff, 2008).

For the study of the rigidity of a long bone against torsion, the second moment of area should be replaced by the *polar moment of area*, J, which is calculated using Eq. (7.2.5) if the distance y_i from the neutral axis is replaced by the distance r_i from the center of rotation (Fig. 7.2.8):

$$J = \sum_i r_i^2 \Delta A_i \tag{7.2.9}$$

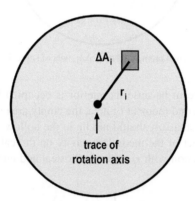

FIGURE 7.2.8 Calculation of the polar moment of area. ΔA_i, area of subregions; r_i, distance from the center of rotation.

For a circular cross section with r_p and r_e periosteal and endosteal radii, the polar moment of area is given by:

$$J = \frac{1}{2}\pi\left(r_p^4 - r_e^4\right) \tag{7.2.10}$$

i.e., it is double the corresponding second moment of area. The polar moment of area can also be calculated as the sum of the perpendicular second moments of area ($J = I_x + I_y$), because when the y axis is perpendicular to the x axis, from the Pythagorean theorem we obtain $x_i^2 + y_i^2 = r_i^2$ and, therefore, $J = I_x + I_y$. This property has been supported as the most representative of a bone's overall mechanical performance (Ruff et al., 1993). Note that some scholars consider J raised to the power of 0.73 as a variable expressing not just torsional rigidity but also overall diaphyseal robusticity (Ruff, 1995, 2000; Sparacello et al., 2011). However, the accuracy of this measure diminishes when the cross sections are markedly noncircular, especially for I_{max}/I_{min} ratios of ~ 1.5 (Daegling, 2002).

At this point it must be stressed that experimental studies have shown that in reality the impact of mechanical loading is more complex than it appears to be using beam theory. Nevertheless, the cross-sectional properties discussed in this section offer an adequate means of assessing mechanical performance. Finally, in addition to geometric properties, bone density also has an impact on rigidity and strength, though this is not as prominent as that of geometry (Woo et al., 1981).

7.2.2 Data Collection

For a thorough study of the mechanical properties of each long bone, cross-sectional data should be collected at 15% intervals from 20% to 80% of the maximum bone length (Fig. 7.2.9) (Macintosh et al., 2013; Ruff and Hayes, 1983). When this is not feasible, a single section taken at the midshaft should be sufficient to express diaphyseal rigidity.

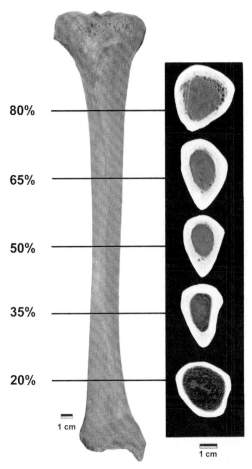

FIGURE 7.2.9 Locations of five section slices.

Cross-sectional long-bone data should ideally be collected using techniques that allow the visualization of both the periosteal and the endosteal contours, such as radiography or computed tomography (CT) (for a brief review of methods see Moore, 2012). However, when such means are not available, a method that captures only periosteal diaphyseal shape should provide accurate data, as explained in the previous section. The most inexpensive, nondestructive method, which does not require specialized equipment and may be easily used in the field, is to obtain periosteal molds from the diaphyses (see Appendix 7.II) (O'Neill and Ruff, 2004). An alternative nondestructive method has been proposed by Davies et al. (2012). This approach employs three-dimensional laser scan data and calculates cross-sectional geometric properties using a custom-built program, AsciiSection, which may be obtained from the authors.

As explained in the previous section, the exclusion of the medullary cavity from the calculations has a small impact on second moments of area, whereas it has no effect whatsoever in the calculation of *TA*. This has been further supported by Sparacello and Pearson (2010), who showed that the thickness of the cortical bone has minimal impact on the mean CSG properties, so the information obtained from periosteal contours can be used for the assessment of bone strength and rigidity (see also Macintosh et al., 2013).

Note that in studies that have used periosteal molds as a means of assessing CSG, *TA* should be favored over *J* as it is the only variable that excludes the medullary cavity by definition, and it is highly correlated with *J* values calculated from CT scans in which the medullary cavity has been taken into account (Stock and Shaw, 2007).

7.2.3 Standardization

Skeletal robusticity expresses the strength/rigidity of a skeletal element in relation to body size. Therefore, biomechanical properties except for ratios I_x/I_y and I_{max}/I_{min} should be standardized according to body size (Ruff, 2008; Ruff et al., 1993; Trinkaus, 1997). Standardization as such allows the comparison of the mechanical properties of bones among individuals of different body sizes and limb proportions (Shaw and Stock, 2009a, 2009b).

Body mass is often used as a measure of body size because it affects axial, bending, and torsional loadings (Ruff et al., 1993). Although the upper limbs are not weight-bearing, the humerus shows the same scaling relationships to body size as the femur (Ruff, 2000). Thus, the same approach can be applied to the upper and lower limbs, using body mass to standardize total area values and (body mass) × (bone length)^2 of the element being analyzed for second moments of area (Ruff, 2008).

If the body mass cannot be estimated, cross-sectional properties can be standardized employing powers of bone length. Specifically, for second moments of area the recommended power is (bone length)$^{5.33}$, whereas for the total area it is (bone length)^3 (Ruff et al., 1993). However, this procedure assumes that the body shape of the individuals compared is equivalent, which is often not a valid assumption (Ruff, 2000). Thus, whenever possible, body mass should be preferred.

7.2.4 Statistical Analysis

All CSG properties are recorded as continuous variables, which may or may not follow the normal distribution. Therefore, they can be statistically analyzed using the standard paired-samples tests to ascertain whether side dominance exists, two independent sample tests to examine differences between males and females and analysis of variance/ Kruskal−Wallis tests for interpopulation comparisons. A case study is presented in Section 9.5.6, Case Study 8. In addition, when the CSG properties do not divert significantly from the normal distribution, GLM and GEE may be adopted. An example using such approaches is given in Case Study 17, Section 9.7.7. Note that the macro Data-creation_CSG, provided in the companion website, may be used to generate artificial data sets that simulate CSG properties, which may then be analyzed using the techniques described in Chapter 9.

7.3 DENTAL WEAR

7.3.1 Mechanisms That Underline Dental Wear

Dental wear is the progressive loss of the tooth crown. Enamel is worn first and the crown becomes shorter and flatter. In more advanced stages, dentine is gradually exposed. Wear progresses more rapidly from that stage onward because dentine consists of comparatively more organic material than enamel. Initially, there is deposition of reparative dentine, but if wear persists, production of new dentine will not keep pace with it. Because of the faster rate of wear in the dentine, the tooth crown exhibits *cupping* (Hillson, 2005). In extreme cases, once the dental pulp is affected, the nerves withdraw toward the root tip and the pulp chamber is filled by dentine (Clarke and Hirsch, 1991). Various degrees of dental wear are shown in Fig. 7.3.1, whereas an extreme case of wear is given in Fig. 7.3.2.

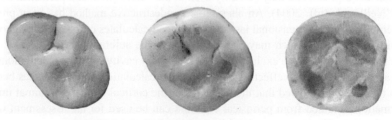

FIGURE 7.3.1 Various degrees of dental wear in molars.

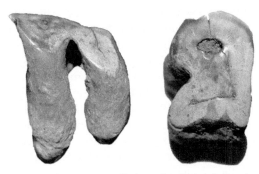

FIGURE 7.3.2 Extreme dental wear on mandibular molar: lingual (left) and occlusal (right) view.

Three main interacting mechanisms are responsible for dental wear: *attrition*, *abrasion*, and *erosion* (Hillson, 2005; Kieser et al., 2001). Attrition results from the direct contact between teeth with no foreign material, dietary or nondietary, intervening (Hillson, 2005; Milner and Larsen, 1991). For example, attrition occurs while grinding the teeth, during swallowing and speech, and when putting effort to perform a physical activity, such as weight lifting (Molnar, 1971, 1972; Roydhouse and Simonsen, 1975). Dental attrition includes: occlusal attrition resulting from contact between the occlusal surfaces of maxillary and mandibular teeth and interproximal attrition resulting from friction between adjacent teeth. It should be stressed that occlusal and interproximal wear are not independent phenomena because the latter is the outcome of the compressive and shearing forces exerted on the occlusal tooth surface (Whittaker et al., 1987). However, overcrowding in the dental arcade has also been shown to play a role in interproximal wear (Oppenheimer, 1964), whereas the shape of each tooth also affects interproximal wear rates. In particular, the bulbous shape of the molar crowns means that interproximal wear can occur only at the widest mesial/distal point, which is the only one where adjacent teeth come into contact, and not along the entire mesial or distal surface of the crown (Deter, 2012). Finally, in contrast to occlusal wear, which increases in rate once the dentine has been affected, the rate of interproximal wear decreases once the contact areas are enlarged up to a certain point, because larger contact areas exhibit greater resistance (Schuurs, 2012). Attrition has certain desirable outcomes because it maintains proper occlusion and helps clean teeth from plaque deposits, thus preventing caries (Hall and German, 1975; Smith, 1986). However, in extreme cases, attrition may become pathogenic and dramatically alters the shape of individual or multiple teeth (Spouge, 1973).

Abrasion is produced by the contact of teeth with dietary and nondietary objects that enter the mouth during masticatory and other mechanical functions (Hillson, 2005; Kaidonis et al., 1998; Schuurs, 2012). Excessive abrasion is common in paleoanthropological and archaeological material (Boldsen, 2005; Young, 1998). Most often it is attributed to the diet of the individuals under study (Grine and Kay, 1988; Kerr, 1988). Food texture and consistency depend upon the intrinsic characteristics of the food (e.g., presence of phytoliths), as well as food preparation techniques (e.g., abrasive inclusions due to the use of grinding stones) (Eshed et al., 2006; Deter, 2009). In addition, abrasion patterns resulting from the use of teeth as tools or from systematically holding nonalimentary items (e.g., pipes) using the teeth are also documented (Molnar, 2011). Fig. 7.3.3 presents a distinctive dental wear pattern, that is, a notable buccal—lingual wear plane in the anterior mandibular teeth, which is likely the result of the use of teeth in a repeated occupational activity.

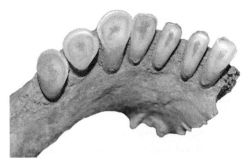

FIGURE 7.3.3 Distinctive buccal—lingual wear plane on the anterior mandibular teeth of a young adult male dating to the seventh to ninth century AD, Southwell, Nottinghamshire (SCSX12 SK2).

Dental erosion is the loss of dental tissue due to chemical processes (Arnadottir et al., 2010; Grippo et al., 2004). It is a multifactorial condition and the acids that produce it may have an intrinsic or extrinsic origin (Silva et al., 2011). Extrinsic erosion is the result of acids originating in an individual's diet, in the work environment, and in other contexts (e.g., acidic water in a swimming pool) (Khan and Young, 2011; Moss, 1998). Intrinsic erosion results from gastric acids that reach the mouth during vomiting and regurgitation (Holbrook et al., 2009; Moss, 1998; Silva et al., 2011; Zero and Lussi, 2000). It should be noted that the critical pH value for dissolving dental enamel is 5.5 and the pH value of gastric acid is 1–1.5 (Meurman and Ten Cate, 1996; Scheutzel, 1996). Saliva plays a very important role in protecting the teeth from erosive processes as it dilutes and neutralizes the acids in the oral cavity. In addition, saliva deposits glycoproteins on the tooth surfaces, which protect hydroxyapatite crystals and reduce decalcification rates (Dawes, 2008). Finally, saliva contains calcium, phosphate, and fluoride, which can remineralize dental tissues (Moss, 1998). It should be noted that although the advanced stages of erosion resemble the dissolution of apatite crystals seen in dental caries, these two phenomena are distinct. Caries is associated with plaque formation, whereas erosion occurs on plaque-free surfaces. Moreover, acidic levels are much higher in erosion than in caries. In particular, plaque microorganisms cannot tolerate low pH values, which is why the two conditions are often mutually exclusive. Finally, erosion affects the dental surfaces, whereas enamel demineralization begins at a subsurface level in dental caries (Meurman and Ten Cate, 1996; Moss, 1998).

Erosion, attrition, and abrasion act synergistically in producing dental wear (Kelleher and Bishop, 1999). For example, once tooth surfaces have become softened by erosion, they are more susceptible to the effects of abrasion and attrition (Holbrook, 2012; Silva et al., 2011).

In addition to the normal gradual loss of dental tissues, there are special types of dental wear. Such a type is *chipping* (Fig. 7.3.4, left). Chipping is an irregular crack of the enamel, and occasionally the dentine, and affects the edge of the crown (Milner and Larsen, 1991; Turner and Cadien, 1969). It may be attributed to jaw mechanics, diet, and food preparation techniques, as well as the use of teeth as tools (Hinton, 1981; Lukacs and Hemphill, 1990). When studying chipping, it is imperative to distinguish between antemortem and postmortem cracks. When chipping has occurred postmortem, the exposed enamel tends to be whiter than adjacent tooth surfaces, and the crack edges are sharp. In contrast, in antemortem chipping the color of exposed enamel is similar to that of the adjacent surfaces and the crack edges are smooth. Finally, if dental calculus has developed on the surface of chipped enamel, then clearly chipping has occurred antemortem (Scott and Winn, 2011).

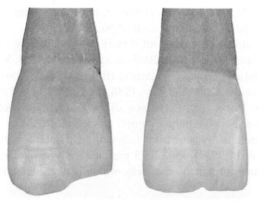

FIGURE 7.3.4 Chipping (left) and notching (right).

Another noteworthy category of special dental wear is *notching* (Fig. 7.3.4, right) Notching manifests as an indentation on the incisal/occlusal tooth surface. This indentation has a greater breadth compared to its depth and its walls are smooth (Bonfiglioni et al., 2004). Circular notches are also occasionally observed in the human dentition and may result from gripping a clay pipe (Anderson, 2002; Hillson, 2005; Ubelaker, 1989), using teeth as pincers (Alt and Pichler, 1998), holding nails between the teeth (Turner and Anderson, 2003), or using a tube to drink (Angel, 1968).

One last special type of dental wear is *interproximal grooving*. Interproximal grooves usually have a horizontal direction; they are located on the mesial and distal surfaces of the crown at or near the cementoenamel junction (Brown and Molnar, 1990; Frayer, 1991; Ubelaker et al., 1969; Wallace, 1974). Many etiologies have been proposed for interproximal grooves but their cause is still controversial. Two theories have gained support. The first attributes interproximal grooves to abrasion caused by the manipulation of objects between the teeth, for instance, during fiber or sinew processing (Blakely and Beck, 1984; Brown and Molnar, 1990; Lukacs and Pastor, 1988; Schulz, 1977). The second identifies as a causative factor the systematic use of toothpicks or probes (Formicola, 1988; Ricci et al., 2016; Ubelaker et al., 1969). Capasso et al. (1999) attribute interproximal grooves with full buccal−lingual extension to fiber or sinew processing, whereas they associate interproximal grooves without full buccal−lingual extension with inter-dental probing with a point or needle. It seems indeed plausible that different types of interproximal grooves have different etiologies, thus the affected teeth and the exact location and number of grooves must be taken into account prior to any interpretation (Formicola, 1991).

7.3.2 Recording Schemes and Statistical Analysis

Various methods have been proposed for the recording of dental wear. The two most common approaches involve (1) recording dental wear using an ordinal scheme based on the extent of exposed dentine and (2) estimating the area of exposed dentine in relation to the overall occlusal/biting surface area. Estimates of exposed dentine area are more time-consuming but preferable, as they generate continuous data and are more objective. Appendix 7.III presents representative ordinal recording schemes, and Appendix 7.IV gives step-by-step instructions on the estimation of the area of exposed dentine. Finally, Appendix 7.V presents the recording of dental wear in Osteoware.

Regarding statistical analysis, because data sets of dental wear may contain either ordinal or continuous data, the statistical tests described in Sections 7.1.3 and 7.2.4 may also apply for testing the extent of dental wear at inter- and intrapopulation levels. A point that must be noted is the normality of the continuous data. When dental wear is calculated as a continuous variable, we employ the ratio between the area of exposed dentine and the overall area of the occlusal surface. Therefore, the values obtained may range from 0 to 1. If many teeth exhibit very little or very pronounced wear, then multiple data values will be 0 and/or 1. In this case the data will not follow the normal distribution because the normal distribution presupposes that sample values may range from $-\infty$ to $+\infty$.[2] Representative nonparametric tests concerning the analysis of dental wear are presented in Section 9.5.6, Case Study 9. This case study is based on artificial data generated by means of the macro DataCreation_DW, provided in the companion website. More advanced statistical techniques, involving GLM and GEE, may also be adopted following the relevant case studies in Section 9.7.7.

REFERENCES

Alt KW, Pichler S. Artificial modifications of human teeth. In: Alt KW, Rösing FW, Teschler-Nicola M, editors. Dental anthropology. Fundamentals, limits and prospects. Wien: Springer-Verlag; 1998. p. 387−415.

Alves Cardoso FA, Henderson CY. Enthesopathy formation in the humerus: data from known age-at-death and known occupation skeletal collections. American Journal of Physical Anthropology 2010;141:550−60.

Anderson T. Unusual dental abrasion from medieval Kent. British Dental Journal 2002;192:2−3.

Angel JL. Human remains at Karataş. American Journal of Archaeology 1968;72:260−3.

Arnadottir IB, Holbrook WP, Eggertsson H, Gudmundsdottir H, Jonsson SH, Gudlaugsson JO, et al. Prevalence of dental erosion in children: a national survey. Community Dentistry and Oral Epidemiology 2010;38:521−6.

Benjamin M, McGonagle D. The anatomical basis for disease localisation in seronegative spondyloarthropathy at entheses and related sites. Journal of Anatomy 2001;199:503−26.

Benjamin M, Evans EJ, Copp L. The histology of tendon attachments to bone in man. Journal of Anatomy 1986;149:89−100.

Benjamin M, Kumai T, Milz S, Boszczyk BM, Boszczyk AA, Ralphs JR. The skeletal attachment of tendons-tendon "entheses". Comparative Biochemistry and Physiology Part A: Physiology 2002;133:931−45.

Benjamin M, Toumi H, Ralphs JR, Bydder G, Best TM, Milz S. Where tendons and ligaments meet bone: attachment sites ("entheses") in relation to exercise and/or mechanical load. Journal of Anatomy 2006;208:471−90.

Benjamin M, Toumi H, Suzuki D, Redman S, Emery P, McGonagle D. Microdamage and altered vascularity at the enthesis-bone interface provides an anatomic explanation for bone involvement in the HLA-B27-associated spondylarthritides and allied disorders. Arthritis and Rheumatism 2007;56:224−33.

Bertram JE, Swartz SM. The "law of bone transformation": a case of crying Wolff? Biological Reviews of the Cambridge Philosophical Society 1991;66:245−73.

Blakely RL, Beck L. Tooth-tool use versus dental mutilation: a case study from the prehistoric southeast. Midcontinental Journal of Archaeology 1984;9:269−84.

Boldsen JL. Analysis of dental attrition and mortality in the medieval village of Tirup, Denmark. American Journal of Physical Anthropology 2005;126:169−76.

---

2. In principle, dental wear data could follow the normal distribution if their mean value was around 0.5 with a very small standard deviation.

Bonfiglioni B, Mariotti V, Facchini F, Belcastro MG, Condemi S. Masticatory and non-masticatory dental modifications in the Epipaleolithic necropolis of Taforalt (Morocco). International Journal of Osteoarchaeology 2004;14:448−56.

Brown T, Molnar S. Interproximal grooving and task activity in Australia. American Journal Physical Anthropology 1990;81:545−53.

Capasso L, Kennedy KAR, Wilczak CA. Atlas of occupational markers on human remains. Teramo: Edigrafital S.p.A; 1999.

Clarke NG, Hirsch RS. Physiological, pulpal, and periodontal factors influencing alveolar bone. In: Kelley MA, Larsen CS, editors. Advances in dental anthropology. New York: Wiley-Liss; 1991. p. 241−66.

Crubézy E, Goulet J, Bruzek J, Jelinek J, Rougé D, Ludes F. Épidémiologie de l'arthrose et des enthésopathies dans une population européenne d'il y a 7700 ans. Revue du Rhumatisme 2002;69:1217−25.

Currey JD. Bones: structure and mechanics. Princeton, New Jersey: Princeton University Press; 2006.

Daegling D. Estimation of torsional rigidity in primate long bones. Journal of Human Evolution 2002;42:229−39.

Davies TG, Shaw CN, Stock JT. A test of a new method and software for the rapid estimation of cross-sectional geometric properties of long bone diaphyses from 3D laser surface scans. Archaeological and Anthropological Sciences 2012;4:277−90.

Davis CB, Shuler KA, Danforth ME, Herndon KE. Patterns of interobserver error in the scoring of entheseal changes. International Journal of Osteoarchaeology 2013;23:147−51.

Dawes C. Salivary flow patterns and the health of hard and soft oral tissues. Journal of the American Dental Association 2008;139(Suppl.):18S−24S.

Deter C. Gradients of occlusal wear in hunter-gatherers and agriculturalists. American Journal of Physical Anthropology 2009;138:247−54.

Deter C. Correlation between dental occlusal wear and approximal facet length. International Journal of Osteoarchaeology 2012;22:708−17.

Djukic K, Milovanovic P, Hahn M, Busse B, Amling M, Djuric M. Bone microarchitecture at muscle attachment sites: the relationship between macroscopic scores of entheses and their cortical and trabecular microstructural design. American Journal of Physical Anthropology 2015;157:81−93.

Eshed V, Gopher A, Galili E, Hershkovitz I. Musculoskeletal stress markers in Natufian hunter-gatherers and Neolithic farmers in the Levant: the upper limb. American Journal of Physical Anthropology 2004;123:303−15.

Eshed V, Gopher A, Hershkovitz I. Tooth wear and dental pathology at the advent of agriculture: new evidence from the Levant. American Journal of Physical Anthropology 2006;130:145−59.

Ferretti JL, Capozza RF, Cointry GR, Garcia SL, Plotkin H, Alvarez Filgueira ML, et al. Gender-related differences in the relationship between densitometric values of whole-body bone mineral content and lean body mass in humans between 2 and 87 years of age. Bone 1998;22:683−90.

Formicola V. Interproximal grooving of teeth: additional evidence and interpretation. Current Anthropology 1988;29:663−4.

Formicola V. Interproximal grooving: different appearances, different etiologies. American Journal of Physical Anthropology 1991;86:85−7.

Frayer DW. On the etiology of interproximal grooves. American Journal of Physical Anthropology 1991;85:299−304.

Frost HM, editor. Bone biodynamics. Boston: Little, Brown; 1964.

Frost HM. Bone "mass" and the "mechanostat." A proposal. Anatomical Record 1987;219:1−9.

Frost HM. Structural adaptations to mechanical usage. A proposed "three-way rule" for bone modeling. Part I. Veterinary and Comparative Orthopaedics and Traumatology 1988a;1:7−17.

Frost HM. Structural adaptations to mechanical usage. A proposed "three-way rule" for bone modeling. Part II. Veterinary and Comparative Orthopaedics and Traumatology 1988b;2:80−5.

Giangregorio L, Blimkie CJR. Skeletal adaptations to alterations in weight-bearing activity: a comparison of models of disuse osteoporosis. Sports Medicine 2002;32:459−76.

Górka K, Romero A, Pérez-Pérez A. First molar size and wear within and among modern hunter-gatherers and agricultural populations. HOMO-Journal of Comparative Human Biology 2015;66:299−315.

Grine FE, Kay RF. Early hominid diets from quantitative image analysis of dental microwear. Nature 1988;333:765−8.

Grippo JO, Simring M, Schreiner S. Attrition, abrasion, corrosion and abfraction revisited: a new perspective on tooth surface lesions. The Journal of the American Dental Association 2004;135:1109−18.

Hall RL, German T. Dental pathology, attrition and occlusal surface form in a prehistoric sample from British Columbia. Syesis 1975;8:275−89.

Havelková P, Villotte S, Velemínský P, Poláček L, Dobisíková M. Enthesopathies and activity patterns in the early medieval great Moravian population: evidence of division of labour. International Journal of Osteoarchaeology 2011;21:487−504.

Hawkey DE. Disability, compassion and the skeletal record: using musculoskeletal stress markers (MSM) to construct an osteobiography from early New Mexico. International Journal of Osteoarchaeology 1998;8:326−40.

Hawkey DE, Merbs CF. Activity-induced musculoskeletal stress markers (MSM) and subsistence strategy changes among ancient Hudson Bay Eskimos. International Journal of Osteoarchaeology 1995;5:324−38.

Henderson CY, Mariotti V, Pany-Kucera D, Villotte S, Wilczak C. Recording specific entheseal changes of fibrocartilaginous entheses: initial tests using the Coimbra Method. International Journal of Osteoarchaeology 2013;23:152−62.

Henderson CY, Mariotti V, Pany-Kucera D, Villotte S, Wilczak C. The new 'Coimbra Method': a biologically appropriate method for recording specific features of fibrocartilaginous entheseal changes. International Journal of Osteoarchaeology 2015. http://dx.doi.org/10.1002/oa.2477.

Hillson S. Teeth. 2nd ed. Cambridge: Cambridge University Press; 2005.

Hinton RJ. Form and patterning of anterior tooth wear among aboriginal human groups. American Journal of Physical Anthropology 1981;67:393−402.

Holbrook WP. Tooth erosion. In: Limeback H, editor. Comprehensive preventive dentistry. New York: John Wiley & Sons, Ltd.; 2012. p. 211−7.

Holbrook WP, Furuholm J, Gudmundsson K, Theodórs A, Meurman JH. Gastric reflux is a significant causative factor of tooth erosion. Journal of Dental Research 2009;88:422−6.

Huiskes R. On the modelling of long bones in structural analyses. Journal of Biomechanics 1982;15:65−9.

Jurmain R, Villotte S. Terminology. Entheses in medical literature and physical anthropology: a brief review. Document published online in 4th February

University of Coimbra, July 2–3, 2009. Coimbra: CIAS–Centro de Investigação em Antropologia e Saúde; 2010. Available: http://www.uc.pt/en/cia/msm/MSM_terminology3.pdf.

Jurmain R, Alves Cardoso F, Henderson C, Villotte S. Bioarchaeology's Holy Grail: the reconstruction of activity. In: Grauer AL, editor. A companion to paleopathology. New York: Wiley-Backwell; 2011. p. 531–52.

Kaidonis J, Richards LC, Townsend G, Tansley GD. Wear of human enamel: a quantitative in vitro assessment. Journal of Dental Research 1998;77:1983–90.

Kelleher M, Bishop K. Tooth surface loss: an overview. British Dental Journal 1999;186:61–6.

Kennedy KAR. Skeletal markers of occupational stress. In: İşcan MY, Kennedy KAR, editors. Reconstruction of life from the skeleton. New York: Liss; 1989. p. 130–60.

Kerr NW. Diet and tooth wear. Scottish Medical Journal 1988;33:313–5.

Khan F, Young WG. The multifactorial nature of tooth wear. In: Khan F, Young WG, editors. Tooth wear: the ABC of the worn dentition. New York: John Wiley & Sons, Ltd; 2011. p. 1–15.

Kieser JA, Dennison KJ, Kaidonis JA, Huang D, Herbison PGP, Tayles NG. Patterns of dental wear in the early Maori dentition. International Journal of Osteoarchaeology 2001;11:206–17.

Klepinger LL. Fundamentals of forensic anthropology. New Jersey: Wiley-Liss; 2006.

Kuorinka I, Forcier L, editors. Work-related musculoskeletal disorders (WMSDs): a reference book for prevention. London: Taylor and Francis; 1995.

Lieberman DE, Polk JD, Demes B. Predicting long bone loading from cross-sectional geometry. American Journal of Physical Anthropology 2004;123:156–71.

Lieverse AR, Bazaliiskii VI, Goriunova OI, Weber AW. Upper limb musculoskeletal stress markers among Middle Holocene foragers of Siberia's Cis-Baikal region. American Journal of Physical Anthropology 2009;138:458–72.

Lieverse AR, Bazaliiskii VI, Goriunova OI, Weber AW. Lower limb activity in the Cis-Baikal: entheseal changes among Middle Holocene Siberian foragers. American Journal of Physical Anthropology 2013;150:421–32.

Lukacs JR, Pastor RF. Activity-induced patterns of dental abrasion in prehistoric Pakistan: evidence from Mehrgarh and Harappa. American Journal of Physical Anthropology 1988;76:377–98.

Lukacs JR, Hemphill BE. Traumatic injuries of prehistoric teeth: new evidence from Baluchistan and Punjab Provinces, Pakistan. Anthropologischer Anzeiger 1990;48:351–63.

Macintosh AA, Davies TG, Ryan TM, Shaw CN, Stock JT. Periosteal versus true cross-sectional geometry: a comparison along humeral, femoral, and tibial diaphyses. American Journal of Physical Anthropology 2013;150:442–52.

Mariotti V, Facchini F, Belcastro MG. Enthesopathies - proposal of a standardized scoring method and applications. Collegium Antropologicum 2004;28:145–59.

Meurman JH, Ten Cate JM. Pathogenesis and modifying factors of dental erosion. European Journal of Oral Sciences 1996;104:199–206.

Michopoulou E, Nikita E, Valakos ED. Evaluating the efficiency of different recording protocols for entheseal changes in regards to expressing activity patterns using archival data and cross-sectional geometric properties. American Journal of Physical Anthropology 2015;158:557–68.

Milella M, Belcastro MG, Zollikofer CPE, Mariotti V. The effect of age, sex and physical activity on entheseal morphology in a contemporary Italian skeletal collection. American Journal of Physical Anthropology 2012;148:379–88.

Milner GR, Larsen CS. Teeth as artifacts of human behavior: intentional mutilation and accidental modification. In: Kelley MA, Larsen CS, editors. Advances in dental anthropology. New York: Wiley-Liss; 1991. p. 357–78.

Molnar S. Human tooth wear, tooth function and cultural variability. American Journal of Physical Anthropology 1971;34:175–9.

Molnar S. Tooth wear and function: a survey of tooth functions among some prehistoric populations. Current Anthropology 1972;13:511–25.

Molnar P. Extramasticatory dental wear reflecting habitual behavior and health in past populations. Clinical Oral Investigations 2011;15:681–9.

Moore MK. Functional morphology and medical imaging. In: DiGangi EA, Moore MK, editors. Research methods in human skeletal biology. San Diego: Academic Press; 2012. p. 397–424.

Moss SJ. Dental erosion. International Dental Journal 1998;48:529–39.

Nagy BLB. Age, activity, and musculoskeletal stress markers. American Journal of Physical Anthropology 1998;26:168–9.

Niinimäki S. What do muscle marker ruggedness scores actually tell us? International Journal of Osteoarchaeology 2011;21:292–9.

Niinimäki S. The relationship between musculoskeletal stress markers and biomechanical properties of the humeral diaphysis. American Journal of Physical Anthropology 2012;147:618–28.

Niinimäki S, Sotos LB. The relationship between intensity of physical activity and entheseal changes on the lower limb. International Journal of Osteoarchaeology 2013;23:221–8.

Nikita E. The use of generalized linear models and generalized estimating equations in bioarchaeological studies. American Journal of Physical Anthropology 2014;153:473–83.

O'Neill MC, Ruff CB. Estimating human long bone cross-sectional geometric properties: a comparison of noninvasive methods. Journal of Human Evolution 2004;47:221–35.

Oppenheimer AM. Tool use and crowded teeth in Australopithecine. Current Anthropology 1964;5:419–21.

Parfitt AM. The attainment of peak bone mass: what is the relationship between muscle growth and bone growth? Bone 2004;34:767–70.

Ricci S, Capecchi G, Boschin F, Arrighi S, Ronchitelli A, Condemi S. Toothpick use among Epigravettian humans from Grotta Paglicci (Italy). International Journal of Osteoarchaeology 2016;26:281–9.

Robb JE. The interpretation of skeletal muscle sites: a statistical approach. International Journal of Osteoarchaeology 1998;8:363–77.

Roydhouse RH, Simonsen BO. Attrition of teeth. Syesis 1975;8:263–73.

. American Journal of Physical Anthropology 1995;98:527

Ruff C. Body size, body shape, and long bone strength in modern humans. Journal of Human Evolution 2000;38:269—90.

Ruff CB. Biomechanical analyses of archaeological human skeletons. In: Katzenberg MA, Saunders SR, editors. Biological anthropology of the human skeleton. New York: Wiley Liss; 2008. p. 183—206.

Ruff CB, Hayes WC. Cross-sectional geometry of Pecos Pueblo femora and tibiae—a biomechanical investigation. I. Method and general patterns of variation. American Journal of Physical Anthropology 1983;60:359—81.

Ruff CB, Larsen CS. Reconstructing behavior in Spanish Florida: the biomechanical evidence. In: Larsen CS, editor. Bioarchaeology of Spanish Florida: the impact of colonialism. Gainesville: University Press of Florida; 2001. p. 113—45.

Ruff CB, Trinkaus E, Walker A, Larsen CS. Postcranial robusticity in *Homo*. I. Temporal trends and mechanical interpretation. American Journal of Physical Anthropology 1993;91:21—53.

Ruff C, Holt B, Trinkaus E. Who's afraid of the big bad Wolff?: "Wolff's Law" and bone functional adaptation. American Journal of Physical Anthropology 2006;129:484—98.

Scheutzel P. Etiology of dental erosion—intrinsic factors. European Journal of Oral Sciences 1996;104:178—90.

Schlecht SH, Pinto DC, Agnew AM, Stout SD. Brief Communication: the effects of disuse on the mechanical properties of bone: what unloading tells us about the adaptive nature of skeletal tissue. American Journal of Physical Anthropology 2012;149:599—605.

Schulz PD. Task activity and anterior tooth grooving in prehistoric California Indians. American Journal of Physical Anthropology 1977;46:87—92.

Schuurs A. Pathology of the hard dental tissues. New York: Blackwell Publishing Ltd; 2012.

Scott EC. Dental wear scoring technique. American Journal of Physical Anthropology 1979;51:213—7.

Scott GR, Winn JR. Dental chipping: contrasting patterns of microtrauma in Inuit and European populations. International Journal of Osteoarchaeology 2011;21:723—31.

Shaibani A, Workman R, Rothschild B. The significance of enthesitis as a skeletal phenomenon. Clinical and Experimental Rheumatology 1993;11:399—403.

Shaw HM, Benjamin M. Structure-function relationships of entheses in relation to mechanical load and exercise. Scandinavian Journal of Medicine and Science in Sports 2007;17:303—15.

Shaw C, Stock J. Intensity, repetitiveness, and directionality of habitual adolescent mobility patterns influence the tibial diaphysis morphology of athletes. American Journal of Physical Anthropology 2009a;140:149—59.

Shaw C, Stock J. Habitual throwing and swimming correspond with upper limb diaphyseal strength and shape in modern human athletes. American Journal of Physical Anthropology 2009b;140:160—72.

Silva JSAE, Baratieri LN, Araujo E, Widmer N. Dental erosion: Understanding this pervasive condition. Journal of Esthetic and Restorative Dentistry 2011;23:205—16.

Skerry TM. One mechanostat or many? Modifications of the site-specific response of bone to mechanical loading by nature and nurture. Journal of Musculoskeletal and Neuronal Interactions 2006;6:122—7.

Smith BH. Patterns of molar wear in hunter-gatherers and agriculturalists. American Journal of Physical Anthropology 1984;63:39—56.

Smith BH. Development and evolution of the helicoidal plane of dental occlusion. American Journal of Physical Anthropology 1986;69:21—36.

Sparacello VS, Pearson OM. The importance of accounting for the area of the medullary cavity in cross-sectional geometry: a test based on the femoral midshaft. American Journal of Physical Anthropology 2010;143:612—24.

Sparacello VS, Pearson OM, Coppa A, Marchi D. Changes in skeletal robusticity in an iron age agropastoral group: the Samnites from the Alfedena necropolis (Abruzzo, Central Italy). American Journal of Physical Anthropology 2011;144:119—30.

Spouge JD. Oral pathology. St. Louis: C.V. Mosby Company; 1973.

Stock JT, Pfeiffer S. Linking structural variability in long bone diaphyses to habitual behaviors: foragers from the southern African Later Stone Age and the Andaman Islands. American Journal of Physical Anthropology 2001;115:337—48.

Stock JT, Shaw CN. Which measures of diaphyseal robusticity are robust? A comparison of external methods of quantifying the strength of long bone diaphyses to cross-sectional geometric properties. American Journal of Physical Anthropology 2007;134:412—23.

Trinkaus E. Appendicular robusticity and the paleobiology of modern human emergence. Proceedings of the National Academy of Sciences United States of America 1997;94:13367—73.

Turner II CG, Cadien JD. Dental chipping in Aleuts, Eskimos and Indians. American Journal of Physical Anthropology 1969;31:303—10.

Turner II CG, Anderson T. Marked occupational dental abrasion from medieval Kent. International Journal of Osteoarchaeology 2003;13:168—72.

Ubelaker DH. Human skeletal remains: excavation, analysis, interpretation. 2nd ed. Washington: Taraxacum; 1989.

Ubelaker DH, Phenice TW, Bass WM. Artificial interproximal grooving of the teeth of American Indians. American Journal of Physical Anthropology 1969;30:145—50.

Villotte S. Connaissances médicales actuelles, cotation des enthésopathies: nouvelle méthode. Bulletins et Mémoires de la Société d'Anthropologie de Paris 2006;18:65—85.

Villotte S. Enthésopathies et Activités des Hommes Préhistoriques-Recherche Méthodologique et Application aux Fossiles Européens du Paléolithique Supérieur et du Mésolithique. Oxford: Archaeopress; 2009.

Villotte S. Practical protocol for scoring the appearance of some fibrocartilaginous entheses on the human skeleton. Document published online on the 23rd of February. 2012. Available: http://www.academia.edu/1427191/Practical_protocol_for_scoring_the_ appearance_of_some_fibrocartilaginous_ entheses_on_the_human_skeleton.

Villotte S, Knüsel CJ. Understanding entheseal changes: definition and life course changes. International Journal of Osteoarchaeology 2013;23:135—46.

Villotte S, Castex D, Couallier V, Dutour O, Knüsel CJ, Henry-Gambier D. Enthesopathies as occupational stress markers: evidence from the upper limb. American Journal of Physical Anthropology 2010a;142:224—34.

Villotte S, Churchill SE, Dutour O, Henry-Gambier D. Subsistence activities and the sexual division of labor in the European Upper Paleolithic and Mesolithic: evidence from upper limb enthesopathies. Journal of Human Evolution 2010b;59:35–43.

Wallace JA. Approximal grooving of teeth. American Journal of Physical Anthropology 1974;30:145–50.

Weiss E. Understanding muscle markers: aggregation and construct validity. American Journal of Physical Anthropology 2003;121:230–40.

Weiss E. Understanding muscle markers: lower limbs. American Journal of Physical Anthropology 2004;125:232–8.

Weiss E. Muscle markers revisited: activity pattern reconstruction with controls in a central California Amerind population. American Journal of Physical Anthropology 2007;133:931–40.

Weiss E. Examining activity patterns and biological confounding factors: differences between fibrocartilaginous and fibrous musculoskeletal stress markers. International Journal of Osteoarchaeology 2015;25:281–8.

Weiss E, Corona L, Schultz B. Sex differences in musculoskeletal stress markers: problems with activity pattern reconstructions. International Journal of Osteoarchaeology 2012;22:70–80.

White TD, Black MT, Folkens PA. Human osteology. 3rd ed. San Diego: Academic Press; 2011.

Whittaker DK, Ryan S, Weeks K, Murphy WM. Patterns of approximal wear in cheek teeth of a Romano-British population. American Journal of Physical Anthropology 1987;73:389–96.

Wilczak CA. Consideration of sexual dimorphism, age, and asymmetry in quantitative measurements of muscle insertion sites. International Journal of Osteoarchaeology 1998;8:311–25.

Wolff J. Das Gesetz der Transformation der Kochen. Berlin: A. Hirschwald; 1892.

Woo SL, Kuei SC, Amiel D, Gomez MA, Hayes WC, White FC, et al. The effect of prolonged physical training on the properties of long bone: a study of Wolff's Law. The Journal of Bone and Joint Surgery 1981;63:780–6.

Yonemoto S. Differences in the effects of age on the development of entheseal changes among historical Japanese populations. American Journal of Physical Anthropology 2016;159:267–83.

Young WG. Anthropology, tooth wear, and occlusion ab origine. Journal of Dental Research 1998;77:1860–3.

Zero DT, Lussi A. Etiology of enamel erosion: intrinsic and extrinsic factors. In: Addy M, Embery G, Edgar WM, Orchardson R, editors. Tooth wear and sensitivity: clinical advances in restorative dentistry. London: Martin Dunitz; 2000. p. 121–39.

APPENDICES

Appendix 7.I: Recording Schemes for Entheseal Changes

This appendix presents the two most broadly adopted recording schemes for ECs, namely the Hawkey and Merbs (1995) and Villotte et al. (2010a) schemes. In addition, the recently proposed Coimbra method (Henderson et al., 2013, 2015) is given.

Recording Scheme by Hawkey and Merbs (1995)

Each enthesis is recorded with respect to:

A. Robusticity
   0. No expression
   1. Slightly elevated bone surface felt when touched; no crests/ridges
   2. Uneven bone surface; mound-shaped elevation; no crests/ridges
   3. Sharp osseous crests/ridges; occasionally depressed bone surface between them
B. Stress
   0. No expression
   1. Pit depth <1 mm
   2. Pit depth 1–3 mm, pit length <5 mm
   3. Pit depth >3 mm, pit length >5 mm
C. Ossification
   0. No expression
   1. Exostosis protruding <2 mm from the bone surface
   2. Exostosis protruding 2–5 mm from the bone surface
   3. Exostosis protruding >5 mm and/or covering a large part of the bone surface

Note 1: The categories of robusticity in tendinous attachment sites are slightly different, as follows: 0, absent; 1, slight indentation; 2, rough bone surface; 3, deep indentation, often with bone crests.

Note 2: Ossification markers are generally avoided, as they appear to relate more to some abrupt traumatic episode than the daily activities of the individual (Hawkey, 1998).

Note 3: The Hawkey—Merbs scoring scheme has been criticized on the basis that it does not take into consideration the anatomical differences between fibrous and fibrocartilaginous entheses (Alves Cardoso and Henderson, 2010; Villotte et al., 2010a).

Recording Scheme by Villotte et al. (2010a) for Fibrocartilaginous Entheses

Expression:

- Present (irregular entheseal surface; enthesophytes; at least three foramina; cystic changes; calcification deposits; osseous defects)
- Absent

Coimbra Method for Fibrocartilaginous Entheses (Henderson et al., 2013, 2015)

Each enthesis is divided into two zones as shown in Fig. 7.I.1, of which zone 1 includes the margin opposite the acute angle of the attachment, and zone 2 includes the surface of the enthesis and the remaining margin. Subsequently, the features described in Table 7.I.1 are recorded per zone.

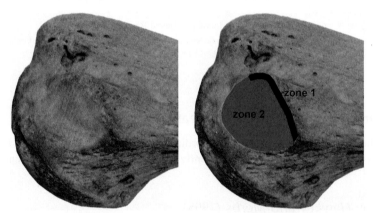

FIGURE 7.I.1   Zones used in the Coimbra method.

TABLE 7.I.1 Coimbra Method

Site	Feature	Ordinal Grades
Zone 1	Bone formation	0. Absent 1. Osseous projection <1 mm from bone surface and extending for <50% of zone 1 2. Osseous projection ≥1 mm from bone surface and extending for ≥50% of zone 1
	Erosion	0. Absent 1. Depressions covering <25% of zone 1 2. Depressions covering ≥25% of zone 1
Zone 2	Textural change	0. Absent 1. Covering >50% of zone 2
	Bone formation	0. Absent 1. Distinct formation >1 mm in any direction and covering <50% of zone 2 2. Distinct formation >1 mm in any direction and covering ≥50% of zone 2

Continued

TABLE 7.I.1 Coimbra Method—cont'd

Site	Feature	Ordinal Grades
	Erosion	**0.** Absent **1.** Depressions covering <25% of zone 2 **2.** Depressions covering ≥25% of zone 2
	Fine porosity	**0.** Absent **1.** Tiny perforations covering <50% of zone 2 **2.** Tiny perforations covering ≥50% of zone 2
	Macroporosity	**0.** Absent **1.** 1—2 small perforations **2.** >2 small perforations
	Cavitation	**0.** Absent **1.** 1 subcortical cavity **2.** >1 subcortical cavities

Appendix 7.II: Estimating Cross-Sectional Geometric Properties From Periosteal Molds

Making the Molds

Step 1. Make a ring of plasticine at the midshaft of all long bones (but at 35% distance from the distal end for humeri to avoid the deltoid muscle attachment).

Step 2. Using a knife, cut this ring in half perimetrically so that its proximal surface is flat and lies on the midshaft of the long bone, or at 35% distance from the distal end for the humerus. For the clavicle, the flat surface should lie toward the medial end of the bone.

Step 3. Mix a small quantity of the base and the catalyst of vinyl polysiloxane impression material in equal proportions (50% base and 50% catalyst), unless otherwise stated in the instructions accompanying the product.

Step 4. Spread the impression material on the flat surface of the plasticine ring perimetrically and let it dry for a couple of minutes.

Step 5. Remove the plasticine and, once the ring made of the impression material is dry enough, mark on the mold the anterior surface of the bone with a marker and cut it. Gently detach it from the bone (Fig. 7.II.1).

Step 6. Glue together the two edges of the mold.

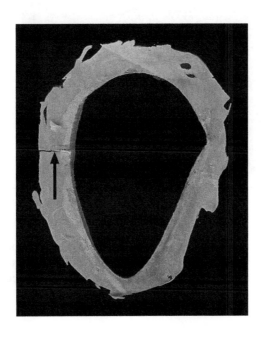

Digitizing the Molds

Step 1. Scan the molds using a minimum resolution of 600 dpi. Be careful to orient all molds in the same direction (this is why we marked the anterior side).

Step 2. Save each image as a .tiff or .jpg file.

Editing in Photoshop

Step 1. Open Photoshop and make the following adjustments: Press "D" on the keyboard to set the default foreground/ background colors, which are black and white, respectively. Alternatively, click on the corresponding icons near the bottom left corner of the Photoshop Tools panel and set the colors using the color palette that appears. In addition, select the Pencil tool by clicking on its icon in the Tools panel and make the following adjustments: set opacity to 100%, flow to 100%, hardness to 100%, and size 2 to 4 px.

Step 2. Open each image in Photoshop and create a new layer from the menu Layer → New → Layer….

Step 3. On the new layer, using the Pencil tool, draw a line that marks the circumference of the bone diaphyseal cross section on the flat surface of the mold, as shown in Fig. 7.II.2. At this point it is necessary to work with increased zoom and move the image around in its window by using the Hand tool, which is activated by holding down the space bar.

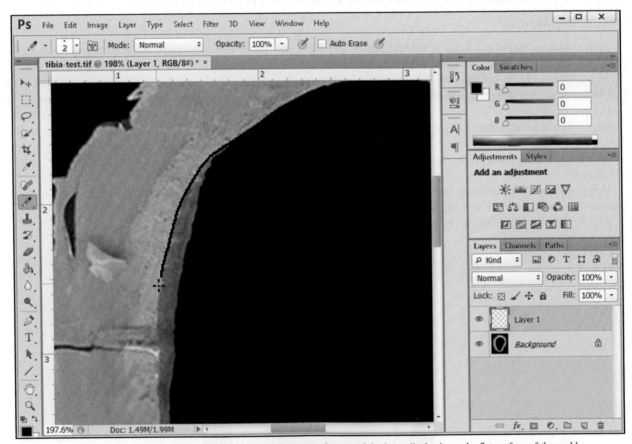

FIGURE 7.II.2 Steps in drawing a line that marks the circumference of the bone diaphysis on the flat surface of the mold.

Step 4. Make sure that the line that marks the circumference of the bone diaphysis is closed. Then select the Bucket tool in the Tools panel. Click once at the exterior of the drawn circumference to make it black. Then press "X" to switch foreground and background colors and click once in the interior of the drawn circumference to make it white. The end result is shown in Fig. 7.II.3.

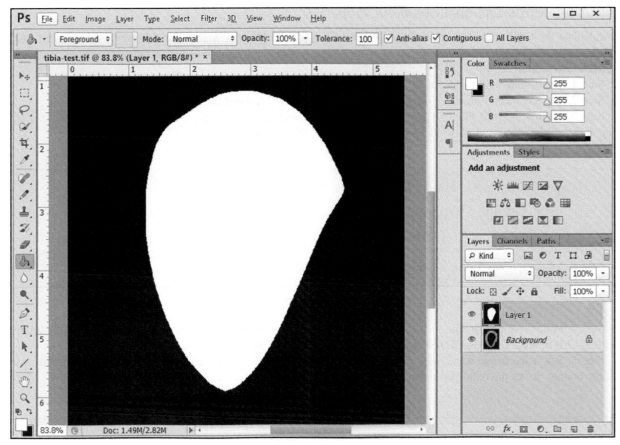

FIGURE 7.II.3   Black and white image of tibial cross-section.

Step 5. Deselect the Background layer (Fig. 7.II.4) and save the final image as a .tiff file.

Step 6. Before closing Photoshop, it is important to check how many pixels are included in each centimeter of the image, as this information will be needed later when we calculate the CSG properties. For this purpose, follow the path Image → Image size. In the dialog box that appears, in the Resolution drop-down menu of panel Document Size, turn the pixels/inch to pixels/cm. In the case of the tibia under examination, we note that each centimeter contains 472.441 pixels.

Alternative to the aforementioned approach, instead of scanning each mold, we may put it on a white piece of paper and draw its interior perimeter using a pencil. Then we scan this figure using a minimum resolution of 600 dpi and follow the same procedure in Photoshop as described above.

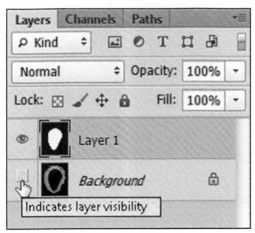

FIGURE 7.II.4   Deselecting the Background layer.

Calculating Cross-Sectional Geometric Properties

To calculate the CSG properties, we need to download ImageJ and Moment Macro. ImageJ can be downloaded free of charge at http://imagej.en.softonic.com, and Moment Macro is also freely downloadable, at http://www.hopkinsmedicine. org/fae/mmacro.html.

Step 1. Open ImageJ (Fig. 7.II.5).

Step 2. Use the menu Plugins → Macros → Install and select "MomentMacroJ_v1_4."

Step 3. Follow the path File → Open and select the .tiff black and white image of the element for which the CSG properties will be calculated. A window appears that shows the selected image.

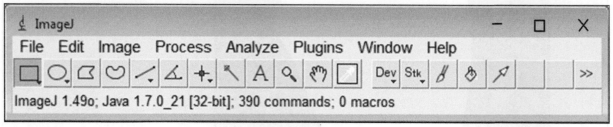

FIGURE 7.II.5 ImageJ interface.

Step 4. Follow the path Image → Adjust → Threshold. After a couple of seconds the interior of the image becomes red (Fig. 7.II.6, left). Close the Threshold window without changing any of the default settings.

Step 5. Select the magic wand, , in the ImageJ tool bar and click on any point at the interior of the mold. A thin yellow outline marks the mold perimeter (Fig. 7.II.6, right).

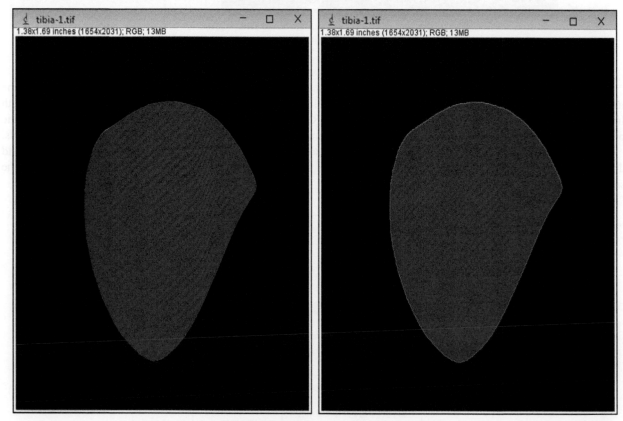

FIGURE 7.II.6 Image processing in ImageJ.

Step 6. Use the menu Plugins → Macros → Moment Calculation. A window asking if the scale should be reset appears (Fig. 7.II.7, left). Click on "Yes" and in the new window that appears type in "mm" (Fig. 7.II.7, right).

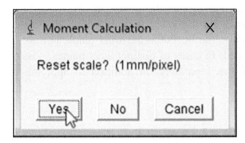
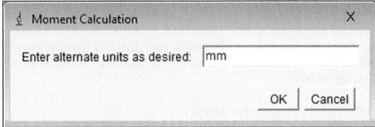

FIGURE 7.II.7   Resetting the scale.

Step 7. In the new window type the number of pixels per millimeter (see step 6 in the Photoshop section, but be careful, as the estimate here is in millimeters, not in centimeters). Based on the value we obtained in the Photoshop section, in the present example we type in "47.2441" (Fig. 7.II.8).

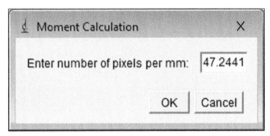

FIGURE 7.II.8   Setting the number of pixels per millimeter.

Step 8. A final window appears and asks if principal axes should be drawn. Click on "No."

Step 9. Type in the name of the sample under study in the new window.

Step 10. Type the value "1" in the dialog box that requests the lower threshold and the value "255" for the upper threshold.

Step 11. The calculations may take some time. When they are completed, the output window of Fig. 7.II.9 appears as well as a window to save the results in .txt format. Save the results.

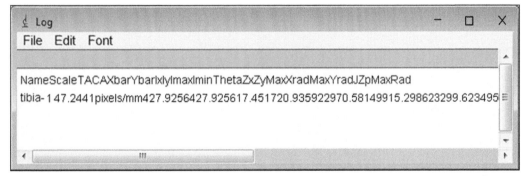

FIGURE 7.II.9   Output window.

Step 12. Open the saved file, copy the two lines, and paste them into an Excel spreadsheet (Fig. 7.II.10).

	A	B	C	D	E	F	G	H	I	J
1	Name	Scale	TA	CA	Xbar	Ybar	Ix	Iy	Imax	Imin
2	tibia-1	47.2441pixels/mm	427.93	427.93	17.452	20.936	22971	9915.3	23300	9586.3
3										

Appendix 7.III: Ordinal Recording Schemes for Dental Wear

There are various qualitative and quantitative methods for recording dental wear. In this appendix, the two most often adopted ones in the literature, Scott (1979) and Smith (1984), are presented. The main limitation of these schemes is that they do not express the plane of wear (e.g., buccolingual, mesiodistal, etc.). For molars this issue can be overcome by dividing each tooth into four quadrants and recording the stage of dental wear separately in each. Similarly, premolars can be divided into a buccal and a lingual half, which will provide information on the buccolingual wear plane, but not the mesiodistal one. For incisors and canines such divisions are more complicated. In cases of distinct wear planes, possibly associated with occupational activities, it is advisable to record such planes separately, in addition to applying the following schemes.

Scott (1979) Scheme for Molars

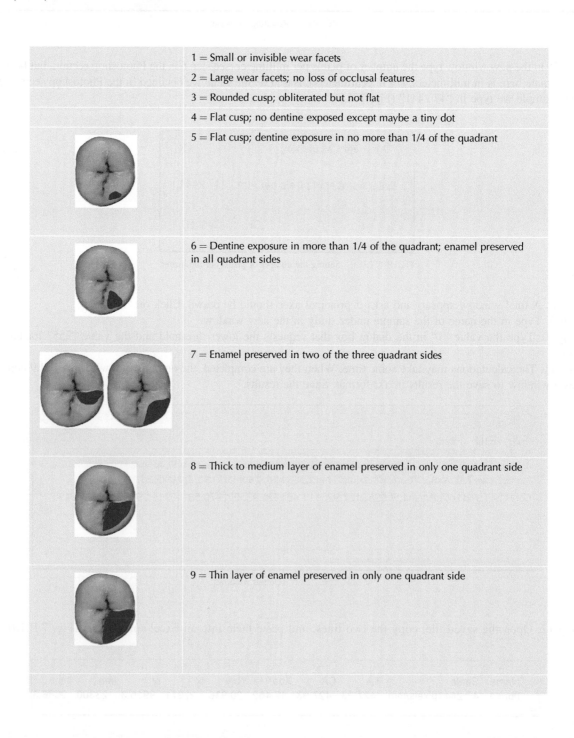

1 = Small or invisible wear facets

2 = Large wear facets; no loss of occlusal features

3 = Rounded cusp; obliterated but not flat

4 = Flat cusp; no dentine exposed except maybe a tiny dot

5 = Flat cusp; dentine exposure in no more than 1/4 of the quadrant

6 = Dentine exposure in more than 1/4 of the quadrant; enamel preserved in all quadrant sides

7 = Enamel preserved in two of the three quadrant sides

8 = Thick to medium layer of enamel preserved in only one quadrant side

9 = Thin layer of enamel preserved in only one quadrant side

—cont'd

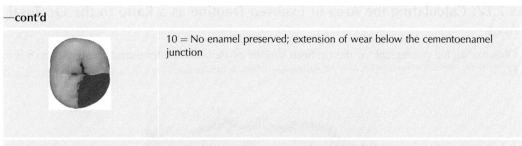

10 = No enamel preserved; extension of wear below the cementoenamel junction

Note: The occlusal surface of each molar is divided into four quadrants and the above scoring system is applied separately to each one. The four quadrant wear scores are then summed to obtain a score of 4–40 per molar.

Smith (1984) Scheme

L, lower; *U*, upper.

	Molars	Premolars		Incisors/Canines	
	L	U	L	U	U
1					
2					
3					
4					
5					
6					
7					
8					

Appendix 7.IV: Calculating the Area of Exposed Dentine as a Ratio to the Occlusal Surface Area

Step 1. Obtain a digital photograph of the occlusal surface of the tooth under examination and save it as a .tiff file (Fig. 7.IV.1).

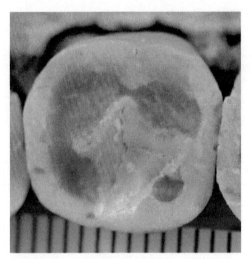

FIGURE 7.IV.1   Digital image of molar occlusal surface.

Step 2. Open this file in ImageJ. A window appears that shows the image.

Step 3. Use the menu Analyze → Set Measurements and select "Area" in the dialog box that appears.

Step 4. Select the Polygon tool, , in the ImageJ Tool bar and, using this tool, select the occlusal surface outline employing a minimum of 30 points (Górka et al., 2015) (Fig. 7.IV.2).

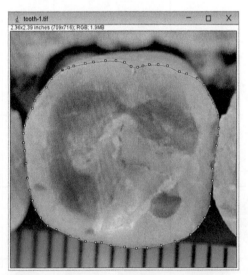

FIGURE 7.IV.2   Selected occlusal surface.

Step 5. Use the menu Analyze → Measure. A window showing the area of the selected region appears (Fig. 7.IV.3).

Step 6. Deselect the selected area by clicking at any point outside it and then select the regions of exposed dentine. To select two or more regions using the Polygon tool, select the perimeter of the first region, press "Shift" on the keyboard, select the perimeter of the second region, and so on (Fig. 7.IV.4).

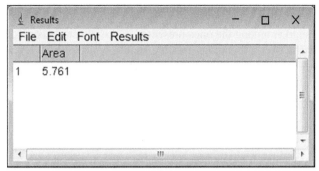

FIGURE 7.IV.3 Area of the selected occlusal surface.

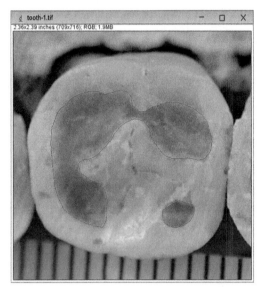

FIGURE 7.IV.4 Selected dentine exposure regions.

Step 7. Use again the menu Analyze → Measure and in the Results window the new area is added (Fig. 7.IV.5).
Step 8. Calculate the ratio of exposed dentine area/occlusal area.

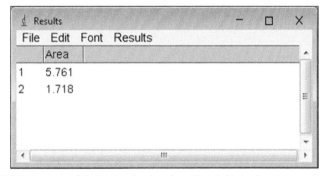

FIGURE 7.IV.5 Area of the total occlusal surface (1) and the dentine exposure regions (2).

Appendix 7.V: Dental Wear Recording in Osteoware

Dental wear is the only activity marker among the ones presented in this chapter recorded in Osteoware. For this purpose, the Dental Inventory, Development, Wear, Pathology module should be used (Fig. 7.V.1). Dental wear can be recorded only in the permanent dentition. To enter the relevant data, select option "Wear" from the Data Category panel. Dental wear is recorded per tooth using the ordinal scheme proposed by Smith (1984) (see Appendix 7.III). An overview of this scheme can be seen by clicking on the "Help" button.

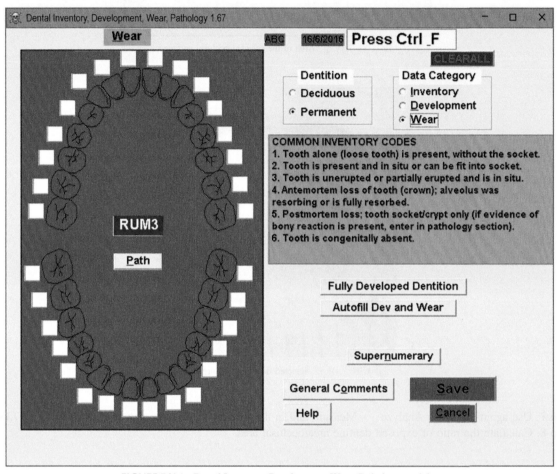

FIGURE 7.V.1   Dental Inventory, Development, Wear, Pathology module.

Chapter 8

Pathological Conditions

Chapter Outline

Chapter Objectives

By the end of this chapter, the reader will be able to:

- appreciate the range of diseases that may affect the human skeleton;
- identify various diseases based on characteristic skeletal lesions;
- record lesions associated with various pathological conditions;
- determine the statistical tests to be adopted depending upon the research questions; and
- acknowledge the limitations of the paleopathological analysis.

In osteoarchaeological contexts, the study of the diseases that afflicted humans as manifested on their skeletal remains is termed *paleopathology*.[1] Paleopathology offers insights into health and disease patterns, life quality, and the antiquity of various pathological conditions, as well as the medical knowledge of past societies. In paleopathology the unit of analysis is the individual, whereas the study of broader patterns at the population level is the subject of *paleoepidemiology*. In forensic contexts, the pathological analysis relies largely on soft tissue remains, whereas the analysis of skeletal manifestations of disease is almost exclusively focused on trauma, as a means of assessing the manner of death of the individual.

This chapter outlines the most common pathological conditions identified on human skeletal and dental remains. Given the large number of conditions that may affect human bones and teeth, only the most frequently encountered ones are presented here, which entails some degree of subjective selection by the author. In addition, skeletal lesions associated with each condition are outlined. The list of lesions presented is not exhaustive, and it should be stressed that the same condition may manifest more or less pronouncedly in different individuals, depending on a number of intrinsic and extrinsic factors. Therefore, not all outlined lesions should be expected to be present in order to identify a condition as present, whereas lesions different from those presented here may also appear. For more information, the reader may consult the seminal works on paleopathology and forensic pathology by Aufderheide and Rodríguez-Martín (1998), DiMaio and DiMaio (2001), Ortner (2003), Roberts and Manchester (2005), and Waldron (2008). At the end of this chapter, suggested recording protocols for the most commonly encountered conditions are given in Appendix 8.I, whereas Appendix 8.II briefly outlines how pathologies are recorded in Osteoware.

8.1 THE OSTEOLOGICAL PARADOX

A serious issue in the paleopathological analysis has been raised by Wood et al. (1992) and it is known as the *osteological paradox*. The authors highlighted three problems that limit paleopathological interpretation: (1) demographic nonstationarity, (2) hidden heterogeneity in frailty, and (3) selective mortality. *Demographic nonstationarity* is mostly relevant in paleodemographic studies. Such studies generally assume that preindustrialized groups were "stationary," that is, characterized by a lack of migration, constant fertility and mortality rates, a zero growth rate, and an equilibrium in age distribution. However, these assumptions are often not met in cemetery assemblages. In "nonstationary" populations the age at death distribution appears to be mostly affected by fertility rather than mortality rates. As such, commonly employed paleodemographic parameters, such as life expectancy, actually represent fertility rather than mortality.

Hidden heterogeneity expresses the fact that the population represented by the skeletal assemblage included individuals with different susceptibilities to disease and death. As such, when drawing conclusions about past health, and especially when performing interpopulation comparisons, it is important to control for this heterogeneity. However, differences in frailty often cannot be identified and controlled for, hence the term hidden heterogeneity.

Selective mortality is directly linked to heterogeneous frailty. Specifically, the skeletal assemblages under study do not consist of the entire population at each age interval, rather they include only the individuals who died at that specific age, who are the individuals exhibiting the highest frailty. As a result, the observed prevalence of pathological conditions overestimates the true prevalence of these conditions in the population under study.

The above issues render the interpretation of skeletal pathologies as stress markers problematic. The response of bone tissue to disease is generally slow; therefore, individuals who carry pathological lesions tend to be those strong enough to endure the disease long enough for their skeletons to be affected. Under this prism, individuals exhibiting pathological lesions were actually healthier and stronger than those who succumbed to disease before it could spread to their bones (Wood et al., 1992). Therefore, increased prevalence of skeletal pathological lesions could actually reflect improved living conditions.

---

1. Paleopathology also includes the study of soft tissues, parasites, animal remains, written and iconographic sources, and any other line of evidence regarding past health and disease. However, the current chapter deals only with skeletal manifestations of disease.

A 2015 review of the impact the Wood et al. (1992) paper had in osteoarchaeological studies is provided by DeWitte and Stojanowski (2015). The authors noted that there has gradually been an increased effort in controlling for heterogeneous frailty and selective mortality by leveraging archaeological contextual information, focusing on subadults as nonsurvivors, and examining the etiology and physiology of skeletal lesion formation.

Regarding the archaeological context, Wood et al. (1992) proposed focusing on egalitarian societies and on sites with short duration of use to minimize the effect of heterogeneous frailty and demographic nonstationarity. In addition, they recommended using archaeological contextual information to identify social clusters, which could relate to group-level variations in frailty. DeWitte and Stojanowski (2015) found no trend toward paleopathological research on egalitarian societies or short-term-use cemeteries; however, they did identify several studies that explored pathology among different social and spatial dimensions, even though few of these addressed the osteological paradox directly.

With respect to the impact of age, certain researchers have compared the prevalence of pathological lesions between those who die in early childhood, a period generally considered precarious, and those who survived to later ages. The goal of such studies was to assess whether more lesions can be identified in the most vulnerable individuals or in older age groups, as in the latter case these would suggest lower frailty. The results of such studies have favored both scenarios (Bennike et al., 2005; Holland, 2013; Perry, 2014).

Finally, DeWitte and Stojanowski (2015) noted the important advances that have been made since 1995 with regard to the etiology of pathological skeletal lesions, as a result of the adoption of biomolecular, histological, and other modern techniques. Such research has offered important insights into the factors producing heterogeneous frailty.

In conclusion, the paper by Wood et al. (1992) has raised some serious issues that cannot be overlooked in studies attempting to explore past life quality by means of paleopathological assessment. Despite its significance, the implications of the osteological paradox have only recently started to be addressed and accounted for in paleopathological studies but there is still room for further consideration. Important in this direction is the incorporation of contextual archaeological and paleoecological information; the adoption of biomolecular, chemical, microscopic, and other advanced techniques of disease diagnosis; the use of epidemiological models; and the application of statistical tests that allow a more effective study of the multifactorial nature of paleopathological conditions.

8.2 MACROSCOPIC PALEOPATHOLOGICAL EXAMINATION

In most studies, the research questions relate to the prevalence of specific conditions within a group, as well as to the various manifestations that a disease may exhibit within a skeleton. To address these issues, the first step is to inventory all skeletal elements available for examination and their degree of preservation, irrespective of whether they are pathologically altered or not. In this way, other scholars can assess how accurate a disease diagnosis is because missing elements may hinder the identification of many conditions. In addition, by inventorying all available elements, disease frequencies can be calculated (Stodder, 2011).

Once a bone inventory has been established, all elements manifesting pathological lesions need to be identified and described (see Appleby et al., 2015; Buikstra and Ubelaker, 1994; Ortner, 2003 for discussions on appropriate terminology). In general, osseous modifications due to pathology will appear as: (1) abnormal bone formation, (2) abnormal bone absence, (3) abnormal bone size, and (4) abnormal bone shape. To identify any of these abnormalities, it is imperative to have a good knowledge of bone morphology and its normal variation. For example, woven bone formation is normal in infants as part of their rapid skeletal growth, whereas in the adult skeleton it is associated with pathological conditions (Ortner, 2003, 2011). Another potentially confounding factor during the identification of pathological lesions is the role of taphonomic processes. Various postmortem modifications produced by scavengers, soil pressure, underground water, careless excavation, and other agents may be mistaken for pathological bone alterations (see Aufderheide and Rodríguez-Martín, 1998).

The next step is the identification of the pathological processes that gave rise to the observed bone modifications. As mentioned earlier, the skeleton has limited means of responding to various insults. Therefore, although it is generally rather easy to attribute lesions to broad pathological categories (e.g., trauma, arthritis), stricter diagnosis is often problematic. In addition, it is imperative to avoid overdiagnosis, that is, providing a diagnosis that is more specific than the evidence justifies (Ortner, 2011). A basic approach in the diagnosis of paleopathological conditions is *differential diagnosis*. In differential diagnosis the expression and distribution of the skeletal lesions is taken into account and various conditions are ruled out as possible causative factors. Considering demographic and contextual information can also assist differential diagnosis because specific conditions preferentially affect men or women of a specific age group and/or manifest under specific climatic and other conditions (Grauer, 2007; Klaus, 2016). An important issue is that the individual may have suffered simultaneously from more than one condition. This phenomenon is known as *disease co-occurrence* and it is important, as the presence of one condition may alter the expression of the other (see Schattmann et al., 2016 for an example of rickets and scurvy co-occurrence).

8.3 DEVELOPMENTAL ANOMALIES

Developmental anomalies are pathological conditions that appeared before birth or at any point during the development of the skeleton. Thus, these abnormalities are either hereditary or acquired during the early life of the individual.

8.3.1 Cranium

Various cranial sutures may fail to develop or they may fuse prematurely. In the former case, the condition is called *sutural agenesis* (Barnes, 2012) and in the latter *craniosynostosis* (Aufderheide and Rodríguez-Martín, 1998). Irrespective of the causative mechanism, when the condition affects the sagittal suture, the end result is *scaphocephaly* and manifests as an abnormally narrow and elongated cranial vault. When the metopic suture is affected, the skull has a triangular appearance from the superior view (*trigonocephaly*), whereas affliction of the coronal or lambdoid sutures results in asymmetry in the cranial vault (*plagiocephaly*). Finally, involvement of the coronal suture results in *acrocephalic* (or *oxycephalic*) individuals with very high and brachycephalic vaults. Other developmental conditions that affect the cranium are *microcephaly*, in which the cranium has an abnormally small size, and *hydrocephaly*, in which the vault is enlarged because of the accumulation of cerebrospinal fluid within the brain ventricles (Barnes, 2012).

8.3.2 Spine and Thorax

Spina bifida is a condition in which the neural arches of S1−S3, and rarely those of other vertebrae, are incompletely fused or fully open (Fig. 8.3.1). It results from genetic factors and deficient maternal folate (vitamin B9) intake during pregnancy (Armstrong et al., 2013 and references therein). Other spinal abnormalities are *hemivertebrae* and *cleft vertebrae*, which result in *scoliosis* and *kyphosis* (Keenleyside, 2015; Merbs, 2004). Finally, the *Klippel−Feil syndrome* manifests as fusion of the bodies and neural arches of the cervical and upper thoracic vertebrae (Larson et al., 2001).

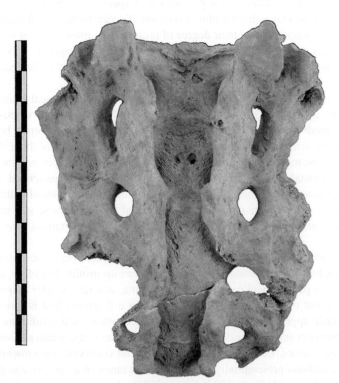

FIGURE 8.3.1 Spina bifida in a young adult male (SCSX12 Sk2) from Southwell (Nottinghamshire, UK), dating to the 7th to 9th century AD. Notice the complete nonunion of all neural arches from S1 to S5.

Rudimentary *supernumerary cervical ribs* may appear as small tubercles or even as riblike extensions. A *supernumerary thoracic rib* may be articulated to a supernumerary hemivertebra, whereas *lumbar ribs* may appear unilaterally or bilaterally (Barnes, 2012).

8.3.3 Conditions Affecting Multiple Anatomical Regions

Two noteworthy conditions in this category are osteogenesis imperfecta and achondroplasia. *Osteogenesis imperfecta* includes a number of conditions characterized by an abnormal fragility of the skeleton due to defective formation of type I collagen (Ortner, 2003). Four types of the condition were originally described by Sillence et al. (1979), but more have been identified since then (Waldron, 2008). Box 8.3.1 outlines the main skeletal manifestations of types I to IV. *Achondroplasia* is the most common form of dwarfism and its skeletal manifestations are given in Box 8.3.2.

BOX 8.3.1 Skeletal Manifestations of Osteogenesis Imperfecta (Ortner, 2003; Waldron, 2008)

- Type I: Osteoporosis, fractures, sutural bones, discolored teeth (dentinogenesis imperfecta)
- Type II: Short limbs and trunk, fractures, sutural bones
- Type III: Multiple fractures, severe bone deformities, dwarfism, kyphoscoliosis
- Type IV: Multiple fractures, small stature, bowed lower limbs

---

BOX 8.3.2 Skeletal Manifestations of Achondroplasia (Ortner, 2003)

- Disproportionately large head (large vault but small face)
- Short limbs but almost normal-sized axial skeleton
- Wide long-bone epiphyses and metaphyses
- Abnormally triangular thorax (short ribs)

8.4 METABOLIC DISEASES

Following Brickley and Ives (2008), the term *metabolic bone disease* will be used here for conditions characterized by a disruption of normal bone modeling and remodeling (see Section 1.5).

8.4.1 Scurvy

Scurvy (Box 8.4.1), also known as *Moller–Barlow disease*, results from the insufficient intake or malabsorption of ascorbic acid (vitamin C) (Halcrow et al., 2014). Humans obtain vitamin C through the consumption of fruits and vegetables, and secondarily from fish, milk, and meat (Mays, 2008). However, vitamin C can be stored in the human body for only a few months; thus regular dietary intake is necessary (Stuart-Macadam, 1989). In scorbutic individuals the collagen produced is of poor quality, which in turn hinders bone formation and calcification and weakens connective tissues, such as vascular walls (Sauberlich, 1994). Subsequently, even slight trauma can cause hemorrhaging. Bleeding generates an inflammatory response that produces bone lesions (Ortner, 2003). The first physical indications of scurvy usually appear 6–12 months after vitamin C deficiency (Brickley and Ives, 2006), but once vitamin C is restored in the diet, healing is rapid (Pimentel, 2003).

8.4.2 Rickets and Osteomalacia

Rickets (Box 8.4.2) is caused by inadequate levels of vitamin D, which is essential for the mineralization of the organic matrix of bone (osteoid). The end result is the accumulation of uncalcified bone (Holick and Adams, 1997). The condition is most prevalent in individuals between ages 6 months and 2 years and only a few cases develop after 4 years of age (Ortner, 2003). In adults, vitamin D deficiency results in *osteomalacia* (Box 8.4.3). As osteomalacia occurs after the cessation of bone growth, its skeletal manifestation is less severe compared to rickets (Brickley et al., 2007).

The main source of vitamin D production is cutaneous exposure to sunlight, though small amounts of vitamin D are also traced in eggs, milk, liver, and oily fishes (Holick, 2003, 2006). Therefore, vitamin D deficiency is usually the

BOX 8.4.1 Skeletal Manifestations of Scurvy (Geber and Murphy, 2012 and references therein; see also Stark, 2014)

- Definite lesions
  - Porosity on sphenoid (greater wings—Fig. 8.4.1) and mandible (medial ramus)
  - Porous bone formation on maxillae (posterior surface), alveolar bone, and palatine processes
- Indicative lesions for juveniles
  - Endocranial new bone formation (frontal bone)
  - Porous bone formation on the sphenoid (lesser wings), zygomatics (orbital surfaces), and maxillae (infraorbital foramina)
  - Periosteal bone formation on the scapulae (supraspinous area), femur (linea aspera), and tibia (diaphysis)
- Indicative lesions for adults
  - Porosity on the maxillae (infraorbital foramina)
  - Bone formation at the long bones of the upper and lower limbs and the os coxae
  - Bilateral ossified hematomas in the lower limbs
  - Periodontal disease
- Suggestive lesions for juveniles
  - Porosity and new bone formation at the cranial vault, orbital roof, and sphenoid (foramina rotundi)
  - Endocranial lesions (occipital, parietals)
- Periosteal bone formation on the scapulae (infraspinous area), os coxae, and long bones of the upper and lower limbs
- Suggestive lesions for adults
  - Endocranial lesions (parietals)
  - Porosity on the sphenoid (lesser wings)
  - New bone formation on the maxillae (infraorbital foramina)
  - Periosteal bone formation on the scapulae (supraspinous area), humeri, and femora

Note 1: At least two indicative lesions need to be present for a probable diagnosis of scurvy, whereas at least one indicative or one suggestive lesion is needed for a possible diagnosis of scurvy.

Note 2: Ortner (2003) also notes among the evidence for juvenile scurvy (1) transverse fractures adjacent to the osteochondral junction of the ribs and enlargement of the rib side of the costochondral joint (*scorbutic rosary*) and (2) metaphyseal fractures. For adults, he notes transverse fractures at the osteocartilaginous junctions of the ribs and inflammatory changes in the alveolar bone.

Note 3: Zuckerman et al. (2014) suggested that cranial vault thickness may also be a useful method in identifying scurvy among subadults, though more research is required.

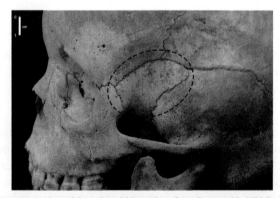

FIGURE 8.4.1 Abnormal porosity on the greater wing of the sphenoid bone in a 5- to 7-year-old child from the Lambayeque Valley Complex (north coast of Peru), dating to 1375—1470 AD. *(From Klaus HD. Subadult scurvy in Andean South America: evidence of vitamin C deficiency in the late pre-Hispanic and colonial Lambayeque Valley, Peru. International Journal of Paleopathology 2014;5:34—45, reprinted with permission.)*

outcome of malnutrition coupled with lack of sunlight exposure (Ives, 2005; Mays et al., 2006). Intestinal malabsorption and genetically resistant forms of vitamin deficiency may also produce rickets/osteomalacia (Berry et al., 2002). Finally, age is also important, as clinical evidence indicates that vitamin D concentrations are reduced in older individuals (Mosekilde, 2005). Rickets and osteomalacia are often interpreted in osteoarchaeological studies as suggestive of malnutrition and overall poor health. The reader may check Snoddy et al. (2016) for a review of the broader implications of vitamin D deficiency.

8.4.3 Osteoporosis

Osteoporosis (Box 8.4.4) is characterized by a reduction in the amount of osseous tissue in the skeleton, resulting in increased fragility of the skeletal elements, often leading to pathological fractures (Rodan et al., 2002). The condition is

BOX 8.4.2 **Skeletal Manifestations of Rickets (Brickley and Ives, 2008; Mays et al., 2006; Ortner, 2003)**

- Skull
  - Craniotabes (thin and soft areas, mainly in the parietals and occipital)
  - Delayed fontanelle closure
  - Subperiosteal bone deposition (thickening) in the vault and facial bones
  - Mandibular deformities
  - Retarded/disordered deciduous tooth eruption and hypoplastic enamel defects
- Spine
  - Decreased vertebral body height
  - Scalloping of vertebral body superior and inferior surfaces (endplates)
  - Possible kyphoscoliosis
- Thorax
  - Forward bending of sternum (*pigeon breast deformity*)

- Flattening of rib curves
- Periosteal bone deposition on ribs
- Rib enlargement at the costochondral junction (*rachitic rosary*)
- Long bones
  - Porous and rough surfaces underlying the epiphyseal growth plates
  - Thinned cortex—narrowed medullary cavity
  - Flared metaphyses
  - Bending deformities and stress fractures
  - Coxa vara (abnormally reduced angle between femoral head and shaft)

Note: Rickets occurring in later childhood and adolescence (late rickets) is characterized by mechanical deformities, which are identical to those seen in osteomalacia (Ortner, 2003).

BOX 8.4.3 **Skeletal Manifestations of Osteomalacia (Brickley and Ives, 2008; Ives and Brickley, 2014)**

- Pseudofractures/pathological fractures (scapular spinous process, ribs, pelvis, femur)
- Decreased rib curvature and inward bending on the lateral rib surface

- Sternum bending
- Vertebral compression fractures
- Pelvic deformities
- Long-bone bowing and femoral coxa vara

BOX 8.4.4 **Skeletal Manifestations of Osteoporosis (Brickley and Ives, 2008)**

- Increased bone porosity
- Thinning of trabecular and cortical bone
- Expansion of medullary cavity

- Increased vulnerability to fractures

Note: Among the above skeletal manifestations, only pathological fractures may be macroscopically visible.

produced by an imbalance between bone resorption and formation (*primary osteoporosis*) or due to nutritional deficiency and pathological factors (*secondary osteoporosis*).

The most common type of primary osteoporosis is *involutional osteoporosis* and includes two syndromes termed *type I* and *type II*. Type I affects postmenopausal women and is connected to lowered estrogen levels, whereas type II affects both elderly men and elderly women and is due to an imbalance in bone remodeling and bone loss with advanced age (Frost, 2003; Riggs et al., 1998).

Secondary osteoporosis occurs primarily as a result of diet, physical activity, and other diseases. For example, calcium and protein deficiency results in bone resorption due to secondary hyperparathyroidism (Rizzoli and Bonjour, 2004). Regarding exercise, physical activity increases bone strength and therefore decreases the probability of osteoporosis-related fractures (Riggs et al., 2006). However, excessive exercise may cause amenorrhea, which generally increases bone resorption (Castelo-Branco et al., 2006). Finally, other pathological conditions, such as genetic anemias and neoplasms, can also produce bone tissue loss (e.g., Eren and Yilmaz, 2005).

8.4.4 Paget's Disease of Bone

Paget's disease of bone (Box 8.4.5) results from an imbalance of bone remodeling rates, although its etiology is still debated (Helfrich, 2003).

BOX 8.4.5 Skeletal Manifestations of Paget's Disease of Bone (Mirra et al., 1995; Saifuddin and Hassan, 2003)

- Skull
  - Lesions mostly in the cranial vault and base
  - Initially lytic lesions but later thickening and sclerosis
- Thorax
  - Thickened ribs
- Spine
  - Enlarged vertebrae

- Compression fractures, possibly resulting in kyphosis
- Pelvis
  - Frequent iliac lesions
  - Severe cases resulting in *protrusio acetabuli*
- Long bones
  - Fractures resulting in bowing deformities (mostly in femur/tibia) and coxa vara

8.5 HEMATOPOIETIC DISEASES

This section deals only with anemias as the most commonly identified hematopoietic diseases in skeletal remains. Anemia is a general term that refers to conditions characterized by either a reduced number of red blood cells or red blood cells of reduced functionality. Etiologically, anemias may be genetic or acquired. Genetic anemias are rare compared to acquired ones. Some of them, such as sickle-cell anemia and thalassemia, are not severe when present in a heterozygous state but at the same time they reduce the severity of the symptoms of malaria (see discussion in Smith-Guzmán, 2015). Acquired anemia has a multifactorial etiology, primarily linked to diet, parasitic infestations, and other causative factors outlined in the following sections (Ortner, 2003).

8.5.1 General Skeletal Manifestations: Cribra Orbitalia and Porotic Hyperostosis

The identification of anemia in skeletal specimens is principally based on lesions on the orbits (*cribra orbitalia*; CO) or on the parietal bones and occipital squama (*porotic hyperostosis*; PH) (Fig. 8.5.1). Macroscopically CO and PH appear as porosity with variable pore dimensions and they are attributed to marrow hyperplasia (Ortner et al., 2001; Schultz, 2001).

These lesions are often treated as evidence of iron-deficiency anemia. The connection between acquired anemia and CO/PH appears to be supported by clinical data (Agarwal et al., 1970; Moseley, 1974) and epidemiological patterns (Blom et al., 2005). However, Wapler et al. (2004) found that only 43.5% of these lesions had the histological structure expected in anemic bone marrow hypertrophy, whereas inflammation and postmortem erosion were identified as more frequent causes. More recently, Walker et al. (2009) argued that iron deficiency actually inhibits bone marrow hypertrophy and proposed hemolytic anemias, such as thalassemias, sickle-cell anemias, and megaloblastic anemias, as more probable causes of PH and CO. In contrast to these results, Oxenham and Cavill (2010) stressed that clinical data do not support the rejection of iron-deficiency anemia as the causative factor of these lesions. A study by McIlvaine (2015) also supported that it may be too early to reject iron deficiency as the cause of PH and CO. The author also stressed that megaloblastic anemias and iron-deficiency anemia have similar etiologies, both being the outcome of reduced consumption of animal protein and

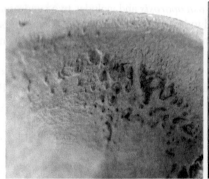 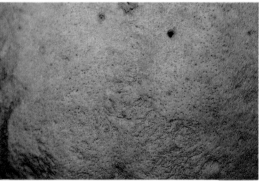

FIGURE 8.5.1 Cribra orbitalia on the left orbital roof of a young adult male (SCSX12 Sk20) from Southwell (Nottinghamshire, UK), dating to the 7th to 9th century AD (*left*) and porotic hyperostosis on the parietals and occipital of an adult female (A2.2003 Sk1364) from St. Peter's Parish (Leicester, UK), dating to the Late Medieval period (*right*). Notice the coalesced foramina and the coexistence of large- and small-sized pores, in the case of the cribra orbitalia, and the microporosity covering the entire visible ectocranial surface in the case of the porotic hyperostosis.

unsanitary living conditions. As a result, if the iron-deficiency anemia hypothesis is refuted, then megaloblastic anemias should also be rejected as causative factors of CO and PH.

8.5.2 Thalassemia

Thalassemia is the result of the deficient synthesis of one of the polypeptide chains of the hemoglobin molecule. As a result, the ability of red blood cells to transport oxygen in the body is reduced. Depending upon its degree of severity, thalassemia may be major, minor, or intermedia. Thalassemia major (Box 8.5.1) results from the inheritance of two thalassemia alleles and requires regular blood transfusions for the patient's survival. Thalassemia minor results from the inheritance of a single thalassemia allele and usually has no symptoms. Finally, in thalassemia intermedia the symptoms are the same as in thalassemia major, but less severe (Ho et al., 1998).

BOX 8.5.1 Skeletal Manifestations of Thalassemia Major (Lagia et al., 2007; Lewis, 2012; Ortner, 2003)

- General
  - Unlikely in paleopathological remains (individuals not surviving past infancy)
  - In children, affliction of the entire skeleton; in adults, affliction of areas of hematopoietic activity
- Skull
  - PH
  - Porosity on the sphenoid, temporals (squamous part), and occipital (lateral and basilar parts)
  - Enlarged facial bones
  - Disorderly dental eruption/malocclusion
- Spine
  - Increased porosity
  - Cortical bone layer destruction
  - Compression fractures

- Thorax
  - Sternal increased porosity and cortical bone erosion
  - Rib widening and cortical bone erosion
- Shoulder girdle
  - Clavicular and scapular cortical bone erosion and increased porosity
- Long bones
  - Delayed epiphyseal closure or premature fusion of growth plate
  - Thinned cortical bone and widening of medullary cavity
  - Pathological fractures
- Hand/foot bones
  - Enlarged metacarpals/metatarsals/phalanges

8.5.3 Sickle-Cell Anemia

Sickle-cell anemia (Box 8.5.2) is due to an amino acid substitution in the b-chain of hemoglobin. Abnormal hemoglobin cannot bind oxygen and results in malformed (sickle-shaped) red blood cells. Homozygotes generally die in infancy or childhood, whereas heterozygotes exhibit symptoms only under hypoxic stress (Ortner, 2003).

BOX 8.5.2 Skeletal Manifestations of Sickle-Cell Anemia (Ballas et al., 2010; Hershkovitz et al., 1997; Ortner, 2003)

- Skull
  - PH
  - Thickened facial bones and orbital roof
- Spine
  - Vertebral body widening and flattening (particularly in the lumbar segment)
  - Depression of central area of vertebral bodies (*fish vertebra appearance*)
- Ribs
  - Enlargement and cortical thickening
- Pelvis
  - Iliac thickening

- Long bones
  - Thickened cortex and narrowed medullary cavity
  - Femoral head necrosis (mostly in adolescents)
  - Slight bowing (mostly in tibia and fibula)
  - Metaphyseal porosity (mostly in upper limbs) and enlarged nutrient foramina
- Metacarpals
  - Widened medullary cavities and enlarged vascular foramina

8.5.4 Iron-Deficiency Anemia

Iron-deficiency anemia results from reduced iron availability in the red blood cells (Box 8.5.3). Iron is an integral component of the hemoglobin molecule and its main function is the transport of oxygen to various bodily tissues. Iron-deficient red blood cells are generally small (microcytic), are pale (hypochromic), have a short life span, and are incapable of transporting oxygen efficiently (Kozłowski and Witas, 2011). The factors that may reduce iron availability include malnutrition, parasitic infestations that inhibit iron absorption, infection that makes the body withhold iron, profuse hemorrhage, or increased iron demands during growth or pregnancy (Holland & O'Brian, 1997; Stuart-Macadam, 1989; Sullivan, 2005).

BOX 8.5.3 Skeletal Manifestations of Iron-Deficiency Anemia (Stuart-Macadam, 1992; Sullivan, 2005)

- Skull
  - Enlarged diploë, thinned cortical bone layer, thickened vault (PH)
  - Porosity of the orbital roof (CO)
- Long bones
  - Osteoporosis

With regard to diet, heme iron is found primarily in meat and it is easily absorbed through the intestine, whereas nonheme iron may be obtained through consumption of cereals, legumes, fruits, and vegetables but it is less bioavailable. Moreover, phytates, tannins, and other food compounds can bind iron into complex formations that cannot be absorbed by the intestine. Finally, calcium consumed together with iron-providing foodstuff inhibits iron absorption, whereas vitamins A and C improve it (Lynch, 1997). With respect to the role of infectious agents, it has been supported that iron-deficiency anemia results from an immune response that binds iron to prevent its use by infectious agents (Stuart-Macadam, 1992). However, although iron withholding may decrease the incidence and intensity of many infections, beyond a certain limit it actually increases host susceptibility to invading organisms (Weinberg, 1992; see also Hadley and DeCaro, 2015 for a lack of association between iron-deficiency anemia and low likelihood of infection). Regarding parasitic infections and their role in iron absorption, infection by whipworms and hookworms causes iron loss through intestinal bleeding, whereas parasites such as giardia and roundworm diminish the intestinal absorption of iron (Brooker et al., 2007; Stoltzfus et al., 1997). Finally, regarding the role of growth, infants require more iron than other age groups because of their high growth rate. As a result, maternal anemia during pregnancy increases the possibility of the offspring becoming anemic too (Allen, 1997).

8.6 ENDOCRINE DISORDERS

The endocrine system synthesizes and secretes various hormones that control a variety of bodily functions (Ortner, 2003). The most important hormones for the skeleton are secreted by the thyroid and pituitary glands. For this reason, only pathological conditions affecting these glands are presented here.

8.6.1 Pituitary Disturbances

The pituitary gland secretes the somatotropic (growth) hormone. Premature obliteration of the hypophysis results in *hypopituitarism*, whereas the opposite condition is known as *hyperpituitarism*. Hypopituitarism may result in *pituitary dwarfism* (Box 8.6.1). Regarding hyperpituitarism, if the condition appears in childhood, the result is great abnormal

---

BOX 8.6.1 Skeletal Manifestations of Pituitary Dwarfism (Ortner, 2003)

- Condition occurring during the growth period
  - Small-sized skeleton
  - Delayed appearance and fusion of secondary ossification centers
  - Cranial sutures open into adult age
- Condition occurring in adulthood
  - Generalized osteoporosis

growth (*pituitary gigantism*), whereas onset toward the end of the growth period will have a smaller impact. A pituitary disturbance that is more common than gigantism is *acromegaly* (Box 8.6.2), which results from reawakened growth in adults, though it has occasionally been reported in children (Ortner, 2003).

BOX 8.6.2 Skeletal Manifestations of Acromegaly (Bartelink et al., 2014; Melmed, 2006; Ortner, 2003)

- Skull
  - Pronounced supraorbital ridges, glabella, external occipital protuberance, mastoid process, temporal and nuchal lines
  - Thickened cranial vault and enlarged facial bones
  - Mandibular elongation, prognathism, dental crowding, and malocclusion
- Spine
  - Enlarged vertebral bodies
  - Osteoarthritic lipping
  - Kyphosis

- Others
  - Marked rib elongation
  - New bone formation at prominent osseous structures (e.g., trochanters) and entheses
  - Enlarged tufts of distal phalanges

8.6.2 Thyroid Disturbances

The thyroid plays a major role in various physiological control mechanisms. *Hypothyroidism* is caused by reduced production of thyroxine, one of the main hormones secreted by the thyroid. The most severe symptoms are seen in cases of congenital hypothyroidism (*cretinism*) (Box 8.6.3). The opposite condition, *hyperthyroidism* (Box 8.6.4), occurs when there is excessive production of thyroxine and affects primarily adults (Ortner, 2003).

BOX 8.6.3 Skeletal Manifestations of Cretinism (Aufderheide and Rodríguez-Martín, 1998)

- Dwarfism (short limbs and disproportionately large cranium)
- Spinal anomalies

- Delayed formation and irregularity of secondary ossification centers

---

BOX 8.6.4 Skeletal Manifestations of Hyperthyroidism (Ortner, 2003)

- Osteoporosis and occasionally stress fractures

- Early epiphyseal fusion and cessation of growth when occurring in the growth period

---

8.7 INFECTIOUS DISEASES

Infectious diseases have had a major impact on the course of human history. The interrelationship between infectious agents and the host population is a complex one and the manifestation of an infectious disease depends upon the pathogenicity of the infectious agent, its mode of transmission, the strength of the host's immune system, and other parameters. It must be noted that all these factors are affected by the natural and social environment in which the agent and the host interact (Roberts, 2000).

8.7.1 Osteomyelitis

Osteomyelitis develops as a result of pyogenic bacteria, mainly *Staphylococcus aureus*, which reach the skeleton (1) directly after trauma, (2) from infected adjacent soft tissues, or (3) through the bloodstream from a remote septic site. If the infection has spread to the bones via a nonhematogenous route, it is usually limited and does not affect the medullary cavity (Labbé et al., 2010). The remainder of this section focuses on hematogenous osteomyelitis, which is the most common type and the one that most often results in pronounced skeletal manifestations (Fig. 8.7.1).

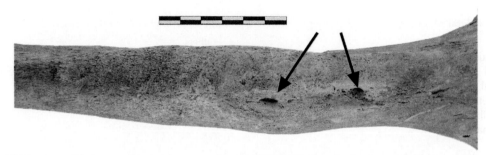

FIGURE 8.7.1 Tibial osteomyelitis in a possible female young adult (A2.2003 Sk108) from St. Peter's Parish (Leicester, UK), dating to the Late Medieval period. Notice the excessive new bone formation giving a swollen appearance to the diaphysis and proximal metaphysis, along with the two draining sinuses *(arrows)*.

Hematogenous osteomyelitis (Box 8.7.1) is more common among juveniles because of their increased growth rate. The infection often results in cortical bone necrosis. The necrotic tissue (*sequestrum*) is removed through a draining abscess (*cloaca*), while new bone (*involucrum*) forms around the infected area (Ikpeme et al., 2010; Labbé et al., 2010). In children large sequestra may cover the entire diaphysis, but the metaphyses usually do not undergo necrosis, as the thin cortical bone layer allows the escape of pus. The epiphyses are generally protected by the intervening growth plate and the fact that their vascular supply is distinct from that of the metaphyses and diaphysis (Ortner, 2003).

BOX 8.7.1 Skeletal Manifestations of Osteomyelitis (Flensborg et al., 2013; Ortner, 2003, 2008a)

- Skull
  - Lytic foci around a sequestrum, surrounded by sclerotic bone
- Spine
  - Rare involvement (mostly in adults)
  - Usually affecting only one vertebra (mainly lumbar)
  - Affecting the body, neural arch, and spinous process (rarely the transverse process), possibly resulting in collapsed vertebrae and spinal angulation
  - Paravertebral abscesses
- Ribs
  - Infection near the junction with the cartilage or at the angle

- Long bones
  - New bone apposition
  - Subperiosteal abscess
- Pelvis
  - Lesions mostly in areas rich in trabecular bone (iliac crest, sacral wings)
- Hands/feet
  - Destruction of cortical bone layer and involucrum formation in young children
  - Bone changes similar to those of other bones in adults

Note that in infants the growth plate that separates the epiphyses from the metaphyses is not yet established; thus there is no barrier between these two anatomical areas. As a result, the long-bone ends may be afflicted. In this age group massive sequestra are rare because the thin and loosely structured cortex permits the escape of pus. However, extensive involucrum formation may occur (Ortner, 2003)

In adults hematogenous osteomyelitis is rare and often the result of continued or recurrent juvenile osteomyelitis (Flensborg et al., 2013). New infections usually appear in the long-bone metaphyses, but inflammation is rather mild. The epiphyses may also be affected, because of the communication between the metaphyses and the epiphyses after the closure of the growth plate (Ortner, 2003).

8.7.2 Tuberculosis

Tuberculosis (TB) (Box 8.7.2) is caused by bacteria of the *Mycobacterium tuberculosis* complex, namely the human type, *M. tuberculosis*, or the bovine type, *M. bovis* (Stone et al., 2009). *M. tuberculosis* is mainly spread among humans during

- Skull
  - Vault lesions: in children, round small lytic foci with minimal marginal new bone formation or large destructive lesions with extensive new bone formation; in adults, single large lesions
  - Facial bones (afflicted in small children): abscesses, small sequestra, destruction of rhinomaxillary region (*lupus vulgaris*)
  - Endocranial lesions
- Spine
  - The most commonly afflicted anatomical area (mainly the lower spine)
  - Usually at least two adjacent vertebrae are affected
  - Lytic lesions on vertebral bodies, resulting in kyphosis (Pott's disease) (Fig. 8.7.2)
  - Paravertebral abscesses
- Thoracic cage
  - Periosteal new bone formation on visceral rib surface
  - Lytic lesions on ribs
  - Rarely lytic lesions on manubrium and corpus sterni
- Pelvis
  - Rare lytic lesions on the ilium, ischium, and pubis, occasionally small sequestra
  - Destruction of sacral wings and osteosclerosis

- Long bones
  - Lesions mostly in metaphyses and epiphyses (diaphysis afflicted in children)
  - Uncommon massive sequestra and limited new bone formation in adults
  - Perforation of the cortical bone layer and extraosseous abscessing in children
- Joints
  - Destruction of articular surface and ankylosis
- Hands/feet
  - *Spina ventosa* (destruction of the cortical bone layer and periosteal new bone formation in the tubular bones, mostly in children)

Note: Holloway et al. (2011) found that the frequency of bone lesions caused by TB has decreased over time from 7250 BC to 1899 AD, whereas lesion distribution has changed, with earlier skeletons manifesting lesions mostly in the spine, and more recent ones having the long bones, joints, hands, and feet also often afflicted.

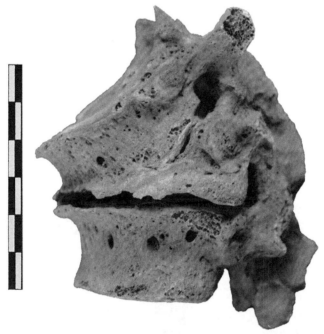

FIGURE 8.7.2   Collapsed 11th thoracic vertebra in tuberculous middle adult female (A2.2003 Sk1008) from St. Peter's Parish (Leicester, UK), dating to the Late Medieval period.

coughing or sneezing, and the principal infection focus is the lungs. *M. bovis* is usually transmitted to humans through the consumption of infected milk, dairy products, and meat (Roberts and Buikstra, 2003), whereas airborne transmission is rare (Thoen et al., 2006).

Primary TB affects individuals without prior exposure to the condition. In most cases it affects only the soft tissues and the lesions heal without further progression of the disease. However, if the initial lesions fail to heal, tubercle bacilli may spread to other body parts (Ortner, 2003). *Secondary TB* manifests later in life if the primary lesion is reactivated or the organism gets reinfected (Roberts, 2011). It must be stressed that in the preantibiotic era, TB manifested skeletally only in 5–7% of the patients (Aufderheide and Rodríguez-Martín, 1998).

8.7.3 Leprosy

Leprosy (or *Hansen's disease*) is caused by the bacillus *Mycobacterium leprae*. The condition is transmitted through prolonged skin contact and droplet infection. The response to the disease is highly variable. In cases of *lepromatous leprosy* (Box 8.7.3) there is little resistance to the mycobacteria and thus more severe expression of the disease, whereas in *tuberculoid leprosy* (Box 8.7.4) the immune response is high (Moschella, 2004). Between these two types of leprosy, there are various intermediate (*borderline*) forms. In addition, certain infected individuals do not develop clinical symptoms at all (*subclinical leprosy*) (Ortner, 2003).

BOX 8.7.3 Skeletal Manifestations of Lepromatous Leprosy (Baker and Bolhofner, 2014; Manchester, 2002; Møller-Christensen, 1978; Ortner, 2003)

- Skull
  - Pitting and resorption of the nasal conchae, vomer, and anterior nasal spine
  - Rounding of nasal aperture margins and resorption of premaxillary alveolar process
  - Porosity and possible perforation of the palate
  - Rare cranial vault erosions and CO
- Long bones
  - Periostitis (mainly in the tibia and fibula)
- Joints
  - Severe osteoarthritis and septic arthritis
- Hands/feet
  - Carpals/tarsals: lytic lesions, bone ridge across the dorsal tarsal surface (*tarsal bar*)
- Metacarpals/metatarsals: thinned diaphyses, resorbed heads, lytic lesions (Fig. 8.7.3)
- Phalanges: bone resorption

Note: The lesions in the nasal and maxillary area are known as *facies leprosa* (Møller-Christensen, 1961), but Andersen and Manchester (1992) have suggested using instead the term *rhinomaxillary syndrome*. These features are exclusive to lepromatous leprosy and traditionally constitute the only unequivocal diagnosis of leprosy in paleopathological data (Andersen et al., 1994; Manchester, 2002). However, it has been argued that other diseases may produce similar changes (Collins Cook, 2002).

BOX 8.7.4 Skeletal Manifestations of Tuberculoid Leprosy (Jopling and McDougall, 1988; Manchester, 2002)

- Same osseous changes as in lepromatous leprosy but occurring earlier and more pronouncedly
- Lesions characteristic of the rhinomaxillary syndrome are absent

---

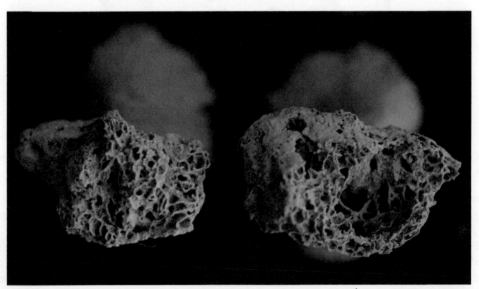

FIGURE 8.7.3 Lytic lesions with subchondral destruction on the heads of the first metatarsals in a lepromatous young adult female from Cyprus, dating to the 15th century. (*From Baker BJ, Bolhofner KL. Biological and social implications of a medieval burial from Cyprus for understanding leprosy in the past. International Journal of Paleopathology 2014;4:17 24, reprinted with permission.*)

8.7.4 Treponemal Diseases

Treponemal diseases are caused by an infection with spirochetes of the genus *Treponema* and include four different disease categories: pinta, yaws, bejel (endemic syphilis), and venereal syphilis (Mitchell, 2003). Pinta is caused by the spirochete *Treponema carateum*, whereas the three remaining diseases are associated with subspecies of *Treponema pallidum* (Klaus and Ortner, 2014).

T. pallidum is genetically, clinically, and epidemiologically complex, which renders the study of the origin of treponematoses difficult. Overall, paleopathological and epidemiological evidence supports the presence of treponemal diseases in the New World before Columbus, whereas evidence of treponemal diseases in the Old World during this period is inconclusive (see extensive discussion in Armelagos et al., 2012).

The expression of treponemal diseases falls into three stages: primary, secondary, and tertiary. Distinctive skeletal lesions occur only in the tertiary stage in all treponemal conditions except for pinta, which does not affect the skeleton (Box 8.7.5) (Aufderheide and Rodríguez-Martín, 1998; Hackett, 1976). Although slight differences in the type and distribution of bone lesions may exist between the three syndromes, their skeletal manifestation is so similar that differential diagnosis is very difficult (Ortner, 2003).

BOX 8.7.5 Skeletal Manifestations of Treponemal Diseases (Ostendorf Smith et al., 2011 and references therein)

Pathognomonic Lesions

- Progressive cranial lesion series: discrete superficial cranial lesion → circumvallate cavitating lesion → stellate scarring → caries sicca (see *Note 1*)

Indicative Lesions

- Anterior true and pseudobowing of the tibiae (*saber shins*)
- Nodes with cavitating lesions on any long bone
- Noncavitating nodal lesions on multiple bones

Lesions Consistent with Treponemal Diseases

- Noncavitating surface nodes and advanced periostitis on long-bone diaphyses

Note 1: Discrete superficial cranial lesions are superficial cavities the base of which reaches the diploë. As these gradually heal, they give rise to circumvallate cavitations whereby new bone forms in the perimeter of the lesions but minor changes occur in the interior lesion surface. Continued healing results in new bone filling the cavity until only a shallow depression is visible with a radial pattern of lines from the center of the depression (stellate scarring). Finally, caries sicca lesions appear as crater-like lesions, whereby a central destruction focus is surrounded by reactive bone (Hackett, 1976).

Note 2: Although gross nasopalatal remodeling (goundou/gangosa) is considered a diagnostic criterion of treponemal disease (Hackett, 1976), Ostendorf Smith et al. (2011) considered it as only corroborating pathognomonic lesions.

Note 3: Long-bone treponemal lesions may be gummatous or nongummatous. Nongummatous lesions manifest as periostitis (Lefort and Bennike, 2007), whereas gummatous lesions appear as lytic lesions circumscribed by woven bone (Ortner, 2003).

Yaws is typically found in rural populations of the humid tropics (Hackett, 1967). It occurs during childhood when the child becomes mobile. However, it may afflict individuals even earlier, from the first year of life, through transmission from the mother or the siblings (Dooley and Binford, 1976). *Venereal syphilis* is transmitted during sexual intercourse and has no climatic restrictions. Transmission may also occur nonsexually but it is exceptionally rare (Ortner, 2003). *Endemic syphilis* is found only in warm arid regions and subtropical climates and is usually acquired during childhood under unhygienic living conditions (Hackett, 1967). Finally, in *congenital syphilis* the infection is transmitted transplacentally from the mother to the fetus. The condition may lead to abortion or delivery either of a stillborn fetus or of a living infected infant (Fiumara et al., 1952).

8.7.5 Nonspecific Infections

Periostitis (Box 8.7.6) describes the production of periosteal new bone and it is often interpreted by osteoarchaeologists as a nonspecific stress marker (see review in Weston, 2011). It must be noted that the term "periostitis" implies an inflammatory response. However, many different mechanisms, for instance, trauma, joint disease, tumors, skeletal dysplasias,

---

BOX 8.7.6 Skeletal Manifestations of Periostitis (Weston, 2011)

- Affecting primarily long bones, especially the tibia
- Periosteal new bone formation (woven bone gradually remodeling to lamellar bone)

nutritional imbalances, and others, can generate periosteal bone formation (Chen et al., 2012; Weston, 2011). In this section the term "periostitis" will be adopted because we are dealing with this phenomenon as the outcome of infection. However, the reader is advised to use the term "periosteal new bone formation" in the study of dry bone when it is not possible to determine the causative factor.

The new bone formed is originally woven but it may later remodel into lamellar bone (Fig. 8.7.4). In general, smooth lesions with well-defined margins indicate that the process of bone formation was chronic, whereas porous bone with poorly defined margins suggests a rapid formation rate (Lovell, 2000).

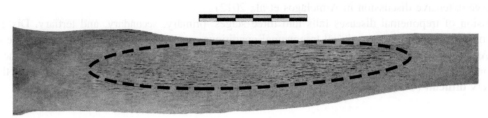

FIGURE 8.7.4 Periostitis on the tibial diaphysis of a male middle adult (A2.2003 Sk1478) from St. Peter's Parish (Leicester, UK), dating to the Late Medieval period. Observe the diffuse new bone formation consisting of moderate pitting and swelling.

8.8 TUMORS

A tumor (or neoplasm) is a mass of tissue with an abnormal growth pattern (Aufderheide and Rodríguez-Martín, 1998). Tumors may be *benign*, if they consist of mature tissue and their growth is slow and localized, or *malignant*, when they are composed of immature bone tissue, are faster growing, and spread to various body parts (Ortner, 2003).

Tumors may originate in the bones (*primary tumors*) but more often they metastasize to the skeleton from another tissue (*secondary tumors*). Note that only malignant tumors can metastasize (Käkönen and Mundy, 2003). Bone metastases can affect several skeletal elements, particularly areas rich in trabecular bone because of hematogenous dissemination, which is the most common way a metastasis may spread to the skeleton (Orr et al., 2000).

8.8.1 Benign Tumors of Bone

Osteomas, especially *button osteomas* (Box 8.8.1), are the most common category of benign tumors. Other benign bone tumors are *osteoblastomas* (Box 8.8.2), *chondromas* (Box 8.8.3), and *osteochondromas* (Box 8.8.4), as well as *giant cell tumors* (*osteoclastomas*) (Box 8.8.5).

BOX 8.8.1 Skeletal Manifestations of Button Osteomas (Eshed et al., 2002; Ortner, 2003)

- Small and smooth circular bony protuberances
- Usually single lesions, occasionally multiple
- Primarily on ectocranial surfaces (mainly on the frontal and parietals); rarely found endocranially

---

BOX 8.8.2 Skeletal Manifestations of Osteoblastomas (Brothwell, 2011; Waldron, 2008)

- Lesions exhibiting osteolysis, osteosclerosis, or a combination of the two
- Mostly affecting the spine, maxillae/mandible, tubular bones of the hands and feet, and long-bone metaphyses

---

BOX 8.8.3 Skeletal Manifestations of Chondromas (Brothwell, 2011; Ortner, 2003)

- Mostly affecting the metaphyses of tubular bones, especially in the hands and feet
- Absent in bones developing through intramembranous ossification
- Usually single lesions, occasionally multiple
- Lesions covered by a thin cortical bone shell

BOX 8.8.4 Skeletal Manifestations of Osteochondromas (Murphy and McKenzie, 2010; Stieber and Dormans, 2005)

- Single or multiple lesions with bulbous (sessile osteo-chondromas) or spurlike (pedunculated osteochondromas) appearance

- Affecting any bone developing by endochondral ossification (most common in long-bone metaphyses)

BOX 8.8.5 Skeletal Manifestations of Giant Cell Tumors (Aufderheide and Rodríguez-Martín, 1998; Brothwell, 2007; Ortner, 2003)

- Multiple symmetrical lytic lesions (most common in long-bone metaphyses)

- Formation of a thin periosteal cortical shell
- Pathological fractures

8.8.2 Primary Malignant Neoplasms

Primary malignant bone tumors are rather rare and occur mostly during the growth of the individual. The most common are *osteosarcomas* (Box 8.8.6), *chondrosarcomas* (Box 8.8.7, Fig. 8.8.1), and *Ewing's sarcoma* (Box 8.8.8). Note that most malignant neoplasms affecting the skeleton are not primary, rather they result from metastasis from other organs. Metastatic tumors affect primarily the axial skeleton and the long-bone epiphyses because of their high content in hematopoietic marrow (Ortner, 2003).

BOX 8.8.6 Skeletal Manifestations of Osteosarcomas (Brothwell, 2011; Ortner et al., 2012)

- Lesions primarily at long-bone metaphyses

- Lesions ranging from purely lytic to producing woven bone; radiating ("sunburst") pattern

BOX 8.8.7 Skeletal Manifestations of Chondrosarcomas (Arnay-de-la-Rosa et al., 2015; Henderson and Dahlin, 1963)

- Mixed lytic and proliferative lesions

- Afflicting mostly long-bone metaphyses, sacrum, and os coxae

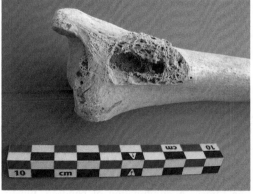

FIGURE 8.8.1 A likely case of chondrosarcoma on the left distal tibia of a possible adult male from the Canary Islands, dating to 1800−1600 years BP. (*From Arnay-de-la-Rosa M, González-Reimers E, Hernández-Marrero JC, Castañeyra-Ruiz M, Trujillo-Mederos A, González-Arnay E, Hernández-León CN. Cartilage-derived tumor in a prehispanic individual from La Gomera (Canary Islands). International Journal of Paleopathology 2015;11:66−9, reprinted with permission.*)

8.9 TRAUMA

The study of trauma in archaeological contexts can offer important insights into past warfare, intragroup violence, and accident rates. In addition, aspects related to the healing process provide information on medical knowledge and social support. In forensic contexts the study of trauma aims primarily at assessing the manner of death and/or assisting in the individuation of the deceased.

Following paleopathological standards, trauma is divided here into *fractures*, *dislocations*, and *surgical procedures*. It must be kept in mind that this classification is arbitrary, as is any trauma classification, but aims at encompassing as many of the traumatic categories discussed in paleopathological contexts as possible. Note that these categories largely avoid the classification of injuries in a manner that implies causation or intent (Lovell, 1997), which is often difficult to discern in archaeological material. However, to conform to forensic anthropological standards, fractures are additionally divided into *blunt force*, *sharp force*, and *high-velocity projectile* trauma (Davidson et al., 2011), though it must be remembered that the borders between trauma classes are not always clear.

8.9.1 Fractures

8.9.1.1 Fracture Types

The term *fracture* refers to the complete or partial break in the continuity of a bone due to abnormal stress applied on the skeleton (see Chapter 7 for a review of the biomechanical properties of bone). This stress can be *dynamic*, meaning sudden high stress, or *static*, whereby the stress is low and applied slowly. Stress in bone results from the application of one or more of the following types of force: (1) tension, (2) compression, (3) torsion, (4) bending, and (5) shear (Fig. 7.2.1). Each stress type yields a different type of fracture; however, many fractures are the outcome of multiple types of stress (Ortner, 2003). The type of fracture also largely depends on whether the trauma was direct or indirect. In *direct trauma* the break occurs at the point of impact, whereas in *indirect trauma* the fracture occurs at a place different from the point of impact (Miller and Miller, 1985).

Tension fractures often occur on sites of tendon–bone attachment and are expressed as a break of the tubercle or process to which the tendon is attached. *Compression fractures* result from force applied in the axial direction, whereas in *torsion fractures* the force has a spiral or twisting direction. In *bending fractures* force is applied on a bone, generating a compressive force on one side of the bone and a tensile force on the other side, and *shearing fractures* occur when opposite forces are applied perpendicular to the diaphysis in slightly different planes (Ortner, 2003).

In addition to the above dynamic types of stress, static stress can cause microcracks, which eventually coalesce and result in so-called *fatigue* or *stress fractures*. A final category of fractures based on causative factors is *pathological fractures*. Such fractures occur on bones that have been weakened by other pathological conditions, and as a result, they break under even minimal stress (Lovell, 2008).

Depending on their severity, fractures may be simple or comminuted. In *simple fractures* the bone has broken at one point only, whereas in *comminuted fractures* there are many broken bone segments. In cases in which the broken bone protrudes through the skin, the fracture is called *open* (Harkess et al., 1996). Finally, if the break does not extend across the bone, the fracture is *incomplete* (*greenstick*), whereas in the opposite case, it is *complete* (Lovell, 1997).

According to their shape, fractures may be transverse, oblique, spiral, or impacted (Fig. 8.9.1). These categories are mostly applicable in the case of tubular elements, such as the long bones, and the shape of the fracture depends upon the type of dynamic stress inflicted on the elements, as briefly outlined earlier. *Transverse fractures* are caused by bending forces or forces applied perpendicular to the long-bone axis; *spiral fractures* are produced by twisting forces, and *impacted fractures* are the result of compressive forces. A combination of bending, twisting, and compressive forces generates *oblique fractures* (Lovell, 1997).

In the cranium, vertebrae, and other anatomical areas rich in trabecular bone, *crush fractures* may occur. These are classified into depressed, compressed, and pressure fractures. In *depressed fractures*, force is applied on only one side of

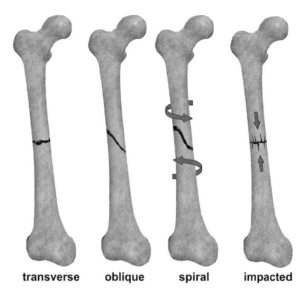

transverse   oblique   spiral   impacted

FIGURE 8.9.1   Transverse, oblique, spiral, and impacted fractures.

the bone, whereas in *compressed fractures* both sides of the bone are affected. Finally, *pressure fractures* are the result of bone adaptation to forces applied usually in the context of cultural bone modifications (Lovell, 1997).

The healing stages of a typical fracture are described in Box 8.9.1, along with possible complications that may arise. Such evidence can offer important information regarding the medical knowledge of past societies.

BOX 8.9.1 Fracture Repair and Possible Complications

Once a bone fractures, blood vessels are ruptured and the blood that accumulates in the injured area forms a hematoma, which gradually coagulates. Subsequently, the blood clot is permeated by fibrous connective tissue and a primary bony callus is formed. Fiber bone is gradually replaced by lamellar bone and, eventually, the callus is eliminated (Lovell, 2008).

malalignment is seen in the radius in the figure, where the midshaft fracture has healed as indicated by the remodeled callus; however, there is marked angulation.

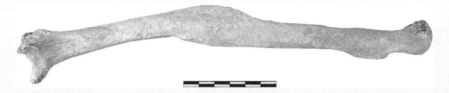

The time required for fracture healing depends on several variables, such as the bone affected, the fracture severity, the stability of the involved elements, the age and dietary patterns of the individual, and the presence of infection or other complicating conditions (Ogden, 2000).

If a fracture is left unaided, it may heal with little deformity; however, complications may also occur, most notably infections and deformities. Infection is seen primarily in open fractures. Long-bone deformities include shortening, lengthening, angulation, and rotation (Lovell, 2008). A case of

In cases of inadequate immobilization, bony union may never occur, but a *pseudarthrosis* may form (Lovell, 2008; Ortner, 2003). A bone fracture may also destroy blood vessels, leading to bone necrosis (Waldron, 2008). Traumatic arthritis may be seen in joints directly or indirectly affected by a traumatic episode, or damage to the overlying muscles may produce *myositis ossificans traumatica*, whereby injured muscle tissue becomes ossified (Aufderheide and Rodriguez-Martin, 1998; Lovell, 2008; Waldron, 2008).

8.9.1.2 Violent Versus Accidental Trauma

By examining the various types of fractures, their distribution in the skeleton, as well as the social, historical, and/or environmental context of the human remains, we can draw conclusions on whether the lesions were the result of a violent encounter or accidental. The reader may consult Galloway (1999) for a detailed account of blunt force trauma, as well as Lovell's (2008) review chapter, which presents the most common types of fractures per skeletal element and associated causative factors.

Trauma resulting from violent encounters is mostly seen in the cranium, ribs, scapula, forearm, and hands, and affects mainly young males (Brickley and Smith, 2006; Lovell, 2008). Skull fractures due to interpersonal violence are found primarily around the frontal bone and secondarily on the facial bones, especially at the nose (Ambade and Godbole, 2006). In the postcranial skeleton a fracture traditionally associated with interpersonal violence is the so-called *parry fracture* on the distal ulna, which is likely to be sustained after raising the arm to protect one's head from a blow (Galloway, 1999; Milner et al., 2015). However, such fractures may also occur accidentally by falling on an outstretched arm or when trying to protect oneself from a falling object (Lessa & Mendonça De Souza, 2004). In contrast to parry fractures, whose etiology is rather ambiguous though still largely connected with interpersonal violence, a *Colles' fracture* usually results from accidentally falling on an outstretched arm and occurs in the distal radial metaphysis (Lovell, 1997, 2008). A special case of violence is child abuse. Modern clinical cases suggest that fractures in the ribs, long bones, and cranium are often associated with violence toward children, although few osteoarchaeological studies have dealt with this issue (Gaither, 2012; Wheeler et al., 2013). Even rarer are osteoarchaeological studies on elder abuse, as discussed by Gowland (2016).

8.9.1.3 Vertebral Fractures Possibly Associated With Repetitive Activity

Two types of vertebral fractures have been associated with repetitive loading of the spine. The first is *spondylolysis*; it is characterized by the separation of the neural arch from the vertebral body at the pars interarticularis, and affects primarily the lumbar vertebrae (Fig. 8.9.2, left) (Merbs, 1996). Regarding its etiology, it has been associated with chronic repetitive stress (Chosa et al., 2004; Sakai et al., 2010; but see Soler and Calderon, 2000), bipedality (Fibiger and Knüsel, 2005; Merbs, 1996), genetic factors (Fredrickson et al., 1984), and lumbosacral morphological variation (Mays, 2006). It seems likely that a combination of age, sex, activity, and genetic predisposition underlies the expression of this condition (see, for example, Pilloud and Canzonieri, 2014). Occasionally, the body of the vertebra affected by spondylolysis may slip forward—a condition known as *spondylolisthesis* (Mays, 2006; Merbs, 2001).

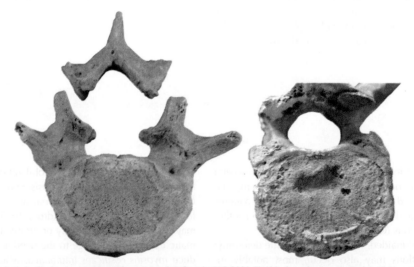

FIGURE 8.9.2 Spondylolysis in the lumbar vertebra of a young adult female (A2.2003 Sk433) from St. Peter's Parish (*left*) and Schmorl's node in a lower thoracic vertebra of a middle adult male (A22/A24.2003 Sk134) from St. Michael's Parish (*right*), both Late Medieval Leicester, UK. In the case of the spondylolysis, observe the complete and bilateral separation of the posterior part of the neural arch from the rest of the vertebra due to a defect in the pars interarticularis. In the case of the Schmorl node, observe the distinct depression at the posterior part of the inferior surface of the thoracic vertebral body.

Another type of vertebral stress fracture are *Schmorl's nodes* (Fig. 8.9.2, right). These manifest as depressions with sclerotic margins on the upper or lower vertebral body surface (vertebral endplate) and result from compressive loads, which cause intervertebral disc herniation (Faccia and Williams, 2008). The etiology of Schmorl's nodes is controversial, with mechanical stress, metabolic deficiencies, increased body weight, trauma, vertebral morphology, and congenital predisposition implicated (e.g., Cholewicki and McGill, 1996; Dar et al., 2010; Plomp et al., 2015; Williams et al., 2007).

8.9.2 Dislocations

A *dislocation* (or *luxation*) occurs when the bones comprising a joint have lost contact (Nikitovic et al., 2012). Less serious cases in which there is only partial loss of contact between joint elements are referred to as *subluxation*. Dislocation is usually caused by trauma, though congenital abnormalities in joint development also increase its likelihood. It may occur in most joints but the two most frequently afflicted are the shoulder and hip because of their great degree of mobility (Ortner, 2003).

For as long as a joint remains dislocated, the articular cartilage cannot be nourished by the synovial fluid, and blood supply to the subchondral bone may be restricted. The cartilage therefore begins to degenerate and arthritic changes may be produced (Ortner, 2003), as well as bone necrosis (Lovell, 2008). Bone atrophy secondary to immobility and infection are also possible outcomes (Rodríguez-Martín, 2006). To be detected in skeletal remains, dislocation must have persisted enough to generate alterations in subchondral bone (Miles, 2000). Therefore, in cases of dislocations that can be put back into place easily (e.g., digits) or that may cause immediate death (e.g., vertebrae), there will be no identifiable skeletal sign of the condition (Lovell, 2008).

8.9.3 Surgical Procedures and Mutilation

Trephination involves the intentional removal of part of the neurocranium ante- or postmortem. This practice has been performed in many areas of the world, from Mesolithic to modern times (e.g., Juengst and Chávez, 2015; Nikita et al., 2013; Weber and Wahl, 2006). Regarding its purpose, it appears that trephination acted as a medical technique to relieve endocranial pressure and headaches, or had a magical/ceremonial role (Capasso and Di Tota, 1996; Moskalenko et al., 2008). In cases in which trephinations occurred postmortem, bone discs were used as amulets.

Trephinations may be produced by four main techniques: (1) drilling using a trephine/drill, (2) scraping using an abrasive instrument (Fig. 8.9.3), (3) cutting using an incisive instrument, and (4) boring and cutting using a drill and an incisive instrument. Multiple methods, however, may have been used during the same operation (Verano, 2016). The main complications that may arise from trephination include brain injury, hemorrhage, and infection (Ortner, 2003). It is noteworthy that although trephinations require great precision, success rates have been particularly high from prehistoric to modern times (Arnott et al., 2003; Moghaddam et al., 2015).

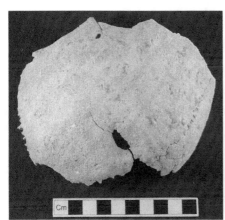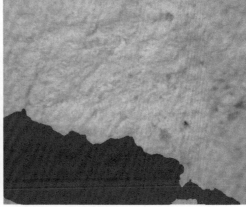

FIGURE 8.9.3 Trephination on the left parietal bone of a Late Garamantian cranium (Libyan Sahara). General view (*left*) and detail showing scraping marks (*right*). (*From Nikita E, Lahr MM, Mattingly D. Evidence of trephinations among the Garamantes, a late Holocene Saharan population. International Journal Osteoarchaeology 2013;23:370–7, reprinted with permission.*)

Circumstances under which *amputations* occurred in antiquity include punishment, accidental and war injuries, surgery, and ritual (Stuckert and Kricun, 2011; Zäuner et al., 2013). Observable signs of healing appear 1 to 2 weeks after the amputation in the form of vascular erosion of the bone ends and adjacent diaphysis. By the end of the second post-amputation week, an endosteal callus becomes apparent and gradually obliterates the medullary cavity at the bone end (Aufderheide and Rodríguez-Martín, 1998).

Decapitation is identified on skeletal remains by cut marks on the basicranium, cervical vertebrae, and/or mandible (Kanjou et al., 2015), whereas *scalping* manifests skeletally as cut marks on the frontal bone or circumferentially around the crown. Additional bone changes associated with healed scalping include bone necrosis of the outer table, new bone formation, and porosity (Toyne, 2011).

8.9.4 Forensic Distinction of Trauma

In forensic analysis emphasis is placed on identifying the manner of death; thus the categories of traumatic injury are defined based on the type of force and instrument that produced the lesions: *blunt force trauma, sharp force trauma,* and *ballistic trauma/high-velocity projectile trauma.* In osteoarchaeological contexts, these types of trauma would be classified under *fractures.*

8.9.4.1 Blunt Force Trauma

Blunt force trauma (BFT) results from broad instruments impacting a rather large surface area at low energy (Galloway, 1999). It may be produced by various objects, such as hammers, clubs, bats, and fists, or even falls (Komar and Buikstra, 2007). Identifying the specific implement used is problematic because several factors, such as magnitude, duration, direction, and focus of the applied force, as well as the type of load and the rate at which it was applied, influence wound morphology (Byers, 2010; Kimmerle and Baraybar, 2008).

In BFT to the cranial vault, the bone typically bends internally, producing radiating fractures, as well as concentric fractures around the site of impact (Fig. 8.9.4) (Frankel and Nordin, 2001; Hart, 2005; but see Kroman et al., 2011). Fracture propagation generally follows the path of least resistance, a property particularly useful in determining the sequence of BFT impacts in cases of two or more blows (Berryman and Symes, 1998). Specifically, fractures from successive impacts will terminate into fractures from earlier impacts (*Puppe's law of sequence*) (Fig. 8.9.5) (Berryman and Symes, 1998). In skulls with open sutures, fractures may travel along them (*diastatic fractures*) (DiMaio and DiMaio, 2001).

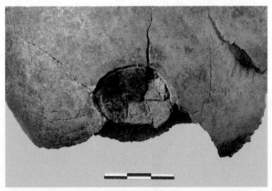

FIGURE 8.9.4 Unhealed circular depressed fracture on the left parietal bone of a middle adult male from prehistoric Anatolia. Observe the fracture lines radiating from the point of impact, as well as the concentric fracture lines. *(From Erdal YS, Erdal ÖD. Organized violence in Anatolia: a retrospective research on the injuries from the neolithic to early bronze age. International Journal of Paleopathology 2012;2:78–92, reprinted with permission.)*

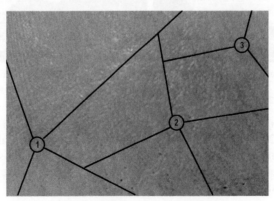

FIGURE 8.9.5   s law of sequence.

Fractures of the facial skeleton are characterized by the so-called *Le Fort fracture patterns* (Fig. 8.9.6) (Le Fort, 1901). Le Fort I (or horizontal) fractures separate the alveolar part from the body of the maxilla, and result from force applied to the lower face. Le Fort II (or pyramidal) fractures affect the nasal bridge, inferior orbits, and posterior maxillae, and are the outcome of force applied to the midface. Le Fort III (or transverse) fractures separate facial from vault bones and result from trauma to the upper face. DiMaio and DiMaio (2001) identified two more facial trauma categories: *dentoalveolar fractures* and *sagittal fractures*. Dentoalveolar fractures result in the separation of part of the mandible, whereas sagittal fractures run sagittally across the maxillae.

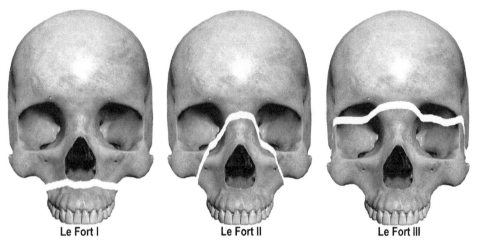

Le Fort I   Le Fort II   Le Fort III

FIGURE 8.9.6 Le Fort fracture patterns.

Regarding the cranial base, *hinge fractures* are caused by forces applied to the side of the head or the tip of the chin, and transverse the cranial base (DiMaio and DiMaio, 2001). *Ring fractures* encircle the foramen magnum and are produced by forces applied on the top of the head and the tip of the chin, or during falls on the buttocks (Voigt and Skold, 1974).

In the long bones, when force is applied perpendicular to the diaphysis, compressive forces develop on the impacted side and tensile forces on the opposite side (Frankel and Nordin, 2001). As bone is able to withstand compression better than tension, the resulting fractures appear cross-sectionally as a butterfly; thus they are described as *butterfly fractures* (Fig. 8.9.7) (Symes et al., 2012).

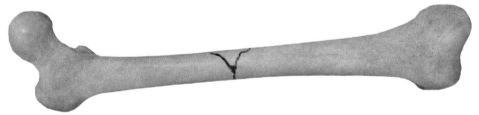

FIGURE 8.9.7 Butterfly fracture.

In the thorax, anteroposterior loadings break the rib angles, whereas lateral forces fracture the sternal and vertebral rib ends. Sternal fractures result from forces applied on the anterior chest, or from anteroposterior chest compression, and they usually transverse the corpus sterni (DiMaio and DiMaio, 2001).

A debatable issue in forensic pathology is the etiology of fractured hyoids. Although it has traditionally been assumed that such fractures result from strangulation (Ubelaker, 1992), hyoid fractures have also been associated with sports injuries and profuse vomiting (Dalati, 2005; Gross and Eliashar, 2004). Currently, fractured hyoids are interpreted as suggestive of trauma to the anterior neck, not necessarily due to strangulation, unless otherwise supported by soft tissues or contextual information (Symes et al., 2012).

8.9.4.2 Sharp Force Trauma

Sharp force trauma (SFT) is produced when a sharp object impacts bone producing incisions (Kimmerle and Baraybar, 2008; Symes et al., 2012). As such, SFT results in linear lesions, with well-defined borders and a smooth cut surface

(Fig. 8.9.8) (Boylston, 2000). Instruments that may cause SFT include knives, machetes, axes, ice picks, scalpels, and others (Kimmerle and Baraybar, 2008).

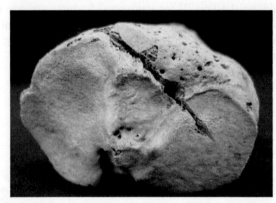

FIGURE 8.9.8 Perimortem sharp force trauma on the right tibia of a >50-year-old male from a mortuary cave site in Chihuahua (Mexico), dating to 1280–1400 AD. *(From Anderson CP, Martin DL, Thompson JL. Indigenous violence in Northern Mexico on the eve of contact. International Journal of Paleopathology 2012;2:93–101, reprinted with permission.)*

There are typically three types of lesions associated with SFT, though more categories may be devised: *stab wounds*, *incised wounds*, and *chop wounds*. Stab wounds have greater depth than width and result from forces applied perpendicular to the bone surface. In incised or cut wounds the lesion length is greater than its depth and the force is applied parallel or tangential to the bone surface (Kimmerle and Baraybar, 2008). Chop wounds combine characteristics of SFT and BFT and are produced by sharp-edged objects that forcefully impact the bone (DiMaio and DiMaio, 2001).

8.9.4.3 High-Velocity Projectile Trauma/Ballistic Trauma

High-velocity projectile trauma is produced when force is rapidly applied on a small surface area. Such trauma is usually generated by bullets. Note that projectiles, such as arrows, do not reach the velocities required for the resulting trauma to be classified as high-velocity projectile trauma; rather the resulting lesions should be categorized as BFT. An excellent discussion on gunshot wounds is provided in Berryman and Symes (1998) and Whiting and Zernicke (2008).

In the cranium, the lesions produced include radiating and concentric fractures (Kimmerle and Baraybar, 2008). However, in contrast to BFT, in which concentric fractures are associated with internal bone beveling, the concentric fractures produced in high-velocity projectile trauma are externally beveled because of the intracranial pressure generated as the bullet transverses the brain (Berryman and Gunther, 2000; Hart, 2005). Because of the very high velocity of the projectile, there is little or no plastic deformation, but greater fragmentation compared to other types of trauma. Exit wounds, absent in BFT, are larger than entry wounds, are irregular in shape, and exhibit external beveling. In the case of multiple ballistic traumas to the same individual, trauma order can be determined using Puppe's law of sequence (described above). The shape and size of the entrance and exit wounds depend on various factors, including the projectile type and the angle of impact (Kimmerle and Baraybar, 2008). Round wounds usually indicate that the impact of the projectile is roughly perpendicular to the bone surface, whereas in other cases the wounds are oval or keyhole-shaped (Symes et al., 2012).

Regarding postcranial bones, in areas rich in trabecular bone, such as long-bone epiphyses and vertebrae, entrance wounds are usually round, whereas in areas of cortical bone, such as the diaphysis, high-velocity projectile trauma usually results in comminuted fractures (Whiting and Zernicke, 2008).

8.9.5 Identifying Perimortem Trauma

Antemortem trauma can be easily identified in most cases as it is characterized by some degree of healing in the form of new bone formation and remodeling. Although the healing process begins almost immediately after trauma, it takes between 1 and 3 weeks for evidence of healing to be visible (Ortner, 2008b). However, as mentioned in Box 8.9.1, the rate of healing depends upon many factors, such as the type of trauma and bone affected, the age and nutritional status of the individual, and others.

What is particularly challenging is the discrimination between perimortem and postmortem trauma. Note that by definition *perimortem trauma* refers to injuries that occurred around the time of death. However, in practice we record as perimortem trauma injuries that occur when the bone is still in a *fresh* state, meaning that it still retains the properties that would make it fracture like living bone. Therefore, the perimortem interval extends into the postmortem period (Christensen et al., 2014).

Perimortem trauma is difficult to differentiate from postmortem damage because in both cases there is no evidence of bone healing; however, some general principles may be applied. Overall, perimortem fractures are identified on the grounds that fresh bone is more likely to splinter or fracture, producing irregular edges, instead of breaking into small pieces, because the collagen that is still present increases the bone's tensile strength, and the water absorbs and dissipates some energy (viscoelasticity) (Christensen et al., 2014; Ortner, 2008b). In contrast, dry bone is much more brittle than fresh bone; thus it tends to break into small pieces rather than splinter, and produces straight regular fractured edges (Ortner, 2008b; Sauer, 1998). In addition, perimortem fractures usually show no color difference between the broken bone area and the surrounding area, whereas postmortem fractures usually have lighter-colored edges compared to surrounding bone (Ubelaker and Adams, 1995).

8.10 JOINT DISEASE

Joint diseases are among the most common pathologies found in human skeletal remains. They are often differentiated into *proliferative* and *erosive* depending upon whether their primary skeletal manifestation is new bone formation or resorption (Ortner, 2003).

8.10.1 Proliferative Arthropathies

8.10.1.1 Osteoarthritis

Osteoarthritis (OA) is the most common joint disease found in archaeological material. It affects the synovial joints, that is, joints where the articulating elements are enclosed in a fibrous joint capsule and great mobility is allowed between them, such as the knee and shoulder. OA results from the destruction of articular cartilage and the subsequent direct contact between articular surfaces. According to its etiology, OA is classified as *primary* or *secondary*. Primary OA occurs later in life as a result of a combination of factors that include sex, age, mechanical stress, genetic predisposition, and others. In contrast, secondary OA develops earlier in life in joints that are abnormal because of other pathological conditions, such as trauma or infection (Rogers, 2000; Weiss and Jurmain, 2007). Box 8.10.1 presents the skeletal manifestations of OA, and a case of knee OA is given in Fig. 8.10.1.

BOX 8.10.1 Skeletal Manifestations of Osteoarthritis (Ortner, 2003; Rogers, 2000)

- Marginal osteophytes (bony lipping around the joint surface)
- Porosity or pitting on the joint surface
- Surface osteophytes (new bone formation on the joint surface)
- Alteration of the joint contour (e.g., widening and/or flattening)
- Eburnation (polished, ivory-like joint surface, occasionally with parallel grooves)

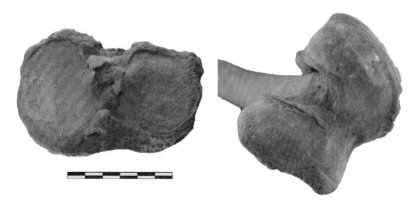

8.10.1.2 Spinal Osteoarthritis

The degenerative changes seen in the intervertebral joints are not actually OA, because OA by definition affects synovial joints, whereas intervertebral joints are amphiarthrodial, that is, cartilaginous joints that allow very limited mobility of the articulating elements (Jurmain, 1999). However, the skeletal response is very similar in both cases; thus spinal degenerative changes will also be classified as *osteoarthritis*. *Spinal OA* (Box 8.10.2) affects primarily the lumbar spine, followed by the cervical (Fig. 8.10.2). In contrast, the thoracic spine exhibits limited movement and, therefore, is less affected (Ortner, 2003).

BOX 8.10.2 Skeletal Manifestations of Spinal Osteoarthritis (Jurmain and Kilgore, 1995)

- Bony lipping (osteophytes) around the vertebral body edge
- Porosity on the vertebral body surface
- Bony lipping, porosity, and/or eburnation on the apophyseal joints
- Occasionally ankylosis

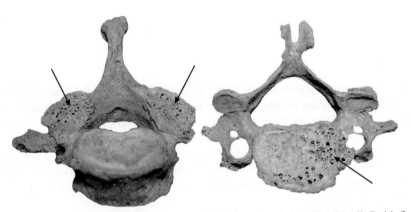

FIGURE 8.10.2 Osteoarthritis on the cervical vertebrae of an old adult male (A24.2003 Sk53) from St. Michael's Parish (Leicester, UK), dating to the Late Medieval period. Observe the extensive porosity/pitting on the apophyseal joint surfaces (left) and on the vertebral body (right), and marginal lipping in both cases.

8.10.1.3 Osteoarthritis as an Activity Marker

The age of onset of OA, as well as the frequency and location of the skeletal changes associated with it, has often been viewed as an activity marker in osteoarchaeological contexts, under the assumption that the development of OA was enhanced by an occupation that involved repetitive movements (see review in Jurmain, 1999). This assumption has been supported by studies of joint disease in athletes and in modern occupational groups; however, such studies have also highlighted the fact that there is no exclusive relationship between a specific form of OA and specific activities (Jurmain, 1999; Waldron, 2011). This is because age, sex, weight, genetic predisposition, nutrition, trauma, and other factors also greatly affect the pathogenesis of OA (see review in Weiss and Jurmain, 2007).

As was the case for OA in the appendicular skeleton, there has been extensive discussion on the extent to which spinal OA can be used to draw conclusions concerning daily activities of past populations. Based on clinical studies, the relationship between spinal OA and specific activity patterns is not a simple one (review in Conaghan, 2002), because spinal OA appears to be related to age, sex, genetic predisposition, body weight, endocrine status, or even bipedal posture (Knüsel et al., 1997; Meulenbelt et al., 2006; Spector and MacGregor, 2004). However, when Robson Brown et al. (2008) imposed compressive loads on cadaveric vertebrae of older individuals, they found a significant positive correlation between age, load bearing, and spinal OA, concluding that spinal OA can be studied as a predictor of load-bearing activities.

8.10.1.4 Diffuse Idiopathic Skeletal Hyperostosis

Diffuse idiopathic skeletal hyperostosis (Fig. 8.10.3 and Box 8.10.3) results from the ossification of the ligaments that run alongside and in parallel with the vertebral column, mainly the anterior longitudinal ligament, though in the thoracic region the condition affects the right side (Rogers and Waldron, 2001). Several etiologies have been proposed for the condition, most connecting it to advanced age and a high body mass index, as well as diabetes mellitus type 2, the metabolic syndrome, and gout (e.g., Kiss et al., 2002; Rogers and Waldron, 2001).

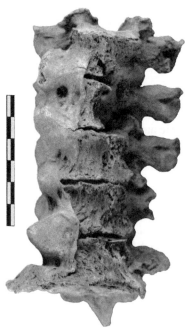

FIGURE 8.10.3 Diffuse idiopathic skeletal hyperostosis in five consecutive lower thoracic vertebrae (anterior view) of an individual (A2.2002 SK1057) from St. Peter's Parish (Leicester, UK), dating to the Late Medieval period. Observe the flowing "candle wax"-appearing bone formation on the right side of the vertebral bodies uniting all successive vertebrae.

BOX 8.10.3 Skeletal Manifestations of Diffuse Idiopathic Skeletal Hyperostosis (Kim et al., 2012)

- Flowing "candle wax"-appearing bone formation uniting at least three successive vertebral bodies
- No ossification in the intervertebral spaces
- No apophyseal joint ankylosis, sacroiliac or costovertebral joint fusion
- Ossification of extraspinal entheses, ligaments, and other soft tissues

---

8.10.2 Erosive Arthropathies

8.10.2.1 Erosive Osteoarthritis

Despite its name, *erosive OA* (Box 8.10.4) actually lies between the proliferative and the erosive forms of joint disease and occurs almost exclusively in females (Pattrick et al., 1989).

8.10.2.2 Rheumatoid Arthritis

Rheumatoid arthritis (Box 8.10.5) is a chronic autoimmune disease. Its cause remains unknown, although it is probably the result of some external stimulus (probably some infection) coupled with a genetic predisposition for the disease (Fox, 2001).

> **BOX 8.10.4 Skeletal Manifestations of Erosive Osteoarthritis (Waldron, 2011)**
>
> - Erosions in the small hand joints, especially the interphalangeal joints
> - Possible ankylosis

> **BOX 8.10.5 Skeletal Manifestations of Rheumatoid Arthritis (Mckinnon et al., 2013)**
>
> - Multiple joint involvement (primarily seen in hand and foot joints)
> - Erosive lesions—joint destruction and reduction of bone density

8.10.2.3 Ankylosing Spondylitis

Ankylosing spondylitis (Box 8.10.6) is a chronic autoimmune condition of unknown etiology. The disease typically affects entheses, producing erosions and bony ankylosis (Sieper et al., 2002).

> **BOX 8.10.6 Skeletal Manifestations of Ankylosing Spondylitis (Ortner, 2003)**
>
> - Ossification beneath and within the ligaments causing fusion of apophyseal, costovertebral, and sacroiliac joints
> - Ossification starting at the sacroiliac joint and lumbar vertebrae and spreading upward by means of syndesmophytes
> - Vertebral fusion can extend throughout the vertebral column or arrest at any point
> - Osteoporosis of vertebral bodies
> - Involvement of the appendicular skeleton (mainly the hips and shoulders) yielding ankylosis without pronounced osseous destruction
>
> *Note:* Syndesmophytes are vertically oriented, whereas osteophytes (typical in OA) have a horizontal orientation (Khan, 2002).

8.10.2.4 Gout

Gout (Box 8.10.7) results from a high concentration of uric acid in the blood (Waldron, 2011). The buildup of uric acid crystals within or around a joint produces inflammation, which results in cartilage and bone erosion (Roberts and Manchester, 2005). The condition is usually associated with obesity, high alcohol consumption, and hypertension (Weaver, 2008).

> **BOX 8.10.7 Skeletal Manifestations of Gout (Ortner, 2003; Rogers, 2000)**
>
> - Mostly affecting small joints and lower extremities (mainly the metatarsophalangeal joint of the great toe)
> - Well-defined lytic lesions with sclerotic margins
> - Penetration into the bone but not reaching the marrow cavity

8.11 DENTAL DISEASES

Because of their highly inorganic content, teeth are least susceptible to taphonomic degradation, therefore they provide permanent records of most of the pathological conditions that afflicted them. The reader may consult Lukacs (2011) for a review of the direction of dental disease research in osteoarchaeology.

8.11.1 Periodontal Disease

Periodontal disease can be classified into *gingivitis* and *periodontitis*. Gingivitis describes the inflammation of the gingivae, whereas periodontitis refers to the inflammation of the tissues attaching the teeth to alveolar bone, eventually resulting in tooth loss and alveolar bone resorption (Soames and Southam, 2005). Therefore, only periodontitis can be identified skeletally (Fig. 8.11.1). Periodontitis may lead to horizontal or vertical bone destruction, manifesting as alveolar septum atrophy and intraosseous pocket formation, respectively (Box 8.11.1) (Lavigne and Molto, 1995).

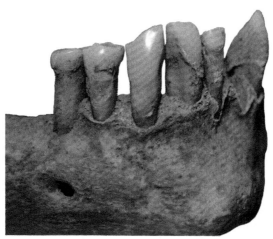

FIGURE 8.11.1   Periodontitis in the anterior mandibular teeth of an adult female (A2.2003 Sk1473) from St. Peter's Parish (Leicester, UK), dating to the Late Medieval period. Observe the combination of root exposure (large cementoenamel junction–alveolar crest distance), horizontal alveolar bone resorption, and porous septa.

BOX 8.11.1 Skeletal Manifestations of Periodontitis (Hillson, 2008)

- Horizontal or vertical bone destruction
- Cancellous bone exposure and rounded alveolar margins

Regarding its etiology, periodontal disease occurs when antigens are produced by microorganisms found in dental plaque. Specifically, the overgrowth of pathogenic species stimulates the production of host-produced inflammatory cytokines, chemokines, and mediators. However, the host leukocytes cannot discriminate between the invading bacteria and the host tissue, resulting in the collateral destruction of soft tissues and alveolar bone. If the condition progresses, it will end in tooth exfoliation (Cekici et al., 2014).

8.11.2 Caries

Caries is characterized by a progressive chemical dissolution of dental tissues (Box 8.11.2 and Fig. 8.11.2). The first macroscopic sign of caries is the appearance of a tiny opaque white or brown spot in the enamel surface. This is gradually enlarged and the enamel surface becomes rough, until a cavity forms. The cavity gradually increases in size until it reaches the dentinoenamel junction. Once the dentine is affected, reparative dentine is formed so that the pulp chamber is protected. Eventually, the infection spreads to the pulp, resulting in an inflammation of the periodontal tissues (Hillson, 2005). It must be noted that the progression of root caries is slightly different from that of the crown. Root caries manifests as a dark stain, which gradually increases in size until a cavity forms. As the cement layer covering the root is very thin, the dentine is easily affected by root caries; however, the pulp chamber is not as easily exposed to infection initiated in the root as it is in the crown (Hillson, 2008).

BOX 8.11.2 Dental Manifestations of Caries (Hillson, 2008; Selwitz et al., 2007)

- Lesions on the crown or root, ranging from slight discolorations to tooth cavities
- Larger lesion diameter within the tooth than on the surface

Note: Some scholars record caries as present only when there is a distinct cavity in the tooth (Belcastro et al., 2007).

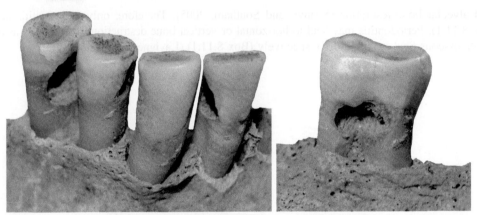

FIGURE 8.11.2 Interproximal caries in a middle adult female (A24.2003 Sk287) from St. Michael's Parish in mandibular anterior teeth (*left*) and root caries in the mandibular molar of a middle adult male (A2.2003 Sk1202) from St. Peter's Parish (*right*), both from Late Medieval Leicester, UK. In both cases observe how the cavity clearly penetrates the dentine, possibly also reaching the pulp chamber.

Carious lesions are the outcome of acids, which are released during the bacterial fermentation of dietary carbohydrates (Selwitz et al., 2007). As such, numerous studies have found an association between caries and diets rich in carbohydrates (e.g., Koca et al., 2006; Temple and Larsen, 2007). However, not all carbohydrates have the same cariogenicity. For example, sucrose is highly cariogenic (Oxenham et al., 2006), whereas starches seem generally to have a low cariogenicity (Hillson, 2008). In contrast, fats, oils, and fish are noncariogenic (Powell, 1988), and protein casein, which is present in milk products, appears to have a protective effect against caries (Mundorff-Shrestha et al., 1994).

Among the nondietary factors that affect caries prevalence are oral hygiene, hormonal levels, pregnancies, lactation, and maternal oral health (Lukacs, 2008; Shearer et al., 2011; Shuler, 2001). Composition and flow rate of the saliva are also influential, as many salivary functions have a protective effect against caries (Lukacs and Largaespada, 2006). At this point it must be stressed that the saliva flow rate is reduced with age, whereas it is generally slower in females compared to males (Dodds et al., 2005). These factors may explain to some extent the higher prevalence of caries among females and older individuals of either sex.

Food preparation also affects caries frequency. For instance, softening food through boiling increases its stickiness and cariogenicity (Larsen, 1995). The amount of time the food stays in the mouth is another important factor (the longer carbohydrates are in the mouth, the more likely they are to cause caries), as is the frequency of eating (more frequent meals imply the more frequent presence of food particles in the mouth). Finally, high levels of tooth wear have been associated with lower levels of caries as they eliminate fissures and mechanically remove food debris from the dental surfaces (Chazel et al., 2005; but see Hillson, 2001).

At this point it must be stressed that calculation of caries prevalence for interpopulation comparisons is often problematic for reasons briefly outlined in Box 8.11.3.

BOX 8.11.3 Caries Correction Factor

Dental caries rates in osteoarchaeological assemblages are usually calculated based on the number of observable carious teeth. However, this underestimates the actual prevalence of caries per assemblage as it does not take into account the number of teeth that have been lost antemortem because of severe caries. Various corrections have been proposed to address this issue, but the one mostly adopted is that suggested by Lukacs (1995):

Step 1. Estimation of the number of teeth lost because of caries:

N1 = (number of teeth lost antemortem) × (proportion of teeth with carious pulp exposure).

Step 2. Estimation of the total number of carious teeth:

N2 = N1 + (number of observed carious teeth).

Step 3. Estimation of the total number of original teeth:

N3 = (number of observed teeth) + (number of teeth lost antemortem).

Step 4. Estimation of the corrected caries rate:

Corrected caries rate = N2 + N3.

8.11.3 Dental Calculus

Dental calculus (Box 8.11.4) is mineralized plaque that accumulates at the deepest layers of a living plaque deposit and adheres to tooth surfaces (Fig. 8.11.3). It may develop above the gum (*supragingival*) or below it (*subgingival*) (Roberts and Manchester, 2005).

BOX 8.11.4 Dental Manifestations of Calculus (Hillson, 2008)

- Mineralized plaque deposits of variable size located above or below the gum
- White to light brown color
- Increasing thickness toward the tooth cervix

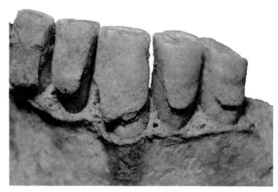

FIGURE 8.11.3   Thick dental calculus deposits on the labial surface of the mandibular anterior teeth of an old adult male (A24.2003 Sk53) from St. Michael's Parish (Leicester, UK), dating to the Late Medieval period.

The formation of calculus deposits is facilitated in alkaline oral environments. Since diets high in protein increase oral alkalinity, the presence of calculus is often interpreted as suggestive of a protein-rich diet (Lillie, 1996). However, high calculus rates have also been associated with high consumption of carbohydrates (Lieverse, 1999; Lillie and Richards, 2000). In any case, numerous factors additional to dietary patterns affect the formation of dental calculus. Such factors include salivary flow rate, calcium and phosphate concentrations in the blood, silicon content in food and water, and others (Lieverse, 1999). In addition, the act of chewing increases salivary flow rate, thus it may promote calculus formation (Dawes, 1970). At the same time chewing foodstuff with abrasive inclusions may mechanically remove calculus deposits. Similarly, dental calculus deposits may be removed by oral hygiene practices and the use of teeth as tools.

8.11.4 Periapical Cavities

Periapical cavities (Fig. 8.11.4) result from bacterial invasion in the exposed pulp cavity, the subsequent infection of the surrounding alveolar bone tissue through the root canal, and the localized collection of pus. Pulp chamber inflammation may be the outcome of excessive attrition, or dental caries, although it may occasionally result from enamel cracks after trauma. The pulp usually dies once it has been exposed to infection, although multirooted teeth may not die at once (Hillson, 2005; Ogden, 2007).

Traditionally, in the literature most periapical cavities have been characterized as *abscesses*. However, Dias and Tayles (1997) highlighted the fact that the term *abscess* is often used wrongly to refer to diverse types of apical cavities. The authors provide a detailed description of the process of periapical inflammation. Specifically, they note that the most common chronic inflammatory response is the formation of a *periapical granuloma*. Over time, the granuloma may develop into an *apical periodontal cyst*. Alternatively, if the infection is severe and involves pyogenic organisms, an *acute periapical abscess* will form. This may result from acute infection of the pulp or, more commonly, establish secondarily in a preexisting granuloma or cyst. If the infection causing an acute abscess is not fully overcome, the *abscess* may become *chronic*. On rare occasions an acute abscess will develop into *acute* or *chronic osteomyelitis* (Box 8.11.5).

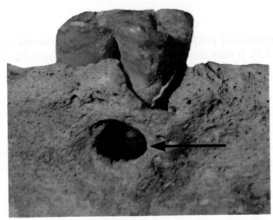

FIGURE 8.11.4 Periapical granuloma associated with a carious mandibular molar in an old adult male (A2.2003 Sk250) from St. Peter's Parish (Leicester, UK), dating to the Late Medieval period. Observe the smooth walls and small diameter of the lesion.

BOX 8.11.5 Skeletal Manifestations of Periapical Cavities (Dias and Tayles, 1997; Dias et al., 2007)

- Periapical granuloma
  - Smooth walls
  - Circumscribed cavity margins
  - Cavity diameter <3 mm
- Periodontal cyst
  - Smooth walls
  - Circumscribed cavity margins
  - Cavity diameter >3 mm
- Acute abscess developing secondarily within a granuloma or cyst
  - Slightly roughened walls

- Primary, chronic abscess
  - Cavity diameter <3 mm
  - Clearly roughened walls and ragged margins
  - Draining sinus leading to the subperiosteal surface or into a maxillary sinus
- Chronic osteomyelitis
  - Cavity with roughened margins, involving a large irregular area
  - Necrotic bone with involucrum
  - Multiple draining sinuses

8.11.5 Antemortem Tooth Loss

Antemortem tooth loss is the exfoliation of teeth while the individual was still alive (Fig. 8.11.5) (Hildebolt and Molnar, 1991). The condition manifests as resorption of the alveolus and it is multifactorial, primarily resulting from the progression of other dental diseases, such as caries and periodontitis, nutritional deficiency, excessive dental wear, trauma, or cultural ablation (Bonfiglioli et al., 2003; Cucina and Tiesler, 2003; Hillson, 2008; Pietrusewsky and Douglas, 1993).

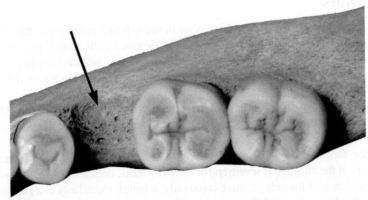

FIGURE 8.11.5 Antemortem loss of right mandibular first molar in a possible young adult female (A2.2003 Sk433) from St. Peter's Parish (Leicester, UK), dating to the Late Medieval period. Observe the extensive bone remodeling that has completely obliterated the alveolus.

8.11.6 Enamel Hypoplasia

Enamel hypoplasia occurs when the growth of the organic matrix, which is subsequently mineralized to form enamel, is disturbed. The resulting defect may take the form of lines (Fig. 8.11.6), furrows, pits, or large areas of missing enamel (Hillson and Bond, 1997). Enamel hypoplasia is not a disease itself but a nonspecific stress indicator because a wide variety of stressors can cause hypoplastic defects, including nutritional stress, infectious diseases, stress associated with weaning, and others (King et al., 2005; Skinner and Goodman, 1992). Malnutrition and disease are the most commonly employed explanatory factors in archaeological material, and between them there is a strong interaction (Ogilvie and Trinkaus, 1990; Skinner and Goodman, 1992).

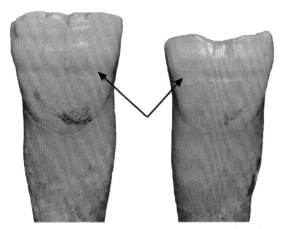

FIGURE 8.11.6 Linear enamel hypoplasia on the maxillary incisors of a young adult male (A2.2003 Sk1607) from St. Peter's Parish (Leicester, UK), dating to the Late Medieval period. Note that more linear hypoplastic defects are visible on the labial enamel surface but only the most pronounced ones are arrowed.

In addition to physiological stress, hereditary anomalies and localized trauma can also lead to enamel hypoplasia (Hillson, 2008). Defects due to systemic stress are likely to affect most teeth developing at the time of the stress; hypoplasia due to trauma or other localized factors will occur on one or adjacent teeth, whereas hereditary defects are usually severe and appear throughout the dentition (Skinner and Hung, 1989).

Because the enamel does not remodel once it is formed, lesions form during that part of childhood when the enamel of the tooth crown is developing (Goodman and Rose, 1991). The position of the enamel defects can subsequently give valuable information on the age at which the defects occurred (Box 8.11.6). In contrast, Hassett (2012) found no clear association between the defect dimensions and the severity and duration of the stressful episode that generated it.

8.12 CALCULATION OF DISEASE PREVALENCE AND STATISTICAL ANALYSIS

Two methods of estimating disease prevalence are adopted in osteoarchaeological studies: the *individual count method* and the *element count method*. The former estimates the ratio of the number of individuals affected by a pathological condition to the number of individuals that constitute the overall skeletal assemblage (number of affected individuals/total number of observable individuals). The latter approach is similar but uses skeletal elements rather than individuals as the unit of analysis (number of affected skeletal elements/total number of observable elements).

Each method gives different information, as the individual one offers insights into overall patterns between males and females, among different age groups, or between population samples, whereas the skeletal element method allows for greater resolution through the study of the patterning of the lesions within each skeleton. Therefore, ideally both approaches should be used and their results will complement each other. However, in cases of particularly poorly preserved remains or in commingled assemblages in which it is not possible to identify which elements belong to a single individual, the skeletal element method is the preferable, or even the only applicable, approach. The specific elements examined in each case will depend upon the pathological condition and the research questions. For example, in a study on OA, each major joint of the upper and lower limbs should be examined, but observations in the temporomandibular joint should also be included in the data set if the research question relates to masticatory stress or extramasticatory repetitive activities that involved the mouth.

BOX 8.11.6 Timing the Age of Formation of Linear Enamel Hypoplasia

Two principal methods have been proposed for aging linear enamel defects. The conventional approach uses the distance of a defect from the cementoenamel junction to estimate the age at time of development based on regression equations that assume a linear model of tooth growth (Goodman and Rose, 1990; Goodman et al., 1984; Rose et al., 1985). This approach has been criticized on the ground that it does not take into account the nonlinear rate of tooth growth, hidden cuspal enamel, and intra- and interpopulation differences in the rate of tooth growth, as well as intertooth crown height variation (Goodman and Song, 1999; King et al., 2005). More recent approaches allocate hypoplastic defects to broad developmental phases, based upon curvilinear models of enamel development (Reid and Dean, 2000, 2006; Reid et al., 2008). The following table is adapted from Reid and Dean (2006) and presents indicative stages of crown formation per age (in days) ± 1 SD, for the anterior teeth of South African and Northern European groups.

Stage of Tooth Growth	I^1	I^2	C^1	I_1	I_2	C_1
South African groups						
Cusp completion	284 ± 18	283 ± 19	339 ± 26	214 ± 23	223 ± 20	327 ± 21
20% of crown height	410 ± 23	416 ± 25	474 ± 35	317 ± 23	337 ± 28	480 ± 33
40% of crown height	569 ± 33	567 ± 31	646 ± 42	444 ± 30	478 ± 30	686 ± 46
60% of crown height	792 ± 36	781 ± 38	871 ± 49	625 ± 31	659 ± 37	961 ± 65
80% of crown height	1094 ± 44	1045 ± 44	1169 ± 48	883 ± 29	932 ± 46	1326 ± 68
Crown completion	1389 ± 30	1367 ± 36	1487 ± 42	1156 ± 31	1226 ± 26	1694 ± 56
Northern European groups						
Cusp completion	289 ± 16	274 ± 16	355 ± 24	256 ± 21	212 ± 21	348 ± 28
20% of crown height	441 ± 31	419 ± 22	515 ± 31	385 ± 28	335 ± 34	524 ± 32
40% of crown height	621 ± 53	583 ± 38	709 ± 42	528 ± 36	496 ± 45	771 ± 44
60% of crown height	913 ± 78	816 ± 47	962 ± 53	735 ± 44	727 ± 77	1119 ± 54
80% of crown height	1293 ± 65	1119 ± 52	1243 ± 63	911 ± 51	1056 ± 85	1581 ± 46
Crown completion	1708 ± 50	1478 ± 49	1672 ± 55	1309 ± 50	1376 ± 46	2066 ± 73

C, canines; I, incisors.

The statistical tests to be applied depend upon the recording scheme used per pathological condition. In general, given the multifactorial etiology of diseases, it is advisable to use multivariate tests that allow the study of the simultaneous impact of multiple factors (e.g., sex, age, ancestry, social status, etc.), such as generalized linear models (including logistic regression and generalized estimating equations). In cases in which the sample sizes are too small to allow for multivariate tests, simpler methods can be adopted, such as χ^2 tests (or Fisher's exact tests), Kruskal—Wallis test, and Mann—Whitney test. All the aforementioned statistical tests and their implementation have been discussed in the previous chapters, as well as in Chapter 9.

REFERENCES

Agarwal KN, Har ND, Shah MM. Roentgenologic changes in iron deficiency anemia. American Journal of Roentgenology 1970;110:635—7.

Allen LH. Pregnancy and iron deficiency: unresolved issues. Nutrition Reviews 1997;55:91—101.

Ambade VN, Godbole HV. Comparison of wound patterns in homicide by sharp and blunt force. Forensic Science International 2006;156:166—70.

Andersen JG, Manchester K. The rhinomaxillary syndrome in leprosy. A clinical, radiological and palaeopathological study. International Journal of Osteoarchaeology 1992;2:121—9.

Andersen JG, Manchester K, Roberts C. Septic changes in leprosy: a clinical, radiological and palaeopathological review. International Journal of Osteoarchaeology 1994;4:21—30.

Anderson CP, Martin DL, Thompson JL. Indigenous violence in Northern Mexico on the eve of contact. International Journal of Paleopathology 2012;2:93—101.

Appleby J, Thomas R, Buikstra J. Increasing confidence in paleopathological diagnosis — application of the Istanbul terminological framework. International Journal of Paleopathology 2015;8:19—21.

Armelagos GJ, Zuckerman MK, Harper KN. The science behind pre-Columbian evidence of syphilis in Europe: research by documentary. Evolutionary Anthropology 2012;21:50—7.

Armstrong S, Cloutier L, Arredondo C, Roksandic M, Matheson C. Spina bifida in a pre-Columbian Cuban population: a paleoepidemiological study of genetic and dietary risk factors. International Journal of Paleopathology 2013;3:19—29.

Arnay-de-la-Rosa M, González-Reimers E, Hernández-Marrero JC, Castañeyra-Ruiz M, Trujillo-Mederos A, González-Arnay E, Hernández-León CN. Cartilage-derived tumor in a prehispanic individual from La Gomera (Canary Islands). International Journal of Paleopathology 2015;11:66—9.

Arnott R, Finger S, Smith C, editors. Trepanation: history, discovery, theory. Lisse: Swets & Zeitlinger; 2003.

Aufderheide AC, Rodríguez-Martín C. The Cambridge encyclopedia of human paleopathology. Cambridge: Cambridge University Press; 1998.

Baker BJ, Bolhofner KL. Biological and social implications of a medieval burial from Cyprus for understanding leprosy in the past. International Journal of Paleopathology 2014;4:17—24.

Ballas SK, Lieff S, Benjamin LJ, Dampier CD, Heeney MM, Hoppe C, Johnson CS, Rogers ZR, Smith-Whitley K, Wang WC, Telen MJ. Definitions of the phenotypic manifestations of sickle cell disease. American Journal of Hematology 2010;85:6—13.

Barnes E. Atlas of developmental field anomalies of the human skeleton: a paleopathological perspective. New York: Wiley-Blackwell; 2012.

Bartelink EJ, Willits NA, Chelotti KL. A probable case of acromegaly from the Windmiller culture of prehistoric Central California. International Journal of Paleopathology 2014;4:37—46.

Belcastro G, Rastelli E, Mariotti V, Consiglio C, Facchini F, Bonfiglioli B. Continuity or discontinuity of the life-style in central Italy during the Roman imperial age-early middle ages transition: diet, health, and behavior. American Journal of Physical Anthropology 2007;132:381—94.

Bennike P, Lewis ME, Schutkowski H, Valentin F. Comparison of child morbidity in two contrasting medieval cemeteries from Denmark. American Journal of Physical Anthropology 2005;128:734—46.

Berry J, Davies M, Mee A. Vitamin D metabolism, rickets and osteomalacia. Seminars in Musculoskeletal Radiology 2002;6:173—81.

Berryman HE, Symes SA. Recognizing gunshot and blunt cranial trauma through fracture interpretation. In: Reichs K, editor. Forensic osteology: advances in the identification of human remains. Springfield: Charles C. Thomas; 1998. p. 333—52.

Berryman HE, Gunther WM. Keyhole defect production in tubular bone. Journal of Forensic Sciences 2000;45:483—7.

Blom DE, Buikstra JE, Keng L, Tomczak P, Shoreman E, Stevens-Tuttle D. Anemia and childhood mortality: latitudinal patterning along the coast of pre-Columbian Peru. American Journal of Physical Anthropology 2005;127:152—69.

Bonfiglioli B, Brasili P, Belcastro MG. Dento-alveolar lesions and nutritional habitus of a Roman Imperial age population (I—IV c.): Quadrella (Molise, Italy). HOMO-Journal of Comparative Human Biology 2003;54:36—56.

Boylston A. Evidence for weapon-related trauma in British archaeological samples. In: Cox M, Mays S, editors. Human osteology in archaeology and forensic science. London: Greenwich Medical Media Ltd.; 2000. p. 357—80.

Boylston A. Recording of weapon trauma. In: Brickley M, McKinley JI, editors. Guidelines to the standards for recording human remains. Reading and Southampton: British Association for Biological Anthropology and osteoarchaeology and Institute of Field Archaeologists; 2004. p. 40—2.

Brickley M, Ives R. Skeletal manifestations of infantile scurvy. American Journal of Physical Anthropology 2006;129:163—72.

Brickley M, Smith M. Culturally determined patterns of violence: biological anthropological investigations at a historic urban cemetery. American Anthropologist 2006;108:163—77.

Brickley M, Ives R. The bioarchaeology of metabolic bone disease. Oxford: Elsevier Academic Press; 2008.

Brickley M, Mays S, Ives R. An investigation of skeletal indicators of vitamin D deficiency in adults: effective markers for interpreting past living conditions and pollution levels in 18th and 19th century Birmingham, England. American Journal of Physical Anthropology 2007;132:67—79.

Bridges PS. Vertebral arthritis and physical activities in the prehistoric southeastern United States. American Journal of Physical Anthropology 1994;93:83—93.

Brooker S, Akhwale W, Pullan R, Estambale B, Clarke SE, Snow RW, Hotez PJ. Epidemiology of plasmodium-helminth co-infection in Africa: populations at risk, potential impact on anemia, and prospects for combining control. American Journal of Tropical Medicine and Hygiene 2007;77:88—98.

Brothwell DR. Tumours and tumour-like processes. In: Pinhasi R, Mays SA, editors. Advances in human palaeopathology. Chichester: John Wiley; 2007. p. 253—81.

Brothwell DR. Tumors: problems of differential diagnosis in paleopathology. In: Grauer AL, editor. A companion to paleopathology. Hoboken: Wiley-Backwell; 2011. p. 420—33.

Buikstra J, Ubelaker D, editors. Standards for data collection from human skeletal remains. Arkansas archaeological Survey research series no. 44. Fayetteville: Arkansas Archaeological Survey; 1994.

Byers SN. Introduction to forensic anthropology. 4th ed. Upper Saddle River: Pearson Education; 2010.

Capasso L, Di Tota G. Possible therapy for headaches in ancient times. International Journal of Osteoarchaeology 1996;6:316—9.

Castelo-Branco C, Reina F, Montivero AD, Colodron M, Vannell JA. Influence of high-intensity training and of dietetic and anthropometric factors on menstrual cycle disorders in ballet dancers. Gynecology and Endocrinology 2006;22:31—5.

Cekici A, Kantarci A, Haturk H, Van Dyke TE. Inflammatory and immune pathways in the pathogenesis of periodontal disease. Periodontology 2000 2014;64:57—80.

Chazel JC, Valcarel J, Tramini P, Pellisier B. Coronal and apical lesions, environmental factors: study in a modern and an archaeological population. Clinical Oral Investigations 2005;9:197—202.

Chen EM, Masih S, Chow K, Matcuk G, Patel D. Periosteal reaction: review of various patterns associated with specific pathology. Contemporary Diagnostic Radiology 2012;35:1—6.

Cholewicki J, McGill S. Mechanical stability of the in vivo lumbar spine: implications for injury and chronic low back pain. Clinical Biomechanics 1996;11:1—15.

Chosa E, Totoribe K, Tajima M. A biomechanical study of lombar spondylolysis based on a three-dimensional finite element method. Journal of Orthopaedic Research 2004;22:158—63.

Christensen AM, Passalacqua NV, Bartelink EJ. Forensic anthropology: current methods and practice. Amsterdam: Elsevier Academic Press; 2014.

Collins Cook D. Rhinomaxillary syndrome in the absence of leprosy: an exercise in differential diagnosis. In: Roberts CA, Lewis ME, Manchester K, editors. The past and present of leprosy: archaeological, historical, palaeopathological and clinical approaches. BAR International Series 1054. Oxford: Archaeopress; 2002. p. 81–8.

Conaghan PG. Update on osteoarthritis part 1: current concepts and the relation to exercise. British Journal of Sports Medicine 2002;36:330–3.

Cucina A, Tiesler V. Dental caries and antemortem tooth loss in the Northern Peten Area, Mexico: a biocultural perspective on social status differences among the Classic Maya. American Journal of Physical Anthropology 2003;122:1–10.

Dalati T. Isolated hyoid bone fracture: review of an unusual entity. International Journal of Oral and Maxillofacial Surgery 2005;34:449–52.

Dar G, Masharawi Y, Peleg S, Steinberg N, May H, Medlej B, Peled N, Hershkovitz I. Schmorl's nodes distribution in the human spine and its possible etiology. European Spine Journal 2010;19:670–5.

Davidson K, Davies C, Randolph-Quinney P. Skeletal trauma. In: Black S, Ferguson E, editors. Forensic anthropology 2000 to 2010. Boca Raton: CRC Press; 2011. p. 183–236.

Dawes C. Effects of diet on salivary secretion and composition. Journal of Dental Research 1970;70:1263–72.

Dawson H, Robson Brown K. Childhood tuberculosis: a probable case from late mediaeval Somerset, England. International Journal of Paleopathology 2012;2:31–5.

DeWitte SN, Stojanowski CM. The osteological paradox 20 years later: past perspectives, future directions. Journal of Archaeological Research 2015;23:397–450.

Dias G, Tayles N. 'Abscess cavity': a misnomer. International Journal of Osteoarchaeology 1997;7:548–54.

Dias GJ, Prasad K, Santos AL. Pathogenesis of apical periodontal cysts: guidelines for diagnosis in palaeopathology. International Journal of Osteoarchaeology 2007;17:619–26.

DiMaio V, DiMaio D. Forensic pathology. 2nd ed. Boca Raton: CRC Press; 2001.

Dobney K, Brothwell D. A method for evaluating the amount of dental calculus on teeth from archaeological sites. Journal of Archaeological Science 1987;14:343–51.

Dodds MWJ, Johnson DA, Yeh CK. Health benefits of saliva: a review. Journal of Dentistry 2005;33:223–33.

Dooley JR, Binford CH. Treponematoses. In: Binford CH, Connor D, editors. Pathology of tropical and extraordinary diseases: an atlas. Washington: Armed Forces Institute of Pathology; 1976. p. 110–7.

Erdal YS, Erdal ÖD. Organized violence in Anatolia: a retrospective research on the injuries from the Neolithic to early bronze age. International Journal of Paleopathology 2012;2:78–92.

Eren E, Yilmaz N. Biochemical markers of bone turnover and bone mineral density in patients with beta-thalassaemia major. International Journal of Clinical Practice 2005;59:46–51.

Eshed V, Latimer B, Greenwald CM, Jellema LM, Rothschild BM, Wish-Baratz S, Hershkovitz I. Button osteoma: its etiology and pathophysiology. American Journal of Physical Anthropology 2002;118:217–30.

Faccia KJ, Williams RC. Schmorl's nodes: clinical significance and implications for the bioarchaeological record. International Journal of Osteoarchaeology 2008;18:28–44.

Fédération Dentaire International. An epidemiological index of developmental defects of dental enamel (DDE). International Dental Journal 1982;32:159–67.

Fédération Dentaire International. A review of the developmental defects of enamel index (DDE index). International Dental Journal 1992;42:411–26.

Fibiger L, Knüsel C. Prevalence rates of spondylolysis in British skeletal populations. International Journal of Osteoarchaeology 2005;15:164–74.

Fiumara NJ, Fleming WL, Downing JG, Good FL. The incidence of prenatal syphilis at the Boston City Hospital. New England Journal of Medicine 1952;247:48–52.

Flensborg G, Suby JA, Martínez G. A case of adult osteomyelitis in a Final Late Holocene hunter-gatherer population, eastern Pampa–Patagonian transition, Argentina. International Journal of Paleopathology 2013;3:128–33.

Fox D. Etiology and pathogenesis of rheumatoid arthritis. In: Koopman W, editor. Arthritis and allied conditions: a textbook of rheumatology. 14th ed. Philadelphia: Lippincott Williams and Wilkins; 2001. p. 1085–102.

Frankel VH, Nordin M. Biomechanics of bone. In: Nordin M, Frankel VH, editors. Basic biomechanics of the musculoskeletal system. 3rd ed. Philadephia: Lippincott Williams and Wilkins; 2001. p. 26–59.

Fredrickson BE, Baker D, McHolick WJ, Yuan HA, Lubicky JP. The natural history of spondylolysis and spondylolisthesis. Journal of Bone and Joint Surgery 1984;66:699–707.

Frost HM. On changing views about age-related bone loss. In: Agarwal S, Stout SD, editors. Bone loss and osteoporosis. An anthropological perspective. New York: Kluwer Academic/Plenum Publishers; 2003. p. 19–31.

Gaither C. Cultural conflict and the impact on non-adults at Puruchuco-Huaquerones in Peru: the case for refinement of the methods used to analyze violence against children in the archeological record. International Journal of Paleopathology 2012;2:69–77.

Galloway A, editor. Broken bones: anthropological analysis of blunt force trauma. Springfield: Charles C. Thomas; 1999.

Garcin V, Velemínský P, Trefný P, Alduc-Le Bagousse A, Lefebvre A, Bruzek J. Dental health and lifestyle in four early mediaeval juvenile populations: comparisons between urban and rural individuals, and between coastal and inland settlements. HOMO – Journal of Comparative Human Biology 2010;61:421–39.

Geber J, Murphy E. Scurvy in the Great Irish famine: evidence of vitamin C deficiency from a mid-19th century skeletal population. American Journal of Physical Anthropology 2012;148:512−24.

Gilmore CC. A comparison of antemortem tooth loss in human hunter-gatherers and non-human catarrhines: implications for the identification of behavioral evolution in the human fossil record. American Journal of Physical Anthropology 2013;151:252−64.

Goodman AH, Rose JC. Assessment of systemic physiological perturbations from dental enamel hypoplasias and associated histological structures. Yearbook of Physical Anthropology 1990;33:59−110.

Goodman AH, Rose JC. Dental enamel hypoplasias as indicators of nutritional status. In: Kelley MA, Larsen CS, editors. Advances in dental anthropology. New York: Wiley-Liss; 1991. p. 279−94.

Goodman AH, Song R. Sources of variation in estimated ages at formation of linear enamel hypoplasias. In: Hoppa RD, FitzGerald CM, editors. Human growth in the past: studies from bones and teeth. Cambridge: Cambridge University Press; 1999. p. 210−40.

Goodman AH, Martin DL, Armelagos GJ, Clark G. Indicators of stress from bone and teeth. In: Cohen MN, Armelagos GJ, editors. Paleopathology at the origins of agriculture. Orlando: Academic Press; 1984. p. 13−49.

Gowland RL. Elder abuse: evaluating the potentials and problems of diagnosis in the archaeological record. International Journal of Osteoarchaeology 2016;26:514−23.

Grauer AL. Macroscopic analysis and data collection in palaeopathology. In: Pinhasi R, Mays S, editors. Advances in human palaeopathology. New York: Wiley; 2007. p. 57−76.

Gross M, Eliashar R. Hyoid bone fracture. Annals of Otology, Rhinology, Laryngology 2004;113:338−9.

Hackett CJ. The human treponematoses. In: Brothwell D, Sandison AT, editors. Diseases in antiquity: a survey of the diseases, injuries and surgery of early populations. Springfield: Charles C. Thomas; 1967. p. 152−69.

Hackett C. Diagnostic criteria of syphilis, yaws and treponarid (treponematosis) and of some other diseases in dry bone (for use in osteoarchaeology). Berlin: Springer-Verlag; 1976.

Hadley C, DeCaro JA. Brief Communication: does moderate iron deficiency protect against childhood illness? A test of the optimal iron hypothesis in Tanzania. American Journal of Physical Anthropology 2015;157:675−9.

Halcrow SE, Harris NJ, Beavan N, Buckley HR. First bioarchaeological evidence of probable scurvy in Southeast Asia: multifactorial etiologies of vitamin C deficiency in a tropical environment. International Journal of Paleopathology 2014;5:63−71.

Harkess J, Ramsey W, Harkess J. Principles of fractures and dislocations. In: Rockwood Jr C, Green D, Bucholz R, Heckman J, editors. Fractures in adults. 4th ed. Philadelphia: Lippincott-Raven; 1996. p. 3−120.

Hart GO. Fracture pattern interpretation in the skull: differentiating blunt force from ballistics trauma using concentric fractures. Journal of Forensic Sciences 2005;50:1276−81.

Hassett BR. Evaluating sources of variation in the identification of linear hypoplastic defects of enamel: a new quantified method. Journal of Archaeological Science 2012;39:560−5.

Helfrich MH. Osteoclast diseases. Microscopy Research and Technique 2003;61:514−32.

Henderson ED, Dahlin DC. Chondrosarcoma of bone - a study of two hundred and eighty-eight cases. The Journal of Bone & Joint Surgery 1963;45:1450−8.

Hengen OP. Cribra orbitalia: pathogenesis and probable etiology. HOMO-Journal of Comparative Human Biology 1971;22:57−76.

Hershkovitz I, Rothschild BM, Latimer B, Dutour O, Léonetti G, Greenwald CM, Rothschild C, Jellema LM. Recognition of sickle cell anemia in skeletal remains of children. American Journal of Physical Anthropology 1997;104:213−26.

Hildebolt CF, Molnar S. Measurement and description of periodontal disease in anthropological studies. In: Kelley MA, Larsen CS, editors. Advances in dental anthropology. New York: Wiley-Liss; 1991. p. 225−40.

Hillson S. Recording dental caries in archaeological human remains. International Journal of Osteoarchaeology 2001;11:249−89.

Hillson S. Teeth. Cambridge: Cambridge University Press; 2005.

Hillson S. Dental pathology. In: Katzenberg MA, Saunders SR, editors. Biological anthropology of the human skeleton. New York: Wiley-Liss; 2008. p. 301−40.

Hillson S, Bond S. Relationship of enamel hypoplasia to the pattern of tooth crown growth: a discussion. American Journal of Physical Anthropology 1997;104:89−103.

Ho YS, Gargano M, Cao J, Bronson RT, Heimler I, Hutz RJ. Reduced fertility in female mice lacking copper-zinc superoxide dismutase. The Journal of Biological Chemistry 1998;273:7765−9.

Holick MF. Vitamin D: a millennium perspective. Journal of Cellular Biochemistry 2003;88:296−307.

Holick MF. Resurrection of vitamin D deficiency and rickets. Journal of Clinical Investigation 2006;116:2062−72.

Holick MF, Adams J. Vitamin D metabolism and biological function. In: Avioli L, Krane S, editors. Metabolic bone disease and clinically related disorders. 3rd ed. San Diego: Academic Press; 1997. p. 123−64.

Holland EJ. Bringing childhood health into focus: incorporating survivors into standard methods of investigation [Ph.D. dissertation]. Toronto: University of Toronto; 2013.

Holland TD, O'Brian MJ. Parasites, porotic hyperostosis and the implications of changing perspectives. American Antiquity 1997;62:183−93.

Holloway KL, Henneberg RJ, de Barros Lopes M, Henneberg M. Evolution of human tuberculosis: a systematic review and meta-analysis of paleopathological evidence. HOMO-Journal of Comparative Human Biology 2011;62:402−58.

Ikpeme IA, Ngim NE, Ikpeme AA. Diagnosis and treatment of pyogenic bone infections. African Health Sciences 2010;10:82−8.

Ives R. Vitamin D deficiency osteomalacia in a historic urban collection. An investigation of age, sex and lifestyle-related variables. Paleopathology Association Newsletter 2005;130:6−15.

Ives R, Brickley M. New findings in the identification of adult vitamin D deficiency osteomalacia: results from a large-scale study. International Journal of Paleopathology 2014;7:45−56.

Jiménez-Brobeil SA, du Souich P, Al Oumaoui I. Possible relationship of cranial traumatic injuries with violence in the south-east Iberian Peninsula from the Neolithic to the Bronze Age. American Journal of Physical Anthropology 2009;140:465−75.

Jiménez-Brobeil SA, Al Oumaoui I, Du Souich P. Some types of vertebral pathologies in the Argar culture (Bronze Age, SE Spain). Internation Journal of Osteoarchaeology 2010;20:36−46.

Jopling WH, McDougall AC. Handbook of leprosy. 4th ed. Oxford: William Heinemann Medical Books; 1988.

Judd MA. Trauma in Ancient Nubia during the Kerma period (ca. 2500−1500 BC) [Ph.D. Dissertation]. University of Alberta; 2000.

Juengst SL, Chávez SJ. Three trepanned skulls from the Copacabana Peninsula in the Titicaca basin, Bolivia (800 BC−AD 1000). International Journal of Paleopathology 2015;9:20−7.

Jurmain R. Stories from the skeleton. Behavioral reconstruction in human osteology. King's Lynn: Gordon and Breach; 1999.

Jurmain R, Kilgore L. Skeletal evidence of osteoarthritis: a palaeopathological perspective. Annals of the Rheumatic Diseases 1995;54:443−50.

Käkönen S, Mundy G. Mechanisms of osteolytic bone metastases in breast carcinoma. Cancer 2003;97:834−9.

Kanjou Y, Kuijt I, Erdal YS, Kondon O. Early human decapitation, 11,700−10, 700 cal BP, within the pre-Pottery Neolithic village of Tell Qaramel, north Syria. International Journal of Osteoarchaeology 2015;25:743−52.

Keenleyside A. Sagittal clefting of the fifth lumbar vertebra of a young adult female from Apollonia Pontica, Bulgaria. International Journal of Osteoarchaeology 2015;25:234−7.

Kerr NW. A method of assessing periodontal status in archaeologically derived skeletal material. Journal of Paleopathology 1988;2:67−78.

Khan MA. Ankylosing spondylitis: introductory comments on its diagnosis and treatment. Annals of the Rheumatic Diseases 2002;61:iii3−7.

Kim MJ, Lee IS, Kim Y-S, Oh CS, Park JB, Shin MH, Shin DH. Diffuse idiopathic skeletal hyperostosis cases found in Joseon Dynasty human sample collection of Korea. International Journal of Osteoarchaeology 2012;22:235−44.

Kimmerle EH, Baraybar JP, editors. Skeletal trauma: identification of injuries resulting from human rights abuse and armed conflict. Boca Raton: CRC Press; 2008.

King T, Humphrey LT, Hillson S. Linear enamel hypoplasias as indicators of systemic physiological stress: evidence from two known age-at-death populations from postmedieval London. American Journal of Physical Anthropology 2005;128:547−59.

Kiss C, Szilágyi M, Paksy A, Poór G. Risk factors for diffuse idiopathic skeletal hyperostosis: a case−control study. Rheumatology 2002;41:27−30.

Klaus HD. Subadult scurvy in Andean South America: evidence of vitamin C deficiency in the late pre-Hispanic and colonial Lambayeque Valley, Peru. International Journal of Paleopathology 2014;5:34−45.

Klaus HD. Paleopathological rigor and differential diagnosis: case studies involving terminology, description, and diagnostic frameworks for scurvy in skeletal remains. International Journal of Paleopathology 2016. http://dx.doi.org/10.1016/j.ijpp.2015.10.002 (in press).

Klaus HD, Ortner DJ. Treponemal infection in Peru's Early Colonial period: a case of complex lesion patterning and unusual funerary treatment. International Journal of Paleopathology 2014;4:25−36.

Knüsel C, Göggel S, Lucy D. Comparative degenerative joint disease of the vertebral column in the medieval monastic cemetery of the Gilbertine Priory of St. Andrew, Fishergate, York, England. American Journal of Physical Anthropology 1997;103:481−95.

Koca B, Guleç E, Gultekin T, Akin G, Gungor K, Brooks SL. Implications of dental caries in Anatolia: from hunting-gathering to the present. Human Evolution 2006;21:215−22.

Komar DA, Buikstra JE. Forensic anthropology. Contemporary theory and practice. Oxford: Oxford University Press; 2007.

Kozłowski T, Witas HW. Metabolic and endocrine diseases. In: Grauer AL, editor. A companion to paleopathology. Oxford: Wiley-Blackwell; 2011. p. 401−19.

Kroman A, Kress T, Porta D. Fracture propagation in the human cranium: a re-testing of popular theories. Clinical Anatomy 2011;24:309−18.

Labbé JL, Peres O, Leclair O, Goulon R, Scemama P, Jourdel F, Menager C, Duparc B, Lacassin F. Acute osteomyelitis in children: the pathogenesis revisited? Orthopaedics & Traumatology, Surgery & Research 2010;96:268−75.

Lagia A, Eliopoulos C, Manolis S. Thalassemia: macroscopic and radiological study of a case. International Journal of Osteoarchaeology 2007;17:269−85.

Larsen CS. Biological changes in human populations with agriculture. Annual Review of Anthropology 1995;24:185−213.

Larson ARU, Josephson KD, Pauli RM, Opitz JM, Williams MS. Klippel-Feil anomaly, omovertebral bone, thumb abnormalities, and flexion-crease changes: novel association or syndrome? American Journal of Medical Genetics 2001;101:158−62.

Lavigne SE, Molto JE. System of measurements of the severity of periodontal disease in past populations. International Journal of Osteoarchaeology 1995;5:265−73.

Le Fort R. Vtude expérimental sur les fractures de la machoire supérieure. Parts I, II, III. Revue de Chirurgie Paris 1901;23:208−27. 360−379, 479−507.

Lefort M, Bennike P. A case study of possible differential diagnoses of a medieval skeleton from Denmark: leprosy, ergotism, treponematosis, sarcoidosis or smallpox? International Journal of Osteoarchaeology 2007;17:337−49.

Lessa A, Mendonça De Souza S. Violence in the Atacama Desert during the Tiwanaku period: social tension? International Journal of Osteoarchaeology 2004;14:374−88.

Lewis ME. Impact of industrialization: comparative study of child health in four sites from medieval and postmedieval England (A.D. 850−1859). American Journal of Physical Anthropology 2002;119:211−23.

Lewis ME. Thalassaemia: its diagnosis and interpretation in past skeletal populations. International Journal of Osteoarchaeology 2012;22:685−93.

Lieverse AR. Diet and the aetiology of dental calculus. International Journal of Osteoarchaeology 1999;9:219−32.

Lieverse AR, Link DW, Bazaliiskiy VI, Goriunova OI, Weber AW. Dental health indicators of hunter-gatherer adaptation and cultural change in Siberia's Cis-Baikal. American Journal of Physical Anthropology 2007;134:323−39.

Lillie MC. Mesolithic and Neolithic populations of Ukraine: indications of diet from dental pathology. Current Anthropology 1996;37:135−42.

Lillie MC, Richards M. Stable isotope analysis and dental evidence of diet at the Mesolithic−Neolithic transition in Ukraine. Journal of Archaeological Science 2000;27:965−72.

Listi GA. Bioarchaeological analysis of diet during the Coles Creek period in the Southern Lower Mississipi Valley. American Journal of Physical Anthropology 2011;144:30−40.

Littleton J. Invisible impacts but long-term consequences: hypoplasia and contact in Central Australia. American Journal of Physical Anthropology 2005;126:295−304.

Lovell NC. Trauma analysis in paleopathology. Yearbook of Physical Anthropology 1997;40:139−70.

Lovell NC. Paleopathological description and diagnosis. In: Katzenberg M, Saunders S, editors. Biological anthropology of the human skeleton. New York: Wiley-Liss; 2000. p. 217−48.

Lovell NC. Analysis and interpretation of trauma. In: Katzenberg M, Saunders S, editors. Biological anthropology of the human skeleton. 2nd ed. New York: Wiley-Liss; 2008. p. 341−86.

Lukacs JR. Dental paleopathology: methods for reconstructing dietary patterns in prehistory. In: İşcan MY, Kennedy KAR, editors. Reconstruction of life from the skeleton. New York: Alan R. Liss; 1989. p. 261−86.

Lukacs JR. The 'caries correction factor': a new method of calibrating dental caries rates to compensate for antemortem loss of teeth. International Journal of Osteoarchaeology 1995;5:151−6.

Lukacs JR. Fertility and agriculture accentuate sex differences in dental caries rates. Current Anthropology 2008;49:901−14.

Lukacs JR. Sex differences in dental caries experience: clinical evidence and complex etiology. Clinical Oral Investigations 2011;15:649−56.

Lukacs JR, Largaespada L. Explaining sex differences in dental caries prevalence: saliva, hormones, and life-history etiologies. American Journal of Human Biology 2006;18:540−55.

Lynch SR. Interaction of iron with other nutrients. Nutrition Reviews 1997;55:102−10.

Manchester K. Infective bone changes in leprosy. In: Roberts CA, Lewis ME, Manchester K, editors. The past and present of leprosy. Archaeological, historical, palaeopathological and clinical approaches. BAR International Series 1054. Oxford: Archaeopress; 2002. p. 69−72.

Matos V, Santos AL. On the trail of pulmonary tuberculosis based on rib lesions: results from the human identified skeletal collection from the Museu Bocage (Lisbon, Portugal). American Journal of Physical Anthropology 2006;130:190−200.

Mays S. Spondylolysis, spondylolisthesis, and lumbo-sacral morphology in a Medieval English skeletal population. American Journal of Physical Anthropology 2006;131:352−62.

Mays S. A likely case of scurvy from early bronze age Britain. International Journal of Osteoarchaeology 2008;18:178−87.

Mays S, Brickley M, Ives R. Skeletal manifestations of rickets in infants and young children in a historic population from England. American Journal of Physical Anthropology 2006;129:362−74.

McIlvaine BK. Implications of reappraising the iron-deficiency anemia hypothesis. International Journal of Osteoarchaeology 2015;25:997−1000.

Mckinnon K, Van Twest MS, Hatton M. A probable case of rheumatoid arthritis from the middle Anglo-Saxon period. International Journal of Paleopathology 2013;3:122−7.

Melmed S. Acromegaly. The New England Journal of Medicine 2006;355:2558−73.

Mensforth R, Lovejoy C, Lallo J, Armelagos G. The role of constitutional factors, diet, and infectious disease in the etiology of porotic hyperostosis and periosteal reactions in prehistoric infants and children. Medical Anthropology 1978;2:1−59.

Merbs CF. Spondylolysis and spondylolisthesis: a cost of being an erect biped or a clever adaptation? Yearbook of Physical Anthropology 1996;39:201−28.

Merbs CF. Degenerative spondylolisthesis in ancient and historic skeletons from New Mexico Pueblo sites. American Journal of Physical Anthropology 2001;116:285−95.

Merbs CF. Sagittal clefting of the body and other vertebral developmental errors in Canadian Inuit skeletons. American Journal of Physical Anthropology 2004;123:236−49.

Meulenbelt I, Kloppenburg M, Kroon HM, Houwing-Duistermaat JJ, Garnero P, Hellio Le Graverand MP, Degroot J, Slagboom PE. Urinary CTX-II levels are associated with radiographic subtypes of osteoarthritis in hip, knee, hand, and facet joints in subject with familial osteoarthritis at multiple sites: the GARP study. Annals of the Rheumatic Diseases 2006;65:360−5.

Miles AEW. Two shoulder-joint dislocations in early 19th century Londoners. International Journal of Osteoarchaeology 2000;10:125−34.

Miller M, Miller JH. Orthopaedics and accidents. London: Hodder & Stoughton; 1985.

Milner GR, Boldsen JL, Weise S, Lauritsen JM, Freund UH. Sex-related risks of trauma in medieval to early modern Denmark, and its relationship to change in interpersonal violence over time. International Journal of Paleopathology 2015;9:59−68.

Mirra J, Brien E, Tehranzadeh J. Paget's disease of bone: review with emphasis on radiologic features, part I. Skeletal Radiology 1995;24:163−71.

Mitchell PD. Pre-Columbian treponemal disease from 14th century AD Safed, Israel and implications for the medieval eastern Mediterranean. American Journal of Physical Anthropology 2003;121:117−24.

Moghaddam N, Mailler-Burch S, Kara L, Kanz F, Jackowski C, Lösch S. Survival after trepanation-early cranial surgery from late iron age Switzerland. International Journal of Paleopathology 2015;11:56–65.

Møller-Christensen V. Bone changes in leprosy. Copenhagen: Munksgaard; 1961.

Møller-Christensen V. Leprosy changes of the skull. Odense: Odense University Press; 1978.

Moore WJ, Corbett ME. The distribution of dental caries in ancient British populations 1. Anglo-Saxon period. Caries Research 1971;5:151–68.

Moschella SL. An update on the diagnosis and treatment of leprosy. Journal of the American Academy of Dermatology 2004;51:417–26.

Mosekilde L. Vitamin D and the elderly. Clinical Endocrinology 2005;62:265–81.

Moseley JE. Skeletal changes in the anemias. Seminars in Roentgenology 1974;9:169–84.

Moskalenko YuE, Weinstein GB, Kravchenko TI, Mozhaev SV, Semernya VN, Feilding A, Halvorson P, Medvedev SV. The effect of craniotomy on the intracranial hemodynamics and cerebrospinal fluid dynamics in humans. Fizlogiya Cheloveka 2008;34:41–8.

Mundorff-Shrestha SA, Featherstone JD, Eisenberg AD, Cowles E, Curzon ME, Espeland MA, Shields CP. Cariogenic potential of foods. II. Relationship of food composition, plaque microbial counts, and salivary parameters to caries in the rat model. Caries Research 1994;28:106–15.

Murphy EM, McKenzie CJ. Multiple osteochondromas in the archaeological record: a global review. Journal of Archaeological Science 2010;37:2255–64.

Nathan H, Haas N. On the presence of cribra orbitalia in apes and monkeys. American Journal of Physical Anthropology 1966;24:351–9.

Nikita E, Lahr MM, Mattingly D. Evidence of trephinations among the Garamantes, a late Holocene Saharan population. International Journal Osteoarchaeology 2013;23:370–7.

Nikitovic D, Janković I, Mihelić S. Juvenile elbow dislocation from the prehistoric site of Josipovac–Gravinjak, Croatia. International Journal of Paleopathology 2012;2:36–41.

Nöbauer I, Uffmann M. Differential diagnosis of focal and diffuse neoplastic diseases of bone marrow in MRI. European Journal of Radiology 2005;55:2–32.

Ogden JA. Skeletal injury in the child. 3rd ed. New York: Springer; 2000.

Ogden A. Advances in the paleopathology of teeth and jaws. In: Pinhasi R, Mays S, editors. Advances in human palaeopathology. Chichester: Wiley; 2007. p. 283–307.

Ogilvie MD, Trinkaus E. Reply to Neiburger. American Journal of Physical Anthropology 1990;82:231–3.

Orr F, Lee J, Duivenvoorden W, Singh G. Pathophysiologic interaction in skeletal metastasis. Cancer 2000;88:2912–8.

Ortner DJ. Identification of pathological conditions in human skeletal remains. 2nd ed. Amsterdam: Academic Press; 2003.

Ortner DJ. Differential diagnosis of skeletal lesions in infectious disease. In: Pinhasi R, Mays S, editors. Advances in human palaeopathology. Chichester: John Wiley & Sons; 2008a. p. 191–215.

Ortner DJ. Differential diagnosis of skeletal injuries. In: Kimmerle E, Baraybar J, editors. Skeletal trauma: identification of injuries resulting from human rights abuse and armed conflict. Boca Raton: CRC Press; 2008b. p. 21–87.

Ortner DJ. Human skeletal paleopathology. International Journal of Paleopathology 2011;1:4–11.

Ortner D, Butler W, Cafarella J, Milligan L. Evidence of probable scurvy in subadults from archeological sites in North America. American Journal of Physical Anthropology 2001;114:343–51.

Ortner DJ, Ponce P, Ogden A, Buckberry J. Multicentric osteosarcoma associated with DISH, in a 19th century burial from England. International Journal Osteoarchaeology 2012;22:245–52.

Ostendorf Smith M, Betsinger TK, Williams LL. Differential visibility of treponemal disease in pre-Columbian stratified societies: does rank matter? American Journal of Physical Anthropology 2011;144:185–95.

Oxenham MF, Cavill I. Porotic hyperostosis and cribra orbitalia: the erythropoietic response to iron-deficiency anemia. Anthropological Science 2010;118:199–200.

Oxenham MF, Nguyen LC, Nguyen KT. The oral health consequences of the adoption and intensification of agriculture in Southeast Asia. In: Oxenham M, Tayles N, editors. Bioarchaeology of Southeast Asia. Cambridge: Cambridge University Press; 2006. p. 263–89.

Pattrick M, Aldridge S, Hamilton E, Manhire A, Doherty M. A controlled study of hand function in nodal and erosive osteoarthritis. Annals of the Rheumatic Diseases 1989;48:978–82.

Perry MA. Tracking the second epidemiological transition using bioarchaeological data on infant morbidity and mortality. In: Zuckerman MK, editor. Modern environments and human health: revisiting the second epidemiological transition. Hoboken: Wiley-Blackwell; 2014. p. 225–41.

Pietrusewsky M, Douglas MT. Tooth ablation in old Hawai'i. Journal of the Polynesian Society 1993;102:255–72.

Pilloud MA, Canzonieri C. The occurrence and possible aetiology of spondylolysis in a pre-contact California population. International Journal of Osteoarchaeology 2014;24:602–13.

Pimentel L. Scurvy: historical review and current diagnostic approach. The American Journal of Emergency Medicine 2003;21:328–32.

Plomp K, Roberts C, Vidarsdottir US. Does the correlation between Schmorl's nodes and vertebral morphology extend into the lumbar spine? American Journal of Physical Anthropology 2015;157:526–34.

Powell ML. Status and health in prehistory. A case study of the Moundville Chiefdom. Washington: Smithsonian Institution Press; 1988.

Reid DJ, Dean MC. Timing of linear enamel hypoplasias on human anterior teeth. American Journal of Physical Anthropology 2000;113:135–9.

Reid DJ, Dean MC. Variation in modern human enamel formation times. Journal of Human Evolution 2006;50:329–46.

Reid DJ, Guatelli-Steinberg D, Walton P. Variation in modern human premolar enamel formation times: implications for Neandertals. Journal of Human Evolution 2008;54:225—35.

Riggs BL, Khosla S, Melton III LJ. A unitary model for involutional osteoporosis: Estrogen deficiency causes both type I and type II osteoporosis in postmenopausal women and contributes to bone loss in aging men. Journal of Bone and Mineral Research 1998;13:763—73.

Riggs BL, Melton III LJ, Robb RA, Camp JJ, Atkinson EJ, Oberg AL, Rouleau PA, McCollough CH, Khosla S, Bouxsein ML. Population-based analysis of the relationship of whole bone strength indices and fall-related loads to age and sex-specific patterns of hip and wrist fractures. Journal of Bone and Mineral Research 2006;21:315—23.

Rizzoli R, Bonjour JP. Dietary protein and bone health. Journal of Bone and Mineral Research 2004;19:527—31.

Roberts CA. Infectious disease in biocultural perspective: past, present and future work in Britain. In: Cox M, Mays S, editors. Human osteology in archaeology and forensic science. London: Greenwich Medical Media; 2000. p. 145—62.

Roberts C. Re-emerging infections: developments in bioarchaeological contributions to understanding tuberculosis today. In: Grauer AL, editor. Companion to paleopathology. New York: Wiley-Blackwell; 2011. p. 434—57.

Roberts CA, Buikstra JE. The bioarchaeology of tuberculosis: a global view on a reemerging disease. Gainesville: University Press of Florida; 2003.

Roberts C, Manchester K. The archaeology of disease. 3rd ed. Gloucestershire: Sutton Publishing; 2005.

Robson Brown K, Pollintine P, Adams MA. Biomechanical implications of degenerative joint disease in the apophyseal joints of human thoracic and lumbar vertebrae. American Journal of Physical Anthropology 2008;136:318—26.

Rodan G, Raisz L, Bilezikian J. Pathophysiology of osteoporosis. In: Bilezikian J, Raisz L, Rodan G, editors. Principles of bone biology. 2nd ed. San Diego: Academic Press; 2002. p. 1275—89.

Rodríguez-Martín C. Identification and differential diagnosis of traumatic lesions of the skeleton. In: Schmitt A, Cunha E, Pinheiro J, editors. Forensic anthropology and medicine: complementary sciences from recovery to cause of death. Totowa: Humana Press; 2006. p. 197—221.

Rogers J. The palaeopathology of joint disease. In: Cox M, Mays S, editors. Human osteology in archaeology and forensic science. London: Greenwich Medical Media, Ltd; 2000. p. 163—82.

Rogers J, Waldron T. DISH and the monastic way of life. International Journal of Osteoarchaeology 2001;11:357—65.

Rojas-Sepúlveda C, Ardagna Y, Dutour O. Paleoepidemiology of vertebral degenerative disease in a Pre-Columbian Muisca series from Colombia. American Journal of Physical Anthropology 2008;135:416—30.

Rose JC, Condon KW, Goodman AH. Diet and dentition: developmental disturbances. In: Gilbert RI, Mielke JH, editors. The analysis of prehistoric diets. London: Academic Press; 1985. p. 281—306.

Saifuddin A, Hassan A. Paget's disease of the spine: unusual features and complications. Clinical Radiology 2003;58:102—11.

Sakai T, Sairyo K, Xuzue N, Kosaka H, Yasui N. Incidence and etiology of lumbar spondylolysis: review of the literature. Journal of Orthopaedic Science 2010;15:281—8.

Sauberlich HE. Pharmacology of vitamin C. Annual Review of Nutrition 1994;14:371—91.

Sauer NJ. The timing of injuries and manner of death: distinguishing among antemortem, perimortem and postmortem trauma. In: Reichs K, editor. Forensic osteology: advances in the identification of human remains. 2nd ed. Springfield: Charles C. Thomas; 1998. p. 321—32.

Schattmann A, Bertrand B, Vatteoni S, Brickley M. Approaches to co-occurrence: scurvy and rickets in infants and young children of 16—18th century Douai, France. International Journal of Paleopathology 2016;12:63—75.

Schultz M. Paleohistopathology of bone: a new approach to the study of ancient diseases. American Journal of Physical Anthropology 2001;33:106—47.

Selwitz RH, Ismail AI, Pitts NB. Dental caries. The Lancet 2007;369:51—9.

Shearer DSDM, Thomson WM, Broadbent JM, Poulton R. Maternal oral health predicts their children's caries experience in adulthood. Journal of Dental Research 2011;90:672—7.

Shuler CF. Inherited risks for susceptibility to dental caries. Journal of Dental Education 2001;65:1038—45.

Sieper J, Braun J, Rudwaleit M, Boonen A, Zinc A. Ankylosing spondylitis: an overview. Annals of the Rheumatic Diseases 2002;61(Suppl. III):iii8—18.

Sillence DO, Senn A, Danks DM. Genetic heterogeneity in osteogenesis imperfecta. Journal of Medical Genetics 1979;16:101—16.

Skinner MF, Hung JTW. Social and biological correlates of localized enamel hypoplasia of the human deciduous canine tooth. American Journal of Physical Anthropology 1989;79:159—75.

Skinner M, Goodman A. Anthropological uses of developmental defects of enamel. In: Saunders SR, Katzenberg MA, editors. Skeletal biology of past peoples: research methods. New York: Wiley-Liss; 1992. p. 153—74.

Smith-Guzmán NE. Cribra orbitalia in the ancient Nile Valley and its connection to malaria. International Journal of Paleopathology 2015;10:1—12.

Snoddy AM, Buckley HR, Halcrow SE. More than metabolic: considering the broader Paleoepidemiological impact of vitamin D deficiency in bioarchaeology. American Journal of Physical Anthropology 2016;160:183—96.

Soames JV, Southam JC. Oral pathology. 4th ed. Oxford: Oxford University Press; 2005.

Sofaer Derevenski JR. Sex differences in activity-related osseous change in the spine and the gendered division of labor at Ensay and Wharram, Percy, UK. American Journal of Physical Anthropology 2000;111:333—54.

Soler T, Calderon C. The prevalence of spondylolysis in the Spanish elite athlete. The American Journal of Sports Medicine 2000;28:57—62.

Spector TD, McGregor AJ. Risk factors for osteoarthritis: genetics. Osteoarthritis Cartilage 2004;12(Suppl. A):S39—44.

Stark RJ. A proposed framework for the study of paleopathological cases of subadult scurvy. International Journal of Paleopathology 2014;5:18—26.

Stieber JR, Dormans JP. Manifestations of hereditary multiple exostoses. Journal of the American Academy of Orthopaedic Surgery 2005;13:110−20.

Stodder ALW. Data and data analysis issues in paleopathology. In: Grauer AL, editor. A companion to paleopathology. Hoboken: Wiley-Backwell; 2011. p. 339−56.

Stoltzfus RJ, Dreyfuss ML, Chwaya HM, Albonico M. Hookworm control as a strategy to prevent iron deficiency. Nutrition Reviews 1997;55:223−32.

Stone AC, Wilbur AK, Buikstra JE, Roberts CE. Tuberculosis and leprosy in perspective. Yearbook of Physical Anthropology 2009;52:66−94.

Strohm TF, Alt KW. Periodontal disease-etiology, classification and diagnosis. In: Alt KW, Rösing FW, Teschler-Nicola M, editors. Dental anthropology. Fundamentals, limits and prospects. New York: Springer; 1998. p. 227−46.

Stuart-Macadam P. Porotic hyperostosis: representative of a childhood condition. American Journal of Physical Anthropology 1985;66:391−8.

Stuart-Macadam P. Nutritional deficiency diseases: a survey of scurvy, rickets, and iron-deficiency anemia. In: İşcan MY, Kennedy KAR, editors. Reconstruction of life from the skeleton. Fayetteville, Arkansas: Arkansas Archaeological Survey Report Number 44; 1989. p. 201−22.

Stuart-Macadam P. Porotic hyperostosis: a new perspective. American Journal of Physical Anthropology 1992;87:39−47.

Stuckert CM, Kricun ME. A case of bilateral forefoot amputation from the Romano-British cemetery of Lankhills, Winchester, UK. International Journal of Paleopathology 2011;1:111−6.

Sullivan A. Prevalence and etiology of acquired anemia in Medieval York, England. American Journal of Physical Anthropology 2005;128:252−72.

Symes SA, L'Abbé EN, Chapman EN, Wolff I, Dirkmaat DC. Interpreting traumatic injury to bone in medicolegal investigations. In: Dirkmaat D, editor. A companion to forensic anthropology. Chichester: Wiley-Blackwell; 2012. p. 340−89.

Temple DH, Larsen CS. Dental caries prevalence as evidence for agriculture and subsistence variation among the prehistoric Yayoi of Japan: biocultural interpretations of an economy in transition. American Journal of Physical Anthropology 2007;134:501−12.

Thoen C, LoBue P, de Kantor I. The importance of Mycobacterium bovis as a zoonosis. Veterinary Microbiology 2006;112:339−45.

Toyne JM. Possible cases of scalping from pre-Hispanic highland Peru. International Journal of Osteoarchaeology 2011;21:229−42.

Ubelaker DH. Hyoid fracture and strangulation. Journal of Forensic Sciences 1992;37:1216−22.

Ubelaker D, Adams B. Differentiation of perimortem and postmortem trauma using taphonomic indicators. Journal of Forensic Sciences 1995;40:509−12.

Verano JW. Differential diagnosis: trepanation. International Journal of Paleopathology 2016;14:1−9.

Voigt GE, Skold G. Ring fractures of the base of the skull. Journal of Trauma 1974;14:494−505.

Waldron T. Palaeopathology. Cambridge: Cambridge University Press; 2008.

Waldron T. Joint disease. In: Grauer AL, editor. A companion to paleopathology. New York: Wiley-Backwell; 2011. p. 513−30.

Walker PL, Bathurst RR, Richman R, Gjerdrum T, Andrushko VA. The causes of porotic hyperostosis and cribra orbitalia: a reappraisal of the iron-deficiency-anemia hypothesis. American Journal of Physical Anthropology 2009;139:109−25.

Wapler U, Crubézy E, Schultz M. Is cribra orbitalia synonymous with anemia? Analysis and interpretation of cranial pathology in Sudan. American Journal of Physical Anthropology 2004;123:333−9.

Weaver A. Epidemiology of gout. Cleveland Clinic Journal of Medicine 2008;75:S9−12.

Weber J, Wahl J. Neurosurgical aspects of trepanations from Neolithic times. International Journal of Osteoarchaeology 2006;16:536−5545.

Weinberg E. Iron withholding in prevention of disease. In: Stuart-Macadam P, Kent S, editors. Diet, demography, and disease: changing perspectives on anemia. New York: Aldine de Gruyter; 1992. p. 105−50.

Weiss E, Jurmain R. Osteoarthritis revisited: a contemporary review of aetiology. International Journal of Osteoarchaeology 2007;17:437−50.

Weston D. Investigating the specificity of periosteal reactions in pathology museum specimens. American Journal of Physical Anthropology 2008;137:48−59.

Weston DA. Nonspecific infection in palaeopathology: interpreting periosteal reactions. In: Grauer AL, editor. A companion to paleopathology. Chichester: Blackwell Publishing; 2011. p. 492−512.

Wheeler SM, Williams L, Beauchesne P, Dupras TL. Shattered lives and broken childhoods: evidence of physical child abuse in ancient Egypt. International Journal of Paleopathology 2013;3:71−82.

Whiting WC, Zernicke RF. Biomechanics of musculoskeletal injury. 2nd ed. Champaign: Human Kinetics; 2008.

Wilczak CA, Jones EB, editors. Osteoware™ software manual: volume II pathology module. Washington: Smithsonian Institution; 2011.

Williams FMK, Manek NJ, Sambrook P, Spector TD, MacGregor AJ. Schmorl's nodes: common, highly heritable, and related to lumbar disc disease. Arthritis and Rheumatism 2007;57:855−60.

Wood JW, Milner GR, Harpending HC, Weiss KM. The osteological paradox. Current Anthropology 1992;33:343−70.

Zäuner SP, Wahl J, Boyadziev Y, Aslanis I. A 6000-year-old hand amputation from Bulgaria-The oldest case from South-East Europe? International Journal of Osteoarchaeology 2013;23:618−25.

Zuckerman MK, Garofalo EM, Frohlich B, Ortner DJ. Anemia or scurvy: a pilot study on differential diagnosis of porous and hyperostotic lesions using differential cranial vault thickness in subadult humans. International Journal of Paleopathology 2014;5:27−33.

APPENDICES

Appendix 8.I: Recording Schemes for Common Pathological Conditions

Given the nonspecific skeletal manifestation of most diseases, it is advisable to record in detail any observable abnormality in the form of new bone formation, bone loss, or abnormal bone shape or size. The categories suggested by Ortner (2003) or Buikstra and Ubelaker (1994) could be used for this purpose. This appendix proposes representative recording standards for rather common skeletal pathological conditions, for which a diagnosis can more readily be reached.

Osteoarthritis

Joint System	Affected Element/Element Part	Expression
Shoulder	Humerus: Head	
	Scapula: Glenoid fossa, clavicular facet of acromion	
	Clavicle: Acromial facet	
Elbow	Humerus: Trochlea, capitulum	
	Radius: Head	
	Ulna: Trochlear notch, radial notch, coronoid process	
Wrist	Radius: Distal articular facet	
	Ulna: Distal articular facet	
	Scaphoid/lunate: Articular facets for radius	
Hand	Hamate: Articular facets	
	Trapezoid: Articular facets	
	Pisiform: Articular facets	
	Capitate: Articular facets	
	Trapezium: Articular facets	
	Triquetral: Articular facets	
	Lunate: Articular facets	
	Scaphoid: Articular facets	
	Metacarpals: Articular facets	
	Phalanges: Articular facets	
Cervical vertebrae	Body: Superior margins	
	Body: Inferior margins	
	Articular facets: Superior	
	Articular facets: Inferior	
Thoracic vertebrae	Body: Superior margins	
	Body: Inferior margins	
	Articular facets: Superior	
	Articular facets: Inferior	
	Costal facets	
Lumbar vertebrae	Body: Superior margins	
	Body: Inferior margins	
	Articular facets: Superior	
	Articular facets: Inferior	
Hip	Os coxa: Acetabulum	
	Femur: Head	
Knee	Femur: Medial/lateral condyles, patellar surface	
	Tibia: Medial and lateral condyles	
	Patella: Articular (posterior) surface	

—cont'd

Joint System	Affected Element/Element Part	Expression
Ankle	Tibia: Distal articular facet, medial malleolus	
	Fibula: Distal articular facet	
	Talus: Articular facets for tibia and fibula	
Foot	Calcaneus: Articular facets	
	Talus: Articular facets	
	Cuboid: Articular facets	
	Navicular: Articular facets	
	First cuneiform: Articular facets	
	Second cuneiform: Articular facets	
	Third cuneiform: Articular facets	
	Metatarsals: Articular facets	
	Phalanges: Articular facets	

The expression should be recorded as either present or absent or using degrees of severity. Regarding presence/absence, according to Waldron (2008), if eburnation is present, then the condition can be classified as present even if no other diagnostic lesions are observable. If eburnation is not present, then two of the other diagnostic criteria (marginal osteophytes, surface osteophytes, porosity, alteration of joint contour) must be present. Other scholars, however, record the condition as present if any one of the aforementioned skeletal manifestations is observed. Regarding the degree of severity, the following scheme may be adopted (adapted from Buikstra and Ubelaker, 1994; Rojas-Sepulveda et al., 2008; Sofaer Derevenski, 2000):

Osteoarthritis

A. Marginal lipping
  0. None
  1. Barely visible and/or extending <1/3 of the joint circumference
  2. Sharp osseous ridge and/or extending 1/3 to 2/3 of the joint circumference
  3. Pronounced spicules and/or extending >2/3 of the joint circumference
  4. Ankylosis
B. Pitting
  0. None
  1. Small pits (<0.5 mm diameter) and/or covering <1/3 of the joint surface
  2. Medium pits (0.5–1.0 mm diameter) and/or covering 1/3 to 2/3 of the joint surface
  3. Large pits (>1.0 mm diameter) and/or covering >2/3 of the joint surface
C. Eburnation
  0. None
  1. Barely discernible and/or covering <1/3 of the joint surface
  2. Polish only and/or covering 1/3 to 2/3 of the joint surface
  3. Polish with grooves and/or covering >2/3 of the joint surface
D. Surface osteophytes
  0. None
  1. Barely visible
  2. Clearly visible

Spinal Osteoarthritis

Vertebral body

A. Marginal lipping
   0. None
   1. Barely visible and/or extending <1/3 of the vertebral body circumference
   2. Sharp osseous ridge and/or extending 1/3–2/3 of the vertebral body circumference
   3. Pronounced spicules and/or extending >2/3 of the vertebral body circumference
   4. Ankylosis
B. Pitting
   0. None
   1. Small pits (<0.5 mm diameter) and/or covering <1/3 of the vertebral body surface
   2. Medium pits (0.5–1.0 mm diameter) and/or covering 1/3–2/3 of the vertebral body surface
   3. Large pits (>1.0 mm diameter) and/or covering >2/3 of the vertebral body surface

Apophyseal joints

A. Marginal lipping
   0. None
   1. Barely visible and/or extending <1/3 of the joint circumference
   2. Sharp osseous ridge and/or extending 1/3–2/3 of the joint circumference
   3. Pronounced spicules and/or extending >2/3 of the joint circumference
   4. Ankylosis
B. Pitting
   0. None
   1. Small pits (<0.5 mm diameter) and/or covering <1/3 of the joint surface
   2. Medium pits (0.5–1.0 mm diameter) and/or covering 1/3–2/3 of the joint surface
   3. Large pits (>1.0 mm diameter) and/or covering >2/3 of the joint surface
C. Eburnation
   0. None
   1. Barely discernible and/or covering <1/3 of the joint surface
   2. Polish only and/or covering 1/3–2/3 of the joint surface
   3. Polish with grooves and/or covering >2/3 of the joint surface
D. Surface osteophytes
   0. None
   1. Barely visible
   2. Clearly visible

Note: After recording arthritis for all joint surfaces present, the maximum value is taken as the score for any specific articulation. For example, after scoring the inferior C2 vertebral body and the superior C3, the maximum value is taken as the score for the C2/C3 articulation (Bridges, 1994).

Schmorl's Nodes

Vertebral Segment	Affected Area	Location (Fig. 8.I.1)	Degree of Expression
Cervical	Superior endplate	Canal	
		Center	
		Periphery	
	Inferior endplate	Canal	
		Center	
		Periphery	
Thoracic	Superior endplate	Canal	
		Center	
		Periphery	

—cont'd

Vertebral Segment	Affected Area	Location (Fig. 8.I.1)	Degree of Expression
	Inferior endplate	Canal	
		Center	
		Periphery	
Lumbar	Superior endplate	Canal	
		Center	
		Periphery	
	Inferior endplate	Canal	
		Center	
		Periphery	

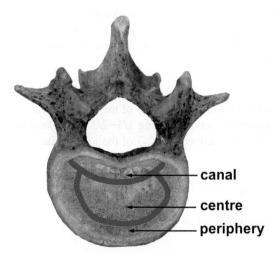

FIGURE 8.I.1 Location of Schmorl's nodes.

For the degree of expression, the following stages may be adopted (adapted from Jiménez-Brobeil et al., 2010; Knüsel et al., 1997):

Stage 0: None
Stage 1: Lesions <2 mm in depth and/or covering <1/2 of the anteroposterior length of the endplate
Stage 2: Lesions >2 mm in depth and/or covering >1/2 of the anteroposterior length of the endplate

Cribra Orbitalia and Porotic Hyperostosis

Location	Severity	State of Healing

For the severity and state of healing, the following stages may be adopted (adapted from Buikstra and Ubelaker, 1994; Hengen, 1971; Mensforth et al., 1978; Nathan and Haas, 1966; Stuart-Macadam, 1985):

Severity

1. Shallow furrows and microporosity
2. Deeper grooves and tiny pores (diameter ≤ 1 mm)
3. Even deeper grooves or furrows, pores with diameter $1-2$ mm
4. Pores of various sizes (some coalescing), minimal osteophytic formation
5. Well-developed osteophytes

State of Healing

1. Unremodeled lesions (sharp margins; microporosity)
2. Remodeled lesions (lamellar bone formation within the pores, eliminating microporosity)
3. Mixed lesions

Periostitis

Skeletal Element	Anatomical Location	Lesion Type	Bone Type	% of Bone Surface Affected	Severity	Type of Reaction

The following categories may be used for recording the above variables (adapted from Weston, 2008):

Lesion Type

1. Focal
2. Diffuse

Bone Type

1. Woven
2. Mixed
3. Lamellar

Severity

1. Mild pitting and swelling
2. Moderate pitting and swelling
3. Large swelling and heavy pitting

Type of Periosteal Reaction

1. Surface modifications
2. Bone destruction

Dental Diseases

MAXILLA

MANDIBLE

Periodontal Disease (Adapted From Kerr, 1988; Listi, 2011; Strohm and Alt, 1998)

A. Cementoenamel junction (CEJ)–alveolar crest (AC) distance
   0. 0–2 mm
   1. 2–5 mm
   2. >5 mm

B. Extent of alveolar bone resorption
   0. None
   1. <1/2 of the root exposed
   2. >1/2 of the root exposed
   3. Complete resorption

C. Septal form
   0. No grooves or foramina
   1. Foramina, grooves, and ridges on the cortical surface
   2. Breakdown of septal contour
   3. Deep septal defect

Antemortem Tooth Loss (Adapted From Gilmore, 2013)

0. None
1. Socket depth >2 mm, irregular socket walls
2. Socket depth <2 mm, irregular socket walls, large pores on alveolar bone
3. Complete socket obliteration

Periapical Cavities (Adapted From Buikstra and Ubelaker, 1994; Dias and Tayles, 1997; Hillson, 2008)

A. Location
   1. Buccal/labial
   2. Lingual

B. Size
   1. <3 mm diameter
   2. >3 mm diameter

C. Cavity wall
   1. Smooth
   2. Rough

D. Etiology
1. Severe caries
2. Excessive tooth wear
3. Unspecified

Dental Caries (Adapted From Buikstra and Ubelaker, 1994; Garcin et al., 2010; Hillson, 2001, 2008; Lukacs, 1989; Moore and Corbett, 1971)

A. Location
0. Absent
1. Occlusal
2. Interproximal
3. Buccal/labial
4. Lingual
5. Root
6. Gross

B. Degree of expression
Occlusal/buccal/lingual/interproximal caries
0. No caries
1. Small enamel cavity but no penetration to the dentine
2. Cavity penetrates the dentine
3. Cavity penetrates the pulp chamber
Root surface caries
0. No caries
1. Shallow cavity following the line of the CEJ or confined to the root surface
2. Cavity penetrates the pulp chamber/root canal
Gross caries
0. No caries
1. Cavity too large to determine if it originated in the crown or root
2. Same as stage 1 but penetrating the pulp chamber or root canal

Dental Calculus (Adapted From Buikstra and Ubelaker, 1994; Dobney and Brothwell, 1987; Hillson, 2008)

A. Location
1. Supragingival
   a. Buccal/labial
   b. Lingual
   c. Mesial
   d. Distal
2. Subgingival
   a. Buccal/labial
   b. Lingual
   c. Medial
   d. Distal

B. Size
0. Absent
1. <1/3 of the crown covered
2. 1/3 to 2/3 of the crown covered
3. >2/3 of the crown covered

C. Thickness
0. 0 mm
1. 1–2 mm
2. 2–4 mm
3. >4 mm

Enamel Hypoplasia (Adapted From Buikstra and Ubelaker, 1994; Fédération Dentaire International, 1982, 1992)

A. Type of defect
   0. Absence
   1. Enamel opacity
   2. Linear horizontal grooves
   3. Linear horizontal pits
   4. Arrays of pits
   5. Single pits
   6. Altogether missing enamel
   7. Other
B. Location
   1. Cusp
   2. Midcrown
   3. Neck

Note 1: To be reasonably certain that the lesions recorded represent a systemic stress event, some scholars record enamel hypoplasia only when present on antimeric teeth (e.g., Lewis, 2002; Lieverse et al., 2007) or if the hypoplasia manifests on two or more teeth during the same developmental stage (Littleton, 2005).

Note 2: The anterior dentition is more susceptible to hypoplastic defects and generally preferred in relevant studies if it is not possible to examine all teeth.

Trauma

Long-Bone Fractures

Bone Affected	Location	Type	Dimensions	Severity	Time of Occurrence	Healing Stage	Complications	Etiology

The following categories may be used for recording the manifestation of long-bone fractures (adapted from Buikstra and Ubelaker, 1994; Judd, 2000; Lovell, 1997):

Location	1. Proximal epiphysis
	2. Proximal metaphysis
	3. Proximal diaphysis
	4. Middiaphysis
	5. Distal diaphysis
	6. Distal metaphysis
	7. Distal epiphysis
Type	1. Complete
	2. Partial
	3. Spiral
	4. Transverse
	5. Oblique
	6. Other

Continued

—cont'd	
Severity	1. Simple 2. Comminuted/butterfly
Time of occurrence	1. Antemortem 2. Perimortem 3. Unspecified
Healing stage	1. Callus formation, woven bone 2. Callus formation, sclerotic bone 3. Complete healing
Complications*	1. Nonunion 2. Angulation 3. Rotation 4. Shortening/lengthening 5. Tissue necrosis 6. Infection 7. Traumatic arthritis 8. Traumatic myositis ossificans 9. Ankylosis 10. Pseudarthrosis
Etiology	1. Blunt force 2. Sharp force 3. High-velocity projectile force 4. Unspecified

Conventionally, when describing length, apposition, rotation, and angulation the distal fragment is measured in relation to the proximal one (Lovell, 1997).

Cranial Fractures

The following categories may be used for recording the manifestation of cranial fractures (adapted from Boylston, 2004; Jiménez-Brobeil et al., 2009; Lovell, 1997):

Bone Affected	Surface Affected	Type	Severity	Time of Occurrence	Healing Stage	Etiology

Surface affected

1. Ectocranial
2. Endocranial
3. Both ectocranial and endocranial

Type

1. Linear
2. Depressed
3. Compressed
4. Pressure fractures

Severity

1. Major trauma (>4 cm length/diameter, >0.5 cm depth)
2. Minor trauma (small, shallow)

Time of occurrence

1. Antemortem
2. Perimortem
3. Unspecified

Etiology

1. Blunt force
2. Sharp force
3. High-velocity projectile force
4. Unspecified

Healing stage

1. Unhealed
2. Healing
3. Healed

Appendix 8.II: Recording Pathological Conditions in Osteoware

Osteoware provides a number of options for recording pathological conditions and the reader may check the accompanying manual describing the various categories in detail and providing ample photographic documentation (Wilczak and Jones, 2011).

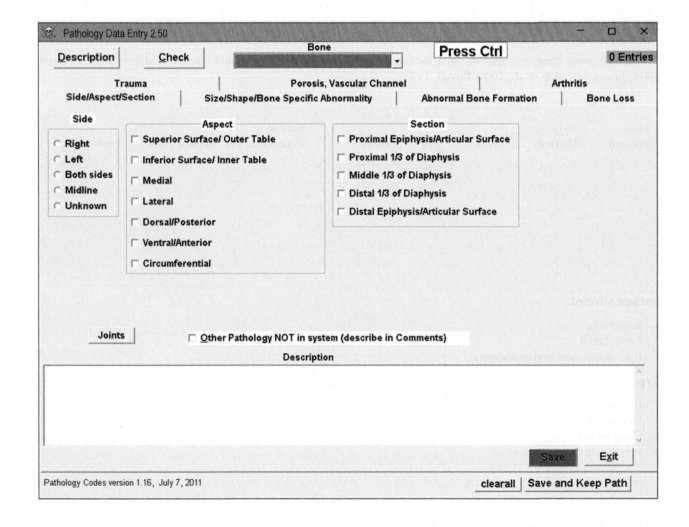

Pathologies can be recorded through the Pathology module. This module consists of numerous data entry screens. At the top center of the Pathology module, a Bone drop-down menu appears, which allows the user to specify the affected element.

The Side/Aspect/Section screen appears first by default and allows the specification of the exact anatomical area of the element involved (Fig. 8.II.1). Note that if a joint is involved, by clicking on the "Joints" button, a drop-down list of joints appears and the user can select the afflicted one.

The Size/Shape/Bone Specific Abnormality tab allows the user to specify the bone changes observed on each affected element. Note that depending on the element specified in the Bone drop-down menu, a different set of options appears in this tab. For instance, compare Fig. 8.II.2, which shows the options for cranial elements, to Fig. 8.II.3 for long bones.

The Abnormal Bone Formation tab allows the specification of the type, appearance, form, location, and size of osteoblastic lesions, whereas the Abnormal Bone Loss tab allows the user to specify the location, size, and form of osteolytic lesions. Trauma and arthritis are entered in tabs separate from the generic bone formation/bone loss tabs. The

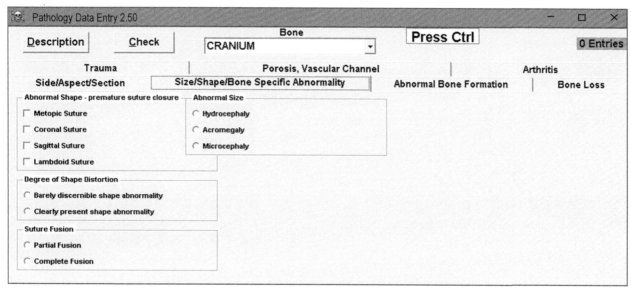

FIGURE 8.II.2 Part of the Size/Shape/Bone Specific Abnormality tab for crania.

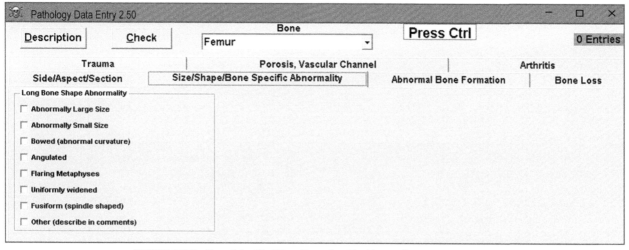

FIGURE 8.II.3 Part of the Size/Shape/Bone Specific Abnormality tab for long bones.

Trauma tab divides trauma into two broad categories, fractures and dislocations, and allows the recording of the type, characteristics, timing, healing stage, and possible complications of fractures, as well as the etiology of dislocations. The Arthritis tab allows the detailed recording of lipping, pitting (porosity), eburnation, erosion, and surface osteophytes on each joint surface. Finally, the Porosis, Vascular Impressions tab is primarily used for the detailed recording of porotic lesions in the cranium (PH, CO), although the same tab can be used for porosity seen on any skeletal element.

Note that dental diseases may be recorded using the Dental Inventory, Development, Wear, Pathology module. By clicking on the "Path" button (Fig. 1.III.9), information regarding dental caries, abscesses, and hypoplasia may be entered per tooth.

Chapter 9

Statistical Methods in Human Osteology

Chapter Outline

Chapter Objectives

By the end of this chapter, the reader will be able to:

- present data concisely using graphs, summary statistics, and contingency tables;
- determine the statistical tests required to address diverse osteoarchaeological and forensic anthropological questions;
- perform a broad range of univariate and multivariate tests; and
- interpret and report the obtained results.

Osteoarchaeologists and forensic anthropologists often have to analyze large data sets to obtain answers regarding whether certain variables in a data set are intercorrelated and if such an intercorrelation can be used for prediction (of, for example, sex, age, stature, etc.), whether clusters with common properties can be identified within a data set, how such clusters relate to one another, and whether the existence of a relationship among clusters is due to random processes or the result of underlying factors.

Statistics is the scientific discipline that can provide answers to these questions as well as to many more. For this reason, this chapter is intended as an introduction to basic statistical principles and techniques. The application of these techniques is facilitated via proper statistical packages. Here, the statistical analyses are mainly performed using SPSS, except for data modeling, in which both SPSS and Microsoft Excel are used. Appendix 9.I briefly presents the SPSS working environment, while Appendix 9.II describes the Excel 2010—2016 configuration for data analysis and macros.

9.1 BASIC STATISTICAL CONCEPTS

Statistics is the scientific field that deals with the collection, organization, evaluation, and presentation of data. The main branches of statistics are *descriptive statistics* and *inferential statistics*. Descriptive statistics includes methods for the succinct description and presentation of data, whereas inferential statistics includes methods for data processing and analysis.

The concepts of *population* and *sample* are fundamental in statistics. A population is an entire set of data concerning people or things that have something in common that we are studying. A sample is part of a population. For example, the lengths of a group of femora and the presence or absence of osteoarthritis in each individual within a group of skeletons constitute two different samples of data. The entire group (known or unknown) of femora or skeletons from which the above samples came is the corresponding population. In these examples, length and the existence of osteoarthritis are *variables,* whereas each femur or skeleton is a *case.*

A variable may be *quantitative* or *qualitative/categorical*. A quantitative variable takes numerical values and corresponds to properties that can be measured, such as weight, length, diameter, time, etc. A quantitative variable may be a *ratio* or an *interval* depending on whether the zero value implies a lack of the quantity under study or not. A typical example of an interval variable is temperature, for which 0°C does not mean that there is "no temperature." In addition, a quantitative variable may be *continuous* or *discrete/discontinuous*. A continuous variable can take any value within a certain range, e.g., height, whereas a discontinuous variable takes only certain values, usually integers, e.g., the most likely number of individuals in an incomplete skeletal assemblage.

Qualitative or categorical variables do not correspond to measurable quantities; rather they express qualitative properties. The values that a categorical variable may take are the categories into which the qualitative property it expresses are divided. For example, entheseal changes may be absent (0) or present (1) in a bone. Accordingly, a variable that expresses entheseal changes takes the value "absent" or "present," or 0 or 1. Qualitative variables may be *nominal* or *ordinal*. In nominal variables, there is no order among their values/categories, e.g., a variable that expresses the sex of an individual and takes the value "male" or "female." Note that the values/categories of a nominal variable may also be coded using numbers, for example, the variable "sex" may take the value "1" for males and "2" for females. Ordinal variables express an ordinal relationship among their values, e.g., in paleopathological data the expression of osteoarthritis may take the values 1 (=mild), 2 (=moderate), 3 (=extreme). When a nominal or an ordinal variable takes only two values, for example, "male" or "female," or 0 or 1, it is called a *binary* variable.

9.2 DESCRIPTIVE STATISTICS

Descriptive statistics are used for the effective presentation of data by means of *graphs*, *summary statistics*, and *contingency tables*. Graphs are used for the visualization of the data properties. The most appropriate graphs for various types of variables and research questions are described throughout this chapter. Summary statistics are adopted to express the properties of a sample of continuous data in a more succinct way, whereas for the same purpose contingency tables are used for samples of nominal or ordinal data.

9.2.1 Summary Statistics

The properties of a sample of continuous data may be expressed by means of *measures*. In summary statistics there are many measures, the most common of which are presented in Table 9.2.1. It is seen that these are classified in *measures of central tendency* and *measures of variability*. The measures of central tendency give information concerning the position of the data when these are arranged along an axis, whereas the measures of variability show how dispersed the data are along this axis.

TABLE 9.2.1 Basic Measures of Summary Statistics

Measures of Central Tendency	Measures of Variability
Mean	Variance
Median	Standard deviation
First quartile	Interquartile range
Third quartile	

The *mean* or *average value* of a sample consisting of m values is defined by:

$$\bar{x} = \frac{x_1 + x_2 + \cdots + x_m}{m} \tag{9.2.1}$$

where $x_1, x_2, \ldots, x_m$ are the sample values. For example, consider the following sample consisting of the femoral lengths in centimeters of 10 adults discovered in a certain archaeological site:

Femoral Length:	43	45	39	41	44	52	44	39	44	42

In this sample, x_1 is the first value, x_2 is the second value, ..., x_m is the last value, and $m = 10$. Based on the data, the mean value of the femoral lengths is 43.3 cm.

The *median* is the value that lies in the middle of the sample values, that is, 50% of the sample values are smaller than or equal to the median and 50% of the sample values are larger than or equal to the median. To find the median, we arrange the sample values from the smallest to the largest and select the middle value. In this example, in which the number of values is an even number, the median is equal to the mean value of the two middle values: (43 + 44) / 2 = 43.5 cm.

Both the mean and the median have the same meaning; they are the values around which all others cluster. However, this strictly holds when there are no *outliers* among the data, i.e., extreme values that differ significantly from the rest. If a sample contains one or more outliers, then the mean does not represent the central sample value. For example, consider the sample (2, 3, 65, 4, 6, 2, 4, 3, 4, 3). The mean is 9.6 because of the extreme (and possibly wrong) value 65. Because of this outlier, 9.6 is not really the value around which the other sample values cluster. In contrast, in this sample the median, which is 3.5, represents the value around which all sample values, except for the outlier, are gathered.

In general, the median is not affected by outliers and this is why it is often used in place of the mean when the data contain extreme values.

The *variance* shows the extent of dispersion of the sample values around the mean provided that there are no outliers. It is calculated from:

$$s^2 = \frac{(x_1 - \bar{x})^2 + (x_2 - \bar{x})^2 + \cdots + (x_m - \bar{x})^2}{m - 1} \tag{9.2.2}$$

If the value of the variance is high, then the distribution of the sample values is substantially spread out. The variance has the disadvantage that it is not expressed in the same units as the sample values. For example, in the femoral length data, the variance is expressed in centimeters squared. To overcome this problem, we calculate the *standard deviation, s*, which is the square root of the variance and also expresses the dispersion of the sample values around the mean. In the sample of femoral lengths, the variance is 13.8 cm^2 and the standard deviation 3.7 cm.

For samples coming from *normal populations*, 68% of the sample values lie within 1 standard deviation from the mean, i.e., in the range from $\bar{x} - s$ to $\bar{x} + s$ (see Section 9.3.3). In the present example, this range is from (43.3 − 3.7 = 39.6) to (43.3 + 3.7 = 47) and contains 70% of the sample values.

To distinguish the mean $\bar{x}$, variance s^2, and standard deviation s of a sample from those of the corresponding population, the mean, variance, and standard deviation of the population are denoted by μ, σ^2, and σ, respectively.

Every sample can be divided into three *quartiles*. The first quartile (Q_1) is the sample value below which 25% of the sample values lie, and the third quartile (Q_3) is the sample value below which 75% of the sample values lie. The second quartile (Q_2) is the median. The difference between the third and the first quartile ($Q_3 - Q_1$) is called the *interquartile range*. When no sample value corresponds to Q_1 or Q_3, then different methods have been proposed for the calculation of these measures. This is why different software packages might give slightly different results.

9.2.2 Boxplots and Histograms

Quartiles are primarily used in drawing *boxplots* (Fig. 9.2.1). A boxplot consists of a rectangle with two antennas, one at the lower base and the other at the upper one. The antennas are usually T and inverse T shaped, respectively. The lower base of the rectangle lies on Q_1 and the upper base marks Q_3. The median is represented by a horizontal line in the interior of the rectangle. The antennas are called *whiskers* and extend to the largest value that is smaller than or equal to $Q_3 + 1.5(Q_3 - Q_1)$ and to the smallest value that is larger than or equal to $Q_1 - 1.5(Q_3 - Q_1)$. If the maximum value is smaller than $Q_3 + 1.5(Q_3 - Q_1)$ and/or the minimum value is greater than $Q_1 - 1.5(Q_3 - Q_1)$, then the whiskers shift to the maximum and/or the minimum sample values (Fig. 9.2.1).

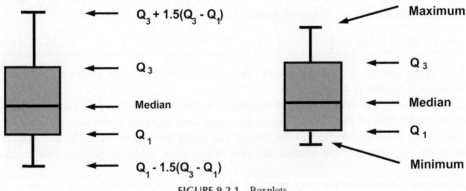

FIGURE 9.2.1 Boxplots.

Histograms are often used to obtain a picture of the shape of the distribution of the sample values, provided that the sample size (number of cases) is large enough ($m > 100$). To draw a histogram, we first define *classes* as follows: If x_{min} and x_{max} are the minimum and maximum sample values, we divide the range $x_{max} - x_{min}$ into k sectors with width equal to $\Delta x = (x_{max} - x_{min})/k$. These sectors are called *classes* or *bins*. Subsequently, we count the number of sample values that fall within each class. This number is called *class frequency*. Once the class frequencies have been calculated, we may plot the histogram; the classes are placed on the horizontal axis and a rectangular column is attached to each class with height proportional to the class frequency.

For example, Table 9.2.2 depicts the humeral lengths of 50 adult individuals. The histogram and the corresponding boxplot are shown in Fig. 9.2.2. It is seen from the histogram that there is a rather symmetrical distribution of the sample values around the mean value, which is 36.1 cm. This symmetry is also evident in the boxplot, which additionally shows that the values 29.5 (2nd case) and 44.3 (17th case) of the sample lie outside the whiskers. This is an indication that these values may be outliers. Stricter criteria about the existence of outliers in a data set are discussed in Section 9.9.1. The presence of outliers in a sample is a critical issue because it determines the statistical methods that will be adopted for its statistical analysis, as discussed in the following inferential statistics sections.

TABLE 9.2.2 Humeral Lengths (in cm) of 50 Adult Individuals[1]

36.8	35.3	36.1	38.2	34.0	36.8	36.8	39.5	37.9	38.3
29.5	36.7	35.1	44.3	36.0	33.3	36.1	40.9	30.1	33.9
33.9	38.8	34.6	34.9	36.3	38.2	35.6	41.3	35.0	37.4
39.5	35.1	35.0	34.8	34.2	34.4	40.0	40.7	33.9	33.7
35.6	36.7	35.7	36.0	37.2	36.4	35.8	32.1	34.2	34.3

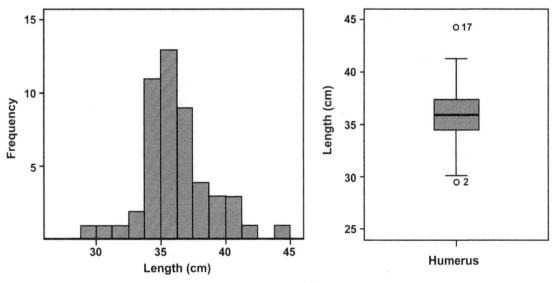

FIGURE 9.2.2   Histogram and boxplot of the sample of Table 9.2.2.

Fig. 9.2.3 shows the histogram and the boxplot of the basion−prosthion length (BPL) values presented in Table 5.VIII.1. It is interesting to observe that this histogram is rather abnormal, indicating that there is not a unique distribution of the data in this sample. This suggests that the sample is probably not homogeneous. Indeed, in this case, we know that the sample values come from different populations. We need to stress that information regarding sample homogeneity based on histograms is valid only when the sample size is large.

To sum up, a visual inspection of the samples through histograms (if the samples are relatively large) and boxplots (irrespective of the sample size) may offer useful information about the distribution of the sample values and the potential

---

1. All data sets used in this chapter are artificial, unless otherwise specified, and are provided in the companion website in the file Datasets/ DataForStatistics.

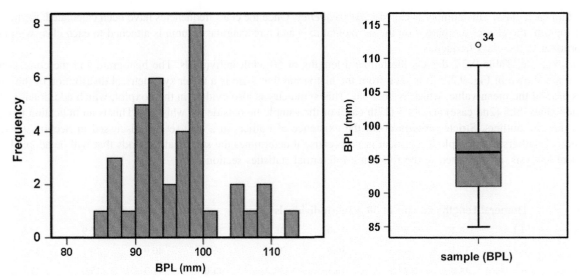

FIGURE 9.2.3 Histogram and boxplot of the basion–prosthion length (BPL) values of Table 5.VIII.1.

existence of outliers. If more than one distribution is identified within a single sample, as in Fig. 9.2.3, this sample cannot be further statistically analyzed without first detecting its subclusters, if possible. When outliers are traced in the sample, they need to be taken seriously into consideration as they may have an important impact on the results obtained from a statistical treatment. In such cases, we first need to check that these outliers represent actual sample values and not some typographical error. After this check, we should use more advanced statistical tests to determine whether these values are indeed outliers. Such a test is discussed in Section 9.9.1.

9.2.3 Contingency Tables

When a variable is nominal or ordinal, we cannot calculate the aforementioned summary statistics. In such cases we calculate *frequencies*. Suppose that x_1, x_2, ..., x_m are the values of a variable in a sample. We call *frequency of value x_i* the integer v_i that shows how many times x_i appears in the sample. For example, in the sample (2, 5, 3, 5, 8, 9, 6, 2, 5, 8, 7) the frequency of value 5 is 3. In this case, the *percentage frequency* of 5 is $100 \times 3/11 = 27.3\%$.

A *contingency table,* also known as *cross tabulation* or *cross tab,* is a table that displays the frequency of the values of a nominal/ordinal variable. For example, the contingency table for the trait *supranasal suture* of Table 5.XI.1 is given in Table 9.2.3. We observe that in sample 1 the presences are greater than the absences, whereas the opposite is valid for all other samples. The question that arises in this case is whether this observation is statistically significant and, therefore, whether it expresses a genetic trait or is the result of random factors. To tackle this problem, we have to use inferential statistics, and the appropriate methods are described in Section 9.6.1.

TABLE 9.2.3 Contingency Table for the Trait Supranasal Suture of Table 5.XI.1

Sample	1	2	3	4
Presence (1)	8	3	2	4
Absence (2)	2	7	9	8

9.2.4 Case Studies on the Calculation of Summary Statistics

Case Study 1: Descriptive Statistics

As an example of how to perform descriptive statistics, consider the data set of Table 9.2.4. The sample consists of 19 females and 31 males, all adults of known age and sex from the Athens Collection at the Department of Biology, National and Kapodistrian University of Athens, Greece. In this sample the femoral physiological length (FPHL) and the height, i.e.,

TABLE 9.2.4 Skeletal Sample of Female and Male Femoral Physiological Length and Height Values (in cm)

Code	Sex	FPHL	Height	Code	Sex	FPHL	Height	Code	Sex	FPHL	Height
WLH-2	M	42.6	163.6	WLH-53	F	41.45	156.7	ABH-104	F	40.3	153.3
WLH-4	F	42.7	160.5	WLH-54	M	40.4	154.1	ABH-105	M	51.25	186.1
WLH-8	M	44	167.1	WLH-55	M	44.7	167.9	ABH-108	M	45.5	170.3
WLH-9	M	43.25	160.1	WLH-60	F	41	150.1	ABH-109	M	43.8	161.6
WLH-10	F	40.05	152.9	WLH-63	M	46.2	167.6	ABH-111	M	47.25	174.5
WLH-11	M	41.75	159.9	WLH-67	M	46.1	171.5	ABH-114	F	38.9	149.0
WLH-12	F	41.85	152.4	WLH-68	M	46	168.7	ABH-138	F	41.3	155.4
WLH-17	M	44.45	162.9	WLH-70	M	45.7	169.2	ABH-139	M	38.35	155.7
WLH-20	M	42.45	161.0	ABH-73	M	46	166.3	ABH-141	M	42.3	161.1
WLH-21	M	46.8	171.1	ABH-74	M	48.1	174.6	ABH-144	F	39.95	150.2
WLH-22	M	45.1	163.6	ABH-75	F	38.4	140.5	ABH-146	M	39.95	154.7
WLH-23	M	43.55	163.2	ABH-77	F	44.65	163.1	ABH-151	F	46.3	168.6
WLH-24	M	45.25	166.9	ABH-78	M	44.7	160.3	ABH-155	M	45.75	167.2
WLH-26	M	43	165.3	ABH-79	F	41.6	155.5	ABH-156	M	44.05	166.1
WLH-30	F	43.55	161.7	ABH-80	F	42.2	157.2	ABH-158	M	42.25	161.7
WLH-33	F	41.35	155.3	ABH-81	M	42.7	161.3	ABH-167	F	39.45	149.6
WLH-37	F	40.55	152.9	ABH-83	M	45.45	167.4	ABH-176	F	40.35	147.6
WLH-40	F	39.6	153.5	ABH-84	F	40.05	148.2	ABH-179	F	39.2	148.3
WLH-41	F	44.3	159.4	ABH-86	F	39.1	148.1	ABH-180	F	36.45	141.0
WLH-44	M	44.35	166.4	ABH-87	M	45.55	165.2	ABH-183	F	38.3	148.4
WLH-45	M	45.1	165.7	ABH-91	F	42.4	156.4	ABH-192	M	49.5	179.1
WLH-46	M	45.8	170.7	ABH-95	F	39.8	152.1	ABH-200	M	44.6	168.8
WLH-47	F	38.4	148.5	ABH-96	F	38.85	150.2	ABH-209	M	46.25	168.2
WLH-49	M	46.9	171.5	ABH-98	F	40.45	151.3	ABH-213	M	44.7	165.6
WLH-50	M	44.9	169.0	ABH-103	M	45.7	168.9	ABH-221	M	47.75	177.7

F, female; *FPHL*, femoral physiological length; *M*, male.

stature, of the individuals (Height) are measured in centimeters. Calculate the summary statistics for the variable FPHL and discuss the results.

Because the data of Table 9.2.4 concern both male and female individuals, the correct approach is to separate the sample of FPHL values into two subsamples, one for males and the other for females, and compute summary statistics separately for these two groups. In SPSS we place the variables Sex and FPHL in two columns and use the menu Analyze → Descriptive Statistics → Explore. In the Explore dialog box we click on the variable FPHL and then click on the "arrow" button to transfer it in the Dependent List panel. Similarly, we transfer the variable Sex into the Factor List panel (Fig. 9.2.4). Next, we click on the "Statistics" button and in the Explore: Statistics dialog box we select "Descriptives," whereas from the "Plots" button we select "Factor levels together" and "Histogram." Some of the obtained results are presented in SPSS Output 9.2.1 and in Figs. 9.2.5 and 9.2.6.

From the summary statistics presented in SPSS Output 9.2.1 we observe some interesting patterns. For example, we see that the bulk of the female sample values lies in the range $\bar{x} \pm s = 40.736 \pm 2.097 = 40.7 \pm 2.1$, whereas that of males is 44.8 ± 2.4. These results show that there is a notable difference in the FPHL values in the two samples, as the range of the female sample values exhibits a small overlap with the corresponding range of the male sample values.

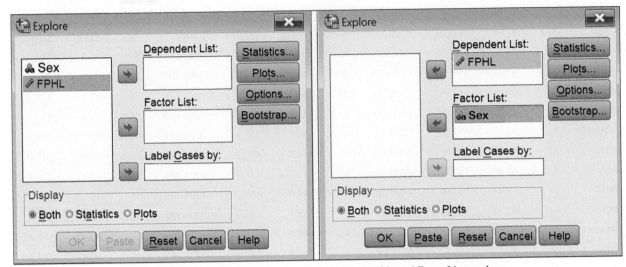

FIGURE 9.2.4   Transferring variables to the Dependent List and Factor List panels.

SPSS OUTPUT 9.2.1 Part of the Descriptives Table

	Sex		Statistic
FPHL	F	Mean	40.736
		Median	40.350
		Variance	4.398
		Standard deviation	2.097
	M	Mean	44.768
		Median	45.000
		Variance	5.646
		Standard deviation	2.376

F, female; *FPHL*, femoral physiological length; *M*, male.

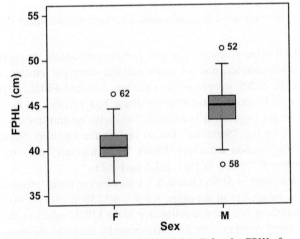

FIGURE 9.2.5   Boxplots of the female and male FPHL values of Table 9.2.4. *F*, female; *FPHL*, femoral physiological length; *M*, male.

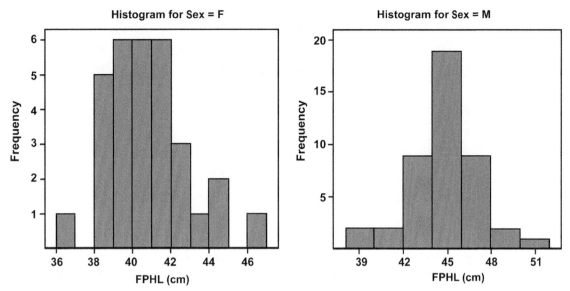

FIGURE 9.2.6 Histograms for the female and male FPHL values of Table 9.2.4. *F*, female; *FPHL*, femoral physiological length; *M*, male.

This difference between males and females is visualized in the boxplots of Fig. 9.2.5 and raises the following question: Is this difference statistically significant, indicating a genetic trait, or is it due to random reasons? The test of the statistical significance is performed in Section 9.4.3, Case Study 3, in which it is shown that the probability of the differences in femoral dimensions between males and females being due to random factors is negligible. As a result of this finding, we cannot pool the male and female data of FPHL and analyze them as a single sample.

In regard to the histograms, they do not exhibit any distinct trend (Fig. 9.2.6). The histogram for males shows a more symmetric distribution of sample values compared to the histogram for females. However, this may be due to the relatively small sample sizes.

An alternative way to plot boxplots in SPSS is from the menu Graphs → Legacy Dialogs → Boxplot. In the dialog box Boxplot that appears we select "Simple" and "Summaries for groups of cases," because the two samples (male and female FPHL values) are arranged in one column, whereas their grouping into the male and female categories is done by means of another (grouping) variable, the variable Sex in our example. We click on "Define" and in the dialog box that appears we transfer the variable FPHL into the Variable panel and the variable Sex into the Category Axis panel. Similarly, the histograms may be obtained from the menu Graphs → Legacy Dialogs → Histogram. In the Histogram dialog box we transfer the variable FPHL into the Variable box and the variable Sex into the Columns panel.

Case Study 2: Contingency tables

Prove that Table 9.2.3 is the contingency table for the trait supranasal suture of Table 5.XI.1.

We transfer the binary data of Table 5.XI.1 to an SPSS spreadsheet and, for simplicity, we name the variables as Trait1, Trait2, …, Trait7. In addition, we define that value 3 in the data set indicates missing values. For this purpose, in the Variable View window we click on the third cell of column Missing, i.e., on the cell that corresponds to Trait2, and then click on the small square that appears on the right of this cell. In the dialog box that pops up we activate the option "Discrete missing values" and type in "3" in the first box (Appendix 9.I).

Because the frequencies will be calculated separately for males and females, we use the *split file* function: Data → Split File. We select "Compare groups" and transfer the variable Sample to the box labeled Groups Based on. Subsequently, we click Analyze → Descriptive Statistics → Frequencies and transfer the variable Trait2, which corresponds to the supranasal suture, to the Variable(s) box. We activate the option "Display frequency tables" (if it is not preselected) and click on "OK." We obtain the table shown in SPSS Output 9.2.2, which is an extension of Table 9.2.3.

SPSS OUTPUT 9.2.2 The Contingency Table for Trait2 (Supranasal Suture)

	Sample			Frequency	Percentage	Valid Percentage	Cumulative Percentage
1	Valid	1		8	66.7	80.0	80.0
		2		2	16.7	20.0	100.0
		Total		10	83.3	100.0	
	Missing	3		2	16.7		
	Total			12	100.0		
2	Valid	1		3	30.0	30.0	30.0
		2		7	70.0	70.0	100.0
		Total		10	100.0	100.0	
3	Valid	1		2	18.2	18.2	18.2
		2		9	81.8	81.8	100.0
		Total		11	100.0	100.0	
4	Valid	1		4	28.6	33.3	33.3
		2		8	57.1	66.7	100.0
		Total		12	85.7	100.0	
	Missing	3		2	14.3		
	Total			14	100.0		

9.3 INFERENTIAL STATISTICS: STATISTICAL HYPOTHESIS TESTING

9.3.1 Introductory Concepts

In the previous section it was shown that boxplots and contingency tables can be used to explore and visualize potential differences among samples. However, when such differences are relatively small, it is difficult to know whether they are due to random factors or represent statistically significant patterns.

To address this issue, we need to employ *inferential statistics*. In inferential statistics, we make *hypotheses* and then test them. A very important hypothesis is called the *null hypothesis* and is symbolized by H_0. This hypothesis accepts that any difference between two or more samples is due to random factors, i.e., it is not statistically significant. For every null hypothesis, there is at least one *alternative hypothesis,* H_1.

The statistical hypotheses we can adopt and test are specific and depend on the type of problem we are examining. In other words, for every problem we select the statistical hypotheses that have already been proposed for the study of that specific problem. For example, in Chapter 5 we examined the calculation of biodistances, d, usually expressed as d^2, and stressed that it is useful to know not just the value of d^2 but also whether this value is statistically significant. In this case the null hypothesis is:

$$H_0: d^2 = 0$$

and the alternative hypothesis is:

$$H_1: d^2 > 0$$

It should be stressed that the null and the alternative hypotheses are always stated using population (not sample) terms. Thus, d^2 in these expressions refers to the squared distance between the populations from which the samples under study originated and not to the distance between the samples themselves.

As another example, consider two samples with mean values $\bar{x}_1$ and $\bar{x}_2$. A question that may arise is whether $\bar{x}_1$ and $\bar{x}_2$ are significantly different. These values will be statistically the same if the samples come from populations with equal means, $\mu_1 = \mu_2$, and different if $\mu_1 \neq \mu_2$ or $\mu_1 > \mu_2$ or $\mu_1 < \mu_2$. Therefore, the statistical hypotheses we can make are:

H_0: The samples come from populations with the same mean

and, for the alternative hypothesis, H_1, the following options:

H_1: The samples come from populations with $\mu_1 \neq \mu_2$
H_1: The samples come from populations with $\mu_1 > \mu_2$
H_1: The samples come from populations with $\mu_1 < \mu_2$

In addition, the null hypothesis may be stated as:

H_0: the samples come from the same population

whereas for the alternative hypothesis, H_1, we have the options:

H_1: The samples come from different populations
H_1: The samples come from different populations with $d_1 > d_2$
H_1: The samples come from different populations with $d_1 < d_2$

where d_1 and d_2 are the medians of the two populations.

9.3.2 One- and Two-Tailed Tests

When the alternative hypothesis, H_1, is expressed using the symbol $\neq$, the test is called *two-tailed*. For example, if we compare the stature of male skeletons from two contemporary sites, we do not know in advance which one of the samples comes from a population with taller males. Therefore, the alternative hypothesis may be stated as:

H_1: The samples come from populations with $\mu_1 \neq \mu_2$ or
H_1: The samples come from different populations

If the alternative hypothesis, H_1, is expressed using the symbol $>$ or $<$, the statistical test is *one-tailed*. For example, if we compare the stature between males and females in a population, we know in advance that males are expected to be taller than females but we want to test whether this difference is statistically significant. In this case the alternative hypothesis may be expressed as:

H_1: The samples come from populations with $\mu_1 > \mu_2$ or
H_1: The samples come from populations with $d_1 > d_2$

where subscript 1 denotes males and 2 females.

9.3.3 The Concept of Distribution

Statistical hypothesis testing is based on the concept of *statistical distribution*. A statistical distribution describes the manner in which the sample values spread around the mean or median.

As mentioned previously, histograms offer a visualization of the distribution of sample values, provided that the sample size is large. From the study of histograms, it has been found that the distribution of sample values is never random but always determined by some law. For example, very often the sample values are symmetrically spread around the mean, forming a bell-shaped distribution in which 68% of the sample values lie within 1 standard deviation from the mean, 95% of the sample values lie within 1.96 standard deviations from the mean, and 99% of the sample values lie within 2.576 standard deviations from the mean. A sample that exhibits such a distribution is called *normal*. More accurately, such a sample is said to come from a *normal population*.

The histogram of a normal sample is given in Fig. 9.3.1. In this figure the depicted curve is called a *normal distribution curve* and depends on the mean and the standard deviation of the sample. Similarly, the normal distribution curve of a population depends on the mean μ and the standard deviation σ of the population. This curve is usually symbolized as $N(\mu, \sigma)$. When $\mu = 0$ and $\sigma = 1$, then the sample comes from a population that follows the *standardized normal distribution*, $N(0,1)$.

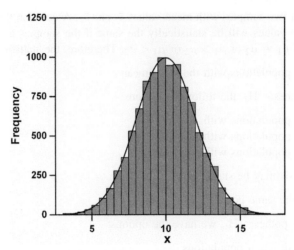

FIGURE 9.3.1   Histogram of a sample following the normal distribution and the curve of the normal distribution.

Because the standardized normal distribution is a limiting case of the normal distribution, in a sample originating from a population that follows the standardized normal distribution, 68% of the values lie within the interval -1 to 1, 95% of the values are in the interval -1.96 to 1.96, and 99% of the values lie within -2.576 to 2.576 (Fig. 9.3.2).

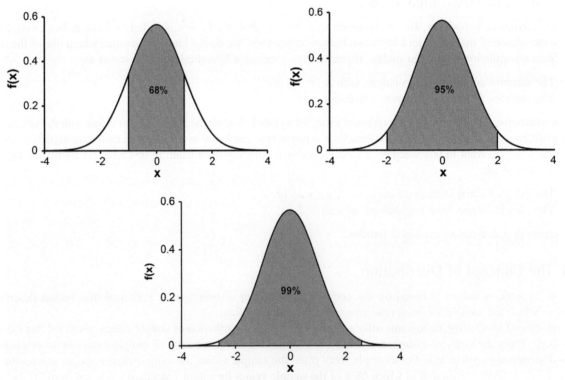

FIGURE 9.3.2   Properties of the standardized normal distribution.

Experimental and theoretical studies have shown that there are many different distributions in addition to the normal distribution. Among them, particularly interesting in inferential statistics are the t or *Student* (t_ν), χ^2 (χ^2_ν), and F or *Fisher* (F_{ν_1, ν_2}) distributions. The t and χ^2 distributions depend upon the *degrees of freedom, ν,* that is, the number of values in a statistical calculation that are free to vary, whereas F depends on two degrees of freedom, ν_1 and ν_2. These distributions cannot be found in natural samples; rather they are mathematically constructed and are very useful in testing statistical hypotheses. For example, as mentioned in Chapter 5, the F distribution is used to test the statistical significance of the squared Mahalanobis distance. Fig. 9.3.3 depicts representations of the Student and χ^2 distributions.

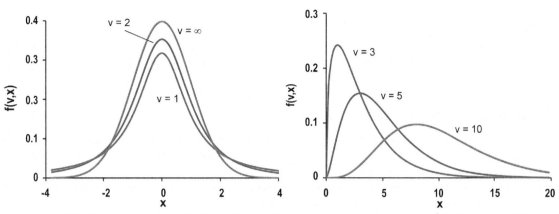

FIGURE 9.3.3 Plots of the Student distribution with different degrees of freedom ($\nu = 1, 2, \infty$) (*left*) and the χ^2 distribution with different degrees of freedom ($\nu = 3, 5, 10$) (*right*). Note that the curve with $\nu = \infty$ in the Student distribution coincides with the standardized normal distribution.

9.3.4 Testing the Null Hypothesis: The *p*-value

To test the null hypothesis, we first define the *significance level*, which is symbolized by α and expresses the probability of wrongly rejecting a valid null hypothesis. The value usually employed for the significance level is $\alpha = .05$, which means that the probability of wrongly rejecting a correct null hypothesis is 5%. Subsequently, we calculate the *p-value*. When this value is smaller than the significance level, i.e., *p*-value $< \alpha$, we reject the null hypothesis. The smaller the *p*-value in comparison to the significance level, the more confident we can be that our decision to reject the null hypothesis is correct.

For example, to decide whether the biological distance MMD (mean measure of divergence) between two samples is significant, we test H_0, MMD $= 0$, with alternative H_1, MMD > 0. The theoretical study of the MMD has shown that when the null hypothesis is valid, i.e., when MMD $= 0$, the variable z defined from the ratio $z = $ MMD$/s$ follows the standardized normal distribution, Eq. (5.2.6). Variable z is called the *test statistic*. From the properties of the standardized normal distribution we know that 95% of the sample values lie within -1.96 to 1.96, thus merely 2.5% of the values are greater than 1.96. This means that the probability of a z value being greater than 1.96 is smaller than .025. Consider now that we have calculated the MMD between two samples and found that $z = 3$. Because this value is greater than 1.96, the probability of this result being the outcome of random factors is less than .025. Therefore, we may reject the null hypothesis H_0, MMD $= 0$, which means that the value of the MMD is statistically significant, bearing in mind that the probability of being mistaken in our conclusion is less than 2.5%.

This example shows the steps we follow in every statistical test:

1. We define the null hypothesis, the alternative hypothesis, and the significance level.
2. For every null hypothesis there is at least one test statistic, say X, that follows a certain distribution when the null hypothesis is valid. The distribution curve of X may be symmetric or asymmetric, as in Fig. 9.3.3.
3. Based on the sample(s) involved in the null hypothesis, we calculate the value of X, say X $= c$, and then calculate the *p*-value (Fig. 9.3.4). For a two-tailed test, the *p*-value is twice the area under the distribution curve to the right of c, whereas for a one-tailed test, the *p*-value is equal to the area under the distribution curve to the left or to the right of c, depending on whether the alternative hypothesis is expressed by the inequality "$<$" or the inequality "$>$". In all cases the null hypothesis is rejected when *p*-value $< \alpha$.

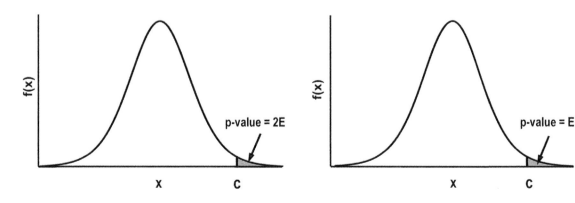

When we reject the null hypothesis, there is an $\alpha\%$ probability that we are making a mistake. However, if our results do not allow us to reject the null hypothesis, then we have to accept it. In this case there is no way of knowing the probability of making a mistake. In other words, **if the null hypothesis is retained, it has not been proven that it is true; it has merely not been demonstrated to be false**.

9.3.5 Parametric and Nonparametric Tests

Statistical tests may be *parametric* or *nonparametric*. Parametric tests presuppose that the samples under study come from populations that follow a known distribution, usually the normal distribution. In other words, in most parametric tests the samples should come from normal populations.

When the samples come from populations of unknown distribution, we have to apply nonparametric tests because these tests do not require any assumptions concerning the distribution of the data. An interesting differentiation between parametric and nonparametric tests is that in nonparametric tests we do not analyze the raw data. Instead, the raw data are usually transformed into *ranks*. If $(x_1, x_2, \ldots, x_m)$ is a sample of quantitative data, we call the *rank* of value x_i the number r_i of sample data that are smaller than or equal to x_i. For example, the sample (0.12, 0.09, 0.11, 0.1) is transformed to (4, 1, 3, 2). In this way, outliers have no effect on the results. Note that nonparametric tests also include the general methods *bootstrap* and *Monte Carlo tests with permutations*.

Parametric methods generally produce more accurate estimates, i.e., they have more statistical *power*, where the power of a statistical test is the probability that it correctly rejects the null hypothesis when the null hypothesis is false. However, this holds provided that the assumptions on which they are based are met. If these assumptions are not met, parametric methods can produce misleading results.

Finally, we should note that although each statistical test is based on a certain test statistic, these test statistics are not given in the following sections to avoid compiling complex mathematical formulas that are automatically calculated by statistical software packages. The reader may find them in many statistical textbooks, such as the ones provided as Suggested Readings at the end of this chapter, as well as on the Internet. The aim of this chapter is to examine when and how each statistical test is applied and how the obtained results may be interpreted.

9.3.6 Test of Normality

The majority of parametric statistical tests presuppose that the data under study follow the normal distribution. For this reason, the test of normality is the first and most important test before proceeding to any further analysis. In this test the null hypothesis and the alternative hypothesis are:

H_0: The sample comes from a normal population
H_1: The sample does not come from a normal population

Various criteria have been proposed for testing the null hypothesis, among which the *Shapiro—Wilk* test has the most *power*. As an example, let us examine whether the samples of male and female FPHL values given in Table 9.2.4 come from populations that follow the normal distribution. In SPSS we arrange the variables Sex and FPHL in two columns and use the menu Analyze → Descriptive Statistics → Explore. In the Explore dialog box we transfer the variable FPHL into the Dependent List panel and the variable Sex into the Factor List panel, as in Fig. 9.2.4. If we had been testing a single sample, the Factor List panel would have been left empty. Next, we click on "Plots" and in the dialog box that appears we activate only the option "Normality plots with tests." After clicking on "Continue" and "OK," we obtain, among others, the table Tests of Normality (SPSS Output 9.3.1). It is seen that the program performs two tests, the Kolmogorov—Smirnov and the Shapiro—Wilk. **Note that in SPSS the *p*-value is denoted as Sig.**

SPSS OUTPUT 9.3.1 Tests of Normality

	Sex	Kolmogorov—Smirnov[a]			Shapiro—Wilk		
		Statistic	df	Sig.	Statistic	df	Sig.
FPHL	F	0.116	31	0.200[b]	0.965	31	0.401
	M	0.107	44	0.200[b]	0.973	44	0.394

It is seen that for the male sample *p*-value = .394 and for the female sample *p*-value = .401, that is, both *p*-values are greater than .05. This means that the null hypothesis cannot be rejected at least at the significance level $\alpha = .05$. Note that this does not mean that the null hypothesis is correct, i.e., we cannot conclude that the samples of the FPHL values for females and males come from normal populations. The correct conclusion is that a lack of normality in these samples has not been demonstrated. Based on this conclusion, parametric tests may be used for these samples.

Important note: Parametric tests can be used even when small deviations from normality are observed, that is, when *p*-values are smaller but close to the .05 limit. Parametric tests are mostly avoided when a sample includes outliers or is very small.

9.3.7 Point and Interval Estimation

One of the main tasks of inferential statistics is to estimate the population parameters from those of a sample. For example, when we calculate a certain biodistance between two samples, we make the (silent) assumption that this biodistance is, in fact, the biodistance between the populations from which the samples come. This approach is called *point estimation* of the properties of a population and it is strictly valid when the parameter under consideration is an *unbiased estimator*. By this term we mean that the sample parameter has the following property. If we take a plethora of samples from the same population, compute the value of this parameter in each sample, and then average all these values, this average value tends to the parameter value in the population. The mean value and the sample variance are unbiased estimators, whereas the sample standard deviation is a biased estimator of the population standard deviation. In regard to biodistances, unbiased estimators of population distances are the corrected squared Mahalanobis distance (CMD) and the MMD, whereas the squared Mahalanobis distance (MD) and the Mahalanobis-type distances TMD and RMD, as defined in Chapter 5, are biased estimators (Nikita, 2015; Sjøvold, 1975, 1977).

An alternative approach to estimating population parameters from samples is by means of *confidence intervals*. The P% confidence interval for a parameter is the range of values that includes the unknown population parameter with a probability equal to P%. The P% probability can also be written as $P = 100(1 - \alpha)$, where α is, in fact, the significance level, defined in the previous section, and signifies the probability that the population parameter lies outside the estimated confidence interval. For instance, when P = 95, then $\alpha = .05$. In this case, the population parameter under study has a 95% probability of lying within the confidence interval and 5% probability of lying outside this interval.

9.4 TESTS OF SIGNIFICANCE BETWEEN TWO SAMPLES

Two or more samples may be independent or dependent. The samples are *independent* when each of them has been obtained independently of the other(s). A main characteristic of such samples is that they may have different sizes (number of cases). The samples are *dependent* if we know in advance that each observation in one sample is directly related to a specific observation in the other sample(s). Therefore, dependent samples always have the same number of observations (cases). Two dependent samples are usually called *paired* or *matched samples*.

9.4.1 Independent Samples Tests

The most common test between two independent samples examines whether the differences in their mean values are statistically significant. The parametric test is called an *independent samples t test* and the null hypothesis and the alternative hypothesis are $H_0, \mu_1 = \mu_2$, and $H_1, \mu_1 \neq \mu_2$, or $H_1, \mu_1 < \mu_2$, or $H_1, \mu_1 > \mu_2$, depending on whether we perform a two-tailed or a one-tailed test.

An interesting feature of the parametric *t* test is that the test statistic used depends on whether the samples come from populations that have the same or different variances. Therefore, we first examine the null hypothesis, $H_0, \sigma_1^2 = \sigma_2^2$, with alternative hypothesis $H_1, \sigma_1^2 \neq \sigma_2^2$, and then we test the hypothesis $H_0, \mu_1 = \mu_2$. The basic precondition for applying an independent samples *t* test is that the two samples come from normal populations, although small deviations from normality do not affect the results, as already mentioned.

For nonparametric tests the statistical hypotheses are:

H_0: The samples come from the same population
H_1 (two-tailed): not H_0
H_1 (one-tailed): The first population exhibits larger (or smaller) values than the second one, which is equivalent to H_1, $d_1 > d_2$, or H_1, $d_1 < d_2$

where d , d are the medians of the two populations. There are several nonparametric tests, the most powerful of which is

9.4.2 Paired Samples Tests

As described in the previous section, when two independent samples are being compared, we are testing whether the samples come from the same population or from populations with the same mean. In contrast, when we compare two dependent (paired) samples, what we are actually testing is whether the difference between the paired values of the two samples is statistically significant. Consider the paired samples $x_1, x_2, ..., x_m$ and $y_1, y_2, ..., y_m$, in which each observation x_i is directly related to observation y_i. Based on these original values, we form the sample $\Delta_1, \Delta_2, ..., \Delta_m$ where $\Delta_1 = x_1 - y_1, \Delta_2 = x_2 - y_2, ..., \Delta_m = x_m - y_m$. To test if the difference between paired values is statistically significant, we need to assess whether the constructed sample of differences $\Delta_1, \Delta_2, ..., \Delta_m$ comes from a population with mean, μ_d, or median, d, equal to zero.

Therefore, in the parametric *paired samples t test* the hypotheses tested are:

$$H_0: \mu_d = 0 \text{ and } H_1: \mu_d \neq 0 \text{ or } H_1: \mu_d < 0 \text{ or } H_1: \mu_d > 0$$

An important precondition for this test is that the sample of differences, $\Delta_1, \Delta_2, ..., \Delta_m$, follows the normal distribution. For nonparametric tests the statistical hypotheses are the following:

$$H_0: d = 0 \text{ and } H_1: d \neq 0 \text{ or } H_1: d > 0 \text{ or } H_1: d < 0$$

From the various nonparametric tests proposed for these hypotheses, the most powerful one is the *Wilcoxon test*.

9.4.3 Case Studies on Statistical Tests Between Two Samples

Case Study 3: Independent Samples (p-value < α)

Examine whether the samples of male and female FPHL values in Table 9.2.4 exhibit a statistically significant difference. In other words, test whether these two samples come from populations with different mean values or from different populations.

In Section 9.3.6 we found that for these samples the null hypothesis regarding normality cannot be rejected, at least not at the significance level $\alpha = .05$. Therefore, the parametric t test may be used for their comparison. However, we should first recode the variable Sex for the following reason. In general, in SPSS, when we compare two or more independent samples, we should adopt the following arrangement: The samples are placed in a single column and in another column a *grouping variable* is created with values 1, 2, ..., n, which denote the first, second, ..., nth sample. Thus, in the present case the variable Sex should be recoded from F, M to 1, 2.

To recode the variable Sex, we may use the menu Transform → Recode into Same Variables. In the dialog box that appears we transfer the variable Sex to the panel labeled Variables and click on the "Old and New Values" button. In the new dialog box we type "F" in the Old Value box and "1" in the New Value box and click on "Add." Similarly, we type "M" in the Old Value box and "2" in the New Value box and click on "Add." We note that the values F, M are replaced by 1, 2, respectively, although the format of the variable remains *string*. At this point it is helpful to assign descriptive labels to each value of the grouping variable. This can be done from the Values column in the Variable View window (Fig. 9.4.1), as described in Appendix 9.I.

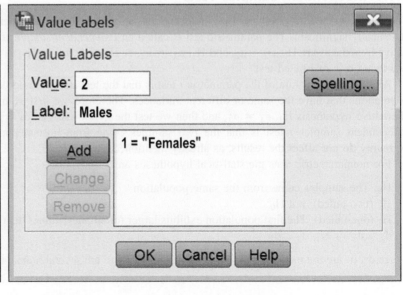

	Sex	FPHL	var
1	2	42.60	
2	1	42.70	
3	2	44.00	
4	2	43.25	
5	1	40.05	
6	2	41.75	
7	1	41.85	
8	2	44.45	
9	2	42.45	
10	2	46.80	
11	2	45.10	
12	2	43.55	

After data arrangement and recoding, we may perform the parametric t test using the menu Analyze $\rightarrow$ Compare Means $\rightarrow$ Independent-Samples T Test. In the dialog box that appears we transfer the variable FPHL to the box labeled Test Variable(s) and the variable Sex to the Grouping Variable box and click on "Define Groups." In the new dialog box we type in the value "1" for Group 1 and the value "2" for Group 2 (Fig. 9.4.2). In addition to the t test, we may apply the bootstrap method. This technique uses the same test function as the parametric t test, but it does not require the samples to follow the normal distribution. It is conducted from Bootstrap $\rightarrow$ Perform bootstrapping. Part of the main results tables concerning the parametric t test is given in SPSS Output 9.4.1.

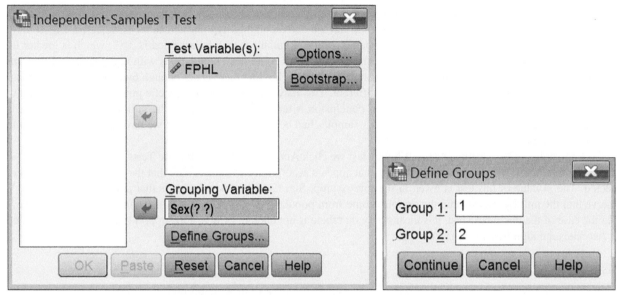

FIGURE 9.4.2 Data input and definition of groups for t test.

SPSS OUTPUT 9.4.1 Part of the Independent Samples T Test Table

		Levene's Test for Equality of Variances		t-test for Equality of Means		
		F	Sig.	t	df	Sig. (two-tailed)
FPHL	Equal variances assumed	0.117	0.733	−7.59	73	0.000
	Equal variances not assumed			−7.76	69.273	0.000

FPHL, femoral physiological length.

We observe that the program uses *Levene's criterion* to test the hypothesis H_0, $\sigma_1^2 = \sigma_2^2$, and the value Sig. $= .733$ shows that this hypothesis cannot be rejected. For this reason, only the results shown in the upper row of the table in SPSS Output 9.4.1 are valid (Equal variances assumed). If there had been a significant difference between variances, we would have to check the lower row of this table (Equal variances not assumed). In the upper row we observe that Sig. (two-tailed) $= .000 < .05$. In fact, a Sig. $= .000$ value in SPSS means a p-value smaller than $.0005$.

It is seen that for $\alpha = .05$, the null hypothesis that the samples come from populations with equal mean values should be rejected. In other words, the mean values of female and male FPHL are statistically different and the probability that this is due to random reasons is practically equal to zero (p-value $< .0005$).

Case Study 4: Independent samples (p-value $> \alpha$)

Consider the following two samples of maximum femoral lengths (in cm) obtained from two different archaeological sites:

Sample 1:	43	45	39	41	44	52	44	39	44	42

Examine whether these samples are statistically significantly different and draw conclusions.

As stressed above, in SPSS the two samples are placed in a single column, and in another column we create a grouping variable with values 1 and 2, which denote the first and the second sample, respectively. We first test the normality of these two samples and the Shapiro—Wilk test gives the p-values .0874 and .687 for samples 1 and 2, respectively. Both p-values are greater than .05 and, therefore, for these samples the null hypothesis for normality cannot be rejected. Thus, parametric tests may be used for their comparison. However, because of the small sample sizes, for more confidence, we should additionally apply nonparametric tests, because in the case of samples with small sizes the test of normality, like every other test, is not reliable when the null hypothesis is not rejected.

The parametric tests are performed as in the previous case study and give the following results: For the equality of variances, p-value (Levene's test) = .727, indicating that the corresponding hypothesis cannot be rejected. Based on this result, the p-value of the t test for equal means when equality of variances may be assumed is .083, which is greater than .05. It is seen that for $\alpha = .05$, the null hypothesis that the samples come from populations with equal mean values cannot be rejected. This does not mean that we accept the null hypothesis, but that there is not enough evidence to support that the femoral lengths in the two sites are significantly different. This may indicate a similar genetic potential for skeletal growth for the populations in the two sites; however, this conclusion is tentative because when the null hypothesis is retained, it does not mean that it is necessarily true. Only if our samples had been large enough could we have been confident that this conclusion is valid.

To conduct the nonparametric Mann—Whitney test we click Analyze → Nonparametric Tests → Legacy Dialogs → 2 Independent Samples... and fill in the dialog box that appears accordingly. We make sure that the Mann—Whitney U test is selected. The p-value of this test is given in the row Asymp. Sig. (2-tailed), which shows that p-value = .087 > .05. We observe that the null hypothesis that the samples come from populations with equal medians cannot be rejected. However, as in the case of the parametric test, this means only that there is not enough evidence to support that the femoral lengths in the two sites are significantly different.

Case Study 5: Paired Samples

Based on the data shown in Table 9.4.1, assess whether the right and left humeral midshaft diameters of 15 female individuals are significantly different.

TABLE 9.4.1 Paired Samples of Right and Left Humeral Midshaft Diameters (in cm)

Individual	Right Side	Left Side
1	5.61	5.58
2	5.96	5.92
3	7.99	8.20
4	6.37	6.13
5	6.12	6.00
6	5.90	5.89
7	6.02	5.97
8	6.87	6.72
9	7.14	7.03
10	7.68	7.50
11	6.73	6.66
12	7.03	6.79
13	6.57	6.44
14	5.78	5.94
15	7.32	7.01

First, we need to create a new variable that expresses the difference between the two samples, Δ_1, Δ_2, ..., Δ_m, and assess whether this variable follows the normal distribution. The normality of the variable of differences is tested as described in previous examples and the Shapiro−Wilk test gives p-value = .452 > .05, which shows that lack of normality in this sample is not demonstrated. Therefore, we may apply the parametric paired samples t test testing the hypotheses H$_0$, $\mu_d = 0$, and H$_1$, $\mu_d \neq 0$. This test is performed as follows.

We place the two dependent samples in two separate columns, Right_side and Left_side, and click Analyze → Compare Means → Paired-Samples T Test. In the dialog box that appears we transfer the two variables to the panel Paired Variables, as shown in Fig. 9.4.3. We obtain various tables of results, the most important of which is the Paired Samples Test (SPSS Output 9.4.2). This table shows that Sig. = .03 < .05, which suggests that there are statistically significant differences between the two sides of the body. The mean value of the difference Right side − Left side is positive and equal to 0.087, which means that the mean for the right side is greater than that for the left side. By combining these results, we can conclude that the daily activities of the population under study involved primarily the right side of the upper body.

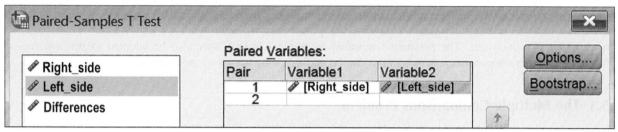

FIGURE 9.4.3 Part of the Paired-Samples T Test dialog box.

SPSS OUTPUT 9.4.2 Part of the Paired Samples Test Table

| | | Paired Differences | | | | | | | |
| | | Mean | Std. Deviation | Std. Error Mean | 95% CI of the Difference | | t | df | Sig. two-tailed |
					Lower	Upper			
Pair 1	Right_side − Left_side	0.0873	0.1401	0.0362	0.0097	0.1649	2.41	14	0.030

If the data had violated the assumption of normality, we would have to run the Wilcoxon test from the menu Analyze → Nonparametric Tests → Legacy Dialogs → 2 Related Samples. In the dialog box that appears we transfer the variables Right_side and Left_side to the Test Pairs box, as in the parametric test. In the Test Type panel we select "Wilcoxon," if it is not preselected. We click on "Exact" and select "Monte Carlo" with number of samples 10,000. We click on "Continue" and "OK." In the table Test Statistics (SPSS Output 9.4.3) we observe that all two-tailed tests give p-values < .05, in complete agreement with the parametric test.

SPSS OUTPUT 9.4.3 Test Statistics[a,b]

			Left_side − Right_side
Z			−2.159[c]
Asymp. Sig. (two-tailed)			0.031
Monte Carlo Sig. (two-tailed)	Sig.		0.029
	99% confidence interval	Lower bound	0.024
		Upper bound	0.033
Monte Carlo Sig. (one-tailed)	Sig.		0.015
	99% confidence interval	Lower bound	0.012
		Upper bound	0.018

We should point out that boxplots often provide a good visualization for the comparison between two or more samples, as shown, for example in Fig. 9.2.5. However, in paired or dependent samples, they may lead to misleading conclusions, because in this case we are not interested in comparing the original sample values. Instead, we are examining whether the mean or median of the variable expressing the difference between the original sample values is different from zero.

9.5 STATISTICAL TESTS AMONG MANY SAMPLES

Depending on the type of test (parametric or nonparametric), the type of samples (independent or dependent), and the number of factors that affect the variables, there are many tests of significance when three or more samples are to be compared. In this section, we restrict the analysis only to tests that are a direct extension of the tests between two samples, examined in the previous section.

The parametric test used to examine whether there are any significant differences between the means of three or more independent samples is called *one-way analysis of variance* (ANOVA). Many different criteria have been proposed for the corresponding nonparametric test, the most powerful of which is the *Kruskal−Wallis test*. The extension of the parametric paired *t* test to three or more dependent samples is the *parametric repeated-measures ANOVA* and its nonparametric version is the *Friedman test*. The parametric repeated measures ANOVA may also be adopted to perform *two-way ANOVA*, whereas its nonparametric version may also be performed by means of the Friedman test.

9.5.1 The Multiple Comparisons Problem

When two samples are being compared, samples 1 and 2, there is only one comparison, 1−2. If the number of samples is increased to 3, the number of comparisons also increases to 3, 1−2, 1−3, and 2−3, whereas for five samples, the comparisons become 10: 1−2, 1−3, 1−4, 1−5, 2−3, 2−4, 2−5, 3−4, 3−5, and 4−5. The statistical problem that arises when we have to perform multiple comparisons is the increase in the probability of falsely rejecting the null hypothesis in one of these tests.

In particular, if N is the number of pairwise comparisons between samples, then the probability of falsely rejecting the null hypothesis in one of the N comparisons increases from α to $1 - (1 - \alpha)^N$. For example, when five samples are tested, resulting in 10 pairwise comparisons, the probability of falsely rejecting the null hypothesis in 1 of the 10 comparisons increases from $\alpha = .05$ to $1 - 0.95^{10} = .401$. In other words, the probability of making a mistake increases from 5% to 40.1%!

Therefore, when multiple comparisons are made, it is imperative either to lower the significance level, α, or to correct the obtained *p*-values. A common approach is to apply the *Bonferroni* correction, where the significance level is corrected by:

$$\alpha = \frac{0.05}{N} \tag{9.5.1}$$

For instance, for 10 comparisons, α should be corrected to $.05/10 = .005$; thus the probability of falsely rejecting the null hypothesis in 1 of the 10 comparisons is $1 - (1 - .005)^{10} = 1 - 0.995^{10} = 0.04889 = 4.9\%$, instead of 40.1%. The Bonferroni correction is equivalent to preserving the significance level to $\alpha = .05$ and multiplying all obtained *p*-values by N.

A better approach is the *Holm−Bonferroni* method. According to this method, the *p*-values are arranged from the smallest to the largest, *p*-value(1) < *p*-value(2) < *p*-value(3) < ... < *p*-value(N). Subsequently, starting from the smallest, these values are multiplied by N, N − 1, N − 2, ..., 1, respectively. The obtained results give the corrected *p*-values, which may be indicated as *p*-HB. If a corrected value is greater than 1, it is turned to 1. Moreover, if *p*-value(k − 1) < *p*-value(k) and the *p*-HB(k) is smaller than the *p*-HB(k − 1), then the *p*-HB(k) is set as equal to the *p*-HB(k − 1).

For an easy application of the Holm−Bonferroni method, we may use the macro Holm−Bonferroni either from the Excel file Holm−Bonferroni through the menu Developer → Macros or from the Excel file OSTEO using the menu Add-Ins → OSTEO → Data Analysis → Holm−Bonferroni correction.

9.5.2 Independent Samples: One-Way Analysis of Variance

One-way ANOVA is a statistical test used to compare the means of three or more independent samples. The null hypothesis is:

$$H_0: \mu_1 = \mu_2 = \mu_3 = ... = \mu_K$$

where K is the number of samples. The alternative hypothesis states that at least one mean is different from another mean. There are three main preconditions to apply ANOVA:

1. There must be homogeneity of variance, i.e., there should be no statistically significant difference in the variance of the populations from which the samples come.
2. Samples should follow the normal distribution. If there is a small deviation from the normal distribution, we can still apply ANOVA.
3. Samples must be independent.

When the null hypothesis is rejected, we conclude that there is a statistically significant difference between the mean values of the samples under study. However, we do not know between which specific pairs of samples the significant differences are traced. Thus, we should perform *post hoc tests*. If the criterion of homogeneity of variance is valid, the *Tukey test* is the best option, whereas in the opposite case, the *Games—Howell test* should be preferred.

9.5.3 Independent Samples: Kruskal—Wallis Test

When one or more of the preconditions to apply ANOVA are violated, we should apply nonparametric tests. Among these tests, the Kruskal—Wallis has the most power. The statistical hypotheses are:

H_0 : All samples come from the same population

H_1 : Not H_0

A limitation of the nonparametric tests for many samples is that no effective post hoc tests are available. In this case, we can draw boxplots to get an idea of the possible differences between samples and perform Mann—Whitney tests for all pairwise comparisons. In the latter case, we should correct the *p*-values by means of the Holm—Bonferroni correction.

9.5.4 Dependent Samples: Repeated-Measures ANOVA

The repeated-measures ANOVA is the extension of the parametric paired *t* test to three or more dependent samples. This test also examines whether the samples come from populations of equal means. Therefore, if we test *K* samples, the null hypothesis states that the population means are equal. The alternative hypothesis states that at least one mean is different from another mean.

The assumptions of repeated-measures ANOVA are similar to those of the simple one-way ANOVA, except for the independence of the samples. Thus, there must be homogeneity of variance and the samples should follow the normal distribution. An additional critical assumption is known as the assumption of *sphericity*. According to this assumption, the variances of the differences between all combinations of related groups must be equal. Repeated-measures ANOVA is particularly sensitive to violations of the sphericity assumption, which may be tested using *Mauchly's test*.

9.5.5 Dependent Samples: Friedman Test

The Friedman test is the nonparametric version of the repeated-measures ANOVA. Therefore, it should be adopted when we have doubts about the validity of the various assumptions on which the parametric repeated-measures ANOVA is based.

9.5.6 Case Studies on the Comparison of Many Samples

Case Study 6: ANOVA and Kruskal—Wallis Test

The body mass (BM) of male adults from three archaeological sites has been estimated from regression equations using the pelvic girdle and stature, and the results are presented in Table 9.5.1. Assess whether the BM is significantly different among the three archaeological sites.

We place all sample values in one column, BM, and in another column, Site, we use numbers 1, 2, and 3 to discriminate the samples. Subsequently, we test the normality of the three samples. Thus, we use the menu Analyze → Descriptive Statistics → Explore. In the Explore dialog box we transfer the variable BM to the Dependent List box and the variable Site to the Factor List box. We click on "Plots" and in the dialog box that appears we select the options "Normality plots with tests" and "Factor levels together."

TABLE 9.5.1 Body Mass (in kg) of Male Adults From Three Archaeological Sites

Site 1	Site 2	Site 3
71	55	69
73	60	74
68	70	70
65	63	80
60	59	68
78	61	62
80	67	64
66		66
		65

We click on "Continue" and "OK" and obtain, among others, the table Tests of Normality in SPSS Output 9.5.1 and the boxplots of the samples in Fig. 9.5.1. We observe that statistically significant deviations from normality are not demonstrated and, therefore, we may proceed to apply ANOVA. However, this result may be unreliable because of the very small sample sizes, so the application of nonparametric techniques is recommended. In regard to the boxplots, they show a substantial differentiation of the second sample from the other two. Whether this is significant will be determined by ANOVA.

SPSS OUTPUT 9.5.1 Tests of Normality

	Site	Kolmogorov–Smirnov			Shapiro–Wilk		
		Statistic	df	Sig.	Statistic	df	Sig.
Body mass	1	0.128	8	0.200	0.972	8	0.916
	2	0.161	7	0.200	0.973	7	0.918
	3	0.183	9	0.200	0.929	9	0.469

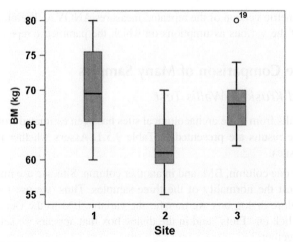

FIGURE 9.5.1 Boxplot of the samples of Table 9.5.1. *BM,* body mass.

To perform one-way ANOVA, we click Analyze → Compare Means → One-Way ANOVA. In the dialog box One-Way ANOVA that appears we transfer the variable BM to the box labeled Dependent List and the variable Site to the Factor box, and from Options we select "Homogeneity of variance test." In the dialog box One-Way ANOVA we click on "Post Hoc" and select the "Tukey" criterion. We click on "Continue" and "OK" and obtain the results presented in SPSS Outputs 9.5.2—9.5.4.

SPSS OUTPUT 9.5.2 Test of Homogeneity of Variances

Body Mass			
Levene statistic	df1	df2	Sig.
0.471	2	21	0.631

SPSS OUTPUT 9.5.3 ANOVA

Body Mass					
	Sum of Squares	df	Mean Square	F	Sig.
Between groups	266.768	2	133.384	3.903	0.036
Within groups	717.732	21	34.178		
Total	984.500	23			

SPSS OUTPUT 9.5.4 Multiple Comparisons

Dependent Variable: Body Mass

Tukey HSD

(I) Site	(J) Site	Mean Difference (I − J)	Std. Error	Sig.	95% Confidence Interval	
					Lower Bound	Upper Bound
1	2	7.982[a]	3.026	0.039	0.36	15.61
	3	1.458	2.841	0.866	−5.70	8.62
2	1	−7.982[a]	3.026	0.039	−15.61	−0.36
	3	−6.524	2.946	0.092	−13.95	0.90
3	1	−1.458	2.841	0.866	−8.62	5.70
	2	6.524	2.946	0.092	−0.90	13.95

[a]The mean difference is significant at the .05 level.

In the table Test of Homogeneity of Variances (SPSS Output 9.5.2) we observe that, based on the Levene criterion, the null hypothesis concerning the homogeneity of variances cannot be rejected (Sig. = .631 > .05). The ANOVA p-value is Sig. = .036 < .05 (SPSS Output 9.5.3), so there is an overall significant difference in the BM of the individuals from the sites under study.

To explore among which archaeological sites significant differences are traced, we examine the table Multiple Comparisons (SPSS Output 9.5.4). From this table we note that the only significant pairwise difference is between sites 1 and 2 (p-value = .039).

As already noted, the very small sample sizes may raise doubts about the aforementioned conclusions. Thus, it may be helpful to verify them by means of nonparametric techniques. To run the Kruskal–Wallis test, we use the menu Analyze → Nonparametric Tests → Legacy Dialogs → K Independent Samples. In the dialog box that appears, we transfer the variable BM to the box labeled Test Variable List and the variable Site to the Grouping Variable box. We click on "Define Range" and in the new dialog box we type in the value "1" for Minimum and the value "3" for Maximum. In the Test Type panel we select "Kruskal–Wallis H" if it is not preselected. We click on "Exact" and select "Monte Carlo" with number of samples 10,000. We click on "Continue" and "OK" and obtain the results given in SPSS Output 9.5.5.

SPSS OUTPUT 9.5.5 Test Statistics[a,b]

			Body Mass
Chi-Square			6.132
df			2
Asymp. Sig.			0.047
Monte Carlo	Sig.		0.043[c]
	99% confidence interval	Lower bound	0.038
		Upper bound	0.049

[a]Kruskal–Wallis test.
[b]Grouping variable: Site.
[c]Based on 10,000 sampled tables with starting seed 299,883,525.

We again observe that the null hypothesis that all samples come from the same population may be rejected at a significance level equal to .05 (Asymp. Sig. = .047 and Monte Carlo Sig. = .043). However, the test gives no information regarding the samples between which a significant difference is traced. To obtain this information we may use the boxplot of Fig. 9.5.1, which shows that Site 2 is different from the other two, or run pairwise Mann–Whitney tests and correct the obtained p-values for multiple comparisons. The uncorrected p-values obtained from the pairwise Mann–Whitney tests are given in Table 9.5.2. To apply the Holm–Bonferroni correction, we arrange the raw p-values in one column in an Excel spreadsheet and run the macro Holm–Bonferroni either from the Excel file Holm–Bonferroni using the menu Developer → Macros or from OSTEO using the menu Add-Ins → OSTEO → Data Analysis → Holm–Bonferroni correction. In the dialog box that appears we enter the range of the raw p-values, click on "OK," and select the output cell. The results obtained are also presented in Table 9.5.2, which shows that there are no significant pairwise differences, in complete disagreement with the results of the Kruskal–Wallis test. In such cases it is up to the researcher to decide how to interpret these findings. In this example, taking into account the boxplot of Fig. 9.5.1, the post hoc results in SPSS Output 9.5.4, and the Kruskal–Wallis test, we may conclude that the only significant pairwise difference is between sites 1 and 2.

TABLE 9.5.2 Uncorrected Mann–Whitney Pairwise p-values and Corrected p-values Using the Holm–Bonferroni Method

Pair	Mann–Whitney p-values	Holm–Bonferroni p-values
1–2	0.032	0.096
1–3	0.630	0.630
2–3	0.034	0.096

Case Study 7: Repeated-Measures ANOVA

The maximum cranial breadth (XCB) is defined as "the maximum cranial breadth perpendicular to the median sagittal plane taken above the supramastoid crests" (Howells, 1973, p. 172). We want to test how clear this definition is for undergraduate students who have no previous experience in craniometry. For this purpose, this definition was given to three students without further clarification. The students were asked to measure the XCB in nine different crania and the data obtained are given in Table 9.5.3.

TABLE 9.5.3 Maximum Cranial Breadth of Nine Crania (in cm) Measured by Three Students

Cranium	Student 1	Student 2	Student 3
1	13.9	13.5	13.5
2	12.5	12.2	12.0
3	14.3	14.4	14.0
4	14.0	13.9	13.5
5	13.2	13.0	12.7
6	13.0	13.2	13.0
7	13.6	13.6	13.4
8	12.7	12.8	12.4
9	13.4	13.4	13.1

In SPSS we arrange the data in three columns titled Student1, Student2, and Student3, and apply repeated-measures ANOVA because the same crania have been measured by three different individuals; thus the samples are dependent. For this purpose, we use the menu Analyze → General Linear Model → Repeated Measures. In the dialog box that appears we define the name of the repeated-measures factor and the number of its levels, which is equal to the number of samples. In our example we name this factor Student and define its three levels as in Fig. 9.5.2. For the program to accept the name and the number of levels, we should click on "Add."

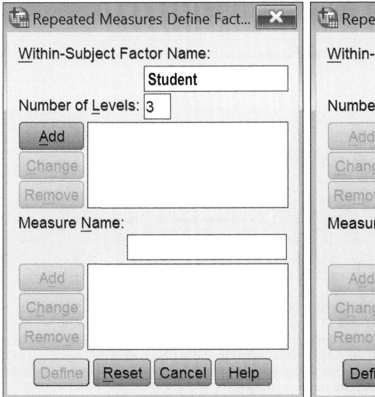
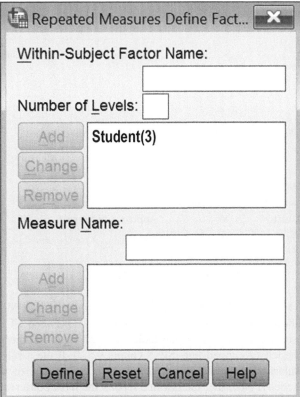

Then we click on "Define" and in the new dialog box that appears we transfer the names of the columns representing the levels of the repeated-measures factor, i.e., the variables Student1, Student2, and Student3, into the Within-Subjects Variables box, as shown in Fig. 9.5.3. Finally, we click on Options and in the corresponding dialog box we transfer the variable Student to the Display Means for box, click on the "Compare main effects" check box, and select "Bonferroni" from the drop-down list. With this latter option, the program will also perform post hoc tests employing the Bonferroni correction for the p-values. Clicking on "Continue" and "OK," we obtain many tables, the most important of which are presented in SPSS Outputs 9.5.6—9.5.8.

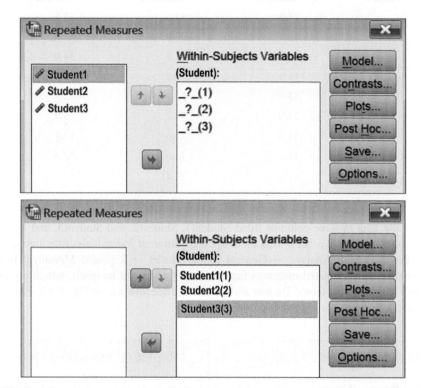

FIGURE 9.5.3 Transferring variables Student1, Student2, and Student3 into the Within-Subjects Variables box.

SPSS OUTPUT 9.5.6 Mauchly's Test of Sphericity

Measure: MEASURE_1								
Within-Subjects Effect	Mauchly's W	Approx. Chi-Square	df	Sig.	Epsilon			
					Greenhouse–Geisser	Huynh–Feldt	Lower Bound	
Student	0.789	1.660	2	0.436	0.826	1.000	0.500	

Mauchly's Test of Sphericity presents the results of Mauchly's test (SPSS Output 9.5.6). It is seen that the null hypothesis that the variances of the differences between all combinations of related groups are equal cannot be rejected. Based on this result, in the table Tests of Within-Subjects Effects, we check the Sig. value that corresponds to the Sphericity Assumed line (SPSS Output 9.5.7). If the assumption of sphericity did not hold, we would report one of the p-values (Sig.) from the second, third, or fourth line of this table. Each of them performs an adjustment for lack of sphericity. Note that the last line reports the most conservative adjustment.

SPSS OUTPUT 9.5.7 Tests of Within-Subjects Effects

Measure: MEASURE_1

Source		Type III Sum of Squares	df	Mean Square	F	Sig.
Student	Sphericity assumed	0.560	2	0.280	19.765	0.000
	Greenhouse–Geisser	0.560	1.651	0.339	19.765	0.000
	Huynh–Feldt	0.560	2.000	0.280	19.765	0.000
	Lower bound	0.560	1.000	0.560	19.765	0.002
Error (student)	Sphericity assumed	0.227	16	0.014		
	Greenhouse–Geisser	0.227	13.211	0.017		
	Huynh–Feldt	0.227	16.000	0.014		
	Lower bound	0.227	8.000	0.028		

SPSS OUTPUT 9.5.8 Pairwise Comparisons

Measure: MEASURE_1

(I) Student	(J) Student	Mean Difference (I − J)	Std. Error	Sig.[a]	95% Confidence Interval for Difference[a]	
					Lower Bound	Upper Bound
1	2	0.067	0.067	1.000	−0.134	0.268
	3	0.333[b]	0.055	0.001	0.167	0.500
2	1	−0.067	0.067	1.000	−0.268	0.134
	3	0.267[b]	0.044	0.001	0.134	0.400
3	1	−0.333[b]	0.055	0.001	−0.500	−0.167
	2	−0.267[b]	0.044	0.001	−0.400	−0.134

Based on estimated marginal means.
[a] Adjustment for multiple comparisons: Bonferroni.
[b] The mean difference is significant at the .05 level.

In SPSS Output 9.5.7 we observe that all tests give p-values lower than .002 and, therefore, there are significant differences between the mean XCB values obtained by the three students. From the table Pairwise Comparisons we note that the measurements of Student 3 are significantly differentiated from those of Students 1 and 2 (SPSS Output 9.5.8).

These results are valid provided that the assumptions of normality and homogeneity of variance are met. Normality is tested following the usual procedure. That is, we click on Analyze → Descriptive Statistics → Explore; in the Explore dialog box we transfer the three variables Student1, Student2, and Student3 in the Dependent List panel; we click on "Plots"; and in the dialog box that appears we activate the option "Normality plots with tests." After clicking on "Continue" and "OK" we obtain the p-values of the Shapiro–Wilk tests for the three samples, which are .923, .999, and .915, respectively, and therefore, statistically significant deviations from normality are not demonstrated for any of the compared samples.

In regard to the homogeneity of variance, this assumption can again be tested from the menu Analyze → Descriptive Statistics → Explore. However, for this test the data of the three samples should be arranged in a single column, Samples, whereas in another column, Student, a grouping variable with values 1, 2, and 3 should be formed to discriminate the samples. In the Explore box we transfer the variable Samples to the Dependent List box and the variable Student to the Factor List box; we click on "Plots," and in the dialog box that appears we select only the option "Untransformed." We obtain the table Test of Homogeneity of Variance, which presents the p-values based on several variations of Levene's test. It is seen that all tests support that the assumption of the homogeneity of variance is not violated (SPSS Output 9.5.9).

SPSS OUTPUT 9.5.9 Test of Homogeneity of Variance

		Levene Statistic	df1	df2	Sig.
Samples	Based on mean	0.004	2	24	0.996
	Based on median	0.008	2	24	0.992
	Based on median and with adjusted df	0.008	2	23.032	0.992
	Based on trimmed mean	0.004	2	24	0.996

If there are doubts about the validity of the assumptions necessary to apply parametric repeated-measures ANOVA, for example, because of small sample sizes, we may run the Friedman test through the menu Analyze → Nonparametric Tests → Legacy Dialogs → K Related Samples. In the dialog box that appears we transfer the variables Student1, Student2, and Student3 to the box labeled Test Variables, and in the Test Type panel we select "Friedman" if it is not preselected. Then we click on "Exact" and select "Monte Carlo" with number of samples 10,000. We click on "Continue" and "OK" and obtain the results given in SPSS Output 9.5.10.

SPSS OUTPUT 9.5.10 Test Statistics[a]

N			9
Chi-Square			12.063
df			2
Asymp. Sig.			0.002
Monte Carlo Sig.	Sig.		0.001
	99% confidence interval	Lower bound	0.000
		Upper bound	0.001

[a]Friedman test.

We again observe that the null hypothesis may be rejected at a significance level equal to .05. However, the results presented in SPSS Output 9.5.10 give no information about the pairs of samples between which statistical differences are traced. As mentioned, for this purpose we need to perform pairwise comparisons using the Wilcoxon test and subsequently correct the obtained p-values for multiple comparisons.

Case Study 8: Statistical Analysis of Cross-Sectional Geometry

The spreadsheet Dataset_CSG in the Excel file DataCreation_CSG provided in the companion website contains artificial data that represent values for the total subperiosteal area (TA), and ratios of different second moments of area (I_{max}/I_{min}, I_x/I_y), for the right and left humeri of males and females from four populations. The same data are also provided in the Excel file DataForStatistics. Analyze this data set using ANOVA/Kruskal–Wallis tests for interpopulation comparisons, whereas for intrapopulation comparisons, use two independent samples tests to examine differences between males and females, and paired samples tests to ascertain whether side dominance exists.

Here, we restrict the analysis to the TA data (Fig. 9.5.4), whereas similar statistical tests can be applied to I_{max}/I_{min} and I_x/I_y. Note that for simplicity, the TA data have not been standardized based on BM, although, in any real study, this step is essential. In contrast, no standardization for BM is required for I_{max}/I_{min} and I_x/I_y because these quantities are ratios of two variables.

dataset_CSG															
TA data															
population 1				population 2				population 3				population 4			
sex: M	M	F	F	M	M	F	F	M	M	F	F	M	M	F	F
side: R	L	R	L	R	L	R	L	R	L	R	L	R	L	R	L
432	394.5	388.8	394.2	430.4	416.5	410	416.9	453.8	422.4	391.4	372.7	401	399.3	360.2	411.7
422.4	389	377.4	360.4	455.5	453	407.2	405.7	416.6	417.7	406.4	378	387.2	402.5	393.1	384.6
431.1	414.7	387.6	394.5	420.1	466.3	391.4	379.9	451.8	424.6	385.6	411.2	397.5	388	396.1	377.8
406.1	403.6	378.7	361.6	450.1	433.9	423.1	389.3	410.2	422.4	401.5	392.6	435.4	405.2	409.9	394.5
430.1	412.5	377.7	398.1	432.8	469.4	411.7	404.5	451.4	435	407.2	379.1	393.4	405.7	400	371.3
429.8	388.5	393.9	376.3	468.2	437.4	390.5	373.7	433.4	407	399.5	393.8	409.4	446.2	396.2	388.7
412.6	372.1	404.8	389.1	465.6	436.8	414.3	409.4	423.8	496.2	428.4	405.8	398.1	404.9	358	370.9
420.2	423.8	397.5	398.4	453.4	440.1	435.3	418.1	417.5	396.7	365.4	399	405.2	414.1	418.2	397.7
386.1	401.2	395.2	382.3	456.3	460.9	401.6	400.5	440.6	445.2	391.8	374.6	421.4	407.1	406.1	407.1
419.7	383.9	372.4	378.3	477.4	462.9	429.4	427.5	439.9	424.5	416.9	412.1	391	401.6	416.4	390.9
418.5	379.3	379.5	396.6	454.9	444	413.2	375.5	410.1	399.5	406.2	407.4	438.5	392.8	439.9	401.9
393.8	380.9	362.7	385.5	421.1	449.2	406.9	388.5	438.1	418.4	406	407.6	410.2	411.1	334.7	384.2
429.3	379.6	378	371.4	450.4	441.4	426	398.7	447	430.4			406.7	403.3	379.1	414.3
424.3	399.3	388.1	377.5	438.9	440	431.7	387.3	443.4	447.7			404.3	411.7	385.9	388.1
428.8	384.2	371.3	397.8	457.1	433.7	409.8	370.3	435.1	404.1			447.2	376.5		
433.7	378.6			460.2	462.4							404.9	406		
408.9	402.1			457.7	445.7							402.3	408.1		
443.3	417.5											410.5	390		
411.8	385.4											400.3	380.1		
423.5	387.4											412.8	410.2		
417.5	400.2											429.6	372.7		
454.1	378.7											401.4	396.9		

FIGURE 9.5.4 Dataset_CSG (cross-sectional geometry) with total subperiosteal area (TA) values.

We first test the normality of these data using the Shapiro—Wilk test. To examine all samples of Fig. 9.5.4 simultaneously, we arrange the 16 samples in 16 separate columns in SPSS and click on Analyze → Descriptive Statistics → Explore; in the Explore dialog box we transfer all 16 variables to the Dependent List panel and click on "Plots" and in the dialog box that appears we activate the option "Normality plots with tests." In addition, we click on Options and select "Exclude cases pairwise." When the samples exhibit different sample sizes, this selection is necessary for the program to recognize as valid all the cases of each sample. We obtain that in all samples the p-values are higher than .05, indicating that there is no evidence of lack of normality, except for three samples, sample (M, L) of population 3 and samples (M, R) and (M, L) of population 4, for which p-value = .023, .029, and .037, respectively. However, these values do not show strong deviations from normality and, therefore, we may proceed to use parametric tests. For educational reasons, in this case study we will also adopt nonparametric tests.

Table 9.5.4 shows the p-values obtained from the application of ANOVA and Kruskal—Wallis tests to the samples that correspond to the right side of males and females of the four populations. Both tests show clearly that there are statistically significant differences among the four populations for both males and females. From the pairwise comparisons presented in Table 9.5.5, we observe that statistically significant differences are traced between populations 1—2, 2—3, 2—4, and 3—4 for males and 1—2 and 2—4 for females. Note that the p-values obtained from Tukey's test do not agree with those obtained from the application of the Mann—Whitney test (Table 9.5.5). However, because all findings indicate that ANOVA can be applied to the data set under consideration, the Tukey results are more reliable.

TABLE 9.5.4 ANOVA and Kruskal—Wallis Test for Equal Means/Medians

	ANOVA	Levene's Test	Kruskal—Wallis Test
Right male	8.77×10^{-11}	0.96	4.6×10^{-8}
Right female	0.000344	0.04	0.00012

TABLE 9.5.5 *p*-values of Post Hoc Comparisons

| Sample Pair | Right Male | | Right Female | |
	Tukey's Test	Mann–Whitney HB Correction	Tukey's Test	Mann–Whitney HB Correction
1–2	1.8×10^{-6}	0.0001	0.0002	0.0001
1–3	0.0863	0.0270	0.0861	0.0200
1–4	0.0518	0.0208	0.5581	0.2323
2–3	0.0265	0.0208	0.2635	0.0829
2–4	6.4×10^{-11}	8.8×10^{-6}	0.0147	0.0829
3–4	5.8×10^{-5}	0.0005	0.6673	0.4715

HB, Holm–Bonferroni.

The boxplot of Fig. 9.5.5 visualizes TA differences between males and females for right-side data. These have been plotted in SPSS as follows. The data need to be arranged in SPSS in four columns (variables): Population with values 1, 2, 3, 4; Sex with values 1, 2; Side with values 1, 2; and TA. To select the TA values for the right side alone, we select the cases for which Side = 1 from the path: Data → Select Cases. To draw the boxplot, we use the menu: Graphs → Legacy dialogs → Boxplot. In the window that opens, we activate the options "Clustered" and "Summaries for groups of cases." We click on "Define" and in the new window we transfer TA to the Variable box, Population to the Category Axis box, and Sex to the Define Clusters by box.

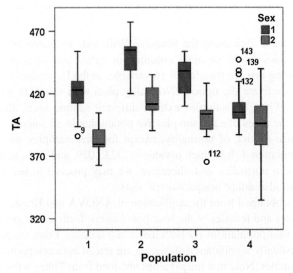

FIGURE 9.5.5 Boxplot for right-side humeral total subperiosteal area (TA) for males (1) and females (2).

Representative intrapopulation comparisons for population 1 are given in Tables 9.5.6 and 9.5.7. These comparisons focus on sexual dimorphism and bilateral asymmetry. In particular, Table 9.5.6 gives the sexual dimorphism results and it can be seen that the difference in TA values between males and females is statistically significant for the right side and close to the limit of statistical significance for the left side. Note that *Levene's test for equality of variances* showed no significant difference between male and female data. With respect to bilateral asymmetry (Table 9.5.7), the parametric

TABLE 9.5.6 *p*-values for Sexual Dimorphism in Population 1

	t Test	Levene's Test	Mann—Whitney Test
Right	8.6×10^{-10}	0.572	1.9×10^{-6}
Left	0.052	0.554	0.07

TABLE 9.5.7 *p*-values for Bilateral Asymmetry in Population 1

	t Test	Wilcoxon Test	Monte Carlo ($n = 99999$)
Male	2.3×10^{-6}	0.00016	0
Female	0.893	0.842	0.853

(paired *t* test), nonparametric (Wilcoxon test), and Monte Carlo permutations support a significant effect for males and a nonsignificant one for females.

An alternative approach to treating cross-sectional geometry (CSG) data under the prerequisite that they follow the normal distribution is by means of generalized linear models (GLM). This approach is described in Section 9.7.4 and in Case Study 17.

Case Study 9: Statistical Analysis of Dental Wear Data

Data sets of dental wear contain either ordinal or continuous data. A point that must be noted is that, as argued in Section 7.3.2, dental wear data recorded as continuous variables are unlikely to follow the normal distribution. Therefore, all nonparametric statistical analyses described earlier for CSG may also apply for testing the extent of dental wear at the inter- and intrapopulation levels.

Representative nonparametric tests concerning the analysis of dataset_DW1, which is given in the Excel files DataCreation—DW and DataForStatistics, provided in the companion website, are shown in Tables 9.5.8—9.5.10. Table 9.5.8 gives the *p*-values of the Kruskal—Wallis tests for equal medians of the right- and left-side samples coming from four populations. It can be seen that the difference in dental wear expression among the four populations is statistically significant overall on the right and the left side. However, from the pairwise comparisons we realize that this difference is statistically significant only between populations 1 and 4 (Table 9.5.9). Finally, with respect to bilateral asymmetry, no significant effect is traced among populations (Table 9.5.10).

TABLE 9.5.8 Kruskal—Wallis Tests for Equal Medians for Dataset_DW1

Side	*p*-value
Right	0.004
Left	0.008

TABLE 9.5.9 *p*-values of Pairwise Comparisons Using Mann–Whitney Tests and Holm–Bonferroni Correction for Dataset_DW1

	Right Side		Left Side	
Pair	Uncorrected	HB	Uncorrected	HB
1–2	0.820	1	0.651	1
1–3	0.013	0.067	0.524	1
1–4	0.0009	0.005	0.0007	0.004
2–3	0.104	0.311	0.771	1
2–4	0.032	0.130	0.013	0.065
3–4	0.934	1	0.065	0.260

HB, Holm–Bonferroni.

TABLE 9.5.10 *p*-values for Bilateral Asymmetry for Dataset_DW1

Population (Sample)	Wilcoxon Test	Monte Carlo (*n* = 99999)
1	0.086	0.086
2	0.301	0.315
3	0.288	0.300
4	0.092	0.092

9.6 TESTS FOR CATEGORICAL DATA

The tests examined in the previous sections deal with quantitative data. However, on many occasions we have to analyze qualitative/categorical data. As already noted in Section 9.2.3, these are data that can be organized into mutually exclusive categories. For example, the variable Sex is a categorical variable, which takes the values "male" and "female." Similarly, the variable Supranasal suture in Table 5.XI.1 is categorical and may take the values "1" or "presence" and "2" or "absence."

As also discussed in Section 9.2.3, when a variable is categorical, we calculate *frequencies*. The frequencies of a variable that is categorized according to two attributes are usually presented in the form of a *contingency table*. An example of a contingency table is given in Table 9.2.3. The usefulness of contingency tables is that they help one to draw conclusions about the existence of differences among samples. However, to test if the observed differences are statistically significant, we have to use inferential statistics, and the appropriate methods are described in this section. Note that apart from the methods discussed here, binary and ordinal data can be effectively analyzed by means of GLM and generalized estimating equations (GEE). These two techniques belong to data modeling and for this reason they are described in Section 9.7.4, and case studies are given in Section 9.7.7.

9.6.1 Chi-Square and Fisher's Exact Tests

A strict criterion used to evaluate if any observed difference in a contingency table arises by chance or not is *Pearson's Chi-Square* (χ^2) *test*. The χ^2 test is used when the percentage of cells with expected frequency below 5 is smaller than 20%. If more cells have small frequencies, then the results of the χ^2 test may not be valid. In cases in which we suspect that the results of the χ^2 test may not be accurate, we apply Fisher's exact test or its variant using Monte Carlo permutations. Fisher's exact test is usually adopted in 2×2 tables, whereas the Monte Carlo variant is used in larger tables.

9.6.2 Correspondence Analysis

When the contingency table has many rows and columns, the χ^2 test is not particularly helpful because it is likely that there are correlations among the variables. In such cases we are interested in finding clusters of data that intercorrelate. For this purpose, we may apply *correspondence analysis (CA)*. CA is a statistical exploratory tool, which graphically represents the dependence between rows and columns of contingency tables. This visual display of data may allow patterns to emerge.

9.6.3 Case Studies on Categorical Data Analysis

Case Study 10: Chi-Square and Fisher's Exact Tests

Assess whether the frequency of the trait supranasal suture is statistically significantly different among the samples of Table 5.XI.1 for which the contingency table is Table 9.2.3.

We arrange the data of the contingency table, Table 9.2.3, as in Fig. 9.6.1, in which the variable Expression represents the presence/absence of the trait, and use the menu Data → Weight cases. In the dialog box that appears we transfer the variable Frequency to the Frequency Variable box after selecting the option "Weight cases by." Then we use the menu Analyze → Descriptive Statistics → Crosstabs and transfer the variable Sample into the Row(s) panel and the variable Expression into the Column(s) panel. Subsequently, we click on "Statistics" and select "Chi-square." In addition, we click on "Exact" and activate the option "Exact" or, alternatively, we select "Monte-Carlo" and increase the number of samples to 10,000. We click on "Continue" and "OK." We obtain the table Chi-Square Tests (SPSS Output 9.6.1).

	Sample	Expression	Frequency
1	1	1	8
2	1	2	2
3	2	1	3
4	2	2	7
5	3	1	2
6	3	2	9
7	4	1	4
8	4	2	8

FIGURE 9.6.1 Data arrangement in SPSS for χ^2 and Fisher's exact tests.

SPSS OUTPUT 9.6.1 Chi-Square Tests

	Value	df	Asymp. Sig. (2-Sided)	Exact Sig. (2-Sided)	Exact Sig. (1-Sided)	Point Probability
Pearson chi-square	9.521[a]	3	0.023	0.023		
Likelihood ratio	9.780	3	0.021	0.029		
Fisher's exact test	8.973			0.027		
Linear-by-linear association	4.663[b]	1	0.031	0.039	0.021	0.011
N of valid cases	43					

[a]*Four cells (50.0%) have an expected count less than 5. The minimum expected count is 3.95.*
[b]*The standardized statistic is 2.159.*

In the table Chi-Square Tests we observe that all tests and especially the Pearson Chi-Square and the Fisher exact test give *p*-values lower than the level of significance .05. Therefore, we may reject the null hypothesis and thus, we confirm our earlier observation, that there is a statistically significant correlation between sample and the expression of the supranasal suture. Unfortunately, these tests cannot clarify between which samples the statistically significant differences are traced. In this case the contingency table may be helpful. Thus, from Table 9.2.3 we observe that sample 1 is the one that differs significantly from the rest.

Case Study 11: Correspondence Analysis

Based on the contingency table, Table 9.6.1, assess whether there is an association between tomb orientation and the age of the deceased.

TABLE 9.6.1 Contingency Table for the Association Between Tomb Orientation and Age of the Deceased

Tomb typology	Age			
	1	2	3	4
1	0	3	4	10
2	2	8	4	4
3	11	2	2	1

Age: 1 = subadult (SA), 2 = young adult (YA), 3 = middle adult (MA), 4 = old adult (OA).
Tomb typology: 1 = cist, 2 = tholos, 3 = pit.

We arrange the data of Table 9.6.1 in three columns, Tomb, Age, Frequency; i.e., similar to Fig. 9.6.1, assign labels to the values of the variables Tomb and Age using the "Values" option in the Variable View window, and click on Data → Weight cases. We transfer the variable Frequency to the Frequency Variable box. Then we use the menu Analyze → Dimension Reduction → Optimal Scaling and in the dialog box that appears we select "All variables are multiple nominal" and "One set." We click on "Define" and in the new dialog box we transfer the variables Tomb and Age to the box labeled Analysis Variables. Finally, we click on the "Variable" button, transfer Age and Tomb to the Joint Category Plots box, and activate "Display plot" (Fig. 9.6.2).

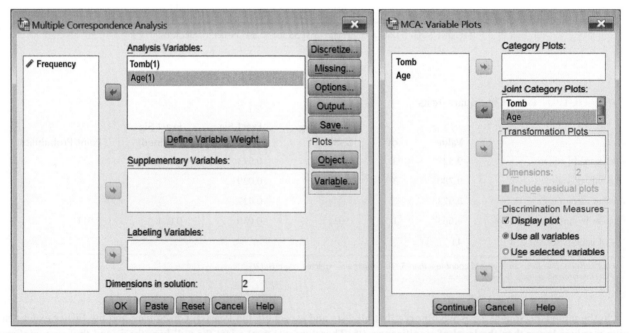

FIGURE 9.6.2 Transferring the variables Tomb and Age to the Analysis Variables box and then to the Joint Category Plots box activating the option "Display plot."

In the Joint Plot of Category Points (Fig. 9.6.3) we observe that there is indeed some differentiation in the tomb typology according to the age of the deceased. Specifically, old adults are mostly buried in cist tombs, young adults in tholos tombs, and subadults in pits, whereas middle adults do not appear to be associated with a particular tomb type.

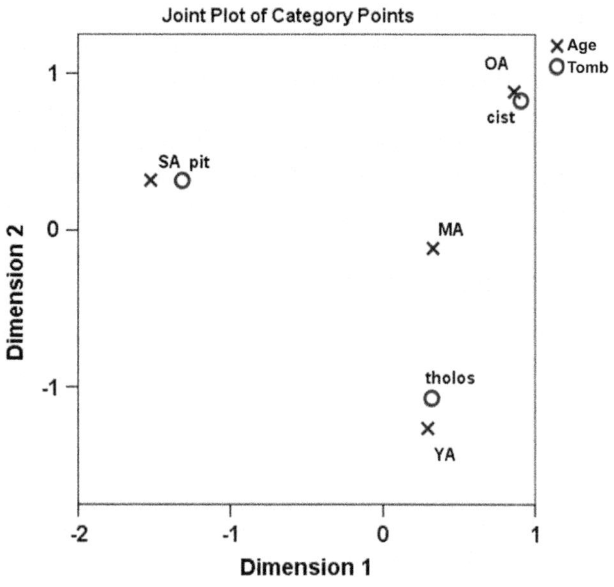

Joint Plot of Category Points

FIGURE 9.6.3 Joint plot of category points.

9.7 DATA MODELING

In many studies we need to find the equation that describes the relationship between two quantitative variables. *Regression* is one of the basic procedures used to find the mathematical expression of this relationship. The criterion used for the determination of the best equation (model) that describes (x, y) data is called the *least-squares criterion*. According to this criterion, the best model corresponds to the minimum of the sum of the squared residuals, where a *residual* is the difference between the experimental and the calculated from the model y value at a certain x value (Fig. 9.7.1).

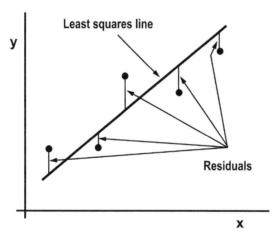

FIGURE 9.7.1 Residuals definition.

Regression is based on very few assumptions. If we are interested only in modeling the experimental data, the basic prerequisite is the absence of outliers. The presence of outliers is very easily traced in the *y* vs *x* plot and is likely to produce an unreliable model. If we are additionally interested in statistical inference, for example, if we want to identify statistically nonsignificant terms in the model, then the assumption of the normality of residuals is necessary.

When two or more models have been determined by means of the least-squares method, the optimum model may be selected based on the *standard error of estimate (SEE)*. This measure is defined by:

$$SEE = \sqrt{\frac{\sum_{i=1}^{N} (y_i(exp) - y_i(calc))^2}{N - q}} \tag{9.7.1}$$

where $y_i(exp)$ is the experimental and $y_i(calc)$ the calculated from the model y value at a certain x_i value, N is the number of experimental points, and q is the number of terms in the regression model. Thus, SEE gives, in fact, the average scatter of the experimental points around the regression curve and, therefore, the best model corresponds to the minimum SEE value.

Among the software packages described in this chapter, Excel is the most flexible in plotting graphs, which is an essential feature in data modeling, whereas SPSS offers the best algorithms for determining the optimum model as well as options for performing advanced regression models, like GLM. Note that the capabilities of Excel are increased by writing proper VBA macros, such as the macros of the Regression file provided in the companion website.

9.7.1 Models Adopted in the Least-Squares Method

The simplest application of the least-squares method is the determination of the coefficients of the linear model:

$$y = a + bx \tag{9.7.2}$$

or

$$y = bx \tag{9.7.3}$$

If the relationship between two variables is not linear, we examine whether a *quadratic* or a *cubic* model can be used. The mathematical expression for the quadratic model is:

$$y = a + bx + cx^2 \tag{9.7.4}$$

whereas that of the cubic model is:

$$y = a + bx + cx^2 + dx^3 \tag{9.7.5}$$

Note that all these models are limiting cases of a polynomial of degree p:

$$y = b_0 + b_1x + b_2x^2 + \ldots + b_px^p \tag{9.7.6}$$

In all these models parameters a, b, c, $\ldots$, b_0, b_1, $\ldots$, b_p are called *adjustable parameters*; they are initially unknown and they are determined based on the least-squares criterion.

A generalization is the *multilinear regression* or *multilinear fitting*, in which we have one dependent and many independent variables. Therefore, the model may have the following form:

$$y = b_0 + b_1x_1 + b_2x_2 + \ldots + b_px_p \tag{9.7.7}$$

The determination of the adjustable parameters is again done by means of the least-squares criterion, but it may be useful to assess which of them are significant and which can be eliminated, as discussed next.

9.7.2 Number of Adjustable Parameters

In general, the least-squares method allows the estimation of the adjustable parameters b_0, b_1, $\ldots$, b_p when the model is given from the relationship:

$$y = b_0 + b_1f_1(x) + b_2f_2(x) + \ldots + b_pf_p(x) \tag{9.7.8}$$

where $f_1(x)$, $f_2(x)$, $\ldots$, $f_p(x)$ are functions of x. When the model is known, the number of the adjustable parameters is also known. However, there are cases in which the model is an empirical relationship or a polynomial of degree p. In such cases, it is necessary to determine the statistically significant terms of the model or the degree of the polynomial, that is, the optimum degree that should be used for the model.

This issue can be easily solved if the p-values of the adjustable parameters are known. Consider that the p-value of the parameter b_k is known. This value corresponds to the null hypothesis H_0, $b_k = 0$, with alternative H_1, $b_k \neq 0$. Therefore, when p-value $> .05$, the null hypothesis cannot be rejected ($b_k = 0$) and therefore parameter b_k may be eliminated from the model. Based on this observation, when we know the model but want to remove the nonsignificant parameters, we calculate the p-values of all parameters and remove the parameter with the greatest p-value, provided that p-value $> .05$. Then we reapply the least-squares method, without the eliminated parameter in the model. We check if there are parameters with p-values $> .05$ and repeat the above process until all the adjustable parameters of the model are statistically significant, i.e., with p-values $< .05$.

If we want to determine the optimum degree of the polynomial, we may use the *forward* or *backward* method. In the forward method we start from a polynomial of a small degree, for example $y = a + bx$, and increase the degree of the polynomial by one at a time, that is, $y = a + bx + cx^2$, $y = a + bx + cx^2 + dx^3$, ... In every step we check if the adjustable parameters are statistically significant (*p*-value $< .05$). Once we find a polynomial in which at least one of the adjustable parameters is nonsignificant, we stop this process and select the previous polynomial as optimum. The inverse of this process is the backward method. In this case we start from a large degree polynomial, say $p = 10$, and reduce the degree of the polynomial by one at a time. At each step we check if at least one of the adjustable parameters is nonsignificant. We stop this process when all parameters are statistically significant and select this polynomial as the optimum one.

9.7.3 General Linear Models (Analysis of Covariance)

Analysis of covariance (ANCOVA) or *general linear models* is an extension of the previous models that includes nominal and/or ordinal variables as independent variables. Thus, ANCOVA generates prediction equations for the various levels of a categorical variable. The continuous independent variables are called *covariates*, whereas the categorical independent variables are called *factors*.

From a statistical point of view, ANCOVA may be considered as a combination of ANOVA and regression. For this reason, ANCOVA assumes the normality of residuals but there are three important additional assumptions: (1) the error variance of the dependent variable is equal across groups (homogeneity of variance), (2) the dependent variable varies linearly with each covariate at each level of the categorical variable, and (3) the lines of the aforementioned relationships have the same slope (homogeneity of regression slopes). The origin of the last two assumptions will be clarified later in Case Study 15.

9.7.4 Generalized Linear Models (GLM) and Generalized Estimating Equations (GEE)

GLM extend linear regression to include dependent variables that may have nonnormal distributions. In particular, GLM are applied when the dependent variable comes from any exponential family distribution, i.e., normal, binomial, Poisson, etc., and it is recorded as a function of p independent variables, i.e., X_1, X_2, ..., X_p, which can be continuous and/or categorical.

The mathematical expression of GLM may be written as:

$$\eta = b_0 + b_1X_1 + b_2X_2 + ... + b_pX_p \tag{9.7.9}$$

where $\eta = f(\mu)$, f being any smooth monotonic *link* function of the mean (μ) of the distribution function of the dependent variable y. This function is called the *link* function.

There are several options for the dependent variable y. For example, y may be a scale, an ordinal, or a binary variable. If y is a scale variable that follows the normal distribution, then the link function is the *identity function* and, therefore, $\eta = y$, where y is the predicted by the model y value. In this case, GLM become identical to a general linear model (ANCOVA). When the response is an ordinal variable taking the values 0, 1, ..., J, the link function η is a *cumulative logit function*. Because this function results in J models, the modeling of ordinal y data using the cumulative logit function is quite complicated. However, in a 2014 study (Nikita, 2014) it was shown that the application of GLM to ordinal data that code an underlying continuous variable assuming an ordinal response gives results that converge satisfactorily with those obtained from GLM assuming a scale response. Thus, the modeling of ordinal y data that code an underlying continuous variable may be done by means of GLM using a scale y variable and this approach simplifies the model considerably, because the variable η in Eq. (9.7.9) is the predicted by the GLM y value. Finally, when we have a binary y variable, the link function in SPSS may be expressed as:

$$\eta = -\ln\frac{P}{1-P} \tag{9.7.10}$$

where P is the probability that the binary variable takes the value 0. Therefore, in SPSS the mathematical expression of GLM under binary response may be written as:

$$\ln\frac{P}{1-P} = -(b_0 + b_1X_1 + b_2X_2 + ... + b_pX_p) \tag{9.7.11}$$

GLM may assess the impact of multiple factors simultaneously, examine the effects of interactions, and model the data. When a GLM is used to model data, the best model is usually determined as follows. We start from the *saturated model* or from any model that includes all the independent variables and several of their interactions, i.e., terms of the form $b_j X_k X_q$ or $b_j X_k X_q X_w$, etc. Then we remove the nonsignificant factors and interactions one by one. The statistically best model corresponds to the smallest *Akaike information criterion* (AIC) and the corresponding *corrected AIC (AICC)* value. Both these criteria are measures of the relative quality of a model, that is, they assess the quality of a model relative to other models.

A basic prerequisite for the application of GLM is the lack of any correlation between outcomes (the values of the dependent variable). If this condition is not met, we should apply GEE. That is, GEE is a version of GLM, appropriate when a possible correlation exists between outcomes, for example, when there are more than one measurement for each individual. This is the case when bilateral asymmetry is examined.

9.7.5 Logistic Regression

Logistic regression, or, more precisely, *binary logistic regression,* is a special case of GLM, where the dependent variable is binary, whereas the independent variables are discrete and/or continuous. However, in most cases, the discrete independent (explanatory) variables are treated as covariates. Therefore, the regression model is given by Eq. (9.7.11).

9.7.6 Reduced Major Axis Regression

When the regression model is obtained by minimizing the sum of the squared residuals, the procedure is called *ordinary least-squares fitting (OLS)*. The underlying assumption of this choice is that we control the independent variable x and measure the dependent (response) variable y, so that measurement errors concern exclusively variable y. When both variables, x and y, are subject to experimental errors, the OLS, called also *model 1 regression*, is not reliable.

In this case the regression procedure should minimize the errors in both variables, *model 2 regression*. There are several ways to do this. In the *reduced major axis regression* (RMA), also called *standard major axis regression,* we minimize the areas of the triangles formed by the data points and the regression line as shown in Fig. 9.7.2. In biological anthropological research RMA offers the advantage that it provides more accurate results for individuals lying at the two extremes of the sample values (for a brief discussion on anthropological applications see Ruff et al., 2012, whereas for an in-depth presentation of RMA consult Warton et al., 2006 and Smith, 2009).

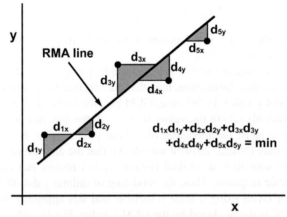

FIGURE 9.7.2 Definition of the reduced major axis regression (RMA) line.

9.7.7 Case Studies on Data Modeling and Applications

Case Study 12: Simple Linear Fitting

Assess whether the age of an infant can be predicted based on its humeral length using the data given in Table 9.7.1. If it can be predicted, find the age of an infant whose humeral length is 50 mm.

In data modeling based on the *residuals least-squares criterion* (*model 1 regression*), the variable that exhibits the most experimental imprecision should be taken as the dependent variable. In this example, it may be difficult to distinguish which

TABLE 9.7.1 Dependence of Humeral Length Upon Age in a Sample of Modern Infants	
Age (weeks)	Humeral Length (mm)
27	45
30	48
30	52
33	59
35	60
35	58
37	62
37	65
39	65
39	67
40	70
40	72
42	72

variable is more error prone. However, what we need to find out is the dependence of age upon humeral length. Therefore, the variable Age may be selected as the dependent variable y and the Humeral length as the independent variable x. Based on this selection, we draw a scatterplot to see how these two variables are interrelated. From the obtained graph (Fig. 9.7.3) we conclude that, despite some scatter of the points, there is a linear relationship between Age and Humeral length.

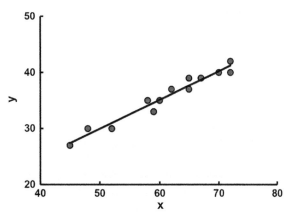

FIGURE 9.7.3 Plot of y = Age versus x = Humeral length and the least-squares line.

To find the equation that describes the least-squares straight line in Excel, that is, the equation that defines the relationship between Age and Humeral length, we may use the menu Data → Data Analysis → Regression. In the Regression box, we click inside the Input Y Range box and then click and drag the cursor in the range of the spreadsheet where the y values have been entered. We repeat the previous step to input the x values in the Input X Range box, leave the option "Constant is zero" unchecked, click on the "Residuals" check box, and click on an output cell, i.e., the cell that will be the upper left corner of the table of results. Part of these results is presented in Fig. 9.7.4.

In SPSS we enter the data in two columns, Humeral length and Age, and use the menu Analyze → Regression → Linear. We transfer the variable Age to the Dependent box and the variable Humeral length to the

	Coefficients	Standard Error	t Stat	P-value
Intercept	4.3259	2.0373	2.1234	0.0572
X Variable 1	0.5129	0.0330	15.5400	7.8E-09

FIGURE 9.7.4 Part of the regression results in Excel.

Independent(s) box. In Method we leave the "Enter" option, click on "Save," and select the options "Predicted Values Unstandardized" and "Residuals Unstandardized." Finally, we click on Options and click on the "Include constant in equation" check box. We obtain, among others, the table Coefficients shown in SPSS Output 9.7.1.

SPSS OUTPUT 9.7.1 Coefficients[a]

	Model	Unstandardized Coefficients		Standardized Coefficients		
		B	Std. Error	Beta	t	Sig.
1	(Constant)	4.326	2.037		2.123	0.057
	Humeral length	0.513	0.033	0.978	15.54	0.000

[a]Dependent variable: Age.

Both tables in Fig. 9.7.4 and in SPSS Output 9.7.1 give precisely the same information. The least-squares linear model is expressed by the equation:

$$y = a + bx = 4.326 + 0.513\,x \tag{9.7.12}$$

where the standard deviations of the constant 4.326 and the slope 0.513 are 2.037 and 0.033, respectively. In addition, these tables provide the p-values .057 and 7.8×10^{-9}, arising from the test of the hypotheses: H_0, $a = 0$, with alternative H_1, $a \neq 0$, and H_0, $b = 0$, with alternative H_1, $b \neq 0$, respectively.

It is seen that the p-value $= 7.8 \times 10^{-9}$ is negligible with respect to .05 and, therefore, the null hypothesis H_0, $b = 0$, should be rejected. Thus, we should accept H_1, $b \neq 0$, which means that the value 0.513 of the slope is statistically significant. In contrast, p-value $= .057$ is slightly greater than .05 and, therefore, the null hypothesis, H_0, $a = 0$, may not be rejected. This result indicates that the constant $a = 4.326$ could be eliminated from the model but this is up to the researcher.

This result is valid under the assumption that the residuals follow the normal distribution. Thus, we should test this assumption. From the selections made earlier, both programs provide the residuals and, therefore, we may use SPSS to test their normality. We obtain that the p-value of the Shapiro–Wilk test is $.551 > .05$, which shows that deviations from normality are not demonstrated.

If the constant term in Eq. (9.7.12) is eliminated from the model, the linear model is expressed as $y = bx$. However, when a is eliminated, b is no longer equal to 0.513. To find the least-squares value of b when $a = 0$, we reapply the least-squares method, as before. However, now in the Regression box of Excel we activate the option "Constant is zero," whereas in the Options box of SPSS we uncheck the "Include constant in equation" check box. The results obtained are $b = 0.582 \pm 0.005$ and p-value $= 1.3 \times 10^{-19}$. Therefore, we deduce that the linear least-squares model is:

$$y = 0.582\,x \tag{9.7.13}$$

Fig. 9.7.3 shows the plot of y = Age versus x = Humeral length and the least-squares line y = 0.582x. We observe that the line y = 0.582x describes the experimental data very satisfactorily. Therefore, the relationship y = 0.582x can be used for the prediction of the age of infants based on their humeral length. Thus, the age of the infant whose humeral length is 50 mm is equal to:

$$y = 0.582 \times 50 = 29.1 \text{ weeks} \tag{9.7.14}$$

The least-squares straight line in Fig. 9.7.3 can be drawn using the predicted y values that both programs, Excel and SPSS, provide. However, in Excel there is a more direct and easier way to add a regression line. After plotting the scatterplot of the data, we right-click on one of these points and in the drop-down menu we select Add Trendline, whereas from the Trendline Format task pane we click on the options "Linear" and "Set Intercept 0." The last option is selected only when the constant, a, in the model is to be 0.

Case Study 13: Polynomial Fitting

Table 9.7.2 shows the variation in human dental size over time. As a proxy for dental size the definition of tooth size given in Brace et al. (1987) has been used. Draw a graph to depict the table values and estimate the age of an individual with tooth size equal to 1300 mm^2.

TABLE 9.7.2 Tooth Size Change Over Time in *Homo*

Thousands of Years Ago	Dental Area (mm^2)	Thousands Years Ago	Dental Area (mm^2)
0	1120	7	1180
0	1128	7	1138
0	1141	10	1220
0	1078	20	1235
0	1149	30	1355
0	1140	50	1415
7	1196	100	1631

Adapted from Brace CL, Rosenberg KR, Hunt KD. Gradual change in human tooth size in the Late Pleistocene and Post-Pleistocene. Evolution 1987;41, 705–720.

As in the previous case study, we draw a scatterplot to assess if the relationship between the two variables is linear, quadratic, or cubic. Moreover, because we need to assess age based on tooth size, we select Age as the dependent variable (y) and Tooth size as the independent one (x). In the obtained graph we observe that the relationship between the two variables is not linear (Fig. 9.7.5). For this reason, we should test whether these data are described best by the quadratic or the cubic model.

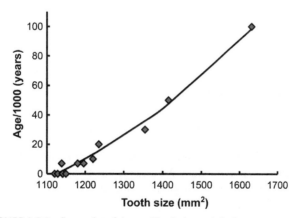

FIGURE 9.7.5 Scatterplot of Age vs Tooth size and the least-squares curve.

To test the quadratic model, we should create a new variable, x^2, whereas for the cubic model we should create variables x^2 and x^3. In Excel variables x, x^2, and x^3 should be in adjacent columns, whereas this is not necessary in SPSS. To determine the most appropriate model, we work as follows.

In Excel we examine first the quadratic model with and without a constant term and repeat this procedure for the cubic model. Thus, we use the menu Data → Data Analysis → Regression. In the Regression box we click inside the Input Y

Range box and select the range of the y values. In the Input X Range box we input not the range of the x values but the rectangular range of the x and x^2 values. In this way the program will apply the quadratic model. We leave the option "Constant is zero" unchecked, click on the "Residuals" check box, and click on the output cell. Part of the obtained results is presented in Fig. 9.7.6, top. We repeat this procedure, activating the option "Constant is zero," and obtain the results of Fig. 9.7.6, bottom. We repeat the whole procedure for the cubic model. In this case, in the Input X Range box we introduce the total range of x, x^2, and x^3 values. The obtained results are shown in Fig. 9.7.7.

	Coefficients	Standard Error	t Stat	P-value
Intercept	136.09226	72.71676	1.87154	0.08809
X Variable 1	-0.33925	0.10993	-3.08604	0.01036
X Variable 2	0.00019	4.084E-05	4.76734	0.00058
Standard Error	3.49060			
	Coefficients	Standard Error	t Stat	P-value
Intercept	0	#Δ/Y	#Δ/Y	#Δ/Y
X Variable 1	-0.13379	0.00626	-21.36363	6.449E-11
X Variable 2	0.00012	4.926E-06	24.10362	1.563E-11
Standard Error	3.83737			

FIGURE 9.7.6 Part of the regression results of the quadratic model when $a \neq 0$ (top) and $a = 0$ (bottom).

	Coefficients	Standard Error	t Stat	P-value
Intercept	806.73280	730.57746	1.10424	0.29535
X Variable 1	-1.86166	1.65384	-1.12566	0.28660
X Variable 2	0.00133	0.00124	1.07957	0.30569
X Variable 3	-2.815E-07	3.051E-07	-0.92260	0.37794
Standard Error	3.51445			
	Coefficients	Standard Error	t Stat	P-value
Intercept	0	#Δ/Y	#Δ/Y	#Δ/Y
X Variable 1	-0.03647	0.05624	-0.64847	0.52998
X Variable 2	-2.741E-05	8.412E-05	-0.32580	0.75069
X Variable 3	5.372E-08	3.088E-08	1.73976	0.10977
Standard Error	3.54932			

FIGURE 9.7.7 Part of the regression results of the cubic model when $a \neq 0$ *(top)* and $a = 0$ *(bottom)*.

From the results presented in Figs. 9.7.6 and 9.7.7 we observe the following. The cubic model with either $a \neq 0$ or $a = 0$ should be rejected because there are adjustable parameters that are statistically nonsignificant (p-value $> .05$) (Fig. 9.7.7). In the quadratic model, when $a \neq 0$, constant a seems to be statistically nonsignificant, whereas when $a = 0$, all the adjustable parameters are statistically significant. Therefore, the quadratic model with $a = 0$ (Fig. 9.7.6, bottom) may be selected as the best. That is, the best model may be expressed as:

$$y = -0.13379\,x + 0.0001187x^2 \tag{9.7.15}$$

This process can be performed automatically by means of the Regression macro provided in the companion website, using option "2" (for finding the optimum polynomial). We arrange the data in two successive columns with the column of the x values at the left of the column of the y values, and run the macro from the Regression Excel file. Note that the obtained results appear in the columns to the right of the y column.

In SPSS we test directly the cubic model with $a \neq 0$, because in this software the Linear procedure tests all polynomials of order 1, 2, and 3 and finds the polynomial of the largest order with all adjustable parameters significant. Before the application of the Linear procedure, we may name the variables as y, x, xx, and xxx, where xx stands for x^2 and xxx for x^3. Then we use the menu Analyze $\rightarrow$ Regression $\rightarrow$ Linear and transfer y to the Dependent box and the variables x, xx, and xxx to the Independent(s) box. In Method we select the "Forward" option, in which the program first inputs the constant (a) and then the coefficient of the variable that exhibits the highest correlation to the dependent variable. The program examines whether this coefficient is statistically significant and then it inputs the coefficient of the variable that exhibits the second highest correlation to the dependent variable, and so on. Alternatively, we could select the "Backward" option. In this case, the program would calculate all parameters and then remove the statistically nonsignificant ones one by one. We click on Options and activate the "Include constant in equation" check box. Finally, we click on "Save" and select the options "Predicted Values Unstandardized" and "Residuals Unstandardized." We obtain, among others, the tables Model Summary and Coefficients shown in SPSS Outputs 9.7.2 and 9.7.3.

SPSS OUTPUT 9.7.2 Model Summary

Model	R	R Square	Adjusted R Square	Std. Error of the Estimate
1	0.992	0.984	0.983	3.668

SPSS OUTPUT 9.7.3 Coefficients[a]

Model		Unstandardized Coefficients		Standardized Coefficients		
		B	Std. Error	Beta	t	Sig.
1	(Constant)	−48.084	2.556		−18.813	0.000
	xxx	3.378×10^{-8}	0.000	0.992	27.361	0.000

[a]Dependent variable: y.

We observe that the program determines an optimum polynomial different from that determined by Excel. In particular, the best model may be now expressed as:

$$y = -48.084 + 3.378 \times 10^{-8} x^3 \tag{9.7.16}$$

This difference is not surprising because the two programs use different algorithms for the selection of the optimum model. In any case, the difference is small, as can be judged from the SEE values. For the quadratic model SEE = 3.8374 (Fig. 9.7.6) and for the cubic model SEE = 3.668 (SPSS Output 9.7.2). Because $3.668 < 3.8374$, the cubic model of Eq. (9.7.16) should be preferred. Note that these results are strictly valid under the assumption that the residuals follow the normal distribution. Thus, a test for the normality of the residuals should be conducted. This test shows that in all cases the null hypothesis that the residuals follow the normal distribution cannot be rejected.

Fig. 9.7.5 shows the scatterplot of the two variables with the least-squares curve determined in SPSS. The curve has been drawn using the values of the variable "Predicted Values Unstandardized" created in the SPSS spreadsheet.

Finally, for the prediction of the age of an individual with tooth size area 1300 mm^2, we obtain:

$$x = 1300 \Rightarrow y = -48.084 + \left(3.378 \times 10^{-8}\right) \times \left(1300^3\right) = 26.1 \text{ thousand years ago}$$

Note that the quadratic model of Eq. (9.7.15) gives the value 26.7 thousand years ago.

Case Study 14: Multilinear Regression

The dependence of the height (h) of adult males upon maximum femoral length (MFL) and maximum tibial length (MTL) in a contemporary population is presented in Table 9.7.3. Assess whether height can be expressed more effectively by the simple linear model $h = a + b \times MFL$ or the multilinear one, $h = a + b \times MFL + c \times MTL$.

In Excel we arrange the data in three columns, h, MFL, and MTL, and use the menu Data → Data Analysis → Regression. In the Regression box we click inside the Input Y Range box and select the range of the h values, and in the Input X Range box we input the range of the MFL and MTL values. Part of the obtained results is presented in Fig. 9.7.8, top. It is seen that the adjustable parameter c does not appear to be statistically significant because p-value $= .091 > .05$, and therefore height may be expressed by the simple linear model $h = a + b \times MFL$. To determine the adjustable parameters a and b of this model, we rerun Regression and in the Input X Range box we input the range of the MFL values only. Part of the obtained results is presented in Fig. 9.7.8, bottom. Thus, height may be predicted from the simple linear model:

$$h = 41.68 + 2.785 \times MFL \tag{9.7.17}$$

TABLE 9.7.3 Dependence of the Height of Adult Males Upon Maximum Femoral Length and Maximum Tibial Length

h	MFL	MTL	h	MFL	MTL
165.1	44.6	37.0	162.7	43.7	37.6
160.3	43.5	37.9	161.2	41.9	36.5
163.8	44.4	37.7	166.9	43.3	35.1
167.5	43.5	37.0	162.3	42.5	35.2
165.9	44.1	36.1	152.9	40.2	35.1
161.2	42.1	34.1	160.7	42.5	34.5
161	42.0	36.3	159.2	41.6	35.8
162.1	43.6	36.7	167.8	46.4	39.7
171	47.8	40.1	170.2	45.3	36.9
149	39.4	33.5	166.9	43.7	37.0
149.9	37.9	33.3	151.4	40.3	34.5
172	47.2	40.7	151.1	40.6	34.0
174.6	47.2	39.0	148.6	40.2	35.1
150.7	39.5	33.5	157.7	42.6	36.2

h, height (cm); *MFL*, maximum femoral length (cm); *MTL*, maximum tibial length (cm).

	Coefficients	Standard Error	t Stat	P-value
Intercept	47.06032	9.25058	5.08728	2.97E-05
X Variable 1	3.56199	0.48670	7.31863	1.14E-07
X Variable 2	-1.06690	0.60739	-1.75653	0.09124
Standard Error	2.63401			

	Coefficients	Standard Error	t Stat	P-value
Intercept	41.68428	9.07294	4.59435	9.81E-05
X Variable 1	2.78507	0.21108	13.19463	4.97E-13
Standard Error	2.73760			

FIGURE 9.7.8 Part of the regression results for the models $h = a + b \times MFL + c \times MTL$ (top) and $h = a + (b \times MFL)$ (bottom) in Excel.

Note that the SEE of the linear model is slightly higher than that of the multilinear model. This is expected because the linear model has one term less. However, if we take into consideration the definition of SEE, the observed difference is negligible.

Precisely the same results are obtained, but in one step, if we apply the Regression macro selecting option "3" (for multilinear fitting with statistically significant parameters). For its application, we arrange the data as above, run the macro, and follow the instructions of the dialog boxes that appear.

In SPSS we may use the menu Analyze → Regression → Linear. We transfer the variable h to the box labeled Dependent and the variables MFL and MTL to the Independent(s) box. From Options we select "Include constant in equation" and in Method we select the method that will be used in the calculation of the adjustable parameters. We select the option "Forward" and obtain, among others, the table of SPSS Output 9.7.4, which again gives the same information as the Excel results of Fig. 9.7.8, bottom. The scatterplot of *h* vs MFL and the least-squares straight line $h = 41.68 + 2.785 \times MFL$ are shown in Fig. 9.7.9.

Case Study 15: ANCOVA

Based on the data of Table 9.7.4 assess whether the TA of the tibia is significantly different among the three samples coming from different archaeological populations and subsequently draw conclusions about the comparative mechanical

SPSS OUTPUT 9.7.4 Coefficients[a]

	Model	Unstandardized Coefficients		Standardized Coefficients		
		B	Std. Error	Beta	t	Sig.
1	(Constant)	41.684	9.073		4.594	0.000
	MFL	2.785	0.211	0.933	13.195	0.000

MFL, maximum femoral length.
[a]*Dependent variable: h.*

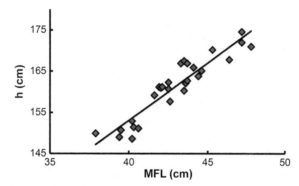

FIGURE 9.7.9   Plot of height (h) vs maximum femoral length (MFL) and the least-squares straight line h = 41.68 + 2.785 × MFL.

TABLE 9.7.4 Data on Tibial Total Subperiosteal Area and Body Mass in Three Samples From Different Archaeological Populations

Pop	BM	TA	Pop	BM	TA
1	75	420	2	71	422
1	72	404	2	72	433
1	68	400	2	75	435
1	81	436	2	79	440
1	79	440	2	83	441
1	77	423	3	67	380
1	73	431	3	69	385
2	77	430	3	65	365
2	80	440	3	70	360
2	83	448	3	72	351
2	76	450	3	78	390
2	75	428	3	77	380

BM, body mass (kg); *Pop*, population; *TA*, total subperiosteal area (mm^2).

loading of the activities in which these populations were involved. Because all cross-sectional geometric properties are also affected by the body mass (BM) of the individual, compare TA in the three samples while controlling for the effect of BM. Note that in Table 9.7.4 the categorical variable indicating the sample is denoted by "Pop," as each sample refers to a different archaeological population.

We first plot the data of Table 9.7.4 as in Fig. 9.7.10. We observe that the dependence of TA upon BM at each of the three levels of the categorical variable Pop is roughly linear, although the lines of these linear relationships do not seem to be parallel. Thus, the assumption of the homogeneity of regression slopes may be questioned. However, there is a stricter criterion for this assumption; if this assumption is violated, the interaction term Pop × BM in the relevant model is statistically significant. Note that the ANCOVA model with interactions is:

$$TA = a + b \times BM + c \times Pop + d \times Pop \times BM \tag{9.7.18}$$

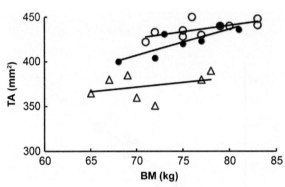

FIGURE 9.7.10 Plot of total subperiosteal area (TA) vs body mass (BM) at the three levels of the categorical variable population (Pop): (●) Pop = 1, (○) Pop = 2, and (Δ) Pop = 3. Lines have been drawn using linear regression.

Therefore, one of the basic prerequisites for the application of ANCOVA on the data of Table 9.7.4 is that the interaction Pop × BM does not make a significant contribution to the values of TA, which means that the p-value of parameter d should be greater than .05.

Excel does not have a macro to perform ANCOVA. Thus, we will use only SPSS. We place the data in three columns, Pop, BM, and TA, and use the menu Analyze → General Linear Models → Univariate. In the dialog box Univariate we transfer the variable TA to the Dependent Variable box, the variable Pop to the Fixed Factor(s) box, and the variable BM to the Covariate(s) box. We click on Model and fill in the relevant dialog box as in Fig. 9.7.11. Thus, we first select "Custom"

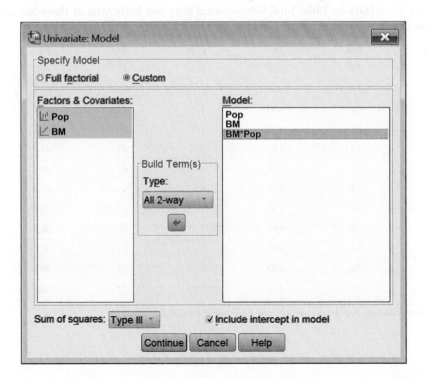

and "Include intercept in the model," and from the drop-down menu in the Build Term(s) panel, we select "Main effects." Then we transfer the variables Pop and BM to the Model box. We proceed, and from the drop-down list we select "All 2-way," and then we select both Pop and BM variables from the Factors & Covariates box and transfer them to the Model panel by clicking on the central arrow. Finally, in the dialog box that appears we click on Options and select "Homogeneity tests." We click on "Continue" and "OK" and obtain, among others, the results presented in SPSS Output 9.7.5. Note that the Levene test presented in the table Levene's Test of Equality of Error Variances gives p-value $= .121$, which shows that the assumption of the homogeneity of variance cannot be rejected. So, the results presented in SPSS Output 9.7.5 appear to be valid. In this table we observe that the contribution from the interaction Pop $\times$ BM does not seem to be statistically significant (p-value $= .312 > .05$) and, therefore, the assumption of the homogeneity of regression slopes does not appear to be violated.

SPSS OUTPUT 9.7.5 Tests of Between-Subjects Effects With Interaction Term

Dependent Variable: TA

Source	Type III Sum of Squares	df	Mean Square	F	Sig.
Corrected model	18,871.660[a]	5	3774.332	36.611	0.000
Intercept	5587.549	1	5587.549	54.199	0.000
Pop	194.335	2	97.167	0.943	0.408
BM	1346.056	1	1346.056	13.057	0.002
Pop × BM	256.505	2	128.253	1.244	0.312
Error	1855.674	18	103.093		
Total	4,130,920.000	24			
Corrected total	20,727.333	23			

BM, body mass; Pop, population; TA, total subperiosteal area.
[a]R Squared $= .910$ (adjusted R Squared $= .886$).

Now, we can proceed to assess the effect of the variable Pop on TA controlling for BM. For this purpose, we again use the menu Analyze $\rightarrow$ General Linear Models $\rightarrow$ Univariate. In the dialog box Univariate that appears we click on Model and then we select the interaction BM $\times$ Pop and click on the central arrow. The interaction BM $\times$ Pop is removed from the model. Subsequently, we click on Options and select "Homogeneity tests," "Parameter estimates," and "Compare main effects." In addition, we transfer the variable Pop to the Display Means by box and select "Bonferroni" from the Confidence interval adjustment.

The option "Parameter Estimates" will give the model parameters, whereas the option "Compare main effects" provides pairwise comparisons of TA in the three samples while controlling for the effect of BM. Finally, we click on "Save" and select "Predicted Values Unstandardized" and "Residuals Unstandardized." These options create two new columns in the SPSS spreadsheet with the predicted from the model TA values and the residuals. The former are used to test how well the model predicts the experimental data, and the latter can be used for the normality test of the residuals. The most important results are as follows.

The table Levene's Test of Equality of Error Variances shows again that the homogeneity of variance assumption cannot be rejected and, therefore, the results in the main table of ANCOVA in SPSS Output 9.7.6 are likely to be valid. In this table we observe that the contributions from both the BM and the Pop variables are statistically significant. This means that TA is statistically different among the three samples.

To clarify between which pairs of samples the significant differences in TA are traced, we consult the results given in SPSS Output 9.7.7. We observe that statistically significant differences exist between samples 1−3 and 2−3. Note that this result is based on the Bonferroni method for adjustment of the p-values for multiple comparisons.

From the results presented in SPSS Output 9.7.8, we may deduce the model that describes the data of Table 9.7.4:

$$TA = 249.745 + 42.317 \times \text{Pop1} + 53.379 \times \text{Pop2} + 1.733 \times \text{BM} \qquad (9.7.19)$$

SPSS OUTPUT 9.7.6 Tests of Between-Subjects Effects Without the Interaction Term

Dependent Variable: TA

Source	Type III Sum of Squares	df	Mean Square	F	Sig.
Corrected model	18,615.154[a]	3	6205.051	58.755	0.000
Intercept	5936.524	1	5936.524	56.212	0.000
Pop	9186.161	2	4593.080	43.491	0.000
BM	1247.921	1	1247.921	11.816	0.003
Error	2112.179	20	105.609		
Total	4,130,920.000	24			
Corrected total	20,727.333	23			

[a]*R Squared = .898 (adjusted R Squared = .883).*
BM, body mass; Pop, population; TA, total subperiosteal area.

SPSS OUTPUT 9.7.7 Pairwise Comparisons

Dependent Variable: TA

(I) Pop	(J) Pop	Mean difference (I − J)	Std. Error	Sig.[a]	95% Confidence Interval for Difference[a] Lower Bound	Upper Bound
1	2	−11.062	5.174	0.135	−24.579	2.455
	3	42.317[b]	5.827	0.000	27.094	57.541
2	1	11.062	5.174	0.135	−2.455	24.579
	3	53.379[b]	5.887	0.000	37.998	68.761
3	1	−42.317[b]	5.827	0.000	−57.541	−27.094
	2	−53.379[b]	5.887	0.000	−68.761	−37.998

Based on estimated marginal means.
[a]*Adjustment for multiple comparisons: Bonferroni.*
[b]*The mean difference is significant at the .05 level.*
Pop, population; TA, total subperiosteal area.

SPSS OUTPUT 9.7.8 Parameter Estimates

Dependent Variable: TA

Parameter	B	Std. Error	t	Sig.	95% Confidence Interval Lower Bound	Upper Bound
Intercept	249.745	36.066	6.925	0.000	174.513	324.977
[Pop = 1]	42.317	5.827	7.262	0.000	30.163	54.472
[Pop = 2]	53.379	5.887	9.067	0.000	41.098	65.660
[Pop = 3]	0[a]	.	.	.	.	.
BM	1.733	0.504	3.438	0.003	0.681	2.784

[a]*This parameter is set to zero because it is redundant.*
BM, body mass; Pop, population; TA, total subperiosteal area.

Note that the variables Pop1 and Pop2 take only the values 0 and 1. In particular, when Pop1 = 1 and Pop2 = 0, then the above equation describes the data that correspond to Pop = 1; when Pop1 = 0 and Pop2 = 1, it describes the data of Pop = 2; and when Pop1 = 0 and Pop2 = 0, this equation describes the data of Pop = 3.

Based on the TA values predicted from Eq. (9.7.19) or using the variable PRE_1 that the program has created, we may plot the experimental and the predicted TA values vs BM at the three levels of the categorical variable Pop. This plot is depicted in Fig. 9.7.12. Note that the model can predict only a linear relationship between the dependent variable, TA, and the covariate, BM, at each level of the categorical variable, and that the lines expressing these linear relationships are always parallel. For this reason, the linearity of the dependence between the dependent variable and the covariates, as well as the homogeneity of the regression slopes, is a basic precondition for the model to describe the experimental data satisfactorily.

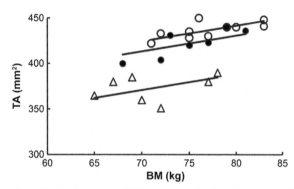

FIGURE 9.7.12 Plot of total subperiosteal area (TA) vs body mass (BM) at the three levels of the categorical variable population (Pop): ($\bullet$) Pop = 1, ($\bigcirc$) Pop = 2, and ($\triangle$) Pop = 3. Lines are model predictions from Eq. (9.7.19).

Finally, an additional important precondition for the p-values of these SPSS outputs to be valid is the normality of the residuals. This precondition can be easily tested because the program has created a new variable, RES_1, which consists of the residuals. Testing the normality of this variable, we obtain a p-value for the Shapiro—Wilk test of .607, which shows that the null hypothesis that the residuals follow the normal distribution cannot be rejected.

Case Study 16: Analysis of Entheseal Changes Using GLM and GEE

As discussed in Section 7.1.3, entheseal changes (ECs) are recorded either as binary dichotomies (present/absent) or using ordinal scales. In this case study we will use the artificial data given in dataset_EC1 and dataset_EC2 in the Excel file DataCreation_EC as well as in the Excel file DataForStatistics provided in the companion website. The first data set expresses ECs as binary dichotomies, and the second employs a four-rank ordinal scheme. Both data sets will be analyzed using GLM and GEE. Traditional statistical tests, like χ^2 and Fisher's exact tests for binary data and Wilcoxon, Mann—Whitney, and Kruskal—Wallis tests for ordinal data, may also be employed. Such tests have already been described in the previous sections of this chapter.

To analyze the data provided in dataset_EC1, we arrange the variables in seven columns, Id, Pop, Sex, Side, Age, FHD, and y, as in the original tables in DataCreation_EC/dataset_EC1 or DataForStatistics/Modeling. These variables express the following: Id is an integer denoting the individual to whom the data of each case belong (this is a necessary parameter for applying GEE but not GLM); Pop takes the values 1, 2, and 3 and denotes the population to which each individual belongs; Sex takes the values 1 and 2 for males and females; Side takes the values 1 and 2 for the right and left side; Age takes the values 1, 2, and 3 for young, middle, and old adults; FHD stands for femoral head diameter and it is a continuous variable used as a proxy for BM; and y is the dependent (response) variable, that is, the EC expression.

To apply GLM, we use the menu Analyze → Generalized Linear Models → Generalized Linear Models. In the dialog box Generalized Linear Models that appears we click on the Type of Model tab and select "Binary logistic" because in this case ECs have been recorded as present/absent. In the Response tab we transfer the variable y to the Dependent Variable box, and in the Predictors tab we transfer the variables Pop, Sex, and Age to the Factor(s) box and the variable FHD to the

Covariates box. Note that at this step we exclude the variable Side from the treatment. Side will be taken into account in the next steps of the analysis. We click on the Model tab and transfer the variables Pop, Sex, Age, and FHD to the Model box as Main effects. We may also select "Robust estimator" from the Estimation tab.

We click on "OK" and obtain, among others, the tables Tests of Model Effects (SPSS Output 9.7.9) and Parameter Estimates (SPSS Output 9.7.10). The first table shows the significance of the various terms of the model and, therefore, whether a certain variable has a significant impact on the EC under study. The second table presents the model parameters, i.e., the values of b_0, b_1, b_2, b_3, b_4 in Eq. (9.7.11); their standard deviations; and the *p*-values. Note that in both tables the impact of each variable on the EC under study is estimated while controlling for the effects of all other variables, i.e., by excluding the effects of all other variables on EC.

SPSS OUTPUT 9.7.9 Tests of Model Effects

| Source | Type III | | |
	Wald Chi-Square	df	Sig.
(Intercept)	0.035	1	0.851
Pop	23.636	2	0.000
Sex	7.307	1	0.007
Age	27.209	2	0.000
FHD	0.305	1	0.581

FHD, femoral head diameter; *Pop*, population.

SPSS OUTPUT 9.7.10 Parameter Estimates

| Parameter | B | Std. Error | 95% Wald Confidence Interval | | Hypothesis Test | | |
			Lower	Upper	Wald Chi-Square	df	Sig.
(Intercept)	−0.148	2.2987	−4.654	4.357	0.004	1	0.9486
[Pop = 1]	−1.096	0.3029	−1.690	−0.502	13.092	1	0.0003
[Pop = 2]	−1.674	0.3939	−2.446	−0.902	18.058	1	2.1×10^{-5}
[Pop = 3]	0						
[Sex = 1]	−0.617	0.2283	−1.064	−0.170	7.307	1	0.0069
[Sex = 2]	0						
[Age = 1]	1.770	0.3539	1.076	2.463	25.013	1	5.7×10^{-7}
[Age = 2]	1.089	0.2797	0.541	1.637	15.162	1	9.9×10^{-5}
[Age = 3]	0						
FHD	0.293	0.5315	−0.748	1.335	0.305	1	0.581
(Scale)	1						

FHD, femoral head diameter; *Pop*, population.

From the Tests of Model Effects table it is seen that all variables have a statistically significant effect on EC except for FHD. That is, in the data set under study, FHD does not seem to affect EC significantly when the effects of Pop, Sex, and Age are removed. The statistically significant impact of Pop, Sex, and Age means that between the classes (categories) of each two of these variables statistically significant differences exist in ECs. For example, such differences exist between males and females. To interpret the results for the variables Pop and Age, each of which exhibits three classes, we should examine the Parameter Estimates table. In particular, in this table the values of Sig. = .0003 and 2.1×10^{-5} that correspond to the lines [Pop = 1] and [Pop = 2] refer to the p-values that test the significance of the difference in EC between populations 1–3 and 2–3, respectively, because in this table population 3 is the reference population. The same holds for Age. Thus, the p-values 5.7×10^{-7} and 9.9×10^{-5} test the null hypothesis that there are no statistically significant differences in EC between age groups 1–3 and 2–3, and because these values are much smaller than .05, this hypothesis is rejected.

It is seen that the table in SPSS Output 9.7.10 does not contain the p-values for the pairs Pop1–Pop2 and Age1–Age2. To obtain these values, we should rerun the GLM; in the Predictors tab we should click on the Options button and select the "Descending" option. Now from the new Parameter Estimates table we obtain the p-values .16 and .031 for pairs Pop1–Pop2 and Age1–Age2, respectively.

At this point we should stress that because we have multiple comparisons, the p-values between population groups as well as those between age groups should be corrected using the Holm–Bonferroni correction. This correction may be performed using the Holm_Bonferroni macro (see Section 9.5.1 as well as Section 9.5.6, Case Study 6) and the obtained results are listed in Table 9.7.5. It is seen that the difference in the EC expression is statistically significant between all age groups. It is also statistically significant between population groups 1–3 and 2–3, whereas this is not the case for groups 1–2.

TABLE 9.7.5 Uncorrected and Holm–Bonferroni Corrected p-values

	Uncorrected	HB Correction
Pop Pair		
1–2	0.160	0.160
1–3	0.0003	0.0006
2–3	2.14×10^{-5}	6.43×10^{-5}
Age Pair		
1–2	0.031	0.031
1–3	5.7×10^{-7}	1.7×10^{-6}
2–3	9.9×10^{-5}	0.0002

HB, Holm–Bonferroni; *Pop*, population.

An alternative approach to computing corrected p-values using the Bonferroni method is via the EM Means tab in the Generalized Linear Models dialog box. In this tab we transfer the variables Pop, Sex, and Age from the Factors and interactions panel to the Display Means for panel and select for each factor the Pairwise contrast. In addition, we select "Bonferroni" from Adjustment for Multiple Comparisons.

In the aforementioned treatment the Side parameter was ignored because, in fact, the two sides were pooled. To treat the data of the right side separately from those of the left side, we may work as follows. From the menu Data → Select Cases we click on "If condition is satisfied" and subsequently click on "If...." In the new dialog box that appears we transfer the variable Side to the box on the right, type in "=1" (Fig. 9.7.13), and click on "Continue" and "OK." The program selects

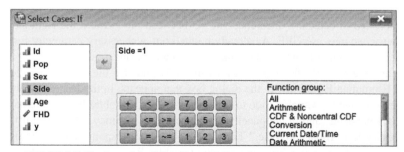

FIGURE 9.7.13 Part of the Select Cases: If dialog box with the selection Side = 1.

only the cases that contain Side $= 1$. Then we run GLM as before. We repeat this procedure for Side $= 2$. The obtained results are presented in SPSS Output 9.7.11 and Table 9.7.6.

It is seen that in this example FHD has a statistically nonsignificant impact on EC, whereas males and females exhibit statistically significant differences in EC only on the right side (p-value $= .044$). In regard to the differentiation of EC among age and population groups, we observe significant differences between Age1—Age3 (right-side data) and Age1—Age3 and Age2—Age3 (left-side data), as well as between Pop1—Pop3 and Pop2—Pop3 (right-side data) and Pop1—Pop2 and Pop2—Pop3 (left-side data).

SPSS OUTPUT 9.7.11 Tests of Model Effects When Side = 1 (Right) and Side = 2 (Left)

| Source | Type III | | | Source | Type III | | |
	Wald Chi-Square	df	Sig.		Wald Chi-Square	df	Sig.
(Intercept)	0.211	1	0.646	(Intercept)	0.617	1	0.432
Pop	12.300	2	0.002	Pop	13.232	2	0.001
Sex	3.329	1	0.068	Sex	4.076	1	0.044
Age	7.540	2	0.023	Age	23.593	2	0.000
FHD	0.023	1	0.879	FHD	1.022	1	0.312

FHD, femoral head diameter; *Pop*, population.

TABLE 9.7.6 Uncorrected and Holm—Bonferroni Corrected p-values for Variables Pop and Age of the GLM Model $\eta = b_0 + b_1Pop + b_2Sex + b_3Age + b_4FHD$

| | Right Side | | Left Side | |
	Uncorrected	HB Correction	Uncorrected	HB Correction
Pop Pair				
1—2	0.827	0.827	0.022	0.044
1—3	0.001	0.004	0.078	0.078
2—3	0.009	0.018	0.0004	0.001
Age Pair				
1—2	0.082	0.164	0.145	0.145
1—3	0.006	0.018	3.5×10^{-6}	1.1×10^{-5}
2—3	0.133	0.164	0.0001	0.0002

FHD, femoral head diameter; *GLM*, generalized linear model; *HB*, Holm—Bonferroni; *Pop*, population.

Finally, if we are interested in detecting differences in EC between the left and the right side, that is, if we want to explore bilateral asymmetry, we may use GEE. As already pointed out, a necessary parameter for applying GEE is the Id, i.e., an integer denoting the individual to whom the data of each case belong.

To apply GEE, we arrange the data the same way as in GLM and use the menu Analyze $\rightarrow$ Generalized Linear Models $\rightarrow$ Generalized Estimating Equations. In the dialog box that appears, in the Repeated tab we transfer the variable Id to the Subject variables box and the variable Side to the Within-subject variables box; in the panel Working Correlation Matrix we may select "Independent," and in the panel Covariance Matrix we may select "Robust estimator." We click on the Type of Model tab and select "Binary logistic." Then we click on the Response tab and transfer the variable y to the Dependent Variable box. In the Predictors tab we transfer the variables Pop, Sex, Side, and Age to the Factor(s) box and the variable FHD to the Covariates box. Note that in this case the variable Side is included in the treatment. We click on the Model tab and transfer all variables to the Model box as Main effects. We click on "OK" and obtain, among others, the table Tests of Model Effects (SPSS Output 9.7.12).

SPSS OUTPUT 9.7.12 Tests of Model Effects for GEE

Source	Type III		
	Wald Chi-Square	df	Sig.
(Intercept)	0.005	1	0.946
Pop	23.233	2	0.000
Sex	7.602	1	0.006
Side	0.664	1	0.415
Age	27.011	2	0.000
FHD	0.187	1	0.666

FHD, femoral head diameter; *Pop*, population.

This table shows that the effect of Side seems to be statistically nonsignificant, i.e., statistically significant differences in EC between the right and the left side are not demonstrated (p-value = .415 > .05). This is the only information that we need to obtain from the application of GEE. The effects of the other variables, Pop, Sex, and Age, may also be obtained from the Model Effects table and the corresponding Parameter Estimates table but these effects have already been explored by means of GLM, as described earlier. Note that, as shown in Nikita (2014), for the study of bilateral asymmetry, GEE is recommended, whereas in all other analyses, GLM is more appropriate.

Dataset_EC2 includes four-rank ordinal data. The analysis of these data using either GLM or GEE may be conducted as for dataset_EC1 but now the "Ordinal logistic" option must be activated in the Type of Model tab. The basic results obtained are summarized in SPSS Outputs 9.7.13 and 9.7.14 and in Table 9.7.7. It is seen that they are quite similar to those obtained from dataset_EC1.

SPSS OUTPUT 9.7.13 Tests of Model Effects

	Both Sides			Right Side			Left Side		
				Type III					
Source	Wald Chi-Square	df	Sig.	Wald Chi-Square	df	Sig.	Wald Chi-Square	df	Sig.
Pop	24.299	2	0.000	17.812	2	0.000	6.411	2	0.041
Sex	0.012	1	0.911	1.165	1	0.280	1.128	1	0.288
Age	35.041	2	0.000	13.460	2	0.001	23.013	2	0.000
FHD	0.532	1	0.466	1.374	1	0.241	0.043	1	0.836

Dependent variable: y.
Model: (Threshold), Pop, Sex, Age, FHD.
Pop, population; *FHD*, femoral head diameter.

Finally, we should again stress that when we may assume that the ordinal data code an underlying continuous variable that follows the normal distribution, then GLM may be applied using a scale response (Nikita, 2014).

Case Study 17: Analysis of Cross-Sectional Geometry Using GLM

Apply GLM to the TA data of the dataset_CSG given in the Excel file DataForStatistics/CSG and compare the results with the corresponding results obtained from the application of traditional tests presented in Section 9.5.6, Case Study 8.

SPSS OUTPUT 9.7.14 Tests of Model Effects for GEE

Source	Type III		
	Wald Chi-Square	df	Sig.
Pop	23.638	2	0.000
Sex	0.009	1	0.923
Side	0.183	1	0.669
Age	37.614	2	0.000
FHD	0.603	1	0.437

FHD, femoral head diameter; *Pop*, population.

TABLE 9.7.7 Uncorrected and Holm−Bonferroni Corrected *p*-values for the GLM Model $\eta = b_0 + b_1 Pop + b_2 Sex + b_3 Age + b_4 FHD$

	Both Sides		Right Side		Left Side	
	Uncorrected	HB	Uncorrected	HB	Uncorrected	HB
Pop Pair						
1−2	0.407	0.407	0.518	0.518	0.649	0.649
1−3	0.000	0.000	0.000	0.000	0.049	0.105
2−3	0.000	0.000	0.001	0.002	0.035	0.105
Age Pair						
1−2	0.000	0.000	0.020	0.040	0.005	0.010
1−3	0.000	0.000	0.000	0.000	0.000	0.000
2−3	0.002	0.002	0.096	0.096	0.007	0.010

HB, Holm−Bonferroni; *Pop*, population.

To apply GLM using a linear scale response, the values of TA should follow the normal distribution. The normality was tested in Case Study 8 and no evidence of lack of normality was found, except for three samples, which, however, did not show strong deviations from normality, and therefore GLM with a linear scale response may be adopted.

For the application of GLM, the data should be arranged similar to those of dataset_EC in the previous case study, i.e., in four columns: Pop, Sex, Side, and TA. Moreover, we move the entire group of population 2 to the bottom of the data set so that we obtain the *p*-values of all possible pairs of populations, 1−2, 1−3, 1−4, 2−3, 2−4, and 3−4, as explained later. Subsequently, we run GLM; in the Type of Model tab we select Linear, in the Response tab we transfer the variable TA to the Dependent Variable box, in the Predictors tab we transfer the variables Pop and Sex to the Factor(s) box, and from the Options button we select "Ascending." We click on the Model tab and transfer the variables Pop and Sex to the Model box as main effects. We may also select "Robust estimator" from the Estimation tab.

From the Parameter Estimates tables we obtain the *p*-values of the pairs of populations 1−4, 2−4, and 3−4. To obtain the *p*-values of the remaining pairs, in the Predictors tab we select "Descending" from the Options button and rerun GLM. Now we obtain the *p*-values of the pairs of populations 1−2 and 1−3, and the already known pair 1−4. Finally, we change again the selection in the Options tab to "Use data order" and obtain the *p*-values of the pairs of populations 2−3, 2−4, and 1−2. All these *p*-values along with their Holm−Bonferroni correction are shown in Table 9.7.8.

It is seen that TA is statistically significant between all pairs of populations except for the pair 1−4 in all cases and the pair 2−3 for the left humeri. Note also that from the Parameter Estimates tables computed when the Side is pooled, as well as when Side = 1 and Side = 2, we obtain that the *p*-values that correspond to [Sex = 1] are equal to .000, indicating that

TABLE 9.7.8 Uncorrected and Holm−Bonferroni Corrected *p*-values for the GLM Model
$TA = b_0 + b_1 Pop + b_2 Sex$

Pop Pair	Pooled Sides		Right Side		Left Side	
	Uncorrected	HB	Uncorrected	HB	Uncorrected	HB
1−2	<0.001	<0.001	<0.001	<0.001	<0.001	<0.001
1−3	<0.001	<0.001	<0.001	<0.001	<0.001	<0.001
1−4	0.546	0.546	0.357	0.357	0.038	0.055
2−3	<0.001	<0.001	<0.001	<0.001	0.028	0.055
2−4	<0.001	<0.001	<0.001	<0.001	<0.001	<0.001
3−4	<0.001	<0.001	<0.001	<0.001	0.001	0.003

HB, Holm−Bonferroni; *Pop*, population.

the effect of Sex is statistically significant under all circumstances. That is, TA is statistically significant between males and females in both right and left humeri.

It is now interesting to compare the results obtained from GLM (Table 9.7.8) to those obtained from ANOVA (Table 9.5.5). We observe that there are some discrepancies. For example, from GLM we find that on the right humeri the only comparison that does not appear to be statistically significant is between populations 1 and 4. In contrast, when ANOVA is used, in males the nonsignificant comparisons additionally include population pair 1−3, whereas for females all comparisons are actually nonsignificant except for pairs 1−2 and 2−4. These differences are due to the fact that the results of the two methods are not directly comparable. **GLM results have been obtained by controlling for the effect of sex, whereas ANOVA treats males and females separately**.

Case Study 18: Data Modeling Using GLM

Table 9.7.9 shows the expression (presence/absence) of osteoarthritis (y) in three samples from modern documented populations, as well as the age of each individual. Model these data and assess whether there are statistically significant differences in the expression of osteoarthritis among these samples, while controlling for the effect of age.

In SPSS we arrange the data in three columns, Pop, Age, and *y*, and use the menu Analyze → Generalized Linear Models → Generalized Linear Models. In the dialog box Generalized Linear Models that appears we click on the Type of Model tab and select "Binary logistic." In the Response tab we transfer the variable y to the Dependent Variable box, and in the Predictors tab we transfer the variable Pop to the Factor(s) box and the variable Age to the Covariates box. We click on the Model tab and fill in the relevant dialog box to include the variables Pop and Age and the interaction Pop × Age. We click on "OK" and obtain, among others, the following: From the table Tests of Model Effects we observe that the interaction term Pop × Age is not significant and, therefore, it may be erased. Moreover, from the table Goodness of Fit we obtain that the AIC and the corresponding AICC values are equal to 38.798 and 41.198, respectively.

We rerun Generalized Linear Models and in the Model dialog box we remove the interaction Pop × Age. Now, we obtain that in the model $\eta = b_0 + b_1 Pop + b_2 Age$ all terms are statistically significant. In addition, from the table Goodness of Fit we obtain that AIC = 38.292 and AICC = 39.373. Finally, if we remove the term $b_1 \times Pop$ from the model, we obtain the values AIC = 48.776 and AICC = 49.084.

It is seen that the AIC and AICC values exhibit a minimum for the model $\eta = b_0 + b_1 Pop + b_2 Age$ and, therefore, this is the optimum model. The Parameter Estimates table of this model is given in SPSS Output 9.7.15. From this table we obtain that the optimum fitting model is:

$$\ln \frac{P}{1-P} = -\eta \Rightarrow P = \frac{1}{1+e^{\eta}} \tag{9.7.20}$$

where

$$\eta = 6.016 - 0.815 \times Pop1 + 3.397 \times Pop2 - 0.123 \times Age \tag{9.7.21}$$

TABLE 9.7.9 Expression of Osteoarthritis in Three Population Samples and Corresponding Age Data

Pop	Age	y	Pop	Age	y	Pop	Age	y
1	75	1	2	80	1	3	33	1
1	72	1	2	75	0	3	41	0
1	28	1	2	45	0	3	50	0
1	81	1	2	24	0	3	60	1
1	79	1	2	57	0	3	72	1
1	45	0	2	49	0	3	78	1
1	73	1	2	55	0	3	65	1
1	37	0	2	79	1	3	65	0
1	25	0	2	65	0	3	55	1
1	52	1	2	60	0	3	48	0
1	29	0	2	38	0	3	28	0
1	38	0	2	72	1	3	28	0
1	45	1	2	65	0	3	45	1
2	61	0	2	60	0	3	66	1

Pop, population; *y,* osteoarthritis.

SPSS OUTPUT 9.7.15 Parameter Estimates

Parameter	B	Std. Error	95% Wald Confidence Interval		Hypothesis Test		
			Lower	Upper	Wald Chi-Square	df	Sig.
(Intercept)	6.016	2.1785	1.746	10.285	7.626	1	0.006
[Pop = 1]	−0.815	1.1410	−3.051	1.422	0.510	1	0.475
[Pop = 2]	3.397	1.2792	0.890	5.904	7.053	1	0.008
[Pop = 3]	0[a]	.	.	.	.	.	.
Age	−0.123	0.0407	−0.203	−0.043	9.165	1	0.002
(Scale)	1[b]						

[a] *Set to zero because this parameter is redundant.*
[b] *Fixed at the displayed value.*
Pop, population.

Note again that the variables Pop1 and Pop2 take only the values 0 and 1, and, therefore, when Pop1 = 1 and Pop2 = 0, these equations describe the data that correspond to the first sample; when Pop1 = 0 and Pop2 = 1, they describe the data of the second sample; and when Pop1 = 0 and Pop2 = 0, these equations describe the data of the third sample.

When *P* in Eq. (9.7.20) is less than .5, then y = 1, otherwise y = 0. The values of *P* and the corresponding predicted y values may be calculated from the program if we click on the "Save" tab and select "Predicted value of mean of response" and "Predicted category" (Fig. 9.7.14).

Based on the original and the predicted y values (Fig. 9.7.14), we may create the contingency table, Table 9.7.10, following the procedure described in Section 9.2.4, Case Study 2. It is seen that the model describes the experimental data very satisfactorily. Thus, the conclusions that can be drawn from SPSS Output 9.7.15 are expected to be valid. These conclusions are the following.

The Age coefficient is negative (−0.123). This means that when age increases, η decreases, resulting in the decrease of *P* and, therefore, the probability of the appearance of osteoarthritis increases. Thus, when controlling for population, i.e., if

		Pop	Age	y	MeanPredicted	PredictedValue
	1	1	75	1	.017	1
	2	1	72	1	.025	1
	3	1	28	1	.852	0
	4	1	81	1	.008	1
	5	1	79	1	.011	1
	6	1	45	0	.414	1
	7	1	73	1	.022	1
	8	1	37	0	.654	0
	9	1	25	0	.893	0
	10	1	52	1	.229	1
	11	1	29	0	.835	0
	12	1	38	0	.626	0
	13	1	45	1	.414	1
	14	2	61	0	.869	0

FIGURE 9.7.14 Part of the SPSS Data View window showing the predicted expression of osteoarthritis (PredictedValue) and the probability P (MeanPredicted).

TABLE 9.7.10 Contingency Table for the Frequency of the Original Variable y and the Predicted One

Pop			Frequency	Frequency (Predicted Category Value)
1	Valid	0	5	5
		1	8	8
		Total	13	13
2	Valid	0	12	13
		1	3	2
		Total	15	15
3	Valid	0	6	6
		1	8	8
		Total	14	14

Pop, population.

we exclude the effect of the Pop variable, Age has a statistically significant impact on the appearance of osteoarthritis, which increases with the increase in age. Similarly, the smaller value of the Pop1 coefficient in comparison to that of Pop2 shows that osteoarthritis is present more frequently in sample 1 than in sample 2.

In regard to the p-values of the coefficients of Pop1 and Pop2, we observe that these are .475 and .008, respectively (SPSS Output 9.7.15). These values correspond to the pairwise comparison of osteoarthritic expression between samples 1–3 and 2–3, respectively. As already explained above, to calculate the p-value for the pairwise comparison between samples 1 and 2, we rerun the program Generalized Linear Models, and in the Predictors dialog box we click on Options, and select "Descending." We find that the p-value for the comparison between samples 1 and 2 is .007. Table 9.7.11 summarizes the raw p-values and those corrected using the Holm–Bonferroni method between all pairs of the three

TABLE 9.7.11 Uncorrected and Corrected *p*-values for Pairwise Comparisons

Sample Pair	*p*-value, Uncorrected	*p*-value, HB Correction
1–2	0.007	0.021
1–3	0.475	0.475
2–3	0.008	0.021

samples. It is seen that when we control for Age, the difference in osteoarthritic expression between samples 1 and 2 and 2 and 3 is statistically significant, whereas this is not the case for samples 1 and 3.

Case Study 19: Logistic Regression

Table 9.7.12 shows the glabella (GL) and mastoid process (MA) scores recorded in a documented collection of male and female crania on the 5-degree ordinal scale proposed by Walker (2008) (see Chapter 3). Determine the logistic regression equation that arises from these data and assess its accuracy.

TABLE 9.7.12 Glabella and Mastoid Process Scores in Males and Females

GL	MA	Sex	GL	MA	Sex	GL	MA	Sex
1	1	F	3	1	F	4	5	M
1	1	F	3	3	M	5	5	M
1	3	F	3	5	M	5	2	M
1	2	F	3	4	M	5	3	M
2	1	F	3	3	F	5	4	M
2	2	F	3	3	M	5	5	M
2	4	M	4	2	F	5	1	F
2	3	M	4	4	M	5	3	M
2	2	F	4	5	M	5	3	F

F, female; GL, glabella; M, male; MA, mastoid process.

Logistic regression with two or more independent (explanatory) variables can be implemented in SPSS as follows: The dependent variable, Sex, may be coded as 0 and 1 for females and males, or as F and M, as in Table 9.7.12. In both cases we may use the menu Analyze → Regression → Binary Logistic. We transfer the variable Sex to the Dependent box and the variables GL and MA to the Covariates box. In Method we leave the "Enter" option, from Save we select "Probabilities" and "Group membership," and we click on "Continue" and "OK." From the results we obtain the following model:

$$P = \frac{1}{1 + e^{-\eta}}$$

where P is the probability of being male and $\eta = -9.299 + 0.696 \times GL + 2.604 \times MA$.

In addition, the model makes the following predictions for the sex, saved as variable PGR_1:

Sex	F	F	F	F	F	F	M	M	F	F	M	M	M	F
Prediction	F	F	F	F	F	F	M	F	F	F	M	M	M	M
Sex	M	F	M	M	M	M	M	M	M	M	F	M	F	
Prediction	M	F	M	M	M	M	F	M	M	M	F	M	M	

It is seen that the accuracy of the prediction is 23/27, i.e., 85.2%, a value also given in the Classification table.

Case Study 20: Reduced Major Axis Regression

Use the data of Table 9.2.4 to determine the dependence of the Height (y) of males upon FPHL using both OLS and RMA.

The RMA method is implemented in the VBA macro Regression if we type in "4" in the Mode Selection dialog box. The x = FPHL, y = Height data should be arranged as in Fig. 9.7.15. The application of this macro is straightforward and the results obtained are also given in Fig. 9.7.15. The macro performs both OLS and RMA fitting and computes the predicted y values, the values of a and b of the model y = a + bx, their standard deviations, and their 95% confidence intervals. The p-values that test the null hypothesis that a parameter is equal to 0 are computed for the OLS method. The

FPHL	y	y(OLS)	y(RMA)	y=a+bx	OLS		RMA	
42.6	163.6	161.32	160.92		**a**	**b**	**a**	**b**
44	167.1	164.71	164.57	parameters:	57.9051	2.4275	49.7805	2.6090
43.25	160.1	162.89	162.62	St.Dev.=	6.6133	0.1475	6.6136	0.1475
41.75	159.9	159.25	158.70	95%-LCI =	44.5589	2.1298	36.4336	2.3282
44.45	162.9	165.81	165.75	95%-UCI =	71.2514	2.7252	63.1274	2.9236
42.45	161.0	160.95	160.53	95%-BLCI =	41.3806	2.0986	34.6937	2.2716
46.8	171.1	171.51	171.88	95%-BUCI =	72.7456	2.8001	65.3188	2.9459
45.1	163.6	167.38	167.44	p-value =	5.07E-11	6.4E-20		
43.55	163.2	163.62	163.40	r(Pearson) =	0.9304			
45.25	166.9	167.75	167.84	R^2 =	0.8657			
43	165.3	162.29	161.97	SEE =	2.2986		2.339677	
44.35	166.4	165.56	165.49	Iterations =	10000			
45.1	165.7	167.38	167.44					

FIGURE 9.7.15 Part of data arrangement and results obtained from the application of the RMA option of the Regression macro.

confidence interval, the parameter is statistically significant. Additionally, the macro computes the Pearson's correlation coefficient r(Pearson) and the R^2, i.e., the square of the *multiple correlation coefficient* (Draper and Smith, 1998).

Note that the confidence intervals are calculated from the relationships presented by Warton et al. (2006) as well as using the bootstrap method. In Fig. 9.7.15 the intervals computed using the Warton et al. relationships are denoted as 95%-LCI and 95%-UCI, and those computed using the bootstrap method as 95%-BLCI and 95%-BUCI.

From the results of the RMA fitting presented in Fig. 9.7.15 we find that the fitting model may be expressed as:

$$y = 49.781 + 2.609 \times \text{FPHL} \tag{9.7.22}$$

Its plot, along with that arising from OLS ($y = 57.905 + 2.4275 \times \text{FPHL}$), is given in Fig. 9.7.16.

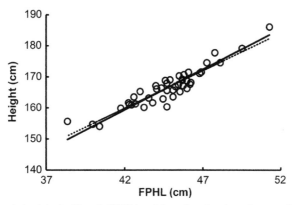

FIGURE 9.7.16 Plot of height vs femoral physiological length (FPHL) and the reduced major axis regression (—) and ordinary least-squares fitting (- - -) straight lines.

9.8 CORRELATION

The concept of correlation is closely related to regression. *Correlation* is any statistical technique that assesses whether two variables exhibit a linear relationship. In other words, it explores whether changes in the values of one variable, x, produce changes in the values of the other variable, y, which can be described by the linear expression $y = a + bx$, where $b \neq 0$. This is the simple *bivariate correlation*. More advanced cases are the *partial correlations* and the *correlation of symmetrical matrices* using the Mantel and partial Mantel tests.

9.8.1 Bivariate Correlation

To assess whether two variables, x and y, are correlated, we may calculate the *Pearson correlation coefficient,* r. This coefficient can take values from -1 to 1. Negative r values suggest that when variable x increases, then variable y decreases, and vice versa. If $r = 0$, there is no correlation between the two variables, whereas if r is positive, when x increases, y increases too.

We should stress that to estimate the statistical significance of the Pearson correlation coefficient, the data need to be continuous and follow the *bivariate normal distribution*. In SPSS we cannot perform a test for bivariate normality. For this reason, we may instead apply simple tests of normality for each of the samples under study, which is a precondition for bivariate normality. If the samples do not appear to come from populations that follow the bivariate normal distribution, we should use the *Spearman correlation coefficient, ρ*. The Spearman correlation coefficient, ρ, also takes values from -1 to 1, it is suitable for continuous and categorical variables, and belongs to the nonparametric tests.

Attention: The Pearson and Spearman correlation coefficients show only whether two variables are intercorrelated, but *correlation* does not imply *causation*.

9.8.2 Partial Correlation

The partial correlation is used to examine the intercorrelation between two variables, while controlling for the effect of one or more other variables. In other words, we assess whether two variables are correlated when the impact of other variables is excluded. The variables may be continuous, categorical, or a combination of continuous and categorical.

9.8.3 Correlation of Symmetrical Matrices

In anthropology, symmetrical matrices are used in different contexts, for example, when we want to assess whether a matrix of biodistances is associated with a matrix of spatial distances and possibly with a matrix of temporal distances. Therefore, it is interesting to examine whether there is a correlation between biodistances and spatial and/or temporal distances. Moreover, in cases in which both spatial and temporal distances are available, we may examine the partial correlation between biodistances and spatial distances controlling for the temporal effect, i.e., when the temporal effect is excluded, and the partial correlation between biodistances and temporal distances controlling for the spatial distances, i.e., excluding the effect of spatial distances.

The correlation between two distance matrices may be performed by means of the *Mantel* test. While the Mantel test allows comparison between only two symmetrical matrices, the *partial Mantel* test can be used to compare two symmetrical matrices while controlling for the effect of another one or more symmetrical matrices. The simple and the partial Mantel tests are implemented in the Mantel option of the macro Correlation in the homonymous Excel file provided in the companion website. An application of this macro is given in the next section.

9.8.4 Case Studies on Correlations

Case Study 21: Bivariate Correlation

Based on the data given in Table 9.8.1, assess whether there is a statistically significant correlation between the age of an individual and the expression of knee osteoarthritis in a modern sample. Determine also whether knee osteoarthritis depends on an individual's BM.

TABLE 9.8.1 Degree of Expression of Knee Osteoarthritis in Relation to Age and Body Mass

Age (years)	Body Mass (kg)	Osteoarthritis
22	61	1
34	70	2
51	62	3
47	75	3
33	60	1
28	72	1
41	77	2
48	85	3
37	82	2
67	70	2

Because one of the variables, Osteoarthritis, is ordinal, we should apply Spearman's correlation. However, for educational purposes, we also apply Pearson's correlation, although it presupposes that the data are continuous and follow the bivariate normal distribution.

In SPSS we arrange the data in three columns and use the menu Analyze → Correlate → Bivariate. We transfer all variables to the Variables box, and in the panel Correlation Coefficients we select "Pearson" and "Spearman," and activate the option "One-tailed" because we already know that Osteoarthritis increases with Age and BM and want to test whether this increase is statistically significant.

We obtain two tables of results, one for the Pearson and the other for the Spearman correlation (SPSS Outputs 9.8.1 and 9.8.2). Both tables present the values of the correlation coefficient (Pearson/Spearman) and the corresponding p-values.

SPSS OUTPUT 9.8.1 Pearson's Correlations

		Age	BM	Osteoarthritis
Age	Pearson correlation	1	0.462	0.709[a]
	Sig. (one-tailed)		0.076	0.007
	N	11	11	11
BM	Pearson correlation	0.462	1	0.550[b]
	Sig. (one-tailed)	0.076		0.040
	N	11	11	11
Osteoarthritis	Pearson correlation	0.709[a]	0.550[b]	1
	Sig. (one-tailed)	0.007	0.040	
	N	11	11	11

BM, body mass.
[a]Correlation is significant at the .01 level (one-tailed).
[b]Correlation is significant at the .05 level (one-tailed).

SPSS OUTPUT 9.8.2 Spearman's Correlations

			Age	BM	Osteoarthritis
Spearman's ρ	Age	Correlation coefficient	1	0.492	0.828[a]
		Sig. (one-tailed)	.	0.062	0.001
		N	11	11	11
	BM	Correlation coefficient	0.492	1	0.574[b]
		Sig. (one-tailed)	0.062	.	0.032
		N	11	11	11
	Osteoarthritis	Correlation coefficient	0.828[a]	0.574[b]	1
		Sig. (one-tailed)	0.001	0.032	.
		N	11	11	11

BM, body mass.
[a]Correlation is significant at the .01 level (one-tailed).
[b]Correlation is significant at the .05 level (one-tailed).

It is seen that the two tests give similar results. Specifically, for the correlation between knee Osteoarthritis and Age, the Pearson correlation coefficient is r = 0.709, the corresponding Spearman coefficient is $\rho = 0.828$, and both these coefficients are statistically significant. Similarly, for the knee Osteoarthritis vs BM correlation, the coefficients are r = 0.55

and $\rho = 0.574$, and they are also both statistically significant. Finally, the correlation between Age and BM is positive ($r = 0.462$, $\rho = 0.492$), i.e., as Age increases, BM also increases; however, in the sample under study this correlation does not appear to be statistically significant (p-value $= .076$ and $.062$ for the Pearson and Spearman test, respectively).

Case Study 22: Partial Correlation

In the previous example we found that the BM exhibits a positive and statistically significant correlation with the expression of osteoarthritis. Based on this result, reexamine the correlation between Age and knee Osteoarthritis while controlling for the effect of BM.

In SPSS we use the menu Analyze → Correlate → Partial and transfer the variables Osteoarthritis and Age to the Variables box and the variable BM to the Controlling for box. In addition, we again activate the option "One-tailed." We obtain the Pearson partial correlation coefficient $r = 0.614$, and it is statistically significant (p-value $= .029$).

SPSS does not have a direct test for the Spearman partial correlation coefficient. This test may be performed by means of the VBA macro Correlation in the homonymous Excel file, provided in the companion website. The advantage of Correlation is that it performs both Pearson's and Spearman's correlation and partial correlation. For the application of partial correlations, each variable should be placed in a column, the controlling variables should be in adjacent columns, and all variables should have labels/titles. All tests are one-tailed.

In the first dialog box we select the type of the correlation (bivariate, partial, or Mantel tests), whereas the second dialog box gives information about the data arrangement. In the third dialog box we input the values and the label for the first variable, in the fourth dialog box we input the values and the label for the second variable, and in the next dialog box we input the values for all controlling variables, including their labels. In the last dialog box we click on the cell that will be the upper left cell of the output area. The obtained results are presented in Fig. 9.8.1 and show a strong correlation between Age and knee Osteoarthritis even if we exclude the effect of BM.

Partial correlation based on regression:				
Partial correlation of Age versus Osteoarthritis controlling for BM				
Pearson Correlation test - 1 tailed				
r=	0.613989			
p-value=	0.029489	Null hypothesis r = 0 may be rejected at level 0.05		
Spearman correlation Non-Parametric test - 1 tailed				
r=	0.765725			
p-value=	0.004912	Null hypothesis r = 0 may be rejected at level 0.05		

FIGURE 9.8.1 Partial correlations from the macro Correlation.

Case Study 23: Correlation Among Biodistances, Spatial Distances, and Temporal Distances

Examine the correlation among the biodistances computed in Appendix 5.XI. In particular, the correlation among the MMD (obtained using six traits; Fig. 5.XI.6) and the RMD and TMD (obtained using seven traits; Fig. 5.XI.7). Next examine the correlation between the MMD and the spatial and temporal distances shown in Fig. 9.8.2.

spatial distance			
0	15	120	100
15	0	55	25
120	55	0	30
100	25	30	0
temporal distance			
0	200	200	100
200	0	1000	1000
200	1000	0	500
100	1000	500	0

FIGURE 9.8.2 Spatial (in km) and temporal (in years) distances.

To apply the "Mantel" option of the macro Correlation, all distances should be arranged in square, symmetrical matrices and each matrix should be accompanied by a label, as in Fig. 9.8.2. We run the macro and in the first input dialog box concerning the Mantel tests we select the "simple" or "partial" Mantel test option. In the following dialog boxes we successively input the range of values for the first, second, and controlling matrix (if the option partial Mantel test has been selected) and the labels of these matrices. In the last dialog box we select the cell that will be the upper left cell of the output area.

The results from the comparisons among the MMD, RMD, and TMD matrices are presented in Fig. 9.8.3. It is seen that these distances are highly correlated. This means that these three distance measures basically provide the same information concerning the biodistances of the populations, at least in the example under study.

Simple Mantel test of MMD versus RMD			
r=	0.981		
p(1-tailed)=	0.0441		
Iterations=	10000		
Simple Mantel test of MMD versus TMD			
r=	0.9613		
p(1-tailed)=	0.0393		
Iterations=	10000		
Simple Mantel test of RMD versus TMD			
r=	0.9647		
p(1-tailed)=	0.0461		
Iterations=	10000		

FIGURE 9.8.3 Simple Mantel tests among the MMD, RMD, and TMD matrices.

The results concerning the correlation between the MMD and the spatial and temporal distances of Fig. 9.8.2 are presented in Fig. 9.8.4. It is seen that there is a strong ($r = 0.900$) and statistically significant (p-value $= .04 < .05$) positive correlation between the MMD and the spatial distances, whereas the corresponding correlation between the MMD and temporal distances is negative ($r = -0.653$) but not statistically significant (p-value $= .169 > .05$). Note also that if we control for the temporal effect, the correlation between the MMD and the spatial distances is still strong and positive ($r = 0.894$) but not statistically significant (p-value $= .09 > .05$).

Simple Mantel test of MMD versus spatial distance					
r=	0.90059				
p(1-tailed)=	0.038				
Iterations=	10000				
Elapsed time =		0.002 min			
Simple Mantel test of MMD versus temporal distance					
r=	-0.6526				
p(1-tailed)=	0.1688				
Iterations=	10000				
Elapsed time =		0.001 min			
Partial Mantel test of MMD versus spatial distance controlling for temporal distance					
r=	0.89365				
p(1-tailed)=	0.08599				
Iterations=	10000				
Elapsed time =		0.002 min			

FIGURE 9.8.4 Simple and partial correlations among the MMD and the matrices of Fig. 9.8.2.

Important note: The Mantel and partial Mantel tests are in fact performed for the accurate estimation of the p-values of the relevant correlations, because the distances in a matrix are not independent of one another. In contrast, the correlation coefficients, r, are the Pearson bivariate or partial correlation coefficients.

9.9 MULTIVARIATE ANALYSIS

Multivariate data analysis refers to any statistical technique for analyzing multivariate data sets. A *multivariate data set* consists of measurements or observations on two or more variables recorded for each case, i.e., item, individual, or experimental trial. Usually a multivariate data set includes an additional variable, the *grouping variable,* that shows the group/sample to which each case belongs. The primary target of multivariate analysis is to identify patterns and relationships between and within groups of cases. For example, we may want to assess if the individuals from two archaeological sites were significantly different based on the linear measurements of their crania.

Multivariate analysis consists of many different techniques. This section focuses on *principal component analysis (PCA), multiple correspondence analysis (MCA), linear discriminant analysis (LDA), multivariate analysis of variance (MANOVA), hierarchical cluster analysis (HCA),* and *multidimensional scaling (MDS).* PCA, MCA, HCA, and MDS have no assumptions on the distribution that the variables should follow. In contrast, LDA and MANOVA are quite sensitive to outliers; they require the variables to follow the multivariate normal distribution within each group of variables and the covariance matrices of each group to be equal. The latter assumption is an extension of the homogeneity of variances required for one-way ANOVA.

9.9.1 Multivariate Normality Test and Outliers

Although multivariate normality is assumed by certain multivariate tests, in practice it is rarely tested. The reason is that, in general, the various statistical tests are quite tolerant to small deviations from normality, whereas more crucial in many statistical methods is the presence of outliers. For the detection of outliers, we may calculate the Mahalanobis distance (MD) of each case from the centroid of the data set. If this distance for a case is statistically significant, i.e., if its p-value is smaller than .05, the case may be considered to be an outlier. Note that the MD of a point from the centroid of points follows the χ^2 distribution with degrees of freedom equal to the number of variables included in the calculation and this property is used for the calculation of its significance. This test is implemented in the macro Outliers, provided in the companion website. In addition, this macro performs the *z test* for outliers in univariate data sets. According to this test, the values of a sample are normalized to *z scores* by means of:

$$z = \frac{x - \bar{x}}{s} \tag{9.9.1}$$

A value is an outlier if the absolute value of z is beyond 2.5.

To apply the macro Outliers, we transfer the data to an Excel spreadsheet, in which the variables are arranged in successive columns, whereas a grouping variable is not necessary. Usually we examine each sample separately. In particular, we run the macro either from its homonymous file or from OSTEO using the menu Add-ins → OSTEO → Data Analysis → Outliers, select the entire range of variable values (excluding the grouping variable), and select an output cell. As an application, consider the data set of Table 5.VIII.1. If we apply this macro to the entire range of data, we observe that there is a suspicious case; case (152, 131, 112, 57) has an MD equal to 10.63 with p-value $= .031 < .05$. However, if we examine only sample 4, where this case belongs to, we find that this case is not an outlier and, therefore, we may proceed to apply the various multivariate techniques, even the ones that are sensitive to outliers, as is done in Section 9.9.8, Case Study 24.

9.9.2 Principal Component Analysis

PCA is a multivariate technique used to reduce multidimensional data to lower dimensions, i.e., to reduce the number of variables while retaining most of the information about the existence of clusters in the data set. For this purpose, PCA transforms the original orthogonal coordinate system to a new one, which is called *principal components (PCs).* The origin of the new orthogonal coordinate system is located in the centroid of the data points. The first axis of the new coordinate system, PC1, is in the direction of the highest variance, the second axis, PC2, is in the direction of the second highest variance, and so on.

To visualize how this is done, consider the simple data set presented in Table 9.9.1. The graphic display of the data presented in this table is given in Fig. 9.9.1, in which we observe that there are two clusters of data points. It is also interesting to note that the values shown in Table 9.9.1 are, in fact, the coordinates of the data points in a two-dimensional scatterplot. Therefore, in general, the values of K variables in a multivariate data set are also coordinates of data points in a K-dimensional scatterplot. However, we can draw scatterplots only for $K = 1$, 2, or 3 and, therefore, there is a need to reduce the number of variables to a maximum of 3, while retaining most of the information about the clusters in the data set.

TABLE 9.9.1 Example Data

	Var1	Var2
Case 1	2	2
Case 2	3	3
Case 3	3	2
Case 4	7	4.5
Case 5	7	4
Case 6	8	5.5

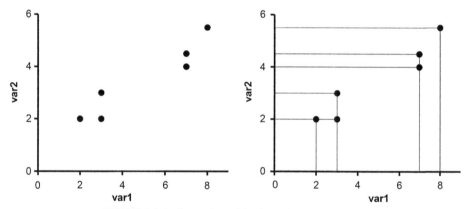

FIGURE 9.9.1 Scatterplots of the data points of Table 9.9.1.

To apply PCA and reduce the variables of Table 9.9.1 from two to one, we first center the variables, i.e., we subtract from the values of each variable the mean variable value. In this way we obtain the centered data of Table 9.9.2. The scatterplot of the centered data is the same as that of the raw values but the origin of the coordinate system is located in the centroid of the data points (Fig. 9.9.2). Now, we may transform this coordinate system to a new one as follows.

TABLE 9.9.2 Centered Data of Table 9.9.1

	Var1	Var2
Case 1	−3	−1.5
Case 2	−2	−0.5
Case 3	−2	−1.5
Case 4	2	1.0
Case 5	2	0.5
Case 6	3	2.0

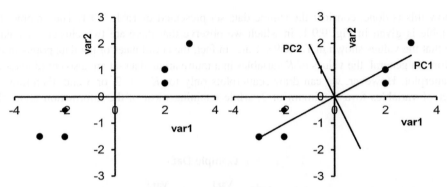

FIGURE 9.9.2 Scatterplots of centered data points of Table 9.9.1 and the axes PC1 and PC2.

We draw an axis, called PC1, through the data points of Fig. 9.9.2 along the greatest dispersal of these points. This axis may be the least-squares straight line. Subsequently, we draw a second axis, PC2, perpendicular to PC1. These two axes form a new coordinate system, which is basically the original coordinate system of Fig. 9.9.1 rotated by a certain angle.

If we project all data points on the new axes, we obtain the coordinates of these points in the new coordinate system of PC1–PC2 axes (Fig. 9.9.3). These coordinates are called *scores* and form a set of data with a number of variables equal to the original data set (Table 9.9.3). However, it is clear from Fig. 9.9.3 that the PC1 axis describes very satisfactorily the data variation, because we observe that the coordinates on this axis, i.e., the values of variable PC1, form two distinct clusters, the same clusters shown in the original scatterplot of Fig. 9.9.1. In contrast, the PC2 axis (in this example) contributes almost no information about the existence of clusters of data. Therefore, variable PC2 may be deleted without losing information. Thus, the original two-dimensional data set of Table 9.9.1 is reduced to one-dimensional data (Table 9.9.3) while retaining most of the information regarding the presence of clusters.

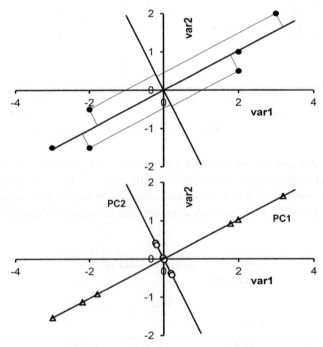

FIGURE 9.9.3 Definition of principal component scores as the coordinates of the centered data points on the PC1 and PC2 axes.

A measure that shows how spread out the data are on a PC axis is the *eigenvalue* of this axis. PC axes with small eigenvalues, usually smaller than 1, provide almost no information about the existence of clusters of data and they may be

TABLE 9.9.3 Scores and Their Reduction to One Variable

	PC1	PC2		PC1
Case 1	−2.982	0.035		−2.982
Case 2	−1.785	0.419		−1.785
Case 3	−2.191	−0.372		−2.191
Case 4	1.988	−0.023	⇒	1.988
Case 5	1.785	−0.419		1.785
Case 6	3.186	0.360		3.186

deleted. Clearly, transforming a two-dimensional table to a one-dimensional data set has no practical value. PCA is useful in cases in which the data table contains many columns (variables).

In statistical software packages this process of reducing the dimensions of a table is performed in a strict mathematical way. For the application of PCA, we should choose either the *covariance* or the *correlation* matrix to find the PC axes. As a rule, the covariance matrix is used when all variables are of similar scale, whereas the correlation matrix is preferred when the scales differ between variables. With the application of PCA, a *score matrix* is produced, which contains the obtained *factors* or PCs (PC1, PC2, …) as variables. In this matrix we usually keep the factors that correspond to eigenvalues greater than 1 and delete the rest. This new table can replace the original one without losing any substantial information regarding possible clusters, that is, uncorrelated data. Such clusters may be visually identified when we draw the scatterplot of PC1 vs PC2 and, in some cases, the three-dimensional plot of PC1 vs PC2 and PC3.

9.9.3 Multiple Correspondence Analysis

PCA is strictly applied on continuous data. When all variables or part of them in a multivariate data set are categorical, and especially nominal categorical, the technique that should be adopted to reduce data dimensionality is MCA. Thus, MCA may be considered as a variant or an extension of PCA to include nominal categorical data.

9.9.4 Linear Discriminant Analysis

Discriminant analysis is used to distinguish clusters of cases and allocate unknown cases to previously defined groups of cases. It is a classification method originally developed as LDA. There are several variants of the method, the simplest of which is the following.

Consider n distinct sets of groups of cases. We calculate the centroids of these groups and then the Mahalanobis distance of each case from these centroids. Each case is allocated to the group from which it exhibits the smallest distance. The same is valid for new (unknown) cases. If the data follow the multivariate normal distribution, we may estimate the probability of a certain case belonging to a certain group from:

$$P = ce^{-d_{MD}^2/2} \tag{9.9.2}$$

where d_{MD} is the Mahalanobis distance between the case and the centroid of the group and c is a constant determined from the condition that the sum of all P-values should be equal to 1. For cross-validation, the *leave-one-out classification* or *jackknife* technique is usually adopted. According to this technique, one case at a time is removed from the analysis and its classification is based on the remaining cases.

9.9.5 Multivariate Analysis of Variance

ANOVA is used to explore statistically significant differences among three or more samples based on one single variable. MANOVA extends this application and explores the existence of statistically significant differences among groups based on multivariate data sets. Like ANOVA, it is a parametric test based on a test statistic. In fact, many test statistics have been proposed and, subsequently, different tests, the most powerful of which are *Pillai's trace* and *Wilks' lambda*.

MANOVA presupposes that the variables follow the multinomial normal distribution, there is homogeneity of variance, and there is equality of the covariance matrices of the dependent variables across groups. If these assumptions are not fulfilled, the simpler approach is to assess the distance among the various groups through their Mahalanobis distances, as described in Appendix 5.VIII. The same procedure may also be followed in the case in which the null hypothesis is rejected and we want to identify the samples between which significant differences are traced.

9.9.6 Hierarchical Cluster Analysis

Cluster analysis comprises several statistical classification techniques in which, according to a specific *measure of similarity* (see Section 9.9.7), cases are subdivided into groups (clusters) so that the cases in a cluster are very similar to one another and very different from the cases in other clusters. HCA is a method of cluster analysis that arranges cases in an hierarchy. The main outcome is a *dendrogram*, which is used to visualize how clusters are formed.

The clustering procedure is usually based on the Euclidean distance, d. This distance between cases (a_{11}, a_{12}, a_{13}, ..., a_{1m}) and (a_{21}, a_{22}, a_{23}, ..., a_{2m}) is calculated from:

$$d = \sqrt{(a_{11} - a_{21})^2 + (a_{12} - a_{22})^2 + \cdots + (a_{1m} - a_{2m})^2} \qquad (9.9.3)$$

However, other measures for the distance between cases may also be adopted, like the squared Euclidean distance, the Pearson coefficient, and a user-defined distance.

To see how Eq. (9.9.3) is used by HCA to cluster data, consider the very simple example of the data of Table 9.9.1. For the application of HCA, we first calculate the Euclidean distances between all pairs of cases. These distances are given in Table 9.9.4, arranged from the smallest to the largest. Now the procedure followed to cluster these data may be the following: The first cluster is formed between cases 4 and 5, which have the smallest Euclidean distance, $d = 0.5$. Then an independent cluster is formed either between cases 1 and 2 or between cases 2 and 3, because in both instances the distance is 1. It is evident that if a cluster is formed between cases 1 and 2, then, in the next step, cases 1, 2, and 3 form a greater cluster. Similarly, if initially a cluster is formed between cases 2 and 3, then, in the next step, again cases 1, 2, and 3 form a greater cluster. The next smallest distance is between cases 1 and 2 and cases 4 and 6. Cases 1 and 2 already belong to a cluster, whereas this does not hold for cases 4 and 6. Therefore, at this step the cluster of cases 4 and 5 is extended to include case 6. Finally, the cluster of cases 1, 2, and 3 and that of cases 4, 5, and 6 are unified to a single cluster, which includes all cases of Table 9.9.1.

TABLE 9.9.4 Euclidean Distances Between the Points (Cases) of Table 9.9.1 Sorted From the Smallest to the Largest

Pair	d	Pair	d
4–5	0.50	2–4	4.27
1–3	1.00	3–5	4.47
2–3	1.00	3–4	4.72
1–2	1.41	1–5	5.39
4–6	1.41	1–4	5.59
5–6	1.80	2–5	5.59
2–5	4.12	3–6	6.10
2–6	4.24	1–6	6.95

These steps for clustering the data of Table 9.9.1 are visualized in the dendrogram of Fig. 9.9.4. In this plot we observe that the first clusters are formed between cases 4 and 5 and cases 2 and 3. Then case 1 is attached to the cluster of cases 2 and 3, forming a greater cluster, and case 6 is attached to the cluster of cases 4 and 5, also forming a greater cluster. In the final step the two previous clusters are unified to an even greater cluster that includes all cases.

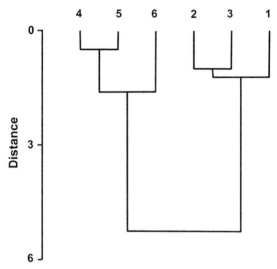

FIGURE 9.9.4 Dendrogram of the data of Table 9.9.1.

In a dendrogram, the vertical axis can show either the distance, d, between two cases when they are joined, as in Fig. 9.9.4, or the *similarity*, s, defined by $s = 100(1 - d/d_{max})$, where d_{max} is the maximum distance between any two cases. Note that in SPSS the actual distances, d, are rescaled to numbers between 0 and 25.

HCA can be applied either to the initial multivariate data set or to the distances calculated from this data set. The first option is preferred when the data set has a rather small number of cases. When this number is large, the dendrogram becomes complicated and difficult to interpret.

9.9.7 Metric and Nonmetric Multidimensional Scaling

MDS comprises a group of techniques that create a map visualizing the relative positions of a number of objects based on the matrix of distances between them. The map may have one, two, or three dimensions. There are two broad categories in MDS: *metric, or classical, MDS* and *nonmetric MDS*.

The goal of metric MDS is to produce a configuration of points, i.e., a map, for which the Euclidean distances, or any other distance used, between the points are as close as possible to the distances used to produce the map. Metric MDS is also known as *principal coordinates analysis.* The objective of nonmetric MDS is to find a map that reproduces not the input distances but the ranks of these distances.

In general, the input data to MDS form a *proximity* matrix, i.e., a symmetrical square matrix, the values of which quantify how "close" or "distant" two objects are. Therefore, its values may be either *dissimilarity* or *similarity* measures. The dissimilarity matrix is, in fact, a distance matrix. The dissimilarity is a measure of distinction; the greater the dissimilarity of two objects, the greater the value of this measure. Therefore, the diagonal elements of a dissimilarity matrix are equal to 0, because the distinction between an object and itself is 0. The concept of *similarity* is the opposite of dissimilarity; the more two objects resemble each other, the larger the similarity of these objects is. For example, the correlation matrix may often be considered as a similarity matrix. Note that in this case the diagonal elements of the similarity matrix are equal to 1.

MDS is similar to other data reduction techniques, like PCA. Thus, MDS attempts to reduce the dimensions (columns) of the proximity matrix to two or three, while preserving most of the information about interpoint distances. The optimum number of dimensions in the MDS model is selected by means of the *stress function*, i.e., a function that measures the difference between the actual distances and their predicted values or between the ranks of actual distances and their predicted values.

9.9.8 Case Studies on Multivariate Analyses

Case Study 24: Multivariate Analysis of Cranial Morphology by Means of Metric Traits

Considering that cranial dimensions are largely controlled genetically, assess the biological affinities among the population samples of the multivariate data set of Table 5.VIII.1.

The first step in biodistance studies using craniometrics is to explore the potential existence of clusters in the data set. For this purpose, we may initially apply PCA. To examine how effectively the samples are discriminated and subsequently confirm the conclusions drawn from PCA, we may apply LDA. To gain a more quantitative idea about the overall difference among the various samples, as well as the difference between each two pairs of samples, we may use MANOVA. For the visualization of clusters among the groups that comprise the data set, we may perform HCA and/or MDS on the Mahalanobis Distances computed on the original multivariate data set.

Principal Component Analysis

In SPSS we arrange the data as in Fig. 9.9.5 and use the menu Analyze → Dimension Reduction → Factor. In the dialog box that appears we transfer only the variables with cranial dimensions, maximum cranial breadth (XCB), basion–bregma height (BBH), basion–prosthion length (BPL), and nasal height (NLH), to the box labeled Variables. From Rotation we may select "Varimax," although this option is not necessary for the current application. From Extraction we select "Principal Components," "Correlation matrix," and "Eigenvalues over 1" so that we obtain only the significant axes (PCs). Note that, as mentioned above, we use "Correlation matrix" when variables are on different scales and "Covariance matrix" when the variable scales are similar. Finally, from Scores we activate the option "Save as Variables." In this way the values for PC1, PC2, and other significant PCs will be saved in the Data View window as new variables entitled FAC1_1, FAC2_1, and so on. We click on "OK" and the PC scores appear as new variables in the Data View window (Fig. 9.9.5).

	Sample	XCB	BBH	BPL	NHL	FAC1_1	FAC2_1
1	1	127	139	91	51	.01570	-1.11139
2	1	128	132	92	52	-.55816	-.92195
3	1	131	132	99	50	-.32363	.02698
4	1	119	130	98	50	-.56547	-1.00632
5	1	128	145	96	58	1.62312	-1.21111
6	1	137	138	87	55	.02451	-.88487
7	1	141	133	107	48	.06045	1.61442
8	1	124	143	96	48	.46124	-.79871
9	1	131	136	105	57	1.13970	-.04615
10	1	138	132	99	50	-.34038	.59939
11	2	139	143	98	54	1.12719	.16148
12	2	128	134	92	50	-.54223	-.80786
13	2	137	138	93	46	-.46987	.23647
14	2	134	131	109	48	-.00723	1.23056

FIGURE 9.9.5 Data View window with part of the principal component scores created after the application of principal component analysis. *BBH*, basion–bregma height; *BPL*, basion–prosthion length; *NLH*, nasal height; *XCB*, maximum cranial breadth.

Now we use the menu Graphs → Legacy Dialogs → Scatter/Dot, select Simple Scatter and click on "Define." In the new dialog box that appears we transfer the variable FAC1_1 (REGR factor score 1) to X Axis, the FAC2_1 (REGR factor score 2) to Y Axis, and the variable Sample to Set Markers by. In this way the points of each sample will be symbolized differently. We click on "OK" and obtain the graph of Fig. 9.9.6. We observe that the individuals from samples 1 and 2 appear to form one cluster, whereas those of samples 3 and 4 stand apart. This suggests that samples 1 and 2 come from populations that are very close biologically, which in turn implies the existence of gene flow between them, whereas the parent populations of samples 3 and 4 were rather isolated and probably belonged to different marital networks or originated elsewhere.

To assess how valid this picture is, we need to determine how much of the original variation in the data is explained by the first two PC axes, PC1 and PC2. This information is gained from the table Total Variance Explained presented in SPSS Output 9.9.1. It is seen that the first two PCs explain almost 61% of the original variance, so the conclusions drawn from the scatterplot might be biased. For this reason, it is important to analyze the data further using other multivariate tests and/or by calculating the Mahalanobis distances between all pairs of populations.

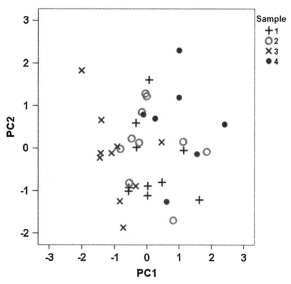

FIGURE 9.9.6 PC1 vs PC2 scatterplot.

SPSS OUTPUT 9.9.1 Total Variance Explained

Component	Initial Eigenvalues			Extraction Sums of Squared Loadings		
	Total	% of Variance	Cumulative %	Total	% of Variance	Cumulative %
1	1.300	32.496	32.496	1.300	32.496	32.496
2	1.142	28.538	61.034	1.142	28.538	61.034
3	0.882	22.062	83.096			
4	0.676	16.904	100.000			

Extraction method: principal component analysis.

Linear Discriminant Analysis

We arrange the data as for PCA and select the option "Discriminant" from the menu Analyze → Classify. In the dialog box that appears we transfer the variables XCB, BBH, BPL, and NLH to the panel Independent and the variable Sample to the box labeled Grouping Variable. We click on "Define Range" and type in value "1" for Minimum and value "4" for Maximum. We click on "Continue" and from Save we activate the options "Predicted group membership" and "Probabilities of group membership." Also, from Classify we select "Summary table" and "Leave-one-out classification." We click on "Continue" and "OK."

Among the tables of results, an important one is the Classification Results (SPSS Output 9.9.2). At the bottom of this table we observe that 75.7% of the cases are correctly classified, whereas if we check the Leave-one-out classification, this percentage drops to 56.8%. Therefore, we can conclude that the overall differentiation among samples is not very satisfactory.

It is also seen that the program creates five new variables in the Data View window entitled Dis_1, Dis1_1, Dis2_1, Dis3_1, and Dis4_1 (Fig. 9.9.7). Dis_1 presents the prediction by the program of the sample to which each case should be attributed, Dis1_1 presents the probability that a case is classified to sample 1, Dis2_1 is the probability a case is classified to sample 2, and so on. We can see that the individuals belonging to samples 1 and 2 are often misclassified, whereas those of samples 3 and 4 are satisfactorily discriminated, which supports the results we obtained from PCA.

MANOVA

We arrange the data as before and select the option "Multivariate" from the menu Analyze → General Linear Model. In the dialog box that appears we transfer the variables XCB, BBH, BPL, and NLH to the panel Dependent Variables and the

SPSS OUTPUT 9.9.2 Part of the Classification Results[a,b] Table

		Sample	Predicted Group Membership				Total
			1	2	3	4	
Original	Count	1	7	2	1	0	10
		2	4	5	0	1	10
		3	0	0	9	1	10
		4	0	1	0	7	7
Cross-validated[c]	Count	1	4	5	1	0	10
		2	4	4	0	2	10
		3	0	1	8	1	10
		4	1	1	0	5	7

[a]75.7% of original grouped cases are correctly classified.
[b]56.8% of cross-validated grouped cases are correctly classified.
[c]Cross-validation is done only for those cases in the analysis. In cross-validation, each case is classified by the functions derived from all cases other than that case.

	Sample	XCB	BBH	BPL	NHL	Dis_1	Dis1_1	Dis2_1	Dis3_1	Dis4_1
1	1	127	139	91	51	1	.5760	.4050	.0179	.0011
2	1	128	132	92	52	1	.5082	.2322	.2571	.0024
3	1	131	132	99	50	1	.5651	.3583	.0723	.0043
4	1	119	130	98	50	1	.8265	.1491	.0243	.0001
5	1	128	145	96	58	1	.4887	.4387	.0027	.0698
6	1	137	138	87	55	3	.1984	.2915	.3808	.1293
7	1	141	133	107	48	2	.3243	.5862	.0240	.0656
8	1	124	143	96	48	1	.5657	.4338	.0004	.0001
9	1	131	136	105	57	1	.4850	.3101	.0152	.1897
10	1	138	132	99	50	2	.3483	.4248	.1850	.0419
11	2	139	143	98	54	2	.2000	.5001	.0061	.2937
12	2	128	134	92	50	1	.5798	.3267	.0925	.0010
13	2	137	138	93	46	2	.3259	.6457	.0257	.0026
14	2	134	131	109	48	1	.5405	.4391	.0129	.0075

FIGURE 9.9.7 Data arrangement and part of the linear discriminant analysis results. *BBH*, basion–bregma height; *BPL*, basion–prosthion length; *NLH*, nasal height; *XCB*, maximum cranial breadth.

grouping variable Sample to the Fixed Factor(s) box. From Options we activate the "Homogeneity tests," and from Model we select "Full Factorial" and activate the option "Include intercept in the model." By clicking on "Post Hoc" we may select many post hoc tests but these tests result in a rather complicated output.

Among the tables of results, the most important ones are given in SPSS Outputs 9.9.3–9.9.5. The first table presents *Box's M test* for equality of the covariance matrices. It is seen that the null hypothesis that the covariance matrices of the variables across samples are equal cannot be rejected. Similarly, Levene's tests for the homogeneity of variance across samples also show that the corresponding null hypothesis cannot be rejected. Therefore, the basic assumptions are fulfilled and, consequently, the results of MANOVA presented in SPSS Output 9.9.5 are valid. In this SPSS output we inspect the Sig. values of panel Sample. It is seen that all tests (Pillai's trace, Wilks' lambda, Hotelling's trace, and Roy's largest root) show that there are statistically significant differences among the samples of Table 5.VIII.1.

SPSS OUTPUT 9.9.3 Box's Test of Equality of Covariance Matrices	
Box's M	27.693
F	0.704
df1	30
df2	2364.006
Sig.	0.883

SPSS OUTPUT 9.9.4 Levene's Test of Equality of Error Variances

	F	df1	df2	Sig.
XCB	0.290	3	33	0.832
BBH	0.829	3	33	0.488
BPL	2.747	3	33	0.058
NLH	2.009	3	33	0.132

Tests the null hypothesis that the error variance of the dependent variable is equal across groups. *BBH,* basion–bregma height; *BPL,* basion–prosthion length; *NLH,* nasal height; *XCB,* maximum cranial breadth.

SPSS OUTPUT 9.9.5 Multivariate Tests

	Effect	Value	*F*	Hypothesis df	Error df	Sig.
Intercept	Pillai's Trace	0.999	14430.14[a]	4	30	0.000
	Wilks' Lambda	0.001	14430.14[a]	4	30	0.000
	Hotelling's Trace	1924.02	14430.14[a]	4	30	0.000
	Roy's Largest Root	1924.02	14430.14[a]	4	30	0.000
Sample	Pillai's Trace	1.124	4.796	12	96	0.000
	Wilks' Lambda	0.206	5.424	12	79.664	0.000
	Hotelling's Trace	2.336	5.580	12	86	0.000
	Roy's Largest Root	1.187	9.497[b]	4	32	0.000

[a]*Exact statistic.*
[b]*The statistic is an upper bound on F that yields a lower bound on the significance level.*

To assess between which pairs of samples the significant differences are traced, we may rerun MANOVA for each pair of samples separately and correct the obtained p-values using the Holm–Bonferroni method. In SPSS the application of MANOVA to a certain pair of samples is straightforward. We first select the samples under consideration from the menu Data → Select Cases, in which we activate the option "If condition is satisfied" and complete the dialog box that appears as in Fig. 9.9.8. Note that the command shown in this figure is used to select samples 1 and 2. Then MANOVA is applied directly via the menu Analyze → General Linear Model → Multivariate, where we simply click on the button "OK." The raw p-values obtained from the pairwise comparisons and their adjustment using the Holm–Bonferroni correction are given in Table 9.9.5, which shows that all pairwise comparisons are statistically significant except that between samples 1 and 2.

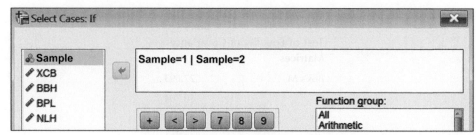

FIGURE 9.9.8 Selection of samples 1 and 2. *BBH,* basion—bregma height; *BPL,* basion—prosthion length; *NLH,* nasal height; *XCB,* maximum cranial breadth.

TABLE 9.9.5 Raw and Corrected *p*-values for Pairwise Comparisons in MANOVA Using the Holm—Bonferroni Method

Pair	Raw *p*-value (Pillai's Trace)	Corrected *p*-value
1—2	0.6255	0.6255
1—3	0.0015	0.0061
1—4	0.0039	0.0118
2—3	0.0006	0.0033
2—4	0.0073	0.0146
3—4	0.0007	0.0037

Alternatively, we may calculate the Mahalanobis distances between the various samples, as described in detail in Appendix 5.VIII. From Fig. 5.VIII.3 we again observe that all distances are statistically significant except that between samples 1 and 2. Note that this result is consistent with the PCA and LDA tests.

Hierarchical Cluster Analysis

As pointed out above, we avoid applying HCA directly to the raw data of Table 5.VIII.1, because the dendrogram obtained will be confusing. For this reason, it is better to apply HCA to the biodistances calculated from the original data.

Consider the CMDs computed in Appendix 5.VIII. To apply HCA in SPSS, we arrange the CMD values in a matrix format as in Fig. 9.9.9 and then use the menu Analyze → Classify → Hierarchical Cluster. In the dialog box that appears we transfer the variables Sample1, Sample2, Sample3, and Sample4 to the box labeled Variable(s), and the variable Samples to the Label Cases by box. We click on "Plots" and select "Dendrogram," while from Methods we choose the method based on which the clusters will be formed; usually we select "Between-groups linkage" or "Ward." Note that in complex samples these options may lead to different dendrograms, which is a drawback of HCA. Finally, in the panel Measure we select the distance or similarity measure to be used in clustering. Because we already use Mahalanobis distances, we select "Interval: Customized." We click on "Continue" and "OK." Fig. 9.9.10 shows the obtained dendrogram. We again observe that samples 1 and 2 form a cluster, whereas samples 3 and 4 stand on separate branches.

	Samples	Sample1	Sample2	Sample3	Sample4
1	Sample1	.0000	.0000	4.0017	6.1293
2	Sample2	.0000	.0000	4.1710	4.5518
3	Sample3	4.0017	4.1710	.0000	6.3001
4	Sample4	6.1293	4.5518	6.3001	.0000

FIGURE 9.9.9 Data arrangement in SPSS.

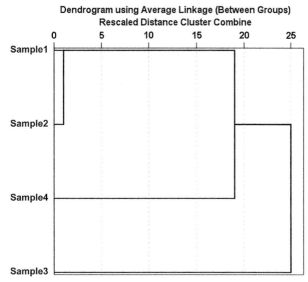

FIGURE 9.9.10   Dendrogram of the squared Mahalanobis distances of Fig. 9.9.9.

Multidimensional Scaling

To perform MDS, we arrange the biodistances as in Fig. 9.9.9, although variable samples may be eliminated, and then we use the menu Analyze → Scale → Multidimensional Scaling (PROXSCAL). In the Data Format dialog box we select "The data are proximities" and "One matrix source," and click on "Define." In the new dialog box that appears we transfer the variables Sample1, Sample2, Sample3, and Sample4 to the Proximities box. Then we click on "Model," select Ratio, Full matrix, Dissimilarities, Dimensions 1 to 3, and click on "Continue." We proceed by clicking on "Plots" and selecting the "Stress" and "Common space" options in the dialog box that appears.

We click on "Continue" and "OK" and obtain, among others, the *scree plot* of Fig. 9.9.11, left, which depicts the variation of the stress function upon the number of dimensions in the MDS model. We observe that the optimum number of dimensions that should be used in MDS is 2 and, therefore, the most appropriate of the Common Space plots is the two-dimensional MDS plot shown in Fig. 9.9.11, right. This plot again shows that samples 1 and 2 tend to form a cluster, whereas 3 and 4 stand apart.

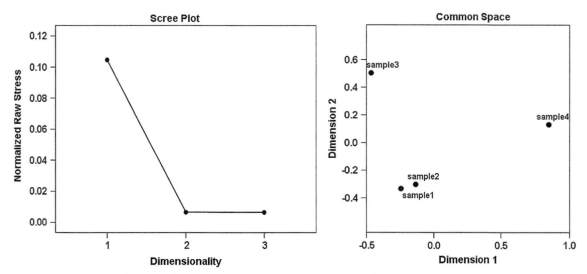

FIGURE 9.9.11   Scree plot (left) and two-dimensional multidimensional scaling plot (right) of Mahalanobis distances.

Case Study 25: Multivariate Analysis of Cranial Morphology by Means of Landmark Coordinates

Apply multivariate techniques to the *Procrustes residuals* obtained from the data set of 3D male cranial landmarks provided in the Excel file DataForStatistics/Multivariate. Note that the groups in this data set come from populations who lived along the Nile River (Fig. 9.9.12), namely the Badari (4400−4000 BC), Naqada (4000−3200 BC), Kerma (2000−1550 BC), and Gizeh (664−343 BC).

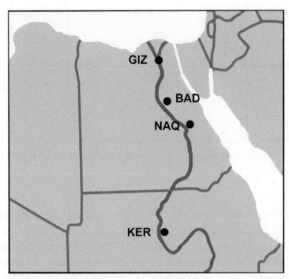

FIGURE 9.9.12   Archaeological sites within the study region. *BAD,* Badari; *GIZ,* Gizeh; *KER,* Kerma; *NAQ,* Naqada.

Appendices 5.III−5.VI outlined the pretreatment of raw 3D data of cranial landmarks up to the application of Generalized Procrustes Analysis (GPA) and the calculation of Procrustes residuals. As a result, the data obtained are the outcome of many steps of data processing and, therefore, the interference of errors cannot be excluded. For this reason, we first need to test for outliers. Thus, we run the macro Outliers, select the entire range of the Procrustes residuals, and define an output cell (Fig. 9.9.13). We observe that there are three suspicious cases: cases 70, 108, and 109. We remove these cases and transfer the remaining values along with the grouping variable to an SPSS spreadsheet.

No	MD	p-value
1	105.777	0.622199
2	103.4786	0.681414
68	119.709	0.269487
69	124.1591	0.185434
70	147.8118	0.011178
71	98.13412	0.803478
106	101.0315	0.740564
107	100.6742	0.748774
108	147.7238	0.011323
109	147.3771	0.011908
110	96.9795	0.826023
111	118.5787	0.2939
112	84.82782	0.969376

FIGURE 9.9.13   Test for outliers using the Outliers macro.

Now we can analyze the residuals using various multivariate tests. However, because of the large number of variables in the data set, certain techniques cannot be applied. For example, we cannot calculate biodistances or apply MANOVA. For this reason, we should first reduce the number of variables using PCA.

We click Analyze → Dimension Reduction → Factor. In the dialog box that appears we transfer all variables except the grouping one to the box labeled Variables. From Rotation we select None and from Extraction we select Principal Components, Covariance matrix, and Eigenvalues over 0 so that we obtain all the PCs. To save these PCs, from Scores we activate the option "Save as Variables."

After PCA is performed, we examine the table Total Variance Explained (SPSS Output 9.9.6). It is seen that the first two PCs explain only 13.8% and 8.3% of the variance, respectively. This is a very small percentage of the total variance and for this reason there is no need to draw the PC1 vs PC2 scatterplot as it will not provide reliable information. However, the PCA procedure is still necessary to reduce the number of variables, as explained earlier. From the Total Variance Explained table we find that the first 32 PCs explain more than 90% of the variance and, therefore, we may use these PCs for further analyses. Thus, we return to the Data View window and erase all the columns with PCs from PC33 (FAC33_1) onward. We may save this file for further analyses. PC1 to PC32 along with the grouping variable are given in the DataForStatistics/Multivariate Excel file.

SPSS OUTPUT 9.9.6 Part of the Total Variance Explained Table

Component		Initial Eigenvalues		
		Total	% of Variance	Cumulative %
Raw	1	0.000	13.822	13.822
	2	0.000	8.296	22.118
	3	0.000	7.712	29.830
	4	0.000	6.138	35.968
	5	0.000	5.686	41.653
	6	0.000	4.728	46.381
	7	0.000	3.999	50.381

We proceed to examine whether LDA suggests the existence of clusters in the data set under study. We use the previous SPSS spreadsheet and click on Analyze → Classify → Discriminant. In the dialog box that appears we transfer the variables FAC1_1 to FAC32_1 to the Independent panel and the grouping variable to the box labeled Grouping Variable, in which we type in the value "1" to box Minimum and the value "4" to box Maximum. From Classify we select "Summary table" and "Leave-one-out classification," and click on "Continue" and "OK."

The table Classification Results is shown in SPSS Output 9.9.7. It is seen that the prediction membership via LDA is rather satisfactory. An overall 91.8% of the original grouped cases are correctly classified and this percentage is reduced to 77.6% after cross-validation. In more detail, for samples 1 to 4 the correct predictions are 12 of 15, 29 of 40, 33 of 44, and 40 of 48. Such a picture should be expected because there is some degree of overlap among the various groups. However, this does not mean that there is no clear differentiation of the four samples, as shown below.

If we apply MANOVA, we find that the null hypothesis that the covariance matrices of the dependent variables across groups are equal should be rejected (Sig. = .003), whereas there are three variables for which Levene's tests for the homogeneity of variance across groups also show that the corresponding null hypothesis should be rejected. Despite these findings, the p-value of the Pillai trace is equal to Sig. = 1.055E-30 = 1.055×10^{-30}, which leaves no doubt that there are statistically significant differences among the groups under study. Table 9.9.6 shows the raw p-values (Pillai's trace) obtained from the pairwise comparisons and their adjustment using the Holm–Bonferroni correction. It is seen that all pairwise comparisons are statistically significant. It is evident that this result does not exclude a partial overlap among groups, as detected in LDA.

A better picture is obtained if we compute the Mahalanobis biodistances among the various groups. We transfer the grouping variable and the 32 PCs from SPSS to an Excel spreadsheet and use the macro Biodistances, as described in

SPSS OUTPUT 9.9.7 Part of the Classification Results[a,b] Table

Group			Predicted Group Membership				
			1.0	2.0	3.0	4.0	Total
Original	Count	1.0	15	0	0	0	15
		2.0	2	33	3	2	40
		3.0	0	0	42	2	44
		4.0	1	0	2	45	48
	%	1.0	100.0	0.0	0.0	0.0	100.0
		2.0	5.0	82.5	7.5	5.0	100.0
		3.0	0.0	0.0	95.5	4.5	100.0
		4.0	2.1	0.0	4.2	93.8	100.0
Cross-validated[c]	Count	1.0	12	3	0	0	15
		2.0	4	29	4	3	40
		3.0	3	2	33	6	44
		4.0	1	3	4	40	48
	%	1.0	80.0	20.0	0.0	0.0	100.0
		2.0	10.0	72.5	10.0	7.5	100.0
		3.0	6.8	4.5	75.0	13.6	100.0
		4.0	2.1	6.3	8.3	83.3	100.0

[a]91.8% of original grouped cases are correctly classified.
[b]77.6% of cross-validated grouped cases are correctly classified.
[c]Cross-validation is done only for those cases in the analysis. In cross-validation, each case is classified by the functions derived from all cases other than that case.

TABLE 9.9.6 Raw and Corrected *p*-values for Pairwise Comparisons in MANOVA Using the Holm–Bonferroni Method

Pairs	Raw *p*-values	Corrected *p*-values
1–2	0.000393	0.000393
1–3	2.34×10^{-5}	4.68×10^{-5}
1–4	2.81×10^{-10}	1.41×10^{-9}
2–3	2.05×10^{-7}	6.15×10^{-7}
2–4	3.59×10^{-11}	2.16×10^{-10}
3–4	3.36×10^{-8}	1.34×10^{-7}

Appendix 5.VIII. Selecting biodistances for continuous data, we obtain the results of Fig. 9.9.14, in which we again observe that all distances are statistically significant.

To visualize these distances, we perform HCA and MDS, as described in the previous case study. The dendrogram and the 2D MDS plot for the CMD are shown in Fig. 9.9.15. We observe that both plots show the existence of two distinct clusters: one between groups 1 and 2, i.e., between Badari and Naqada, and the other between groups 3 and 4, i.e., between Gizeh and Kerma. Note that the same result was obtained in a study that included more samples and many more landmarks (Nikita et al., 2012).

Squared Euclidean and Mahalanobis distances for continuous or ordinal data						
MD pooled matrix determinant = 9.83732298930663E-02						
Missing values indicator = -1						
Pairs	ED	EDN	p-EDN	MD/OMD	CMD/COMD	p-MD/CMD
1-2	5.6861	5.7003	0.0011	10.8991	5.4506	1.81E-05
1-3	8.1023	7.2497	3.84E-06	27.3165	18.1520	5.16E-16
1-4	8.1227	8.4923	1.79E-08	30.7798	20.8767	3.98E-18
2-3	4.1112	4.0678	1E-06	12.9657	8.4464	2.39E-14
2-4	4.3945	3.9473	7.45E-07	16.5644	11.2751	1.51E-18
3-4	3.9054	3.9185	2.06E-07	10.1468	6.4113	2.58E-12

FIGURE 9.9.14   Biodistances calculated using the first 32 principal components.

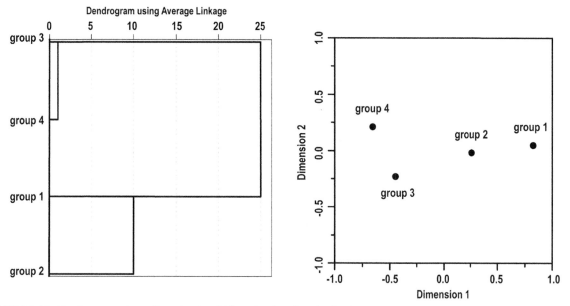

FIGURE 9.9.15   Dendrogram and two-dimensional multidimensional scaling plot for the corrected squared Mahalanobis distances of Fig. 9.9.14.

Case Study 26: Cranial Size Differences

Assess whether there are differentiations in the cranial size of samples 1 to 4 in the aforementioned data set.

In geometric morphometric studies, centroid size is used as a proxy for cranial size. To calculate the centroid size in our data, we use the table of 3D landmarks of male individuals given in the spreadsheet 3D Landmarks of the Cranial data Excel file. We may remove the three outliers detected previously in the corresponding Procrustes residuals (cases 70, 108, and 109). Note that although the data in the spreadsheet 3D Landmarks were obtained after GPA using the Morpheus software, they retain the original cranial size because, during their treatment, we used the option "Restore Scale."

To compute the centroid size, we can run the CentroidSize macro, select the entire rectangular range of the landmark coordinates, and click on an output cell. The calculated centroid sizes constitute a univariate data set with values belonging to the four samples. Thus, we may apply ANOVA or its nonparametric variant, the Kruskal−Wallis test. To perform these tests in SPSS, we work as in Section 9.5.6, Case Study 6. Thus, we enter the grouping variable and the values of the normalized centroid size in two columns and use the menu Analyze → Compare Means → One-Way ANOVA. In the dialog box One-Way ANOVA we transfer the grouping variable to the Factor box and the variable of the normalized centroid sizes to the box labeled Dependent List and select "Homogeneity of variance test." We also click on "Post Hoc" and select the "Tukey" criterion.

We find that the ANOVA p-value (.009) is smaller than the level of significance (.05), indicating the existence of statistically significant differences between samples. From the table Multiple Comparisons we observe that these differences concern only samples 1−3 (p-value = .016). Taking into account that the average normalized centroid sizes of the

Badari and Kerma crania are 74.3 and 76.1, respectively, we can conclude that the size of the Badari crania is significantly smaller than that of the Kerma crania.

Case Study 27: Multivariate Analysis of Cranial Morphology by Means of Nonmetric Traits

Apply multivariate techniques to the TMD calculated in Fig. 5.XI.7.

Once we have calculated a matrix of biodistances, it is useful to visualize them using HCA and MDS. In addition, we may examine possible correlations of the biodistances with temporal and spatial distances, as described in Section 9.8.4, Case Study 23.

To apply HCA and MDS to the TMD data presented in Fig. 5.XI.7, we follow the procedures described in Case Study 24 and obtain the plots of Fig. 9.9.16. It is seen that samples 2 and 4 cluster together, suggesting a genetic proximity between the corresponding populations, whereas samples 1 and 3 come from distant populations.

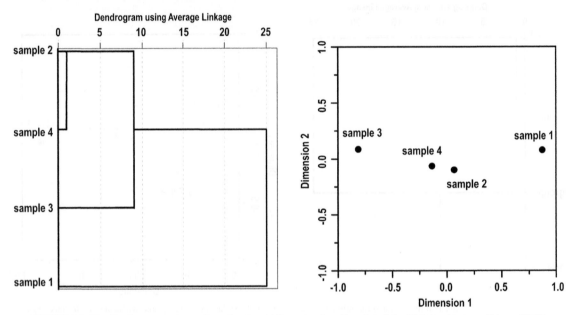

FIGURE 9.9.16 Dendrogram and two-dimensional multidimensional scaling plot of the Mahalanobis-type distance TMD.

Case Study 28: Multiple Correspondence Analysis

Table 9.9.7 presents example data on the sex, profession, and entheseal changes (ECs) of 16 individuals belonging to three groups. In this table Sex is coded as F (female) and M (male), Profession is coded as 0 (manual) and 1 (nonmanual), and ECs are represented by three of the Coimbra method variables (see Appendix 7.I), Bone formation, zone 1 (BFZ1); Bone formation, zone 2 (BFZ2); and Erosion, zone 1 (ERZ1). Determine whether there are distinct clusters in this data set.

Because the data set contains two nominal variables, Sex and Profession, MCA should be applied. We transfer the data of Table 9.9.7 to an SPSS spreadsheet and click on Analyze → Dimension Reduction → Optimal Scaling. In the dialog box that appears we select "All variables multiple nominal" and "One set." Then we click on "Define" and in the new dialog box we transfer the variables Sex, Profession, BFZ1, BFZ2, and ERZ1 to the box labeled Analysis Variables. In addition, we define the number of Dimensions in the solution as 2. We click on "Save" and activate the option "Save object scores to the active dataset." In this way the two significant Dimensions (the equivalent of PCs in PCA) will be saved in the Data View window as new variables titled OBSCO1_1 and OBSCO2_1.

To plot the first two Dimensions, we proceed as in PCA. That is, we use the menu Graphs → Legacy Dialogs → Scatter/Dot, select Simple Scatter and click on "Define." In the new dialog box that appears we transfer the variable OBSCO1_1 to X Axis, OBSCO2_1 to Y Axis, and Sample to Set Markers by. We obtain the graph of Fig. 9.9.17, which shows that the individuals from sample B form a distinct cluster, whereas those of samples A and C appear to form a second cluster.

To assess how valid this picture is, we again need to estimate how much of the original variation in the data is explained by the first two Dimensions. To do this, we may rerun MCA defining the number of Dimensions in the solution as 5, equal

TABLE 9.9.7 Example Data Set Consisting of Three Samples

Sample	Sex	Profession	BFZ1	BFZ2	ERZ1
A	F	1	2	2	1
A	M	1	0	0	0
A	F	0	1	1	0
A	M	1	1	2	1
B	M	0	2	1	0
B	F	0	2	1	0
B	F	0	2	1	2
B	M	0	2	2	1
B	M	0	0	1	0
B	M	0	2	1	2
C	M	0	1	2	0
C	F	0	0	1	0
C	F	1	0	1	0
C	F	0	1	1	1
C	M	1	1	2	1
C	M	1	0	2	1

BFZ1, Bone formation, zone 1; *BFZ2,* Bone formation, zone 2; *ERZ1,* Erosion, zone 1; *F,* female; *M,* male.

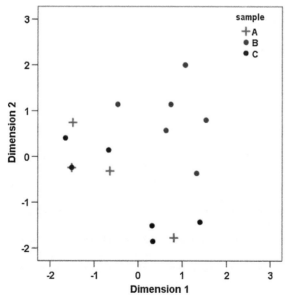

FIGURE 9.9.17 Two-dimensional multiple correspondence analysis plot for the data set of Table 9.9.7.

to the number of variables. From the table Model Summary we obtain the eigenvalues of all Dimensions and their sum. In the example we study, the eigenvalues of the first two Dimensions are 2.731 and 1.29, respectively, whereas the total sum is 6.425. Therefore, the first two Dimensions explain $42.51\% + 20.08\% = 62.6\%$ of the original variance. This percentage is rather low, so the conclusions drawn from the scatterplot might be biased.

REFERENCES

Brace CL, Rosenberg KR, Hunt KD. Gradual change in human tooth size in the Late Pleistocene and Post-Pleistocene. Evolution 1987;41:705–20.

Draper N, Smith H. Applied regression analysis. 3rd ed. New York: Wiley; 1998.

Howells WW. Cranial variation in man. A study by multivariate analysis of patterns of difference among recent human populations. Cambridge MA: Harvard University Press; 1973.

Nikita E. The use of generalized linear models and generalized estimating equations in bioarchaeological studies. American Journal of Physical Anthropology 2014;153:473–83.

Nikita E. A critical review of the mean measure of divergence and Mahalanobis distances using artificial data and new approaches to the estimation of biodistances employing nonmetric traits. American Journal of Physical Anthropology 2015;157:284–9.

Nikita E, Mattingly D, Lahr MM. Three-dimensional cranial shape analyses and gene flow in North Africa during the middle to late Holocene. Journal of Anthropological Archaeology 2012;31:564–72.

Ruff CB, Holt BM, Niskanen M, Sladék V, Berner M, Garofalo E, Garvin HM, Hora M, Maijanen H, Niinimäki S, Salo K, Schuplerová E, Tompkins D. Stature and body mass estimation from skeletal remains in the European Holocene. American Journal of Physical Anthropology 2012;148:601–17.

Sjøvold T. Some notes on the distribution and certain modifications of Mahalanobis generalized distance. Journal of Human Evolution 1975;4:549–58.

Sjøvold T. Non–metrical divergence between skeletal populations. The theoretical foundation and biological importance of C. A. B. Smith's mean measure of divergence. OSSA 1977;4(Suppl. 1):1–133.

Smith RJ. Use and misuse of the reduced major axis for line-fitting. American Journal of Physical Anthropology 2009;140:476–86.

Warton DI, Wright IJ, Falster DS, Westoby M. Bivariate line-fitting methods for allometry. Biological Reviews 2006;81:259–91.

SUGGESTED READINGS

Abdi H. Bonferroni and Šidák corrections for multiple comparisons. In: Salkind NJ, editor. Encyclopedia of measurement and statistics. Thousand Oaks: Sage; 2007.

Aickin M, Gensler H. Adjusting for multiple testing when reporting research results: the Bonferroni vs. Holm methods. American Journal of Public Health 1996;86:726–8.

Agresti A. Analysis of ordinal categorical data. 2nd ed. New York: Wiley; 2010.

Agresti A. Categorical data analysis. 3rd ed. New York: Wiley; 2013.

Casella G, Berger RL. Statistical inference. 2nd ed. Belmont: Duxbury Press; 2001.

Conover WJ. Practical nonparametric statistics. 3rd ed. New York: Wiley; 1999.

Corder GW, Foreman DI. Nonparametric statistics for non-statisticians: a step-by-step approach. 2nd ed. New York: Wiley; 2014.

Cox DR. Principles of statistical inference. Cambridge: Cambridge University Press; 2006.

Davison AC, Hinkley DV. Bootstrap methods and their application. Cambridge: Cambridge University Press; 1997.

deLevie R. Advanced Excel for scientific data analysis. Oxford: Oxford University Press; 2004.

Field A. Discovering statistics using IBM SPSS statistics. 4th ed. Thousand Oaks: Sage; 2013.

Fox J. Applied regression analysis, linear models and related methods. London: Sage; 1997.

Good P. Permutation, parametric and bootstrap tests of hypotheses. 3rd ed. New York: Springer; 2005.

Greenacre M. Correspondence analysis in practice. 2nd ed. London: Chapman & Hall/CRC; 2007.

Hammer Ø, Harper DAT, Ryan PD. PAST: paleontological statistics software package for education and data analysis. Palaeontologia Electronica 2001;4.

Härdle D, Simar L. Applied multivariate statistical analysis. 2nd ed. New York: Springer; 2007.

Howell DC. Statistical methods for psychology. 7th ed. Belmont: Cengage Wadsworth; 2009.

Johnson R, Wichern D. Applied multivariate statistical analysis. 6th ed. London: Pearson; 2007.

Legendre P, Legendre L. Numerical ecology. 3rd ed. Amsterdam: Elsevier; 2012.

McCullagh P, Nelder JA. Generalized linear models. 2nd ed. London: Chapman & Hall; 1989.

Rummel RJ. Understanding correlation. Honolulu: University of Hawaii; 1976.

Stokes ME, Davis CS, Koch GG. Categorical data analysis using the SAS system. 2nd ed. New York: SAS; 2001.

Tabachnick BG, Fidell LS. Using multivariate statistics. 6th ed. London: Pearson; 2012.

Wilcox RR. Basic statistics: understanding conventional methods and modern insights. Oxford: Oxford University Press; 2009.

Young GA, Smith RL. Essentials of statistical inference. Cambridge: Cambridge University Press; 2010.

Ziegler A, Vens M. Generalized Estimating Equations. Notes on the choice of the working correlation matrix. Methods of Information in Medicine 2010;49:419–20.

APPENDICES

Appendix 9.I: IBM SPSS Interface

All analyses in SPSS presented in Chapter 9 were performed using version 21.0. IBM releases a new version each year; however, the modifications that characterize each new edition hardly ever affect the analyses described in this textbook.

SPSS Worksheets

In SPSS there are two main windows: SPSS Data Editor and SPSS Viewer. The SPSS Data Editor is the worksheet in which we input the data we are going to analyze, and the SPSS Viewer is the window that presents the results. The Data Editor consists of two windows: Data View (Fig. 9.I.1) and Variable View (Fig. 9.I.2). In Data View we input the data, whereas in Variable View we may define their properties. The horizontal lines in Data View are called *cases*, whereas the columns correspond to *variables*. For instance, part of the data given in Table 5.XI.1 is presented in Fig. 9.I.3. In this figure each horizontal line (case) represents the data for one specific individual and each column contains one variable.

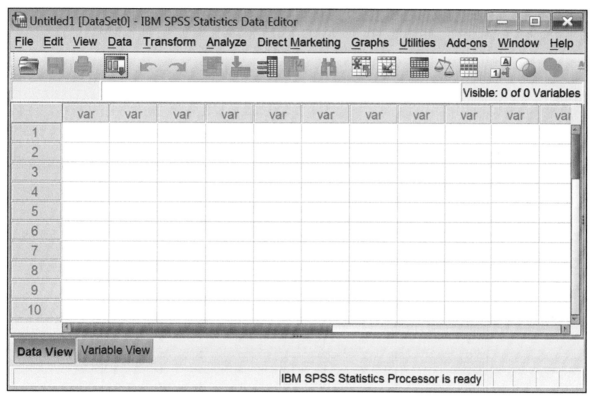

FIGURE 9.I.1 Data View window.

The *menu bar* in Data Editor contains the menus File, Edit, View, Data, Transform, Analyze, Direct Marketing, Graphs, Utilities, Add-ons, Window, and Help. The same menus can be found in SPSS Viewer, which additionally includes the options Insert and Format. The most important of these menus are the following: The File menu, which is used to open a new or an old file, save a file, print, etc.; the Edit menu, for modifying or copying various window features; the Data and Transform menus, which are used to make global changes to SPSS data files and modify the variables; and the Analyze and Graphs menus, which are used to perform various statistical analyses and plot graphs, respectively. Below the menu bar is the *toolbar*, which contains icons as shortcuts to the main commands of the menu bar.

Data Input

The simplest way to input data in an SPSS spreadsheet is to type them directly in the Data View window. In addition, we can transfer data from an Excel spreadsheet to an SPSS file by copying them (using the Ctrl + C command) and pasting them in SPSS (using the Ctrl + V command). In the same way we can transfer data from a .txt file to SPSS, under the precondition that the columns in the .txt file are separated by tabs. Finally, we can input data from Excel or .txt using the menu File → Open → Data.

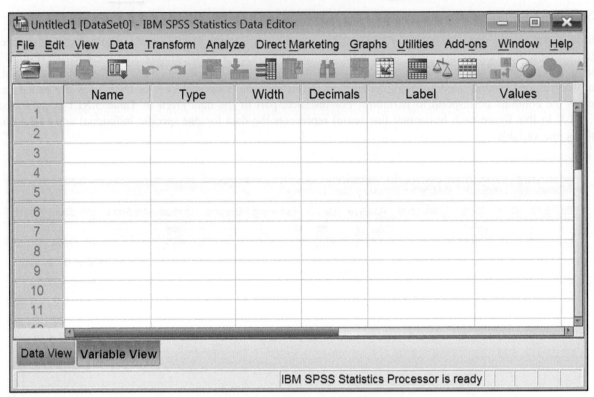

FIGURE 9.I.2 Variable View window.

	Sample	MS	SNS	SOS	PF	EF	CO	SO
1	1	2	1	1	1	1	1	2
2	1	2	1	1	1	1	1	2
3	1	2	1	2	1	2	1	2
4	1	2	1	1	1	1	2	2
5	1	2	2	1	1	2	1	2
6	1	2	1	3	1	1	1	2
7	1	1	1	3	2	1	2	2
8	1	2	1	1	2	1	1	2
9	1	1	2	2	1	2	1	2
10	1	1	1	1	1	1	2	2
11	1	2	3	1	2	1	1	2
12	1	2	3	2	1	2	1	2
13	2	2	1	2	1	3	2	1
14	2	2	2	2	2	3	2	2

FIGURE 9.I.3 Data View window presenting part of the data given in Table 5.XI.1.

Data Editing

Once we have input the data, we may define their format and properties in the window Variable View. The main options are the following:

- We click on the cells of the column Name and type the heading of each column/variable in the Data View window.
- In the second column (Type) we define the type of the variable. If we click on any cell in this column, a small square appears on the right. Once we click on this square, a window pops up in which we may define the variable. The options are Numeric, Comma, Dot, Scientific notation, Date, Dollar, Custom currency, String, and Restricted Numeric. Numeric is any variable for which the values are numbers. We should clarify that even a qualitative variable,

e.g., sex, may be considered numeric when its categories have been coded using numbers, e.g., $1 = $ male and $2 = $ female. Comma is a numeric variable in which the thousands are defined using commas and the decimals using dots, e.g., 5,012.6. Dot is a numeric variable in which the thousands are defined using dots and the decimals using commas, e.g., 5.012,6. Scientific notation suggests that we have used scientific presentation for our variables, e.g., 9.12E2 instead of 912, or 9.12E-2 instead of 0.0912. Date is used when a variable expresses a date. Dollar is used when a variable expresses a dollar amount. For any other currency, we select Custom currency. String represents a qualitative variable denoted with letters or with letters and numbers, e.g., male, yes, F1, 2M. Finally, Restricted Numeric is for integers with leading zeros.

- In the column Width we determine how many characters the name of a string variable can have.
- In the column Decimals we determine the number of decimals for numeric variables.
- In the column Label we can give a small description for each variable. For example, in Fig. 9.I.4 the labels explain the abbreviations for the variables.

	Name	Type	Width	Decimals	Label
1	Sample	Numeric	8	0	
2	MS	Numeric	8	0	metopic suture
3	SNS	Numeric	8	0	supra-nasal suture
4	SOS	Numeric	8	0	supra-orbital structures
5	PF	Numeric	8	0	parietal foramina
6	EF	Numeric	8	0	ethmoidal foramina
7	CO	Numeric	8	0	coronal ossicles
8	SO	Numeric	8	0	squamous ossicles

FIGURE 9.I.4 Labels for the variables of Fig. 9.I.3.

- In the column Values we define the categories of a categorical variable. The preselection is "None" and refers to quantitative variables. For example, in the data set of Fig. 9.I.3 the categorical variable MS (metopic suture) has been coded as $1 = $ presence, $2 = $ absence, or $3 = $ missing value. Because in the Data View window we can see only the numbers 1 to 3, it is helpful to determine what each of these numbers stands for, to avoid confusion when we interpret the results, particularly when we examine data sets with many variables. To do so, we click on the cell in the column Values that corresponds to the variable MS and subsequently click on the small square that appears. The dialog box shown in Fig. 9.I.5, left, pops up, and in the box labeled Value we type in "1," in the Label box we type in "presence," and we click on "Add." The expression $1 = $ "presence" is entered in the large rectangular box. We continue by typing in "2" in the Value box and the word "absence" in the Label box and clicking on "Add." We repeat this process for the missing values and end up with Fig. 9.I.5, right.
- In SPSS we use specific values in the column Missing to define missing values. To define a value as missing, we click on the appropriate cell of this column and then click on the small square that appears on the right. The dialog box shown in Fig. 9.I.6, left, pops up. Note that we have many options for defining missing values. We may use up to three discrete values (e.g., 0, -1, 33), a range of values (e.g., 0 to -10), or a range of values and one additional discrete value (e.g., 0 to -10, 333). In the data set of Fig. 9.I.3 the missing values are indicated by the integer 3. Therefore, in this case we use one discrete value, 3, to denote cells with missing values (Fig. 9.I.6, right).

Select Cases

We use this option when we want to study a subset of a data set, for instance, if we want to analyze only the first sample in the data set of Fig. 9.I.3. In such cases we use the menu Data $\rightarrow$ Select Cases. In the corresponding dialog box we click on "If condition is satisfied" and click on "If...." In the new dialog box that appears we select the variable Sample and transfer it to the box on the right. We type in "$=1$" (Fig. 9.I.7) and click on "Continue" and "OK." The program selects only the cases (lines) that contain the first sample.

If we look at the original Data View window, we observe that all cases belonging to samples 2, 3, and 4 have been marked out. In addition, a new column has been added at the end of the data set, entitled filter_$, with values equal to 0 when Sample $\neq$ 1 and 1 when Sample $= 1$. From this point onward, any analysis we run will include only the cases with

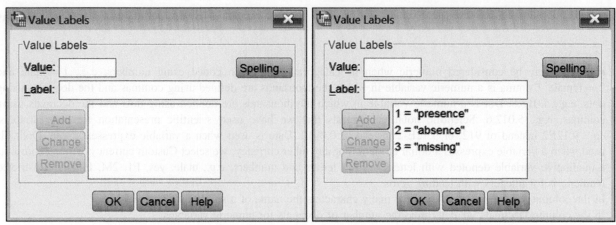

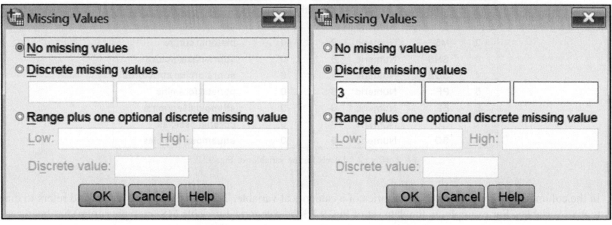

FIGURE 9.1.5 Value Labels dialog box.

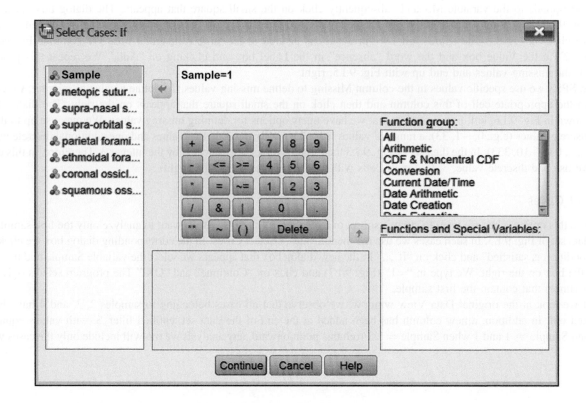

FIGURE 9.1.6 Setting 3 as missing value marker.

Sample = 1. To deactivate this option, we again use the menu Data → Select Cases and in the dialog box that appears we select "All cases." It is also advisable to delete the column filter_$.

Consider now that we want to study two or more samples, say samples 1 and 3. In this case, we use the command Sample = 1 | Sample = 3 (Fig. 9.I.8), in which the symbol | is the OR operator.

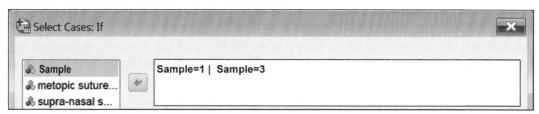

FIGURE 9.I.8   Selection of cases belonging to samples 1 and 3.

Editing Graphs

SPSS allows the plotting of various graphs to present data. Usually these graphs require further editing. If we want to edit a graph, we double-click on it. Then a new window, the Chart Editor, appears, which allows the formatting of the graph. For example, to modify the digits on the axes, we click on one of them. All the digits are selected and a new dialog box, labeled Properties, appears, from which we can change the font, size, color, and number of decimal places, as well as the scale of the axes.

After any change, we must click on Apply. Similarly, if we click on one of the symbols that represent the data points, all similar symbols are selected and a new dialog box appears that allows one to change the type of symbol, color, size, etc. Once we finish formatting the graph, we close the Chart Editor using the menu File → Close.

Open Files

To open a preexisting file, we either double-click on its icon or use the menu File → Open. An interesting feature is that we can open an Excel file in SPSS, as already noted. For this purpose we use the menu File → Open → Data and in the dialog box Open Data in the Files of Type box we select Excel (*.xls, *.xlsx, *.xlsm). Subsequently, we browse to find the specific Excel file and click on it. We click on Open and a new dialog box appears. If in the Excel file the first line contains the variable titles, we click on "Read variable names from the first row of data." Also, we select the spreadsheet we want to open in SPSS and click on "OK." Alternatively, we can copy specific columns from Excel and paste them in SPSS, as already mentioned. We can also do the reverse, that is, copy columns from SPSS and paste them into Excel.

Save Files

To save a file, we use the path File → Save as. A data file in SPSS is saved with the extension .sav, whereas an output file (SPSS Viewer) is saved with the extension .spo. SPSS files can also be saved as Excel documents. For this purpose we use the menu File → Save as and select Excel 97 through 2003 (*.xls) or Excel 2007 through 2010 (*.xlsx) in the box labeled Save as type. We should note that only the data in the Data View window are saved in Excel.

To transfer an SPSS table of results to Excel (or to Word), we right-click on the table, select Copy or Copy Special, and, subsequently, Paste it (or use the Paste Special option) to Excel.

Finally, to save SPSS graphs as image files, we click on the graph and then right-click and select Export. In the dialog box that appears we select None (Graphics Only) in the panel Document: Type and determine the type of image (TIF, JPG, …) in the panel Graphics. Finally, from Browse we define the location in which the new image will be saved.

Appendix 9.II: Excel 2010−2016 Configuration for Data Analysis and Macros

The Analysis ToolPak

To perform complex statistical analyses in Excel, we should use the Analysis ToolPak. This is an Excel add-in program that provides tools for data analysis. If the Data Analysis command does not appear in the ribbon, the Analysis ToolPak is not available and we need to load it as follows. We click on the File tab, click on Options, and then click on the Add-Ins category. In the Manage box we select Excel Add-Ins and then click on "Go." Finally, in the Add-Ins dialog box we select the options "Analysis ToolPak" and "Analysis ToolPak-VBA."

The Developer Tab

The Developer tab is a basic tool that gives access to macros. To add the Developer tab to the ribbon, we execute the following steps: We click on the File tab, click on Options, and then click on the Customize Ribbon category. In the dialog box that appears and in the list of Main tabs, we select the Developer check box.

To run a macro, we click on the Developer tab, we click on Macro Security, and then in the Trust Center dialog box we select the option "Enable all macros." Now, to run a certain macro, we click on the Developer tab, we click on Macros, and then in the dialog box that appears we select the macro and click on "Run."

This procedure may also be followed for the macros of the OSTEO package. However, in this case we may more effectively use the menu Add-ins → OSTEO and select the appropriate macro from the drop-down lists (Fig. 9.II.1).

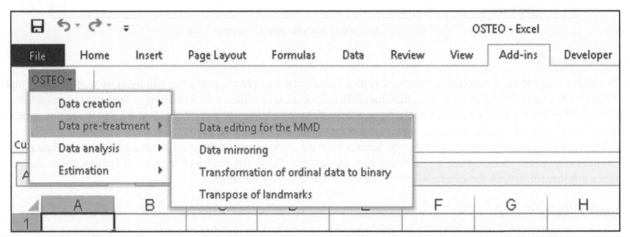

FIGURE 9.II.1 Application of OSTEO for data editing for the calculation of the mean measure of divergence (MMD).

Index

Printed and bound by CPI Group (UK) Ltd, Croydon, CR0 4YY

12/10/2024

01773422-0001